# Kidney Inflammation, Injury and Regeneration 2020

# Kidney Inflammation, Injury and Regeneration 2020

Editors

**Patrick C. Baer**
**Benjamin Koch**
**Helmut Geiger**

MDPI • Basel • Beijing • Wuhan • Barcelona • Belgrade • Manchester • Tokyo • Cluj • Tianjin

*Editors*

Patrick C. Baer
Nephrology
Goethe University
Frankfurt
Germany

Benjamin Koch
Nephrology
Goethe University
Frankfurt
Germany

Helmut Geiger
Nephrology
Goethe University
Frankfurt
Germany

*Editorial Office*
MDPI
St. Alban-Anlage 66
4052 Basel, Switzerland

This is a reprint of articles from the Special Issue published online in the open access journal *International Journal of Molecular Sciences* (ISSN 1422-0067) (available at: www.mdpi.com/journal/ijms/special_issues/kindey_ijms_2020).

For citation purposes, cite each article independently as indicated on the article page online and as indicated below:

LastName, A.A.; LastName, B.B.; LastName, C.C. Article Title. *Journal Name* **Year**, *Volume Number*, Page Range.

**ISBN 978-3-0365-2370-5 (Hbk)**
**ISBN 978-3-0365-2369-9 (PDF)**

# Kidney Inflammation, Injury and Regeneration 2020

Editors

**Patrick C. Baer**
**Benjamin Koch**
**Helmut Geiger**

MDPI • Basel • Beijing • Wuhan • Barcelona • Belgrade • Manchester • Tokyo • Cluj • Tianjin

*Editors*

Patrick C. Baer
Nephrology
Goethe University
Frankfurt
Germany

Benjamin Koch
Nephrology
Goethe University
Frankfurt
Germany

Helmut Geiger
Nephrology
Goethe University
Frankfurt
Germany

*Editorial Office*
MDPI
St. Alban-Anlage 66
4052 Basel, Switzerland

This is a reprint of articles from the Special Issue published online in the open access journal *International Journal of Molecular Sciences* (ISSN 1422-0067) (available at: www.mdpi.com/journal/ijms/special_issues/kindey_ijms_2020).

For citation purposes, cite each article independently as indicated on the article page online and as indicated below:

LastName, A.A.; LastName, B.B.; LastName, C.C. Article Title. *Journal Name* **Year**, *Volume Number*, Page Range.

**ISBN 978-3-0365-2370-5 (Hbk)**
**ISBN 978-3-0365-2369-9 (PDF)**

# Contents

**About the Editors** . . . . . . . . . . . . . . . . . . . . . . . . . . . . . . . . . . . . . . . . . . vii

**Patrick C. Baer, Benjamin Koch and Helmut Geiger**
Kidney Inflammation, Injury and Regeneration 2020
Reprinted from: *Int. J. Mol. Sci.* **2021**, *22*, 5589, doi:10.3390/ijms22115589 . . . . . . . . . . . . . . 1

**Myeongjoo Son, Seyeon Oh, Junwon Choi, Ji Tae Jang, Kuk Hui Son and Kyunghee Byun**
Attenuating Effects of Dieckol on Hypertensive Nephropathy in Spontaneously Hypertensive Rats
Reprinted from: *Int. J. Mol. Sci.* **2021**, *22*, 4230, doi:10.3390/ijms22084230 . . . . . . . . . . . . . . 5

**Jordi Guiteras, Laura De Ramon, Elena Crespo, Nuria Bolaños, Silvia Barcelo-Batllori, Laura Martinez-Valenzuela, Pere Fontova, Marta Jarque, Alba Torija, Oriol Bestard, David Resina, Josep M Grinyó and Joan Torras**
Dual and Opposite Costimulatory Targeting with a Novel Human Fusion Recombinant Protein Effectively Prevents Renal Warm Ischemia Reperfusion Injury and Allograft Rejection in Murine Models
Reprinted from: *Int. J. Mol. Sci.* **2021**, *22*, 1216, doi:10.3390/ijms22031216 . . . . . . . . . . . . . . 19

**Dita Maixnerova and Vladimir Tesar**
Emerging Modes of Treatment of IgA Nephropathy
Reprinted from: *Int. J. Mol. Sci.* **2020**, *21*, 9064, doi:10.3390/ijms21239064 . . . . . . . . . . . . . . 37

**Jixiu Jin, Tian Wang, Woong Park, Wenjia Li, Won Kim, Sung Kwang Park and Kyung Pyo Kang**
Inhibition of Yes-Associated Protein by Verteporfin Ameliorates Unilateral Ureteral Obstruction-Induced Renal Tubulointerstitial Inflammation and Fibrosis
Reprinted from: *Int. J. Mol. Sci.* **2020**, *21*, 8184, doi:10.3390/ijms21218184 . . . . . . . . . . . . . . 53

**Louisa Steines, Helen Poth, Marlene Herrmann, Antonia Schuster, Bernhard Banas and Tobias Bergler**
B Cell Activating Factor (BAFF) Is Required for the Development of Intra-Renal Tertiary Lymphoid Organs in Experimental Kidney Transplantation in Rats
Reprinted from: *Int. J. Mol. Sci.* **2020**, *21*, 8045, doi:10.3390/ijms21218045 . . . . . . . . . . . . . . 67

**You-Jin Kim, Se-Hyun Oh, Ji-Sun Ahn, Ju-Min Yook, Chan-Duck Kim, Sun-Hee Park, Jang-Hee Cho and Yong-Lim Kim**
The Crucial Role of Xanthine Oxidase in CKD Progression Associated with Hypercholesterolemia
Reprinted from: *Int. J. Mol. Sci.* **2020**, *21*, 7444, doi:10.3390/ijms21207444 . . . . . . . . . . . . . . 81

**Lana Nežić, Ranko Škrbić, Ljiljana Amidžić, Radoslav Gajanin, Zoran Milovanović, Eugenie Nepovimova, Kamil Kuča and Vesna Jaćević**
Protective Effects of Simvastatin on Endotoxin-Induced Acute Kidney Injury through Activation of Tubular Epithelial Cells' Survival and Hindering Cytochrome C-Mediated Apoptosis
Reprinted from: *Int. J. Mol. Sci.* **2020**, *21*, 7236, doi:10.3390/ijms21197236 . . . . . . . . . . . . . . 99

**Jean-Paul Decuypere, Shawn Hutchinson, Diethard Monbaliu, Wim Martinet, Jacques Pirenne and Ina Jochmans**
Autophagy Dynamics and Modulation in a Rat Model of Renal Ischemia-Reperfusion Injury
Reprinted from: *Int. J. Mol. Sci.* **2020**, *21*, 7185, doi:10.3390/ijms21197185 . . . . . . . . . . . . . . 117

**Carmen De Miguel, Abigayle C. Kraus, Mitchell A. Saludes, Prasad Konkalmatt, Almudena Ruiz Domínguez, Laureano D. Asico, Patricia S. Latham, Daniel Offen, Pedro A. Jose and Santiago Cuevas**
ND-13, a DJ-1-Derived Peptide, Attenuates the Renal Expression of Fibrotic and Inflammatory Markers Associated with Unilateral Ureter Obstruction
Reprinted from: *Int. J. Mol. Sci.* **2020**, *21*, 7048, doi:10.3390/ijms21197048 . . . . . . . . . . . . . . **131**

**Foteini Moschovaki-Filippidou, Stefanie Steiger, Georg Lorenz, Christoph Schmaderer, Andrea Ribeiro, Ekaterina von Rauchhaupt, Clemens D. Cohen, Hans-Joachim Anders, Maja Lindenmeyer and Maciej Lech**
Growth Differentiation Factor 15 Ameliorates Anti-Glomerular Basement Membrane Glomerulonephritis in Mice
Reprinted from: *Int. J. Mol. Sci.* **2020**, *21*, 6978, doi:10.3390/ijms21196978 . . . . . . . . . . . . . . **149**

**Hee-Yeon Jung, Se-Hyun Oh, Ji-Sun Ahn, Eun-Joo Oh, You-Jin Kim, Chan-Duck Kim, Sun-Hee Park, Yong-Lim Kim and Jang-Hee Cho**
NOX1 Inhibition Attenuates Kidney Ischemia-Reperfusion Injury via Inhibition of ROS-Mediated ERK Signaling
Reprinted from: *Int. J. Mol. Sci.* **2020**, *21*, 6911, doi:10.3390/ijms21186911 . . . . . . . . . . . . . . **165**

**Sebastian Mertowski, Paulina Lipa, Izabela Morawska, Paulina Niedźwiedzka-Rystwej, Dominika Bebnowska, Rafał Hrynkiewicz, Ewelina Grywalska, Jacek Roliński and Wojciech Załuska**
Toll-Like Receptor as a Potential Biomarker in Renal Diseases
Reprinted from: *Int. J. Mol. Sci.* **2020**, *21*, 6712, doi:10.3390/ijms21186712 . . . . . . . . . . . . . . **185**

**Magdalena Nalewajska, Klaudia Gurazda, Małgorzata Marchelek-Myśliwiec, Andrzej Pawlik and Violetta Dziedziejko**
The Role of Endocan in Selected Kidney Diseases
Reprinted from: *Int. J. Mol. Sci.* **2020**, *21*, 6119, doi:10.3390/ijms21176119 . . . . . . . . . . . . . . **213**

**Ewa Kwiatkowska, Katarzyna Stefańska, Maciej Zieliński, Justyna Sakowska, Martyna Jankowiak, Piotr Trzonkowski, Natalia Marek-Trzonkowska and Sebastian Kwiatkowski**
Podocytes—The Most Vulnerable Renal Cells in Preeclampsia
Reprinted from: *Int. J. Mol. Sci.* **2020**, *21*, 5051, doi:10.3390/ijms21145051 . . . . . . . . . . . . . . **223**

**Khai Gene Leong, Elyce Ozols, John Kanellis, David J. Nikolic-Paterson and Frank Y. Ma**
Cyclophilin A Promotes Inflammation in Acute Kidney Injury but Not in Renal Fibrosis
Reprinted from: *Int. J. Mol. Sci.* **2020**, *21*, 3667, doi:10.3390/ijms21103667 . . . . . . . . . . . . . . **235**

**Yu Ah Hong, So Young Jung, Keum Jin Yang, Dai Sig Im, Kyung Hwan Jeong, Cheol Whee Park and Hyeon Seok Hwang**
Cilastatin Preconditioning Attenuates Renal Ischemia-Reperfusion Injury via Hypoxia Inducible Factor-1 Activation
Reprinted from: *Int. J. Mol. Sci.* **2020**, *21*, 3583, doi:10.3390/ijms21103583 . . . . . . . . . . . . . . **249**

**Anja Urbschat, Anne-Kathrin Thiemens, Christina Mertens, Claudia Rehwald, Julia K. Meier, Patrick C. Baer and Michaela Jung**
Macrophage-Secreted Lipocalin-2 Promotes Regeneration of Injured Primary Murine Renal Tubular Epithelial Cells
Reprinted from: *Int. J. Mol. Sci.* **2020**, *21*, 2038, doi:10.3390/ijms21062038 . . . . . . . . . . . . . . **265**

**Anna Gluba-Brzózka, Beata Franczyk, Robert Olszewski and Jacek Rysz**
The Influence of Inflammation on Anemia in CKD Patients
Reprinted from: *Int. J. Mol. Sci.* **2020**, *21*, 725, doi:10.3390/ijms21030725 . . . . . . . . . . . . . . . **283**

# About the Editors

**Patrick C. Baer**

Patrick C. Baer is a Cell Biologist and Associate Professor of Experimental Medicine at the Hospital of the Goethe University in Frankfurt/M. He completed his studies in Biochemistry at the Technical University of Darmstadt and received his doctorate at the Goethe University of Frankfurt/M. P.C.B. has published 101 research articles, including three book chapters and three patents. P.C.B. has been working with cell culture models of proximal and distal tubular epithelial cells of the kidney for 25 years. The research areas of P.C.B. also focus on the isolation, culture and differentiation of mesenchymal stroma/stem cells (MSCs) and the transplantation of MSCs or their derivatives to improve renal regeneration.

**Benjamin Koch**

Benjamin Koch earned an MD with Prof. W. Wels at the Georg-Speyer-Haus, Institute for Tumor Biology and Experimental Therapy, Frankfurt/M., Germany. His thesis work established RNAseq in its early days and integration with ChIPseq in order to identify novel target genes of an important transcription factor in leukemia. He then performed clinical training at the Goethe University Hospital (Division of Nephrology, Prof. Helmut Geiger). In addition to his clinical work in nephrology, he coordinates research projects in the lab of Prof. Patrick C. Baer and is directly involved in researching (1) pathogen-induced acute and chronic kidney injury as well as (2) novel blood filtration devices in inflammation and sepsis. His research tools include RNAseq, proteomics, and translatomics based on general molecular biology.

**Helmut Geiger**

Helmut Geiger is Professor of Medicine and head of the department of nephrology at the University Hospital Frankfurt/M. He has worked as a physician since 1983 in Würzburg, Budapest, Nuremberg-Erlangen and Frankfurt/M. During this time, he has written more than 250 scientific publications and has received funding from the DFG, BMBF, BMWi and several foundations. His main research interests are renal diseases, kidney transplantation and hypertension. H.G. has been awarded the Nils-Alwall Prize of the German Working Group for Clinical Nephrology and the Franz Gross Science Prize of the German High Pressure League.

International Journal of
*Molecular Sciences*

MDPI

*Editorial*

# Kidney Inflammation, Injury and Regeneration 2020

**Patrick C. Baer *, Benjamin Koch and Helmut Geiger**

Division of Nephrology, Department of Internal Medicine III, University Hospital, Goethe-University, 60596 Frankfurt, Germany; b.koch@med.uni-frankfurt.de (B.K.); h.geiger@em.uni-frankfurt.de (H.G.)
* Correspondence: patrick.baer@kgu.de; Tel.: +49-69-6301-5554; Fax: +49-69-6301-4749

check for updates

**Citation:** Baer, P.C.; Koch, B.; Geiger, H. Kidney Inflammation, Injury and Regeneration 2020. *Int. J. Mol. Sci.* **2021**, *22*, 5589. https://doi.org/10.3390/ijms22115589

Received: 29 April 2021
Accepted: 24 May 2021
Published: 25 May 2021

**Publisher's Note:** MDPI stays neutral with regard to jurisdictional claims in published maps and institutional affiliations.



The kidneys play a vital role in the basic physiological functions of the body. Kidney dysfunction impairs these physiological functions and can lead to a wide range of diseases. Damage to the kidney cells can be caused by a variety of ischemic, toxic or immunological complaints that lead to inflammation and cell death, which can lead to organ damage and, ultimately, complete failure. Although the mechanisms underlying acute kidney injury (AKI) and chronic kidney disease (CKD) are quite distinct, clinical evidence suggests that the two conditions are inextricably interconnected [1]. AKI and CKD, regardless of the underlying cause, have inflammation and activation of the immune system as the common underlying mechanisms. Inflammation, a process aimed, in principle, at detecting and fighting harmful pathogens, is, therefore, a major pathogenic mechanism for both AKI and CKD [1]. While the kidney has the remarkable ability to regenerate after an acute injury and can recover completely, depending on the type of kidney lesion, the options for clinical interventions are currently limited to fluid management and extracorporeal kidney support. However, persistent chronic inflammation can trigger renal fibrosis and chronic kidney disease. The investigation of the molecular mechanisms involved in each individual injury is currently insufficiently understood.

In this context, we started a forum for the publication of new results on kidney inflammation, injury and regeneration, as well as for reviewing and discussing existing studies from this interesting research area. In 2019, we initiated the first edition of the Special Edition "Kidney Inflammation, Injury and Regeneration" with 29 articles [2]. The focus of this first edition was more on a summary of current results (represented by 17 review articles), along with 12 original articles from the current research. In the second Special Edition, presented here, the focus is now more on the current research results mainly from in vivo studies. This issue is accompanied by five review articles summarizing the current results on various nephrological diseases or issues. In this current Special Edition, thirteen original research articles are presented: twelve in vivo studies in a murine or rat model and one in vitro study [3]. Seven studies show results from AKI models [4–10], five from fibrosis models (or CKD models) [9,11–14] and two from a transplant rejection model [4,15] (two studies used two different in vivo models).

Steines and coworkers demonstrated that intrarenal tertiary lymphoid organs are sites of humoral immune activation within allografts during chronic rejection and that anti-B-cell activating factor treatment can hinder the formation of tertiary lymphoid organs in allografts [15]. The authors hypothesized that inhibition of the local alloresponses in chronic rejection with an anti-B-cell activating factor antibody represents a potential benefit to kidney transplant patients. Others evaluated the effects of a novel human fusion recombinant protein in two representative kidney inflammatory models: a renal ischemia-reperfusion model (an AKI model) and an allogeneic kidney transplant model [4]. This study shows that targeting with that novel protein offers a good microenvironment profile to protect the ischemic process in the kidney and to prevent kidney rejection.

Another study using a renal ischemia–reperfusion (IR) model showed that preconditioning with cilastatin, a specific inhibitor of renal dehydrodipeptidase-1, attenuates renal IR injury via activation of the main hypoxia factor. The authors confirmed this effect through in vitro studies with immortal tubular epithelial cells [10]. Others used an IR model to show that the NOX1-selective inhibition attenuates kidney IR injuries via the downregulation of oxidative stress-mediated kinase signaling [8] or to investigate the autophagy dynamics during an IR injury, a potential treatment strategy due to removing damaged cells, macromolecules and organelles [6]. The effect of growth differentiation factor 15 (GDF15) was investigated in a murine model of anti-glomerular basement membrane glomerulonephritis [7]. The study showed that GDF15 is required for the regulation of T-cell chemotactic chemokines in the kidneys and demonstrated the protective effects of GDF15. The study revealed a novel mechanism limiting the migration of lymphocytes to the site of inflammation during glomerulonephritis [7]. The findings of Nežić and coworkers investigated the molecular mechanism involved in the reno-protective effects of simvastatin in an endotoxin-induced AKI model [5]. The study indicated that simvastatin, a well-known lipid-lowering medication, has cytoprotective effects on induced tubular apoptosis, mediated by the upregulation of cell survival molecules and inhibition of the mitochondrial proteins. Therefore, the authors hypothesized that simvastatin has significant cell-protective effects in septic AKI [5].

Leong and coworkers showed that cyclophilin A, a damage-associated molecular pattern, promoted inflammation and acute kidney injury in a renal IR model but did not contribute to inflammation or interstitial fibrosis in a model of progressive kidney fibrosis (unilateral ureteric obstruction (UUO)) [9]. Other studies showed the effects of different proteins/peptides against UUO-induced renal injury, inflammation and fibrosis. The 20-amino acid peptide ND-13 protects against UUO-induced damage and is, therefore, a potential new therapeutic approach to prevent renal diseases [14]. Furthermore, the effects of verteporfin on UUO-induced renal tubulointerstitial inflammation, fibrosis and transforming growth factor-β1 regulation were investigated. The study showed that verteporfin decreases the UUO-induced increase in tubular injury, inflammation and extracellular matrix deposition in mice [12]. Son and coworkers investigated the attenuating effects of dieckol on hypertensive nephropathy in spontaneously hypertensive rats and hypothesized that dieckol could be beneficial for decreasing hypertensive nephropathy by decreasing EMT and renal fibrosis [11].

Others investigated the role of xanthine oxidase (XO) in CKD progression associated with hypercholesterolemia [13]. The authors used a murine model of uninephrectomy to induce CKD, in addition to a high-cholesterol diet with a XO inhibitor, and, also, evaluated the results in an in vitro model using immortal tubular epithelial cells. The study clearly showed that XO inhibition exerts reno-protective effects and identifies XO as a novel therapeutic target for hypercholesterolemia-associated kidney injury [13]. Finally, one in vitro study using cisplatin-injured primary tubular epithelial cells focused on the decisive role of the Lipocalin-2 iron load for its pro-regenerative functions [3]. The study detected a positive correlation between the total iron amounts in tubular epithelial cells and cellular proliferation. In conclusion, it was hypothesized that macrophage-released Lipocalin-2-bound iron is provided to tubular epithelial cells during toxic cell damage, whereby the injury is limited and recovery is favored [3].

In addition, five interesting review articles were included in this Special Edition summarizing the current state of knowledge of the treatment of IgA nephropathy [16], the role of endocan in kidney diseases [17] and the influence of inflammation on anemia in CKD patients [18]. It also discusses the mechanism of kidney injury in preeclampsia and the susceptibility of podocytes [19]. Finally, the review summarizes the role of Toll-like receptors in the pathogenesis of glomerulopathy and their role as potential marker molecules for the development of renal diseases [20].

**Author Contributions:** Writing, review and editing, P.C.B. and review and editing, B.K. and H.G. All authors have read and agreed to the published version of the manuscript.

**Funding:** The authors received no funding for this Editorial.

**Conflicts of Interest:** The authors declare no conflict of interest.

## References


1. Andrade-Oliveira, V.; Foresto-Neto, O.; Watanabe, I.K.M.; Zatz, R.; Câmara, N.O.S. Inflammation in Renal Diseases: New and Old Players. *Front. Pharmacol.* **2019**, *10*, 1192. [CrossRef] [PubMed]
2. Baer, P.C.; Koch, B.; Geiger, H. Kidney Inflammation, Injury and Regeneration. *Int. J. Mol. Sci.* **2020**, *21*, 1164. [CrossRef] [PubMed]
3. Urbschat, A.; Thiemens, A.-K.; Mertens, C.; Rehwald, C.; Meier, J.K.; Baer, P.C.; Jung, M. Macrophage-Secreted Lipocalin-2 Promotes Regeneration of Injured Primary Murine Renal Tubular Epithelial Cells. *Int. J. Mol. Sci.* **2020**, *21*, 2038. [CrossRef] [PubMed]
4. Guiteras, J.; De Ramon, L.; Crespo, E.; Bolaños, N.; Barcelo-Batllori, S.; Martinez-Valenzuela, L.; Fontova, P.; Jarque, M.; Torija, A.; Bestard, O.; et al. Dual and Opposite Costimulatory Targeting with a Novel Human Fusion Recombinant Protein Effectively Prevents Renal Warm Ischemia Reperfusion Injury and Allograft Rejection in Murine Models. *Int. J. Mol. Sci.* **2021**, *22*, 1216. [CrossRef] [PubMed]
5. Nežić, L.; Škrbić, R.; Amidžić, L.; Gajanin, R.; Milovanović, Z.; Nepovimova, E.; Kuča, K.; Jaćević, V. Protective Effects of Simvastatin on Endotoxin-Induced Acute Kidney Injury through Activation of Tubular Epithelial Cells' Survival and Hindering Cytochrome C-Mediated Apoptosis. *Int. J. Mol. Sci.* **2020**, *21*, 7236. [CrossRef] [PubMed]
6. Decuypere, J.-P.; Hutchinson, S.; Monbaliu, D.; Martinet, W.; Pirenne, J.; Jochmans, I. Autophagy Dynamics and Modulation in a Rat Model of Renal Ischemia-Reperfusion Injury. *Int. J. Mol. Sci.* **2020**, *21*, 7185. [CrossRef] [PubMed]
7. Moschovaki-Filippidou, F.; Steiger, S.; Lorenz, G.; Schmaderer, C.; Ribeiro, A.; Von Rauchhaupt, E.; Cohen, C.D.; Anders, H.-J.; Lindenmeyer, M.; Lech, M. Growth Differentiation Factor 15 Ameliorates Anti-Glomerular Basement Membrane Glomerulonephritis in Mice. *Int. J. Mol. Sci.* **2020**, *21*, 6978. [CrossRef] [PubMed]
8. Jung, H.-Y.; Oh, S.-H.; Ahn, J.-S.; Oh, E.-J.; Kim, Y.-J.; Kim, C.-D.; Park, S.-H.; Kim, Y.-L.; Cho, J.-H. NOX1 Inhibition Attenuates Kidney Ischemia-Reperfusion Injury via Inhibition of ROS-Mediated ERK Signaling. *Int. J. Mol. Sci.* **2020**, *21*, 6911. [CrossRef] [PubMed]
9. Leong, K.G.; Ozols, E.; Kanellis, J.; Nikolic-Paterson, D.J.; Ma, F.Y. Cyclophilin A Promotes Inflammation in Acute Kidney Injury but Not in Renal Fibrosis. *Int. J. Mol. Sci.* **2020**, *21*, 3667. [CrossRef] [PubMed]
10. Hong, Y.A.; Jung, S.Y.; Yang, K.J.; Im, D.S.; Jeong, K.H.; Park, C.W.; Hwang, H.S. Cilastatin Preconditioning Attenuates Renal Ischemia-Reperfusion Injury via Hypoxia Inducible Factor-1$\alpha$ Activation. *Int. J. Mol. Sci.* **2020**, *21*, 3583. [CrossRef] [PubMed]
11. Son, M.; Oh, S.; Choi, J.; Jang, J.; Son, K.; Byun, K. Attenuating Effects of Dieckol on Hypertensive Nephropathy in Spontaneously Hypertensive Rats. *Int. J. Mol. Sci.* **2021**, *22*, 4230. [CrossRef] [PubMed]
12. Jin, J.; Wang, T.; Park, W.; Li, W.; Kim, W.; Park, S.; Kang, K. Inhibition of Yes-Associated Protein by Verteporfin Ameliorates Unilateral Ureteral Obstruction-Induced Renal Tubulointerstitial Inflammation and Fibrosis. *Int. J. Mol. Sci.* **2020**, *21*, 8184. [CrossRef] [PubMed]
13. Kim, Y.-J.; Oh, S.-H.; Ahn, J.-S.; Yook, J.-M.; Kim, C.-D.; Park, S.-H.; Cho, J.-H.; Kim, Y.-L. The Crucial Role of Xanthine Oxidase in CKD Progression Associated with Hypercholesterolemia. *Int. J. Mol. Sci.* **2020**, *21*, 7444. [CrossRef] [PubMed]
14. De Miguel, C.; Kraus, A.C.; Saludes, M.A.; Konkalmatt, P.; Domínguez, A.R.; Asico, L.D.; Latham, P.S.; Offen, D.; Jose, P.A.; Cuevas, S. ND-13, a DJ-1-Derived Peptide, Attenuates the Renal Expression of Fibrotic and Inflammatory Markers Associated with Unilateral Ureter Obstruction. *Int. J. Mol. Sci.* **2020**, *21*, 7048. [CrossRef] [PubMed]
15. Steines, L.; Poth, H.; Herrmann, M.; Schuster, A.; Banas, B.; Bergler, T. B Cell Activating Factor (BAFF) Is Required for the Development of Intra-Renal Tertiary Lymphoid Organs in Experimental Kidney Transplantation in Rats. *Int. J. Mol. Sci.* **2020**, *21*, 8045. [CrossRef] [PubMed]
16. Maixnerova, D.; Tesar, V. Emerging Modes of Treatment of IgA Nephropathy. *Int. J. Mol. Sci.* **2020**, *21*, 9064. [CrossRef] [PubMed]
17. Nalewajska, M.; Gurazda, K.; Marchelek-Myśliwiec, M.; Pawlik, A.; Dziedziejko, V. The Role of Endocan in Selected Kidney Diseases. *Int. J. Mol. Sci.* **2020**, *21*, 6119. [CrossRef] [PubMed]
18. Gluba-Brzózka, A.; Franczyk, B.; Olszewski, R.; Rysz, J. The Influence of Inflammation on Anemia in CKD Patients. *Int. J. Mol. Sci.* **2020**, *21*, 725. [CrossRef] [PubMed]
19. Kwiatkowska, E.; Stefańska, K.; Zieliński, M.; Sakowska, J.; Jankowiak, M.; Trzonkowski, P.; Marek-Trzonkowska, N.; Kwiatkowski, S. Podocytes—The Most Vulnerable Renal Cells in Preeclampsia. *Int. J. Mol. Sci.* **2020**, *21*, 5051. [CrossRef] [PubMed]
20. Mertowski, S.; Lipa, P.; Morawska, I.; Niedźwiedzka-Rystwej, P.; Bębnowska, D.; Hrynkiewicz, R.; Grywalska, E.; Roliński, J.; Załuska, W. Toll-Like Receptor as a Potential Biomarker in Renal Diseases. *Int. J. Mol. Sci.* **2020**, *21*, 6712. [CrossRef] [PubMed]

International Journal of
*Molecular Sciences*

MDPI

*Article*

# Attenuating Effects of Dieckol on Hypertensive Nephropathy in Spontaneously Hypertensive Rats

**Myeongjoo Son [1,2], Seyeon Oh [2], Junwon Choi [2], Ji Tae Jang [3], Kuk Hui Son [4,*] and Kyunghee Byun [1,2,*]**

[1] Department of Anatomy & Cell Biology, Gachon University College of Medicine, Incheon 21936, Korea; mjson@gachon.ac.kr

[2] Functional Cellular Networks Laboratory, Department of Medicine, College of Medicine, Graduate School and Lee Gil Ya Cancer and Diabetes Institute, Gachon University, Incheon 21999, Korea; seyeon8965@gmail.com (S.O.); choijw88@gc.gachon.ac.kr (J.C.)

[3] Aqua Green Technology Co., Ltd., Smart Bldg., Jeju Science Park, Cheomdan-ro, Jeju 63243, Korea; whiteyasi@gmail.com

[4] Department of Thoracic and Cardiovascular Surgery, Gachon University Gil Medical Center, Gachon University, Incheon 21565, Korea

* Correspondence: dr632@gilhospital.com (K.H.S.); khbyun1@gachon.ac.kr (K.B.)

**Abstract:** Hypertension induces renal fibrosis or tubular interstitial fibrosis, which eventually results in end-stage renal disease. Epithelial-to-mesenchymal transition (EMT) is one of the underlying mechanisms of renal fibrosis. Though previous studies showed that Ecklonia cava extracts (ECE) and dieckol (DK) had inhibitory action on angiotensin (Ang) I-converting enzyme, which converts Ang I to Ang II. It is known that Ang II is involved in renal fibrosis; however, it was not evaluated whether ECE or DK attenuated hypertensive nephropathy by decreasing EMT. In this study, the effect of ECE and DK on decreasing Ang II and its down signal pathway of angiotensin type 1 receptor (AT1R)/*TGFβ*/*SMAD*, which is related with the EMT and restoring renal function in spontaneously hypertensive rats (SHRs), was investigated. Either ECE or DK significantly decreased the serum level of Ang II in the SHRs. Moreover, the renal expression of AT1R/*TGFβ*/*SMAD* was decreased by the administration of either ECE or DK. The mesenchymal cell markers in the kidney of SHRs was significantly decreased by ECE or DK. The fibrotic tissue of the kidney of SHRs was also significantly decreased by ECE or DK. The ratio of urine albumin/creatinine of SHRs was significantly decreased by ECE or DK. Overall, the results of this study indicate that ECE and DK decreased the serum levels of Ang II and expression of AT1R/*TGFβ*/*SMAD*, and then decreased the EMT and renal fibrosis in SHRs. Furthermore, the decrease in EMT and renal fibrosis could lead to the restoration of renal function. It seems that ECE or DK could be beneficial for decreasing hypertensive nephropathy by decreasing EMT and renal fibrosis.

**Keywords:** epithelial-to-mesenchymal transition; E. cava extracts; dieckol; spontaneously hypertensive rats; renal fibrosis; angiotensin II

check for updates

**Citation:** Son, M.; Oh, S.; Choi, J.; Jang, J.T.; Son, K.H.; Byun, K. Attenuating Effects of Dieckol on Hypertensive Nephropathy in Spontaneously Hypertensive Rats. *Int. J. Mol. Sci.* **2021**, *22*, 4230. https://doi.org/10.3390/ijms22084230

Academic Editors: Patrick C. Baer, Benjamin Koch and Helmut Geiger

Received: 1 April 2021
Accepted: 16 April 2021
Published: 19 April 2021



## 1. Introduction

The kidney is a major organ that is affected by hypertensive target organ damage: chronic kidney disease commonly occurs in around 16% of hypertensive patients [1].

The pathological features of hypertensive nephropathy include inflammation, glomerular sclerosis, tubular atrophy, and interstitial fibrosis [2]. The fibrotic tissue replaces the normal functional kidney tissue, which leads to renal failure [3,4]. Thus, renal fibrosis or tubular interstitial fibrosis is the main pathological lesion of hypertensive nephropathy, which induces end-stage renal disease (ESRD) [5]. Renal fibrosis shows the following characteristics: increased massive extracellular matrix (ECM) production, increased recruitment of fibroblasts to tissue injury sites, and increased phenotype changes from fibroblasts to α-smooth muscle actin (α-SMA)-expressing myofibroblasts [6]. The increased α-SMA-expressing myofibroblasts lead to the unnecessarily excessive deposition of collagen and enhance the dysregulation of matrix metalloproteinases, which destroys the basement membrane and further accelerates fibrosis [6].

Recently, many studies have shown that epithelial-to-mesenchymal transition (EMT) is one of the underlying mechanisms of renal fibrosis [7,8]. By undergoing EMT, the epithelial cell gradually loses epithelial markers, such as E-cadherin, which is the main element of cell-to-cell junctions, and gains markers of mesenchymal phenotype, such as α-SMA [9]. By losing the cell junctions, the cells that underwent the EMT process easily move toward the interstitial space [9]. Moreover, the epithelial cells that acquired the properties of myofibroblasts express α-SMA and synthesize ECM proteins, such as collagen, eventually leading to tubular interstitial fibrosis (TIF) [9].

Angiotensin II (Ang II) acts as the main player in hypertension-induced fibrosis. As the main activator of the renin–angiotensin–aldosterone system (RAAS), Ang II causes severe vascular, glomerular, and tubulointerstitial injuries, which are accompanied by the increase in transforming growth factor-beta (TGFβ) via the angiotensin type 1 receptor (AT1R) [10]. The levels of Ang II and its receptor in the kidneys of the spontaneously hypertensive rats (SHRs) were higher than those of Wistar Kyoto (WKY) rats [11]. It is known that Ang II induces EMT via TGFβ-dependent signaling pathways [12]. The Ang II treatment for NRK52E cells (normal rat tubular epithelial cell lines) induces the expression of the TGFβ1/SMAD signaling pathway, which eventually increases the proapoptotic and fibrotic proteins [13]. When Ang II binds with AT1R, the SMAD3 signal pathway is activated and induces EMT in NRK52E cell lines [12].

Polyphenols from marine algae have been reported to function as Ang I-converting enzyme (ACE) inhibitors [14–17]. ACE is involved in the conversion of Ang I to Ang II, and increases Ang II as a potent vasoconstrictor, leading to hypertension [18]. Several phlorotannins, such as phlorofucofuroeckol A, dieckol (DK), and eckol, which are present in extracts from Ecklonia cava or Ecklonia stolonifera, show ACE inhibiting activities; thus, these polyphenols were expected to decrease blood pressure (BP) [15,19]. Even though E. cava extracts (ECE) and DK show ACE inhibiting activities, no report has investigated whether ECE or dieckol is involved in the EMT of the kidney or renal fibrosis that is induced by hypertension. Thus, the effect of ECE and DK on decreasing Ang II and its down signal pathway of AT1R/TGFβ/SMAD2/3, which is related with the EMT of the kidney and restoring renal function in SHRs, was investigated in this study.

## 2. Results

### 2.1. ECE and DK Reduced Systolic BP and Serum Level of Ang II in SHRs

The systolic BP of the SHRs was significantly higher than that of the WKY rats and was significantly decreased by the administration of either ECE or DK. The decreasing effects of 50, 100, and 150 mg/kg/day of ECE and DK administration were not significantly different (Figure 1a). The diastolic and mean BPs of the SHRs were significantly higher than those of the WKY rats. The administration of either ECE or DK did not significantly decrease the diastolic and mean BP (Figure 1b,c).

The serum level of Ang II in the SHRs was significantly higher than that of the WKY rats and was significantly decreased by the administration of either ECE or DK. Moreover, the most prominent decreasing effect was observed in the group treated with 150 mg/kg/day of ECE (Figure 1d).

### 2.2. ECE and DK Attenuated the Expression of AT1R in the Kidney of SHRs

The expression of AT1R was evaluated through qRT-PCR and staining. The mRNA expression of AT1R in the medulla and cortex of the kidney was significantly higher in the SHRs than that of the WKY rats. Such expression was decreased by the administration of either ECE or DK (Figure 2a). In the medulla, the decreasing effect was most prominent in the group treated with DK. In the cortex, 150 mg/kg/day of ECE had the most prominent decreasing effect. The expression level of AT1R in the cortex and medulla of the SHRs, which was evaluated through staining, was significantly increased and was significantly decreased by the administration of either ECE or DK. Moreover, the most prominent decreasing effect was observed in the group treated with DK (Figure 2b,c).

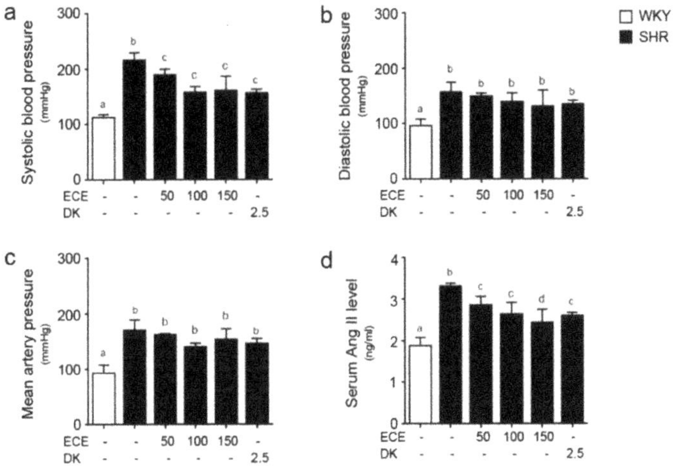


**Figure 1.** Comparative analysis of ECE and DK administration on the reduction of systolic blood pressure and serum angiotensin II level in SHRs. (**a**) Systolic blood pressure, (**b**) diastolic blood pressure, (**c**) mean artery blood pressure, and (**d**) serum angiotensin II level were measured prior to sacrifice. Three doses of ECE (50 mg/kg/day, 100 mg/kg/day and 150 mg/kg/day) were oral administrated for 4 weeks and 2.5 mg/kg/day DK also oral administrated for 4 weeks. Means denoted by a different letter indicate significant differences among groups ($p < 0.05$). - means the same group. ECE, Ecklonia cava extract; DK, dieckol.

To validate ECE and DK attenuation of AT1R expression in kidney tubules, a mouse proximal tubule cell line (TCMK-1) was activated by angiotensin II in an in vitro model [20]. The expression level of AT1R protein in angiotensin II-treated TCMK-1 cells with ECE (5, 25, 50 ug/mL), DK or inhibitor was decreased compared to only angiotensin II treatment (Figure 2d).

### 2.3. ECE and DK Reduced the Expression of TGFβ, SMAD2/3, and Snail2 in the Kidney of SHRs

The expressions of TGFβ in the medulla and cortex of the SHRs were significantly higher than those of the WKY rats, which were decreased by the administration of ECE or DK. In the medulla, the decreasing effect was most prominent in the groups treated with 150 mg/kg/day of ECE and DK. In the cortex, the decreasing effect was most prominent in the group treated with DK (Figure 3a). The expressions of SMAD2 in the medulla and cortex of the SHRs were higher than those of the WKY rats, which were significantly decreased by the administration of ECE or DK. The decreasing effect in the medulla was most prominent in the groups treated with 150 mg/kg/day of ECE or DK. In the cortex, the decreasing effects of 50, 100, and 150 mg/kg/day of ECE or DK were not significantly different (Figure 3b). The expression of SMAD3 in the medulla and cortex of the SHRs was significantly higher than that of the WKY rats, and was significantly decreased by the administration of ECE or DK. The most prominent decreasing effect was observed in the group treated with 150 mg/kg/day of ECE (Figure 3c). The expression of Snail2 in the medulla and cortex of the SHRs was significantly increased by the administration of ECE or DK. The most prominent decreasing effect was observed in the group treated with DK (Figure 3d). In the in vitro model, the expression level of TGFβ and pSMAD2/3 protein in angiotensin II-treated TCMK-1 cells with ECE (5, 25, 50 ug/mL), DK or inhibitor was decreased compared to the only angiotensin II treatment (Figure 3e,f).

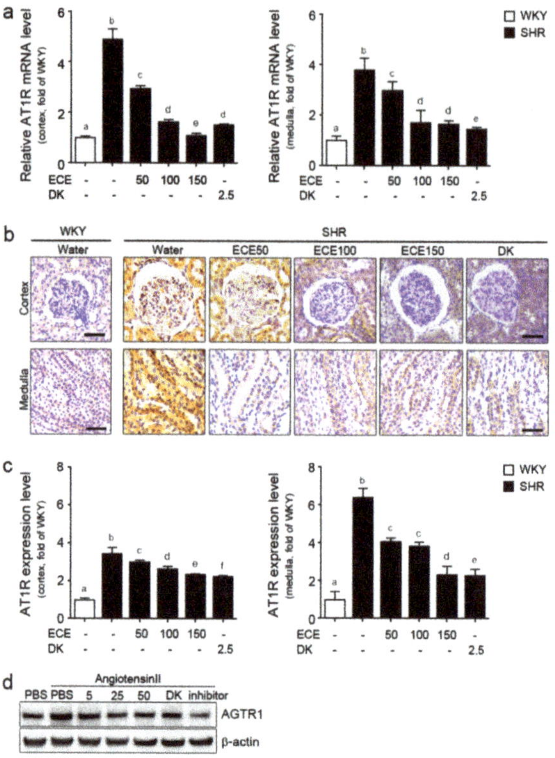


**Figure 2.** Comparative analysis of ECE and DK administration on the reduction of expression of AT1R in the kidney of SHRs and in angiotensin II-treated TCMK-1 cells. (**a**) AT1R mRNA levels in cortex area, and in medulla of the kidney were measured by qRT-PCR analysis. (**b**) AT1R protein expression levels in cortex area, and in medulla of kidney were measured by immunohistochemistry and (**c**) the protein levels were quantified by Image J software. Three doses of ECE (50 mg/kg/day, 100 mg/kg/day and 150 mg/kg/day) were orally administrated for 4 weeks and 2.5 mg/kg/day of DK were also orally administrated for 4 weeks. (**d**) AT1R protein expression levels in angiotensin II-treated TCMK-1 cells (renal epithelial tubular cells) with 5, 25, 50 ug/mL ECE, 2.5 ug/mL DK or inhibitor were measured by Western blotting. Scale bar = 25 μm. Means denoted by a different letter indicate significant differences among groups ($p < 0.05$). - means the same group. ECE, Ecklonia cava extract; DK, dieckol; Inhibitor, 1 μmol/L telmisartan.

### 2.4. ECE and DK Reduced the EMT in the Kidney of the SHRs

The expression of the mesenchymal cell marker, such as vimentin and α-SMA, of the SHRs was significantly higher than that of the WKY rats and was significantly decreased by the administration of either ECE or DK (Figure 4). The decreasing effect on the expression of vimentin in the cortex of the SHRs was most prominent in the group treated with DK, whereas the decreasing effect on the expression of vimentin in the medullas of the SHRs was most prominent in the group treated with 150 mg/kg/day of ECE. Moreover, the decreasing effect on the expression of vimentin in the cortex of the SHRs was most prominent in the group treated with DK (Figure 4a,b). The expression of α-SMA in the cortex and medulla of the SHRs was most significantly decreased in the group treated with 150 mg/kg/day of ECE (Figure 4c,d). The expression of the epithelial cell marker, such as E-cadherin, in the cortex and medulla of the SHRs was significantly lower than that of the WKY rats (Figure S1) and was significantly increased by the administration of either ECE or DK.

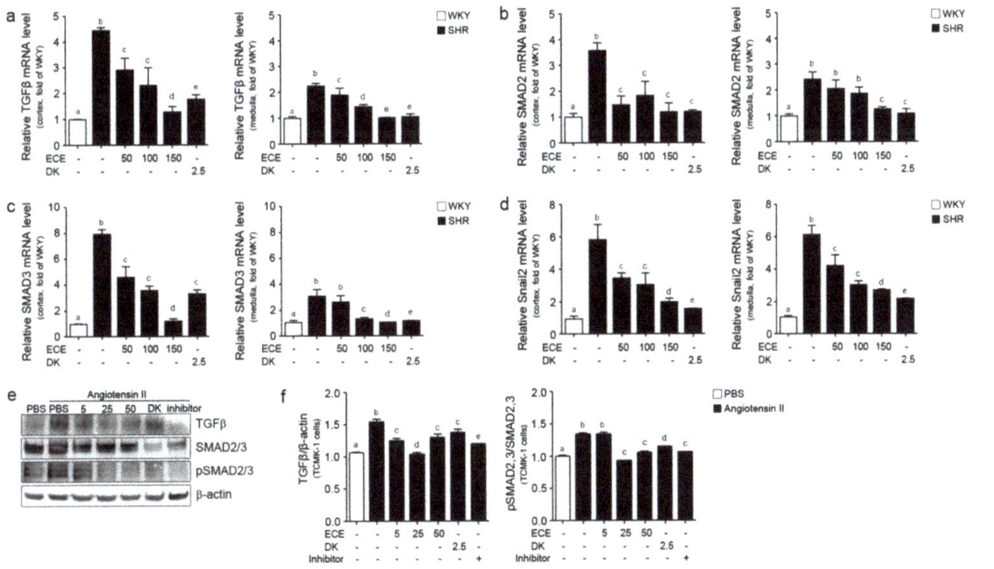

**Figure 3.** Comparative analysis of ECE and DK administration on the reduction of expression of TGFβ, SMAD2/3, and Snail2 in the kidneys of SHRs. (**a**) TGFβ, (**b**) SMAD2, (**c**) SMAD3, (**d**) Snail2 mRNA levels in cortex area, and in medulla of kidney were measured by qRT-PCR analysis. Three doses of ECE (50 mg/kg/day, 100 mg/kg/day and 150 mg/kg/day) were orally administrated for 4 weeks and 2.5 mg/kg/day DK were also orally administrated for 4 weeks. (**e**) TGFβ, SMAD2/3, pSMAD2/3 protein expression levels in angiotensin II-treated TCMK-1 cells (renal tubular epithelial cells) with 5, 25, 50 ug/mL ECE, 2.5 ug/mL DK or inhibitor were measured by Western blotting and (**f**) the protein levels were quantified by Image J software. Means denoted by a different letter indicate significant differences between groups ($p < 0.05$). - means the same group. ECE, Ecklonia cava extract; DK, dieckol; Inhibitor, 1 μmol/L telmisartan.

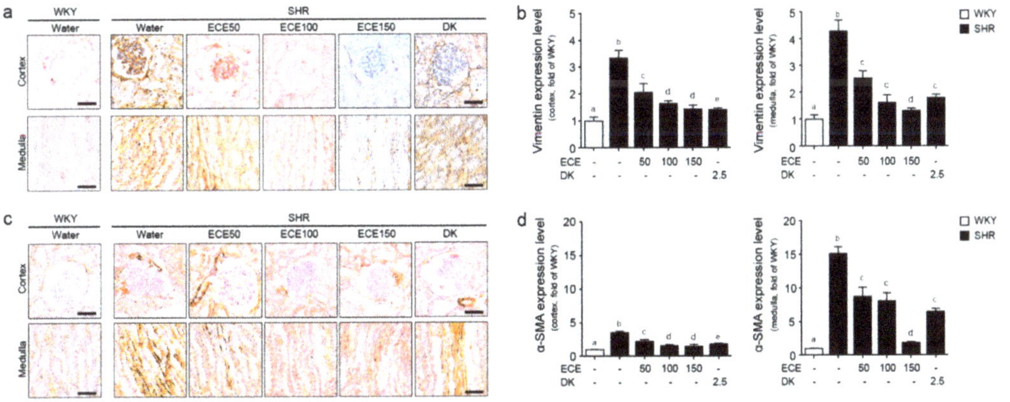

**Figure 4.** Comparative analysis of ECE and DK administration on the reduction of EMT in the kidney of the SHRs. (**a**) Vimentin protein expression levels in cortex area, and in medulla of kidney were measured by immunohistochemistry and (**b**) the protein levels were quantified by Image J software. (**c**) α-SMA protein expression levels in cortex area, and in medulla of kidney were measured by immunohistochemistry and (**d**) the protein levels were quantified by Image J software. Scale bar = 25 μm. Three doses of ECE (50 mg/kg/day, 100 mg/kg/day and 150 mg/kg/day) was oral administrated for 4 weeks and 2.5 mg/kg/day DK also oral administrated for 4 weeks. Means denoted by a different letter indicate significant differences between groups ($p < 0.05$). - means the same group. ECE, Ecklonia cava extract; DK, dieckol.

### 2.5. ECE and DK Reduced the Renal Fibrosis and Glomerular Sclerosis in the Kidney of SHRs

The fibrosis area in the cortex and medulla of the kidney of the SHRs was significantly higher than that of the WKY rats (Figure 5a,b) and was significantly decreased by the administration of either ECE or DK. In the cortex, the most prominent decreasing effect was observed in the group treated with DK, whereas in the medulla, the most prominent decreasing effect was observed in the group treated with 150 mg/kg/day of ECE. The GSI of the SHRs was significantly higher than that of the WKY rats (Figure 5c,d) and was significantly decreased by the administration of ECE or DK. Moreover, the most prominent decreasing effect was observed in the group treated with DK.

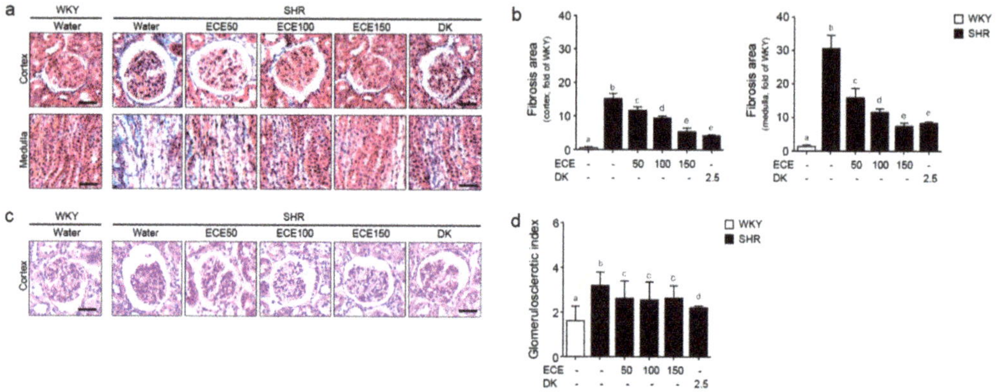


**Figure 5.** Comparative analysis of ECE and DK administration on the reduction of renal fibrosis and glomerular sclerosis in the kidney of SHRs. (**a**) Masson's trichrome stained cortex area and medulla area of kidney showing fibrosis area (blue color) and (**b**) fibrosis area was quantified by Image J software. (**c**) PAS-stained cortex area and medulla area of kidney showing glomerular sclerosis and (**d**) the sclerosis were evaluated using a semi-quantitative scoring method (Grades 0–4). Scale bar = 25 µm. Three doses of ECE (50 mg/kg/day, 100 mg/kg/day and 150 mg/kg/day) were orally administrated for 4 weeks and 2.5 mg/kg/day of DK was also orally administrated for 4 weeks. Means denoted by a different letter indicate significant differences between groups ($p < 0.05$). - means the same group. ECE, Ecklonia cava extract; DK, dieckol; GSI; glomerulosclerotic index.

### 2.6. ECE and DK Attenuated Renal Function Aggravation in SHRs

The amount of water intake within 24 h was not significantly different among all groups (Figure 6a). The urine volume of the SHRs within 24 h was significantly lower than that of the WKY rats (Figure 6b). It was significantly increased by the administration of 100 and 150 mg/kg/day of ECE and DK. The urine sodium/potassium (Na/K) ratio was not significantly different among all groups (Figure 6c). The albumin level in the urine of the SHRs was significantly higher than that of the WKY rats and was significantly decreased by the administration of ECE or DK. The decreasing effects of 50, 100, and 150 mg/kg/day of ECE and DK were not significantly different (Figure 6d). The ratio of urine albumin/creatinine of the SHRs was significantly higher than that of the WKY rats and was decreased by the administration of ECE or DK. The decreasing effects of 50 and 100 mg/kg/day of ECE and DK were not significantly different (Figure 6e).

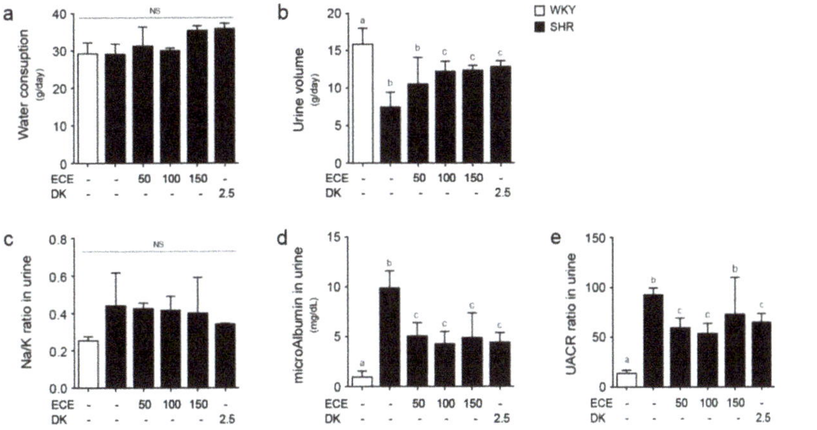


**Figure 6.** Comparative analysis of ECE and DK administration on the attenuation of renal function aggravation in SHRs. (**a**) Water consumption, (**b**) urine volume, (**c**) urine Na/K ratio, (**d**) urine microalbumin level, (**e**) urine albumin-to-creatinine ratio (UACR) were measured prior to sacrifice. Three doses of ECE (50 mg/kg/day, 100 mg/kg/day and 150 mg/kg/day) were orally administrated for 4 weeks and 2.5 mg/kg/day of DK was also orally administrated for 4 weeks. Means denoted by a different letter indicate significant differences between groups ($p < 0.05$). - means the same group. ECE, Ecklonia cava extract; DK, dieckol; NS, not significant.

## 3. Discussion

Hypertension is the second leading etiology of ESRD after diabetes [21]. It is hard to predict the severity of hypertensive renal fibrosis with BP, since renal fibrosis could severely progress even when the patient's BP is not extremely high [21]. Although antihypertensive treatments with ACE inhibitors, such as angiotensin receptor blockers, renin inhibitors, and aldosterone antagonists, could reduce the severity of hypertensive kidney disease, they are not enough to prevent the progression of hypertensive nephropathy [22]. Even though the recommended target BP is achieved at below 130/80 mmHg, the treatment strategy for decreasing BP cannot delay the progression of hypertensive nephropathy [23]. Although hypertensive nephropathy is typically described as nephroangiosclerosis and glomerular hyalinosis [24,25], recently, it was revealed that the interstitium of the kidney, which is involved in TIF, is related to disease progression, as well as the glomerular and vascular compartments [26,27]. Since TIF is a main pathophysiology of hypertensive nephropathy, it is essential to the development of new agents directed to modulate TIF to prevent the progression of hypertensive nephropathy. In recent years, EMT has been known as a crucial player in renal fibrosis [28,29].

Ang II induces vasoconstriction and consequently induces hypertension [30]. In hypertension, RAAS is activated systemically, and the upregulation of RAAS is accompanied in several organs, such as the kidney [31,32]. The hyperactivation of intrarenal RAAS is an important mechanism of hypertension and chronic kidney disease [31,32]. Both TGFβ1 and Ang II induce the activation of the intrarenal RAAS and enhance the expressions of angiotensinogen, renin, ACE, and AT1R, which induce EMT [33]. In our study, the systolic BP of the SHRs was significantly decreased by the administration of either ECE or DK. The serum level of Ang II of the SHRs was significantly decreased by the administration of either ECE or DK. The expression of AT1R in the cortex and medulla of the SHRs was significantly decreased by the administration of either ECE or DK.

The upregulation of RAAS, such as the increased expression of AT1R, activates the down signaling pathway of TGFβ1 [34]. Activated by RAAS, TGFβ1 induces EMT via the SMAD-dependent and SMAD-independent pathways [33]. As the SMAD-dependent signaling pathway, TGFβ1 signaling is transduced via TGFβRII and TGFβRI and leads to the activation of SMAD2/3. [10]. SMAD4 binds to SMAD2/3 and promotes the translocation of the SMAD complex into the nucleus [10]. Translocated SMADs upregulate the expressions of EMT genes, such as Snail, Twist, and ZEB [34]. In our study, the expression of AT1R was significantly higher in the cortex and medulla of the SHRs than that of the WKY rats, and was decreased by the administration of either ECE or DK. The expression of TGFβ and SMAD2/3 in the cortex and medulla of the SHRs was decreased by the administration of either ECE or DK.

The EMT is characterized by the loss of an epithelial marker, such as E-cadherin, and the attainment of mesenchymal markers, such as α-SMA, vimentin, and fibronectin [35]. E-cadherin is the most expressed cadherin in the epithelial cells and is, thus, frequently used as an epithelial marker [36]. α-SMA is a phenotypic marker of myofibroblast cells, and its expression is a feature of the advanced stages of EMT [37]. α-SMA-expressing myofibroblasts, which undergo EMT, induce the synthesis of excessive ECM and abnormal ECM remodeling and renal fibrosis [37].

Hypertensive nephropathy induces glomerulosclerosis and interstitial fibrosis, which induces the decrease in renal function and significant proteinuria [6]. In our study, the expression of vimentin and α-SMA in the medulla and cortex of the SHRs was increased and was decreased by the administration of either ECE or DK. The amount of fibrosis area in the medulla and cortex of the SHRs was increased, and it was decreased by the administration of either ECE or DK. The index of glomerular sclerosis of the SHRs was increased, and it was decreased by the administration of either ECE or DK.

The urine volume of the SHRs progressively decreased as compared with that of the WKY rats of the same age [38]. It is known that the greater the excretion of urine sodium, the less the urinary potassium excretion. Moreover, in human studies, the urine Na/K ratio is associated with the increase in BP and the fast impairment of renal function [39]. In our study, the urine volume of the SHRs was lower than that of the WKY rats, even though the water intake amount was not different between the SHRs and WKY rats. The urine Na/K ratio of the SHRs was significantly different among the WKY rats, SHRs, and ECE- or DK-treated groups. The urine Na/K ratio was used as a marker of dietary sodium and potassium intake in human studies [39]. The BP increased with the increase in sodium intake. However, increased potassium intake decreased the BP by increasing the excretion of sodium into the urine [40]. Therefore, the urine Na/K ratio is associated with the BP in humans [40]. In our study, all animals were not fed with a high-sodium diet, which explains why the urine Na/K ratio among the groups did not show any significant difference.

Hypertension tends to increase proteinuria [37]. It is known that the urine albumin-to-creatinine ratio is associated with the decrease in the glomerular filtration rate [41]. Previous studies have shown that the development of microalbuminuria in SHRs is caused by predominant tubular injury, which induce the urinary loss of low molecular weight proteins [42,43]. In our study, the urine albumin-to-creatinine ratio of the SHRs was higher than that of the WKY rats, and was decreased by the administration of either ECE or DK.

Previous studies showed that several polyphenols have an inhibiting effect on ACE activity [14–17]. However, these studies only reported ACE inhibitory activity as an IC50 value, which is the 50% inhibition concentration of a positive control, and they did not show an antihypertensive effect or protecting effect against hypertensive nephropathy in the animals. One study showed that ECE decreased BP in the 2-kindney 1-clip Goldblatt hypertensive rats [44]. Pyrogallol-phloroglucinol-6,6-bieckol decreased BP in the high fat diet-induced hypertension animal model by modulating vascular dysfunction [45]. However, these studies showed only decreasing BP and did not evaluate whether ECE showed any effect of attenuating hypertensive nephropathy. Our study showed that ECE and DK decreased the expression of AT1R/TGFβ/SMAD2/3 in the kidney and decreased the serum level of Ang II. Additionally, ECE and DK decreased EMT, renal fibrosis and glomerular sclerosis. It seems that ECE and DK might be helpful in attenuating hypertensive nephropathy.

## 4. Materials and Methods

### 4.1. Preparation of ECE and Isolation of DK

The ECE were obtained from the Aqua Green Technology Co., Ltd. (Jeju, Korea). The E. cava was thoroughly washed with pure water and air-dried at room temperature for 48 h. It was ground, and 50% ethanol was added, followed by heating at 85 °C for 12 h. The ECE were filtered and then, when concentrated, sterilized by heating at a high temperature for 40–60 min and then spray-dried. Dieckol, which is one of the representative phlorotannins of E. cava, was then isolated. Briefly, centrifugal partition chromatography was performed using a two-phase solvent system that mixed pure water, ethyl acetate, n-hexane, and a methanol mixture (ratio 7:7:2:3). The organic stationary phase was filled in the column and the mobile phase was filled in the column, following the descending order of flow rate (2 mL per minute) and was used for separation. We followed the methods of Dr. Son et al. (2019) [45].

### 4.2. Hypertension Animal Model

Male SHRs (8 weeks old) and male WKY rats (8 weeks old) were bought from the Orient Bio (Sungnam, Korea) and kept at a constant temperature of approximately 24 °C, relative humidity of 50–55%, and light/dark cycle of 12 h/12 h. The rat sublimation was conducted for 1 week. The rats were randomly divided into six groups (five rats per group):

(i) WKY group, in which the rats were orally administered with drinking water for 4 weeks;

(ii) SHR group, in which the rats were orally administered with drinking water for 4 weeks;

(iii–v) SHR group, in which the rats were orally administered with ECE of (iii) 50 mg/kg/day, (iv) 100 mg/kg/day, and (v) 150 mg/kg/day for 4 weeks;

(vi) SHR group, in which the rats were orally administered with 2.5 mg/kg/day DK for 4 weeks. After 4 weeks, water consumption, urine volume and urine chemical analysis were validated with metabolic cage for 24 h. After completing the metabolic analysis, all rats were sacrificed according to the ethical principles of the Institutional Animal Care and Use Committee of Gachon University (approval number: LCDI-2019-0121).

### 4.3. Immunohistochemistry

Kidney tissue paraffin blocks were sectioned at 8 μm, placed on gelatin-coating slides, and dried at 37 °C for 3 days. The kidney tissue slides were deparaffinized and then incubated with 0.3% hydrogen peroxide (Sigma-Aldrich, MO, USA) for 10 min. Afterward, the slides were rinsed three times with phosphate-buffered saline (PBS), and incubated with an animal serum to inhibit antibody nonspecific binding. Moreover, they were incubated with primary antibodies (anti-AT1R, anti-E-cadherin, anti-α-SMA, and anti-vimentin) and rinsed with PBS three times. The tissue slides were then incubated with the biotinylated secondary antibodies from the ABC kit (Vector Laboratories, Burlingame, CA, USA), incubated for 3 h with a blocking solution, and rinsed with PBS three times. The tissue slides were developed with 3,3-diaminobenzidine as a substrate for 3 min, mounted with a xylene-based DPX solution (Sigma-Aldrich), and visualized via light microscopy (Olympus Optical Co., Tokyo, Japan).

### 4.4. RNA Extraction and Quantitative Real-Time Polymerase Chain Reaction (qRT-PCR)

The RNA from the rat kidney tissues was isolated using the RNAiso Plus reagent (TAKARA, Japan) according to the manufacturer's instructions. The kidney tissues were first divided into two parts, namely, the cortex part and the medulla part. The kidney tissues were finely cut and crushed into powder, and the powders were resuspended with 1 mL of RNAiso Plus reagent, mixed with 0.1 mL of pure glade chloroform (Amresco, Solon, OH, USA), and then centrifuged at 13,000× *g* for 20 min at 4 °C. After centrifugation, the supernatant was mixed with 0.25 mL of pure glade isopropyl alcohol, and the extracted RNA pellets were washed with 70% alcohol and centrifuged at 7500× *g* for 5 min at 4 °C.

The dried pellets were dissolved in 10–30 μl diethylpyrocarbonate-treated pure water, and RNA was quantified and checked using the NanoDrop 2000 (Thermo Fisher Scientific, MA, USA). Complementary DNA (cDNA) was prepared from RNA using a cDNA synthesis kit (PrimeScript™, TAKARA). A quantitative real-time polymerase chain reaction (qRT-PCR) determined the RNA levels from the kidney tissues. The forward and reverse primers were mixed with distilled water, and then 10 μl mixtures were placed in a 384-well qRT-PCR plate. The cDNA and SYBR green (TAKARA) were subsequently added and then validated using a qRT-PCR machine (Bio-Rad, Hercules, CA, USA). The genes of interest are listed in Supplementary Table S1. We followed the methods of Dr. Son et al. 2019 [45].

### *4.5. Enzyme-Linked Immunosorbent Assay (ELISA)*

To confirm the serum Ang II level, an aliquot of the withdrawn blood (1.5 to 1.7 mL) was added in serum separator tubes (Becton Dickinson, Franklin Lakes, NJ, USA) and then centrifuged at 2000× *g* for 20 min at room temperature. Afterward, the separated serum was moved into a new tube and stored in a deep freezer. The Ang II ELISA kit (MyBioSource, San Diego, CA, USA) was used for analyzing the presence of serum according to the manufacturer's instructions. Ang II was measured within 1 week after blood collection from the animals.

### *4.6. Histological Analysis*

#### 4.6.1. Masson's Trichrome (MT) Stain

Masson's trichrome (MT) stain validates the fibrosis of the kidney. Blocks of paraffin-embedded kidney tissue were sectioned to a thickness of 8 μm, placed on a coating slide, and dried at 37 °C for 3 days. The tissue slides were deparaffinized with xylene and alcohol and were re-fixed with Bouin's solution for 24 h and rinsed with running tap water for 3 min. The slides were submerged with Weigert's iron hematoxylin solution for 10 min and Biebrich scarlet-acid fuchsin solution for 15 min and then differentiated with phosphomolybdic–phosphotungstic acid solution for 10 min. Finally, the slides were transferred to aniline blue solution for 3 min and then washed with water. The stained slides were mounted with xylene-based DPX solution (Sigma-Aldrich) and visualized via light microscopy (Olympus). The collagen fiber appears to be blue in color in the fibrosis area, whereas the renal epithelium appears to be red in color. MT-stained fibrosis areas were measured using the ImageJ software. Original images of the MT-stained kidney were converted into RGB images, and then these images were deconvolved using the ImageJ software using the color deconvolution plugin.

#### 4.6.2. Periodic Acid–Schiff (PAS) Stain

A periodic acid–Schiff (PAS) stain validated the glomerular damage of the kidney. Blocks of paraffin-embedded kidney tissue were sectioned to a thickness of 8 μm, placed on a coating slide, and dried at 37 °C for 3 days. The tissue slides were deparaffinized with xylene and alcohol, hydrated with water, oxidized with 0.5% periodic acid solution for 5 min, and washed with water. The slides were submerged with the Schiff reagent for 15 min and then washed with lukewarm tap water for 5 min. Finally, the slides were transferred to Mayer's hematoxylin solution for 1 min and then washed with water. The stained slides were mounted with xylene-based DPX solution (Sigma-Aldrich) and visualized via light microscopy (Olympus).

Glomeruli were randomly selected, and the glomerular damage was evaluated using a semi-quantitative scoring method (Grades 0–4) using PAS-stained kidney tissue slides.

(1) Grade 0: normal glomeruli;
(2) Grade 1: minimal sclerosis (sclerotic area up to 25%);
(3) Grade 2: moderate sclerosis (sclerotic area 25% to 50%);
(4) Grade 3: moderate–severe sclerosis (sclerotic area 50% to 75%);
(5) Grade 4: severe sclerosis (sclerotic area 75% to 100%);

The glomerulosclerotic index (GSI) was calculated using the following equation: $(4 \times n4) + (3 \times n3) + (2 \times n2) + (1 \times n1) / n4 + n3 + n2 + n1 + n0$, where n (x) is the number of renal glomerular sclerosis in each grade [46]. This analysis was carried out in the treatment groups by a masked observer.

### 4.7. Systolic Blood Pressure, Diastolic Blood Pressure, and Mean Arterial Blood Pressure Measurements

The systolic BP, diastolic BP, and mean arterial BP were measured using a noninvasive CODA tail-cuff system (Kent Scientific Corp., Torrington, CT, USA). The rat sublimation was conducted for 20 min for 5 days, and the BP was measured on the last day.

### 4.8. In Vitro Modeling Using TCMK-1 Cells

TCMK-1 cells, a mouse proximal tubule cell line, were purchased from American Type Culture Collection (Washington, DC, USA). High glucose Dulbecco's Modified Eagle's medium (Gibco; Grand island, NY, USA), 10% fetal bovine serum (FBS) and 1% penicillin-streptomycin were used as culture mediums. To validate the inhibitory effects of ECE and DK in angiotensin II-treated TCMK-1 cells, we treated ECE (5, 25, 50 μg/mL) and DK (1.8 μg/mL) with 100 nmol/L angiotensin II (Sigma-Aldrich, St Louis, MO, USA) for 12 h. Telmisartan (1 μmol/L, Sigma-Aldrich) was used for AT1 receptor antagonist and pretreated before angiotensin II for 3 h [47].

### 4.9. Preparation of Protein and Western Blotting

To isolate protein from angiotensin II-treated TCMK-1 cells, the cells were scraped using the RIPA lysis buffer with phosphatase and proteinase inhibitor (EzRIPA; ATTO; Tokyo, Japan) and incubated on ice for 20 min. After centrifuging at 13,000× *g* for 20 min, at 4 °C, clean supernatants were moved to a new tube and the concentration of supernatants was analyzed with a bicinchoninic acid assay kit (BCA kit; Thermo Fisher Scientific, Inc.; Waltham, MA, USA). To validate protein expression from TCMK-1 cells, blotting was conducted. An equal amount of lysate proteins (30 μg/lane) was separated by 10% sodium dodecyl sulfate polyacrylamide gel using electrophoresis. Then, running proteins were transferred to polyvinylidene fluoride membranes, which were incubated with diluted primary antibodies (Anti-β-actin, AGTR1, TGF-β, SMAD2/3 and pSMAD2/3) at 4 °C. The incubated membranes with antibodies were thoroughly washed using Tris-buffered saline with 0.1% Tween 20 and incubated with secondary antibodies for 2 h at room temperature. All membranes were developed by enhanced chemiluminescence (LAS-4000s; GE Healthcare, Chicago, IL, USA). The antibodies information used in this study can be found in Table S2.

### 4.10. Statistical Analysis

The results are presented as mean ± SD, and *p*-values of <0.05 means it is statistically significant. The Kruskal–Wallis test was used to validate the differences among the groups, and the Mann–Whitney U test was used in the SPSS ver. 22 software (IBM Corporation; NY, Armonk, USA) completed post hoc comparisons. Means denoted by a different letter indicate significant differences between groups.

## 5. Conclusions

In conclusion, AT1R was upregulated in the SHRs, and the signal pathway increased TGFβ and SMAD2 or 3, which induced EMT. Either ECE or DK downregulated the signal pathway and decreased EMT. Therefore, ECE or DK decreased the mesenchymal cell markers such as the expression of vimentin and α-SMA, the fibrotic tissue of the kidney, and the ratio of urine albumin/creatinine and attenuated the EMT. Furthermore, renal fibrosis led to the restoration of renal function (Figure 7).

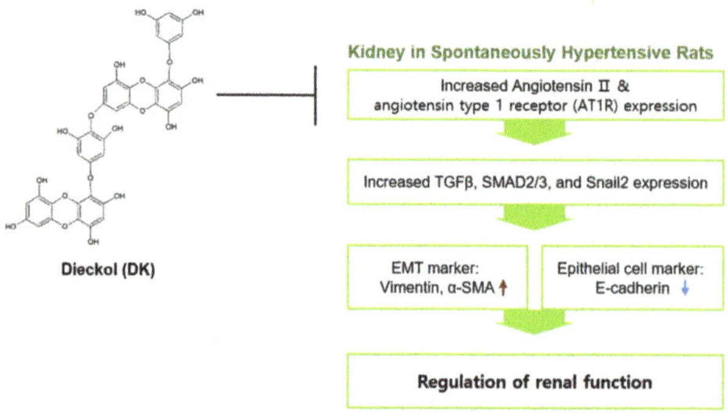


**Figure 7.** Schematic image for effects of ECE and DK administration in SHRs. ECE or DK downregulated AT1R/TGFβ/SMAD2 or three molecule expression and EMT marker expression in SHRs.

**Supplementary Materials:** The following are available online at https://www.mdpi.com/article/10.3390/ijms22084230/s1.

**Author Contributions:** Conceptualization, K.H.S. and K.B.; formal analysis, M.S. and S.O.; funding acquisition, K.B.; project administration, K.B.; resources, J.T.J.; validation, M.S., S.O. and J.C.; writing—original draft, M.S. and K.H.S. All authors have read and agreed to the published version of the manuscript.

**Funding:** This research was part of a project entitled "Development of functional food products with natural materials derived from marine resources" (no. 20170285), which was funded by the Ministry of Oceans and Fisheries, Republic of Korea.

**Institutional Review Board Statement:** The study was conducted according to the guidelines of the Institutional Animal Care and Use Committee and approved by the Institutional Ethics Committee of Gachon University (LCDI-2019-0121).

**Informed Consent Statement:** Not applicable.

**Data Availability Statement:** All data are contained within the article.

**Acknowledgments:** The authors are grateful to Aqua Green Technology Co., LTD (Jeju, South Korea) for assisting in the preparation of the E. cava extract and DK.

**Conflicts of Interest:** The authors declare no competing financial interests by the sponsoring/commercial partners.

## References

1. Whelton, P.K.; Carey, R.M.; Aronow, W.S.; Casey, D.E., Jr.; Collins, K.J.; Dennison Himmelfarb, C.; DePalma, S.M.; Gidding, S.; Jamerson, K.A.; Jones, D.W.; et al. 2017 ACC/AHA/AAPA/ABC/ACPM/AGS/APhA/ASH/ASPC/NMA/PCNA Guideline for the Prevention, Detection, Evaluation, and Management of High Blood Pressure in Adults: A Report of the American College of Cardiology/American Heart Association Task Force on Clinical Practice Guidelines. *J. Am. Coll. Cardiol.* **2018**, *71*, e127–e248. [CrossRef]
2. Mennuni, S.; Rubattu, S.; Pierelli, G.; Tocci, G.; Fofi, C.; Volpe, M. Hypertension and kidneys: Unraveling complex molecular mechanisms underlying hypertensive renal damage. *J. Hum. Hypertens.* **2014**, *28*, 74–79. [CrossRef] [PubMed]
3. Breyer, M.D.; Susztak, K. The next generation of therapeutics for chronic kidney disease. *Nat. Rev. Drug Discov.* **2016**, *15*, 568–588. [CrossRef] [PubMed]
4. Schelling, J.R. Tubular atrophy in the pathogenesis of chronic kidney disease progression. *Pediatr. Nephrol.* **2016**, *31*, 693–706. [CrossRef] [PubMed]
5. Duggan, K.A.; Hodge, G.; Chen, J.; Trajanovska, S.; Hunter, T. Vasoactive intestinal peptide infusion reverses existing renal interstitial fibrosis via a blood pressure independent mechanism in the rat. *Eur. J. Pharm.* **2020**, *873*, 172979. [CrossRef]
6. Chen, D.Q.; Feng, Y.L.; Cao, G.; Zhao, Y.Y. Natural Products as a Source for Antifibrosis Therapy. *Trends Pharm. Sci.* **2018**, *39*, 937–952. [CrossRef]
7. Strutz, F. Pathogenesis of tubulointerstitial fibrosis in chronic allograft dysfunction. *Clin. Transpl.* **2009**, *23*, 26–32. [CrossRef]

8. Hills, C.E.; Squires, P.E. TGF-beta1-induced epithelial-to-mesenchymal transition and therapeutic intervention in diabetic nephropathy. *Am. J. Nephrol.* **2010**, *31*, 68–74. [CrossRef] [PubMed]
9. Iwano, M.; Plieth, D.; Danoff, T.M.; Xue, C.; Okada, H.; Neilson, E.G. Evidence that fibroblasts derive from epithelium during tissue fibrosis. *J. Clin. Investig.* **2002**, *110*, 341–350. [CrossRef]
10. Balakumar, P.; Sambathkumar, R.; Mahadevan, N.; Muhsinah, A.B.; Alsayari, A.; Venkateswaramurthy, N.; Jagadeesh, G. A potential role of the renin-angiotensin-aldosterone system in epithelial-to-mesenchymal transition-induced renal abnormalities: Mechanisms and therapeutic implications. *Pharm. Res.* **2019**, *146*, 104314. [CrossRef]
11. Pan, J.; Zhang, J.; Zhang, X.; Zhou, X.; Lu, S.; Huang, X.; Shao, J.; Lou, G.; Yang, D.; Geng, Y.J. Role of microRNA-29b in angiotensin II-induced epithelial-mesenchymal transition in renal tubular epithelial cells. *Int. J. Mol. Med.* **2014**, *34*, 1381–1387. [CrossRef] [PubMed]
12. Yang, F.; Huang, X.R.; Chung, A.C.; Hou, C.C.; Lai, K.N.; Lan, H.Y. Essential role for Smad3 in angiotensin II-induced tubular epithelial-mesenchymal transition. *J. Pathol.* **2010**, *221*, 390–401. [CrossRef] [PubMed]
13. Kim, C.S.; Kim, I.J.; Bae, E.H.; Ma, S.K.; Lee, J.; Kim, S.W. Angiotensin-(1-7) Attenuates Kidney Injury Due to Obstructive Nephropathy in Rats. *PLoS ONE* **2015**, *10*, e0142664. [CrossRef]
14. Wijesekara, I.; Kim, S.K. Angiotensin-I-converting enzyme (ACE) inhibitors from marine resources: Prospects in the pharmaceutical industry. *Mar. Drugs* **2010**, *8*, 1080. [CrossRef] [PubMed]
15. Athukorala, Y.; Jeon, Y.J. Screening for angiotensin 1-converting enzyme inhibitory activity of Ecklonia cava. *J. Food Sci. Nutr.* **2005**, *10*, 134–139.
16. Wijesinghe, W.A.; Ko, S.C.; Jeon, Y.J. Screening of Extracts from Red Algae in Jeju for Potentials MarineAngiotensin-I Converting Enzyme (ACE) Inhibitory Activity. *Algae* **2006**, *21*, 343–348.
17. Wijesinghe, W.A.; Ko, S.C.; Jeon, Y.J. Effect of phlorotannins isolated from Ecklonia cava on angiotensin I-converting enzyme (ACE) inhibitory activity. *Nutr. Res. Pract.* **2011**, *5*, 93–100. [CrossRef]
18. Gómez-Guzmán, M.; Rodríguez-Nogales, A.; Algieri, F.; Gálvez, J. Potential Role of Seaweed Polyphenols in Cardiovascular-Associated Disorders. *Mar. Drugs* **2018**, *16*, 250. [CrossRef]
19. Jung, H.A.; Hyun, S.K.; Kim, H.R.; Choi, J.S. Angiotensin-converting enzyme I inhibitory activity of phlorotannins from Ecklonia stolonifera. *Fish. Sci.* **2006**, *72*, 1292–1299. [CrossRef]
20. Son, M.; Oh, S.; Choi, C.H.; Park, K.Y.; Son, K.H.; Byun, K. Pyrogallol-Phloroglucinol-6,6-Bieckol from Ecklonia cava Attenuates Tubular Epithelial Cell (TCMK-1) Death in Hypoxia/Reoxygenation Injury. *Mar. Drugs* **2019**, *17*, 602. [CrossRef]
21. Seccia, T.M.; Caroccia, B.; Calò, L.A. Hypertensive nephropathy. Moving from classic to emerging pathogenetic mechanisms. *J. Hypertens.* **2017**, *35*, 205–212. [CrossRef] [PubMed]
22. Liu, Y.; Shen, W.; Chen, Q.; Cao, Q.; Di, W.; Lan, R.; Chen, Z.; Bai, J.; Han, Z.; Xu, W. Inhibition of RAGE by FPS-ZM1 alleviates renal injury in spontaneously hypertensive rats. *Eur. J. Pharm.* **2020**, *882*, 173228. [CrossRef] [PubMed]
23. Udani, S.; Lazich, I.; Bakris, G.L. Epidemiology of hypertensive kidney disease. *Nat. Rev. Nephrol.* **2011**, *7*, 11–21. [CrossRef] [PubMed]
24. Hill, G.S.; Heudes, D.; Bariéty, J. Morphometric study of arterioles and glomeruli in the aging kidney suggests focal loss of autoregulation. *Kidney Int.* **2003**, *63*, 1027–1036. [CrossRef] [PubMed]
25. Hill, G.S. Hypertensive nephrosclerosis. *Curr. Opin. Nephrol. Hypertens.* **2008**, *17*, 266–270. [CrossRef]
26. Seccia, T.M.; Maniero, C.; Belloni, A.S.; Guidolin, D.; Pothen, P.; Pessina, A.C.; Rossi, G.P. Role of angiotensin II, endothelin-1 and L-type calcium channel in the development of glomerular, tubulointerstitial and perivascular fibrosis. *J. Hypertens.* **2008**, *26*, 2022–2029. [CrossRef]
27. Seccia, T.M.; Belloni, A.S.; Guidolin, D.; Sticchi, D.; Nussdorfer, G.G.; Pessina, A.C.; Rossi, G.P. The renal antifibrotic effects of angiotensin-converting enzyme inhibition involve bradykinin B2 receptor activation in angiotensin II-dependent hypertension. *J. Hypertens.* **2006**, *24*, 1419–1427. [CrossRef]
28. Huang, S.; Susztak, K. Epithelial Plasticity versus EMT in Kidney Fibrosis. *Trends Mol. Med.* **2016**, *22*, 4–6. [CrossRef]
29. Lovisa, S.; LeBleu, V.S.; Tampe, B.; Sugimoto, H.; Vadnagara, K.; Carstens, J.L.; Wu, C.C.; Hagos, Y.; Burckhardt, B.C.; Pentcheva-Hoang, T.; et al. Epithelial-to-mesenchymal transition induces cell cycle arrest and parenchymal damage in renal fibrosis. *Nat. Med.* **2015**, *21*, 998–1009. [CrossRef]
30. Satou, R.; Penrose, H.; Navar, L.G. Inflammation as a Regulator of the Renin-Angiotensin System and Blood Pressure. *Curr. Hypertens. Rep.* **2018**, *20*, 100. [CrossRef]
31. Urushihara, M.; Kagami, S. Role of the intrarenal renin-angiotensin system in the progression of renal disease. *Pediatr. Nephrol.* **2017**, *32*, 1471–1479. [CrossRef] [PubMed]
32. Yang, T.; Xu, C. Physiology and Pathophysiology of the Intrarenal Renin-Angiotensin System: An Update. *J. Am. Soc. Nephrol.* **2017**, *28*, 1040–1049. [CrossRef] [PubMed]
33. Meng, X.M.; Nikolic-Paterson, D.J.; Lan, H.Y. TGF-β: The master regulator of fibrosis. *Nat. Rev. Nephrol.* **2016**, *12*, 325–338. [CrossRef] [PubMed]
34. Hao, Y.M.; Yuan, H.Q.; Ren, Z.; Qu, S.L.; Liu, L.S.; Yin, K.; Fu, M.; Jiang, Z.S. Endothelial to mesenchymal transition in atherosclerotic vascular remodeling. *Clin. Chim. Acta* **2019**, *490*, 34–38. [CrossRef] [PubMed]

35. Guan, M.; Li, W.; Xu, L.; Zeng, Y.; Wang, D.; Zheng, Z.; Lyv, F.; Xue, Y. Metformin Improves Epithelial-to-Mesenchymal Transition Induced by TGF-$\beta$1 in Renal Tubular Epithelial NRK-52E Cells via Inhibiting Egr-1. *J. Diabetes Res.* **2018**, *2018*, 1031367. [CrossRef] [PubMed]
36. Zhang, A.; Jia, Z.; Guo, X.; Yang, T. Aldosterone induces epithelial-mesenchymal transition via ROS of mitochondrial origin. *Am. J. Physiol. Renal. Physiol.* **2007**, *293*, F723–F731. [CrossRef]
37. Leader, C.J.; Kelly, D.J.; Sammut, I.A.; Wilkins, G.T.; Walker, R.J. Spironolactone mitigates, but does not reverse, the progression of renal fibrosis in a transgenic hypertensive rat. *Physiol. Rep.* **2020**, *8*, e14448. [CrossRef] [PubMed]
38. Buemi, M.; Nostro, L.; Di Pasquale, G.; Cavallaro, E.; Sturiale, A.; Floccari, F.; Aloisi, C.; Ruello, A.; Calapai, G.; Corica, F.; et al. Aquaporin-2 water channels in spontaneously hypertensive rats. *Am. J. Hypertens.* **2004**, *17*, 1170–1178. [CrossRef]
39. Koo, H.; Hwang, S.; Kim, T.H.; Kang, S.W.; Oh, K.H.; Ahn, C.; Kim, Y.H. The ratio of urinary sodium and potassium and chronic kidney disease progression: Results from the KoreaN Cohort Study for Outcomes in Patients with Chronic Kidney Disease (KNOW-CKD). *Medicine* **2018**, *97*, e12820. [CrossRef]
40. He, J.; Mills, K.T.; Appel, L.J.; Yang, W.; Chen, J.; Lee, B.T.; Rosas, S.E.; Porter, A.; Makos, G.; Weir, M.R.; et al. Urinary Sodium and Potassium Excretion and CKD Progression. *J. Am. Soc. Nephrol.* **2016**, *27*, 1202–1212. [CrossRef]
41. Inker, L.A.; Astor, B.C.; Fox, C.H.; Isakova, T.; Lash, J.P.; Peralta, C.A.; Kurella Tamura, M.; Feldman, H.I. KDOQI US commentary on the 2012 KDIGO clinical practice guideline for the evaluation and management of CKD. *Am. J. Kidney Dis.* **2014**, *63*, 713–735. [CrossRef]
42. Inoue, B.H.; Arruda-Junior, D.F.; Campos, L.C.; Barreto, A.L.; Rodrigues, M.V.; Krieger, J.E.; Girardi, A.C. Progression of microalbuminuria in SHR is associated with lower expression of critical components of the apical endocytic machinery in the renal proximal tubule. *Am. J. Physiol. Renal. Physiol.* **2013**, *305*, F216–F226. [CrossRef]
43. Russo, L.M.; Osicka, T.M.; Brammar, G.C.; Candido, R.; Jerums, G.; Comper, W.D. Renal processing of albumin in diabetes and hypertension in rats: Possible role of TGF-beta1. *Am. J. Nephrol.* **2003**, *23*, 61–70. [CrossRef] [PubMed]
44. Hong, J.H.; Son, B.S.; Kim, B.K.; Chee, H.Y.; Song, K.S.; Lee, B.H.; Shin, H.C.; Lee, K.B. Antihypertensive effect of Ecklonia cava extract. *Korean J. Pharm.* **2006**, *37*, 200–205.
45. Son, M.; Oh, S.; Lee, H.S.; Ryu, B.; Jiang, Y.; Jang, J.T.; Jeon, Y.J.; Byun, K. Pyrogallol-Phloroglucinol-6,6′-Bieckol from *Ecklonia cava* Improved Blood Circulation in Diet-Induced Obese and Diet-Induced Hypertension Mouse Models. *Mar. Drugs* **2019**, *17*, 272. [CrossRef] [PubMed]
46. Maric, C.; Sandberg, K.; Hinojosa-Laborde, C. Glomerulosclerosis and tubulointerstitial fibrosis are attenuated with 17beta-estradiol in the aging Dahl salt sensitive rat. *J. Am. Soc. Nephrol.* **2004**, *15*, 1546–1556. [CrossRef]
47. Wang, J.; Wen, Y.; Lv, L.L.; Liu, H.; Tang, R.N.; Ma, K.L.; Liu, B.C. Involvement of endoplasmic reticulum stress in angiotensin II-induced NLRP3 inflammasome activation in human renal proximal tubular cells in vitro. *Acta Pharm. Sin.* **2015**, *36*, 821–830. [CrossRef] [PubMed]

International Journal of *Molecular Sciences*

MDPI

*Article*

# Dual and Opposite Costimulatory Targeting with a Novel Human Fusion Recombinant Protein Effectively Prevents Renal Warm Ischemia Reperfusion Injury and Allograft Rejection in Murine Models

**Jordi Guiteras [1,2], Laura De Ramon [1], Elena Crespo [1], Nuria Bolaños [1], Silvia Barcelo-Batllori [3], Laura Martinez-Valenzuela [1,4], Pere Fontova [1], Marta Jarque [1], Alba Torija [1], Oriol Bestard [4,5], David Resina [6], Josep M Grinyó [5,*] and Joan Torras [4,5,*]**

[1] Experimental Nephrology Laboratory, Institut d'Investigació Biomèdica de Bellvitge (IDIBELL), L'Hospitalet de Llobregat, 08907 Barcelona, Spain; jguiteras@idibell.cat (J.G.); deramon.laura@gmail.com (L.D.R.); ecrespo@idibell.cat (E.C.); nbolanos@idibell.cat (N.B.); lauramartinezval252@gmail.com (L.M.-V.); pfontova@idibell.cat (P.F.); mjarque@idibell.cat (M.J.); atorija@idibell.cat (A.T.)

[2] Fundació Bosch i Gimpera, University of Barcelona, 08028 Barcelona, Spain

[3] Molecular Interactions Unit, Institut d'Investigació Biomèdica de Bellvitge (IDIBELL) Scientific-Technical Services, L'Hospitalet de Llobregat, 08907 Barcelona, Spain; sbarcelo@idibell.cat

[4] Nephrology Department, Bellvitge University Hospital, L'Hospitalet de Llobregat, 08907 Barcelona, Spain; obestard@bellvitgehospital.cat

[5] Faculty of Medicine, Bellvitge Campus, University of Barcelona, L'Hospitalet de Llobregat, 08907 Barcelona, Spain

[6] Bioingenium S.L., Barcelona Science Park, 08028 Barcelona, Spain; dresina@bioingenium.net

* Correspondence: jgrinyo@ub.edu (J.M.G.); jtorras@bellvitgehospital.cat (J.T.)

check for updates

**Citation:** Guiteras, J.; De Ramon, L.; Crespo, E.; Bolaños, N.; Barcelo-Batllori, S.; Martinez-Valenzuela, L.; Fontova, P.; Jarque, M.; Torija, A.; Bestard, O.; et al. Dual and Opposite Costimulatory Targeting with a Novel Human Fusion Recombinant Protein Effectively Prevents Renal Warm Ischemia Reperfusion Injury and Allograft Rejection in Murine Models. *Int. J. Mol. Sci.* **2021**, *22*, 1216. https://doi.org/10.3390/ijms22031216

Academic Editor: Patrick C. Baer

Received: 30 December 2020

Accepted: 20 January 2021

Published: 26 January 2021



**Abstract:** Many studies have shown both the CD28—D80/86 costimulatory pathway and the PD-1—PD-L1/L2 coinhibitory pathway to be important signals in modulating or decreasing the inflammatory profile in ischemia-reperfusion injury (IRI) or in a solid organ transplant setting. The importance of these two opposing pathways and their potential synergistic effect led our group to design a human fusion recombinant protein with CTLA4 and PD-L2 domains named HYBRI. The objective of our study was to determine the HYBRI binding to the postulated ligands of CTLA4 (CD80) and PD-L2 (PD-1) using the Surface Plasmon Resonance technique and to evaluate the in vivo HYBRI effects on two representative kidney inflammatory models—rat renal IRI and allogeneic kidney transplant. The Surface Plasmon Resonance assay demonstrated the avidity and binding of HYBRI to its targets. HYBRI treatment in the models exerted a high functional and morphological improvement. HYBRI produced a significant amelioration of renal function on day one and two after bilateral warm ischemia and on days seven and nine after transplant, clearly prolonging the animal survival in a life-sustaining renal allograft model. In both models, a significant reduction in histological damage and CD3 and CD68 infiltrating cells was observed. HYBRI decreased the circulating inflammatory cytokines and enriched the FoxP3 peripheral circulating, apart from reducing renal inflammation. In conclusion, the dual and opposite costimulatory targeting with that novel protein offers a good microenvironment profile to protect the ischemic process in the kidney and to prevent the kidney rejection, increasing the animal's chances of survival. HYBRI largely prevents the progression of inflammation in these rat models.

**Keywords:** costimulation; coinhibition; ischemia-reperfusion injury; kidney transplant; SPR; protein binding affinity; innate immunity; adaptive immunity; inflammation

## 1. Introduction

Delayed graft function (DGF) is the clinical manifestation of ischemia-reperfusion injury (IRI) in human renal transplantation. The clinical impact of DGF on transplant-related outcomes is an increase in the risk of rejection, inferior allograft function, difficult management of immunosuppression in the early post-transplant phase, and the need for repeated renal biopsies with their related associated complications [1–3].

IRI causes a series of humoral and cellular responses, producing complex and diverse pathophysiological pathways of damage to the organ [4,5]. The occlusion of the arterial blood supply leads to tissue hypoxia and the imbalance of metabolic demand, thus activating cell death programs, endothelial dysfunction, transcriptional reprogramming, the expression of cytokines, leukocyte-endothelial adhesion, macrophage and lymphocyte activation, and the generation of small amounts of reactive oxygen species (ROS) [6–9]. Additionally, the restoration of blood flow and reoxygenation is frequently associated with an exacerbation of tissue injury and intense inflammatory response [10]. During reperfusion, the restoration of oxygen levels further damages cells exposed to previous ischemia, leading to the production of large amounts of ROS that contribute to cell membrane and DNA damage. Reperfusion damage results in an autoimmune response, which includes mostly natural antibody recognition and complement cascade activation [11]. This induces cell death and the activation of the innate and, afterwards, the adaptive immune system [6]. Regarding adaptive immunity, multiple roles of T cells have been described in studies of ischemia, showing evidences in both antigen-specific and antigen-independent mechanisms of activation [1,12,13].

Given the crucial role that costimulatory signals play in T cell-mediated immune responses, several costimulatory pathways have been targeted using monoclonal antibodies and fusion proteins to induce immunosuppression. Currently, it is well known that the so-called costimulatory pathways constitute a complex set of stimulatory and inhibitory signals which together fine-tune cell responses. To induce immunosuppression, several of these targets have been directed [14–17]. Some studies reported that CTLA4 blocks the costimulatory CD28 pathway by binding to the ligands CD80 and CD86. This blockade prevents the clonal expansion of effector T cells, leading them to an anergy or apoptotic state [18–20]. The costimulatory blocker Belatacept (a mutated version of CTLA4Ig) was approved for immunosuppression in renal transplantation in the early 2000s. The observed advantages of Belatacept over cyclosporine include better graft function, the preservation of renal structure, and improved cardiovascular risk profile [21]. Concerns associated with Belatacept are a higher frequency of cellular rejection episodes, but protocol biopsies at 1 year showed a lower incidence of chronic allograft nephropathy with Belatacept compared to cyclosporine [22]. According to Parsons et al., Belatacept can also reduce Human leukocyte antigen (HLA) class I antibodies in a significant proportion of highly sensitized recipients [23].

Recent studies have shown the immunosuppressive effects of exacerbating the coinhibitory pathway formed by PD-1 and the ligands PD-L1 and PD-L2 [24–28]. Early PD-1 expression has been demonstrated in renal allograft, which was considered essential to modulate T cell expansion and cytokine production. Blocking the PD-1/PD-L1 coinhibitory pathway during the first week after transplantation doubled the number of PD-1–expressing CD8 and CD4 cells infiltrating the graft, mainly in the interstitium [29]. Contrasting to PD-L1, PD-L2 is mainly expressed in the Antigen presenting cells (APC), does not link to CD80, and seems to be more significant in terms of protection against an ischemic or allogeneic insult [24,30–32]. Moreover, this pathway has been recently related to the regulatory T cell induction setting, a cellular subset implicated in the immune and inflammatory response regulation [33–35].

According to these T cell-modulating pathways, the concurrent blockade of the CD28—CD80/86 costimulatory pathway with CTLA4 and the stimulation of the PD-1 coinhibitory pathway with PD-L2 in the cell synapses could exert better immunosuppressive or anti-inflammatory effects [24,36]. In this regard, our group designed a novel human fusion protein construct to target these dual and opposite costimulatory signals. The production of the molecule consists of gen synthesis, cloning, and transient transfection with a stable Chinese hamster ovary (CHO) mammalian cell line. This recombinant protein design consists of an IgG1 FC linked to a CTLA4 molecule which is also bound to two PD-L2 molecules by polypeptide links (Figure 1).

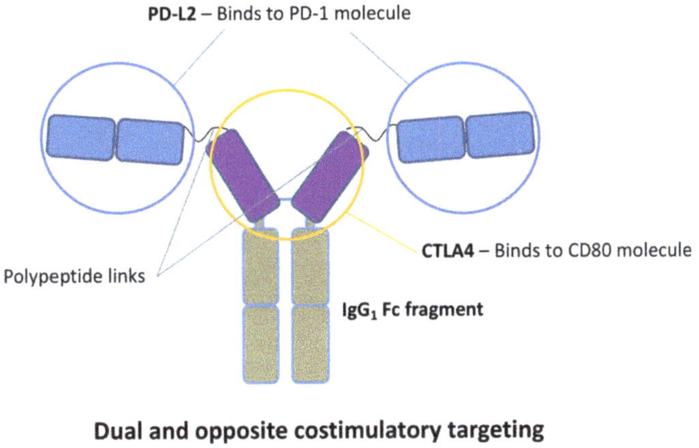


**Figure 1.** HYBRI protein structure.

This dual targeting may promote T cell anergy and apoptosis, enhance T cell exhaustion and T-reg expansion, and downregulate the CD80/86 expression in antigen-presenting cells [37–39]. This might suggest that lower concentrations of CTLA4 would be needed to inhibit the CD28—CD80/86 costimulatory synapsis. This potential dual targeting may close a synergistic circle to exert potent anti-inflammatory and immunosuppressive effects. We studied two experimental settings, the inflammatory environment of renal warm IRI and the renal allogeneic transplantation with cold ischemia, to evaluate the effect of our HYBRI protein.

## 2. Results

### *2.1. Analysis of HYBRI Binding Affinity to Murine CD80 and PD-1 Proteins Using the Surface Plasmon Resonance (SPR) Technique*

SPR analysis was used to characterize the affinity and kinetics between the HYBRI construct and PD-1 and CD80. HYBRI was covalently bound to the CM5 sensor surface and the analytes (CD80 and PD-1) were injected in solution over the surface at concentrations ranging from 15.6 to 2000 nM. Sensorgrams (Figure 2) show a dose-dependent direct interaction between the analytes and HYBRI. Affinity constants determined in the steady state reflected a high affinity for both CD80 and PD1 binding to HYBRI (Table 1). Kinetics analysis revealed rapid association (Ka) and dissociation (Kd) for both CD80 and PD1. From these kinetic constants, affinity constants could be calculated (KD) and were in good agreement with the affinity constants determined from the steady-state analysis. Experiments were also conducted to assess the effect of the presence of PD-1 on CD80 binding to HYBRI, and there was found to be a lack of competition between the two molecules for HYBRI [40].

**Table 1.** CD80 and PD1 bind to HYBRI. Affinity constants (KD) were calculated from SPR analysis in the steady state and from the kinetics analysis.

| | Steady State | | Kinetics | |
|---|---|---|---|---|
| | | ka (1/Ms) | kd(1/s) | KD (M) |
| CD80 | $3.72 \times 10^{-6}$ | $1.57 \times 10^{5}$ | $5.68 \times 10^{-1}$ | $3.62 \times 10^{-6}$ |
| PD-1 | $5.29 \times 10^{-5}$ | $6.37 \times 10^{4}$ | 3.19 | $4.91 \times 10^{-5}$ |

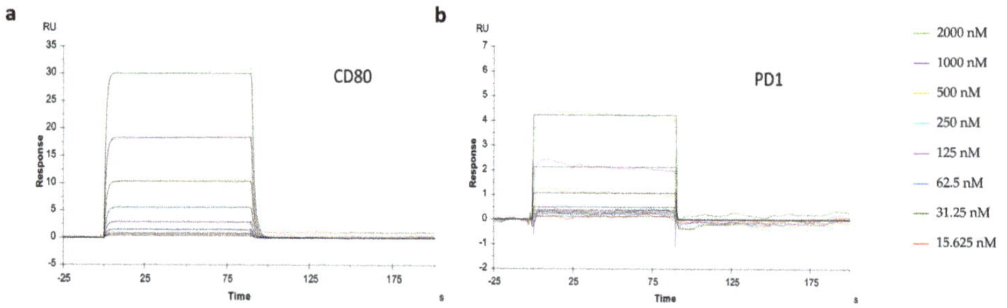


**Figure 2.** Representative sensorgrams of CD80 (**a**) and PD1 (**b**) binding to HYBRI. HYBRI was bound to CM5 chip and CD80 and PD1 serial dilutions (15.625, 31.25, 62.5, 125, 250, 500, 1000, and 2000 nM) represented in distinct colors were injected for 90 s. Experimental data are shown as color traces and black traces represent the fitted data according to the 1:1 Langmuir binding model.

## 2.2. *Bilateral Warm Ischemia Model in Native Rat Kidneys*

### 2.2.1. Effects of HYBRI on Renal Function

HYBRI therapy produced a significant improvement in kidney function the following three days after warm ischemia, with a reduction in creatinine at 24 h from 2.85 mg/dL to 1.5 mg/dL ($p$ = 0.0002) and a reduction in urea from 192.8 mg/dL to 129.2 mg/dL for the non-treated group to the HYBRI group, respectively ($p$ = 0.0335, Figure 3). Interestingly, the major difference between groups was observed on the second day after ischemia, when both parameters began to decrease in the HYBRI group but peaked in the non-treated group. At this point, the creatinine level of the non-treated group increased to 3.02 mg/dL compared to the reduction to 0.89 mg/dL ($p$ = 0.001) for the group treated with the HYBRI protein. Furthermore, in the case of blood urea the slope on the second day continued increasing, with a significant difference from 281.3 mg/dL in the non-treated group to 76.4 mg/dL in the HYBRI group ($p$ = 0.0022). There were no serum creatinine and urea level fluctuations in the sham group.

### 2.2.2. Renal Histopathology and Immunohistochemistry

A significant reduction in histological damage was observed from a total inflammatory score of 6.75 in the non-treated group to 3.2 in the HYBRI group ($p$ = 0.0021), while there was no inflammation in the sham group (Figure 4).

Despite no significant differences, the HYBRI group showed a reduction of almost half in CD3 infiltrating cells (from 13.2 in the non-treated group to 8 in the HYBRI group). An enrichment of FoxP3+ infiltrating cells (Tregs) in the kidney was observed (from 0.7 in the non-treated group to 1.3 in the HYBRI group, with a trend to significance ($p$ value= 0.075)). Even more, creating a ratio between infiltrating FoxP3+ cells and infiltrating CD3+ cells, animals treated with HYBRI showed a percentage of 39.1% in contrast to 8.9% in non-treated animals ($p$ value= 0.069). The treatment also revealed a significant reduction in CD68 infiltrating cells from 3.3 in the non-treated group to 1.8 in the HYBRI group ($p < 0.0001$).

### 2.2.3. Peripheral Blood and Spleen Cell Populations

There were no significant differences between groups in a flow cytometry analysis in spleen cell subpopulations. Regarding the Peripheral blood mononuclear cell (PBMC) analysis, the only differences seen were in the percentage of FoxP3+ cells (Tregs) in the CD4+ cells. These cells were expanded from 5% to 13% the next day after ischemia in the HYBRI group. In contrast, in the non-treated group, the difference was lower, with an initial 4% to 9% twenty-four hours after ischemia. Similar trends were observed in the percentage of CD25+ cells in both the CD3+ and CD4+ cell subsets.

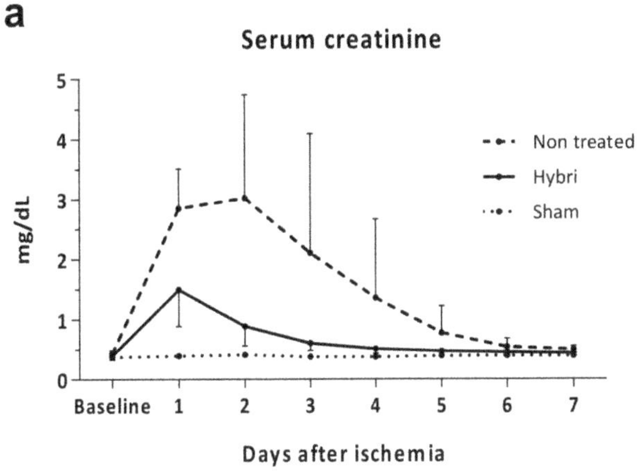


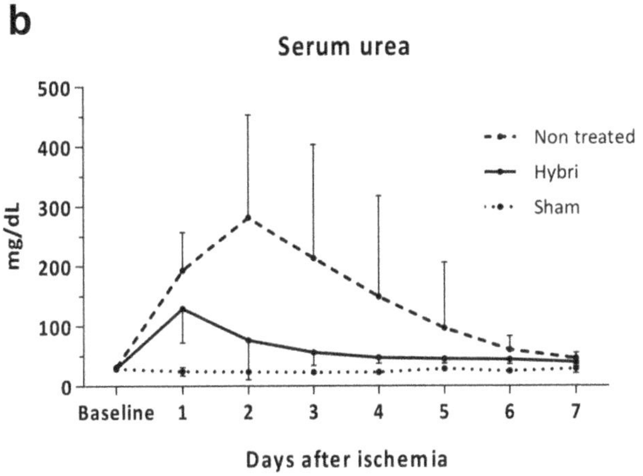


**Figure 3.** Functional renal parameters throughout the ischemia-reperfusion model for all treatments, including serum creatinine (**a**) and serum urea (**b**). Values are expressed in mg/dL. Data are expressed as mean.

### 2.2.4. Circulating Inflammatory Cyto/Chemokines

The serum levels of MCP1 and RANTES (also known as CCL5) at the end of the study decreased significantly with the HYBRI treatment. In addition, concerning the IP-10, IL-12, and MIP-1$\alpha$ levels, treatment with HYBRI in ischemic kidneys significantly reduced those cytokines to values similar to those of sham rats. A partial but non-significant reduction in the serum IL-2 levels was also observed in the HYBRI group compared to the non-treated rats (Figure 5).

### 2.2.5. Renal Gene Expression

After analyzing both the TaqMan low density array (TLDA) and Polymerase chain reaction (PCR) techniques with a CT method analysis, a few significant differences were observed comparing the HYBRI group with the non-treated group. In this regard, the CTLA4 ($p = 0.0133$) and FoxP3 ($p = 0.0435$) gene expression were significantly reduced in the non-treated group compared to the HYBRI group.

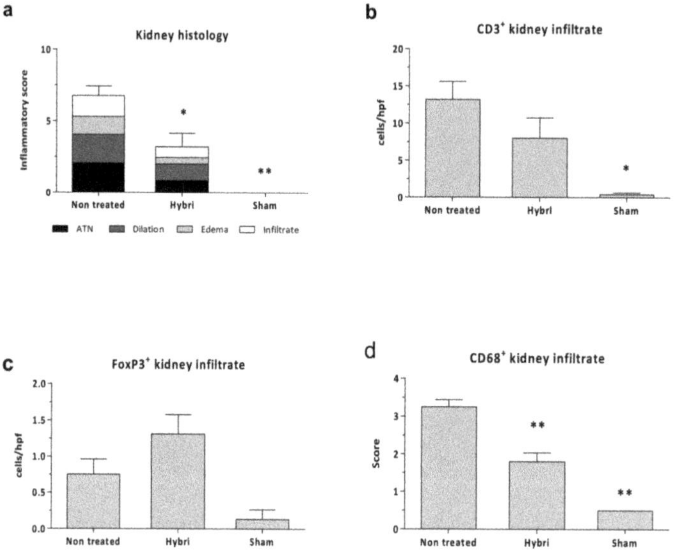


**Figure 4.** Renal histopathology parameters for ischemia-reperfusion injury in the three studied groups. Semi-quantitative inflammatory score values (**a**) for Hematoxylin-Eosin stain. Cells per hpf values for renal immunofluorescence CD3+ (**b**) and FoxP3+ (**c**) kidney infiltrate, and semi-quantitative score for CD68+ surface intensity (**d**). Data are expressed as a mean ± SEM. *, $p < 0.05$ vs. non-treated; **, $p < 0.01$ vs. non-treated.

In HYBRI animals, there was a trend for lower expressions of Ccl7, Ccr5, Cxcl10, Fcnb, Ptprc, S100a6, Trl2, Tlr4, HGF, RORC, and VCAM genes compared to non-treated animals. Interestingly, the degree of reduction in the expression of those genes in the group treated with HYBRI led to values closer to those of the sham group, and, contrarily to non-treated rats, they were not statistically different, thus bringing the treated kidneys closer to a healthier genotype.

The Pathwax database results for all these genes showed that the HYBRI treatment affected nine molecular pathways related to cellular processes, such as apoptosis, necroptosis, and focal adhesion (see Supplementary Material). It also affected twelve environmental information processing-related pathways, such as cytokine–cytokine receptor interaction; cell adhesion molecules; and NF-kappa B, MAPK, JAK-STAT, and TNF signaling pathways as the most relevant. Of note, HYBRI also affected thirty-three pathways related to human diseases, with the PD-1 expression pathway as the most significant. Twenty-one organismal systems-related pathways such as NK cell-mediated cytotoxicity; Th1, Th2, and Th17 cell differentiation; the chemokine signaling pathway; T and B-cell and toll-like receptor signaling pathways were also affected. The gene expression results showed that almost all the analyzed genes are regulated in the IRI setting, but just thirteen of them are significantly addressed by the HYBRI treatment.

### 2.3. *Rat Allogeneic Kidney Transplant Model*

#### 2.3.1. Effects of HYBRI on Renal Function and Survival

HYBRI treatment resulted in an improvement in renal function in the allogeneic transplant model. At the early ischemic peak 24 h after kidney transplantation, despite no significant differences HYBRI treatment reduced the serum creatinine from 1.4 to 1.1 mg/dL and the serum urea levels from 185.8 to 157.2 mg/dL. Furthermore, HYBRI treatment showed a significant reduction in creatinine levels on day 7 after kidney transplantation ($p$ = 0.0171), when kidney function begins to decline due to allogeneic kidney rejection (Figure 6).

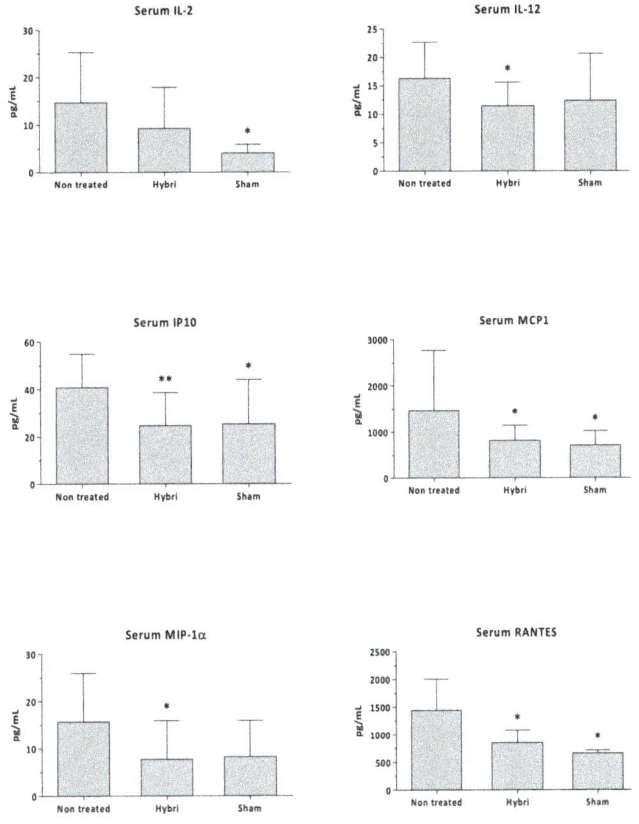


**Figure 5.** Circulating IL-2, IL-12, IP10, MCP1, MIP-1α, and RANTES in renal warm ischemia model measured by Luminex assay. Data are expressed as a mean ± SEM. *, $p < 0.05$ vs. non-treated; **, $p < 0.01$ vs. non-treated.

There were also significant mortality differences between the studied groups. The initial number of twenty-one non-treated animals was reduced to seven at the 21st day, representing a 33% survival rate (Figure 7). Among the surviving animals, only one lived to the end of the study at day 90 (4.8%). The mean survival of this group was 23 days. On the other hand, the administration of the HYBRI protein during the firsts 6 days of the study significantly improved the animal survival up to 57 days, more than double that in the group without treatment. This data was significant in the Log rank Mantel Cox test of the Kaplan Meier curve. On the 21st day of the study, a survival rate of 80% of the group was seen ($p = 0.021$), and this finally decreased to 30% at the end of the study at day 90, a higher percentage than the almost 5% corresponding to the untreated group ($p = 0.005$).

2.3.2. Renal Histopathology and Immunohistochemistry

As seen in Figure 8, conventional kidney histology reflected a significant score reduction from 8.1 in the non-treated group to 3.5 in the HYBRI group ($p < 0.001$). Regarding kidney infiltrating cells, there were significant differences in CD3+, where the mean of 24.9 cells/hpf in the non-treated group was reduced to 10.3 cells/hpf in the HYBRI-treated group ($p = 0.0237$). Macrophage infiltration was also significantly reduced with HYBRI treatment, where the mean semi-quantitative score of 2.97 in the non-treated group was decreased to 1.94 with HYBRI treatment ($p = 0.0015$). Humoral effect was analyzed with

C4d staining, and significant reductions were found with the HYBRI treatment in both studied areas ($p = 0.0287$ for glomeruli and $p = 0.0034$ for peritubular capillary).

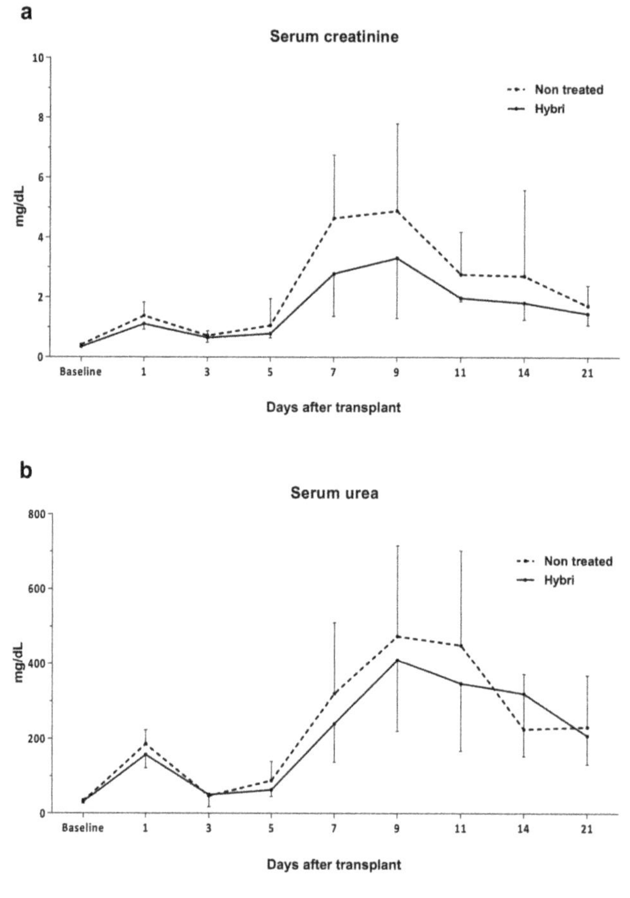


**Figure 6.** Functional renal parameters throughout the allogeneic transplant model for HYBRI treatment and non-treated groups. (**a**) Serum creatinine and (**b**) serum urea levels for the initial 21 days of the study. Values are expressed in mg/dL. Data are expressed as means.

### 2.3.3. Circulating Inflammatory Cyto/Chemokines

A significant reduction of up to three-fold in IP-10, RANTES, and MCP1 was observed in rats treated with HYBRI compared with non-treated rats. Animals treated with HYBRI had reduced MIP1$\alpha$ values, but they were not statistically different because there was a huge dispersal in non-treated rats. Finally, non-significant reduction in IFN$\gamma$ and IL-12 was seen (Figure 9).

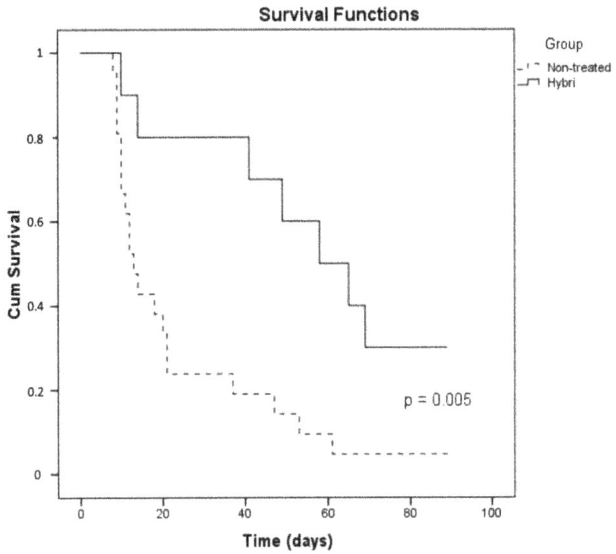


**Figure 7.** Survival differences with the Kaplan Meier analysis of the two studied groups in the rat allogeneic transplant model.

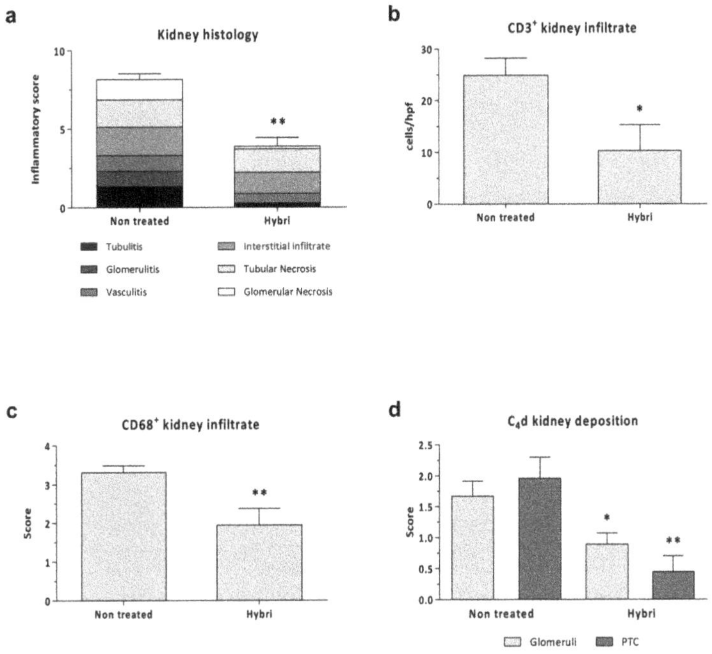


**Figure 8.** Renal histopathology parameters for allogeneic transplant model in the two studied groups. Semi-quantitative inflammatory score values (**a**) for Hematoxylin-Eosin stain. Cells per hpf values for renal immunofluorescence CD3+ (**b**) and semi-quantitative score for CD68+ surface intensity (**c**) and C4d kidney deposition (**d**). Data are expressed as a mean ± SEM. *, $p < 0.05$ vs. Non-treated; **, $p < 0.01$ vs. Non-treated.

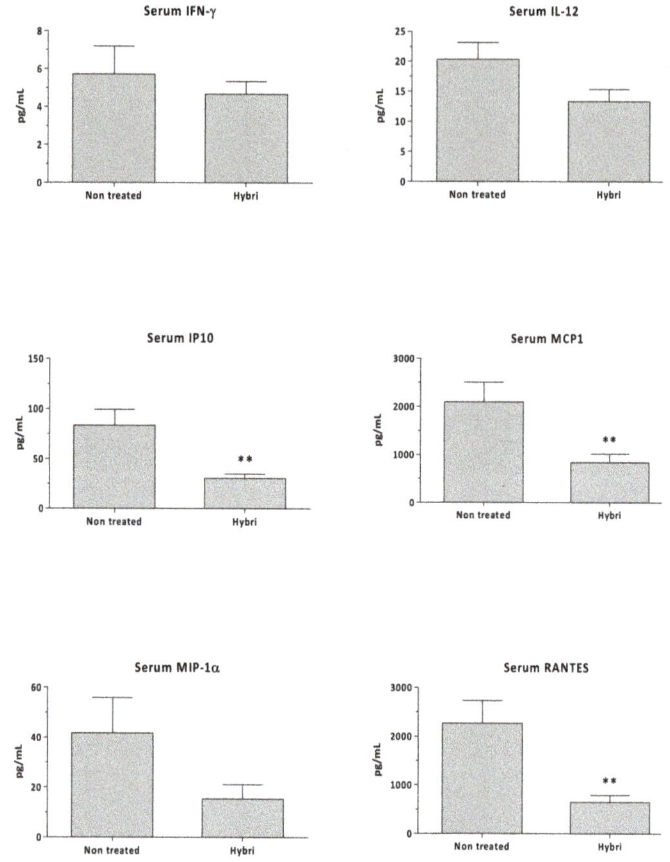


**Figure 9.** Circulating IFNγ, IL-12, IP10, MCP1, MIP-1α, and RANTES in allogeneic transplant model measured by Luminex assay. Data are expressed as a mean ± SEM. **, $p < 0.01$ vs. non-treated.

## 3. Discussion

Ischemia reperfusion damage is a deleterious response in acutely injured kidneys in several clinical situations. In this setting, costimulatory lymphocyte signals have been involved or modulated successfully [41–45]. We here show a positive modulation of both warm renal ischemia and allograft response by means of a dual and opposite costimulatory targeting, combining two coinhibitory receptors, CTLA4 and PDL2.

After the theoretical design of the construct and the genetic transient insertion in the CHO mammalian cell line, HYBRI was synthesized and its in vitro activity was assessed in the mixed lymphocyte reaction [46] with successful inhibition of T cell response. As a first validation, the well-known SPR technique showed the great affinity of our newly designed HYBRI protein with the CD80 and PD-1 targets, thus confirming that the binding sites of the proteins that make up the structure do not condition their binding avidity. In this regard, HYBRI protein presents its effective binding to both CD80 and PD-1 simultaneously, which indicates that HYBRI can block the CD28-CD80 costimulatory pathway while stimulating the PD-1-PD-L2 coinhibitory pathway. These bindings are effective despite the approximately 70% protein homology shared between species, given that HYBRI is a fully human protein [47,48]. Consequently, these results support the protein affinity to its designed targets, appearing as an interesting option in the inflammatory animal models addressed in the present study. Despite the reported similar KD values of the CD80 and

HYBRI CTLA4 interaction, the KD values of the PD-1 and HYBRI's PD-L2 interaction are higher than the values found in the literature [31,49–52]. Similarly to the increased affinity of the modified PD-L2 described by Philips et al. [51], PD-L2 molecules in the HYBRI construct may have suffered conformational changes, which might account for its increased binding to PD-1. Nevertheless, in both rat models HYBRI shows therapeutic efficacy, which suggests that the binding is high enough to exert biological effects.

The dual and opposite costimulatory targeting conferred by HYBRI have induced a protective effect against the kidney warm ischemia model, as the renal function and structure after the insult is greatly improved in the treated rats. This effect may be based on CD80 costimulatory blocking, which reduces the macrophage and T cell migration and, also, may promote T cell apoptosis [19,53–56]. The PD-1/PD-L2 pathway may have also produced Treg clonal expansion and diminished the T effector cell expression [24,34,57]. These pathways appear to be well addressed by the protein, although the expressions of these molecules and their ligands are not exclusive to the APC and T cells and, in some cases, can be bidirectional [34]. For example, renal tubular epithelial cells (RTECs), podocytes, and other renal cells also express CD80 and PD-L2 on their surface [58–60]. This may suggest that the desired homeostatic effect is not specific to APCs but can also be exerted on other semi-professional cells in antigen presentation. As ischemia is present in both groups, it can be seen that the expansion of Tregs promoted by the administration of HYBRI plays an essential role in homeostasis. Thus, the observed reduction in macrophages and T cells in the kidney together with the increase in regulatory T cells indicates the cellular modulation by the HYBRI treatment of post ischemic renal inflammatory damage. In addition, the significant decline in circulating inflammatory-related mediators reflects the efficacy of HYBRI in modulating the inflammatory response at the systemic level [61–64].

A daily peripheral cytometric study showed only changes between study groups for Tregs expansion on the first day after ischemia. The results suggest that the CD25+ population experienced clonal expansion early after ischemia injury, also including the FoxP3+ subset, but that the Tregs subset is additionally expanded with the HYBRI treatment. At the end of the study, peripheral and spleen population assessment did not reveal significant cell differences between the groups despite a significant reduction in renal inflammatory infiltrate being found with HYBRI treatment. Thus, peripheral blood or spleen compartments may not reflect organ parenchymal changes where there is a real inflammatory environment with myriads of attractive and activation signals. The HYBRI treatment modulated the kidney inflammatory status towards a more attenuated inflammatory response and the enrichment of the Tregs population. In the allogeneic setting with a stronger immune response, the effect of HYBRI treatment may have offered two benefits. On the one hand, the reduction in the inflammation derived from cold ischemia reperfusion damage, but also an intense modulation of the adaptive response of T and possibly B cells given the reduction in C4d deposition.

A gene array analysis showed differences between the sham group and ischemia-reperfusion groups, but few significant differences between the non-treated and HYBRI groups. Thus, the regulation of some of the studied genes can be observed. These genes are related to both the inflammation and expression of cell surface proteins such as CD80 and CD86. In this regard, the HYBRI treatment may produce a reduction in CD80 and CD86 cell surface expression, an important point in this immunomodulation strategy [19,53,54]. It is also remarkable that the protein HYBRI modifies only some of the pathways related to IRI, despite showing a large and significant therapeutic effect in vivo.

Regarding early cold ischemia injury in the allogeneic transplant model, a slight amelioration in renal functional parameters is observed in the group treated with HYBRI. In this complex surgical model, it is hard to discern ischemic damage among all surgical attritions, contrarily to the easier native warm ischemia. In this second proposed model, however, the effect of the HYBRI protein plays an essential role in kidney rejection, where the treated group improved the renal function on days 7 and 9 after transplantation and prolonged the survival of animals to more than double that of non-treated rats. Recently, it has been shown that there is early PD-1 expression in renal allograft dynamics. Blocking this PD-1/PD-L1 negative costimulatory pathway during the first week doubled the number of PD-1-expressing CD8 and CD4 cells, causing terminal acute rejection [29]. These findings with an approach completely opposite to our PD-1, which activates this negative pathway, suggest the essential role of this pathway in modulating T cell expansion and cytokine production in the allograft setting. Similar studies with PD-L1 and PD-L2 blocking antibodies in a model of IRI also aggravated the renal damage, again suggesting the protecting role of this coinhibitory pathway [24].

To summarize, the SPR study has shown the exquisite binding affinity of HYBRI to both targets and the advantage of binding simultaneously in vitro. Regarding in vivo studies, the HYBRI protein may effectively mitigate damage from warm ischemia reperfusion. In the context of the kidney transplant model, the HYBRI protein also prevents kidney rejection even by treating animals only during the first week. Therefore, this dual and opposite protein effect on costimulatory pathways can promote several immunomodulatory mechanisms, leading to protecting the kidney from multiple immunoinflammatory states.

## 4. Materials and Methods

### *4.1. HYBRI Characterization and Binding Affinity Assessment with Surface Plasmon Resonance (SPR) Technique*

Surface plasmon resonance (SPR) analyses were performed at 25 °C on a Biacore T200 (GE Healthcare BioSciences AB, Uppsala, Sweden). The HYBRI construct was diluted in acetate buffer pH 5 (50 µg/mL and immobilized on a CM5 chip (GE) by amine coupling in the active flow channels (Fc) at two different ligand densities. Briefly, the surface was activated with a mixture of 1:1 mixture of 0.1 M NHS (N-hydroxysuccinimide) and 0.1 M EDC (3-(N,N-dimethylamino) propyl-N-ethylcarbodiimide) at a flow rate of 5 µL/min, followed by the injection of ligand or buffer for the active or reference channel, respectively. Ethanolamine solution was injected in both channels in order to block the remaining reactive groups of the surface. Analytes (recombinant murine PD-1 and CD80, R&D systems) were prepared in PBS-P in serial dilutions (0, 15.6, 62.5, 125, 250, 500, 1000, and 2000 nM) and were injected in parallel in two active and reference channels at 30 µL/min flow for 90 s and a dissociation time of 240 s. Blanks were included for double referencing. Experiments were also conducted to assess the effect of PD-1 presence on the CD80 binding to Hybri. For this, concentrations series of CD80 (0–2000 nM) in the presence of PD-1 (250 nM) were included. Kinetic and affinity constants were calculated using the Biacore T200 evaluation software 2.0 after reference and blank subtraction, and sensorgrams were fitted according to the 1:1 Langmuir model.

### *4.2. Animals and Surgical Procedures*

All the procedures were performed following the Guidelines of the European Committee on Care and Use of Laboratory Animals and Good Laboratory Practice. Rats from Charles River, Spain, were housed with 12 h dark/light cycles and at a constant temperature. The animals were fed *ad libitum* with standard diet and water. For both ischemia and transplant surgical models, a combined anesthesia based on ketamine (75 mg/kg), atropine (0.05 mg/kg), and valium (5 mg/kg) was used. A single intramuscular injection of ciprofloxacin (5 mg) was administered after the surgery.

### *4.3. Renal Warm Ischemia Model*

In this model, Lewis rats received intraperitoneally one single dose of 20 mg/kg of HYBRI administered 24 h before bilateral renal ischemia of 40 min ($n$ = 10, Hybri). Non-treated animals were used as control group ($n$ = 10, Vehicle), and they received one single intraperitoneal administration of 300 µL of PBS 24 h before the bilateral renal ischemia of 40 min. The sham group received neither treatment nor ischemia and only laparotomy as a technique control group was performed ($n$ = 3, Sham).

Blood samples were obtained from the tail vein at time zero and on daily basis until sacrifice on day 7 after ischemia. Animals were euthanized under anesthesia on the seventh day, blood was obtained by aortic puncture, and the spleen and kidneys were processed.

### 4.4. Allogeneic Transplant Model (Cold Ischemia)

In a model of renal allotransplantation, binephrectomized Lewis rats received a single kidney transplant from a Wistar donor rats. HYBRI group ($n$ = 10) animals were treated with administration of 500 µg of HYBRI intraperitoneally 2 h before transplantation and the six following days. Non-treated ($n$ = 21) animals were used as a control group with the administration of 200 µL of PBS with the same schedule.

Blood samples of both groups were obtained from the tail vein at time zero and on days 1, 3, 5, 7, 9, 11, and 14 and weekly after the transplant. Surviving animals at day 90 were euthanized under anesthesia, blood was obtained by aortic puncture, and the spleen and kidneys were processed.

### 4.5. Renal Function

Renal function was analyzed daily on warm ischemia model and on days 0, 1, 3, 5, 7, 9, 11, and 14 and weekly on the allogeneic transplant model. Serum creatinine and urea measurements were performed following Jaffe's and GLDH reactions (Olympus Autoanalyzer AU400, Hamburg, Germany) in the Veterinary Clinical Biochemistry Laboratory of Universitat Autonoma de Barcelona.

### 4.6. Histological and Immunohistochemistry Studies

Coronal kidney slices 1–2 mm thick were fixed in buffered 4% of formalin, paraffined, and stained with H&E. Kidney sections from the ischemia-reperfusion study were evaluated by a blinded pathologist, examining the tubular necrosis, dilation, interstitial edema, and cellular infiltrate. Abnormalities were scored on semiquantitative scale from 0 to 4 as follows: 0, no abnormalities; 1, changes <25%; 2, changes 25–50%; 3, changes 50–75%; and 4, changes >75%. A mean group score was attained from all the individual parameters.

For the allogeneic study, sections were analyzed by a blinded pathologist for tubulitis, interstitial infiltration, vasculitis, glomerulitis, tubular necrosis and glomerular necrosis following the Banff criteria for acute/active lesions scoring, held at the Ninth Banff Conference on Allograft Pathology in La-Coruna, Spain, on 26 June 2007.

For immunohistochemistry techniques, paraffin tissue sections were stained for CD3 (Abcam, Cambridge, UK), C4d (Hycult Biotech, Uden, Netherlands), CD68 (AbD Serotec, Raleigh, NC, USA), and FoxP3 (Novus Biologicals, CO, USA). Sections were immune peroxidase labeled and revealed by diaminobenzidine (Sigma, Madrid, Spain). For the CD3, CD68, and FoxP3 measurement, at least 10 hpf were taken to analyze and count. For the C4d measurement, a semiquantitative scale from 0 to 3 was employed. Negative controls from immunostained-matched sections without primary antibodies were used.

### 4.7. Peripheral Blood and Spleen Cell Subsets Characterization by Flow Cytometry

Daily peripheral blood from warm ischemia model and blood before transplant and on days 7 and 21 for the transplant model was collected in heparin tubes and separated in cytometry tubes to add the antibodies and lysis buffer needed to continue with the cytometry protocol.

Splenocytes were preserved at −80 °C after its isolation using the Ficoll (GE Healthcare) density gradient. Standard methods were used to thaw, wash, and recover the cells. An incubation of 25 min in the dark at room temperature with different monoclonal antibodies was performed for the cytometry technique using FACS Canto II Cytometer and the subsequent analysis using FACS DIVA software (BD Biosciences, San Jose, CA, USA). The antibodies were titrated, mixed, and formulated for optimal staining performance.

Cocktail T/B/NK (BD 558495) containing anti-CD3 APC, anti-CD45RA FITC, and anti-CD161 PE for T, B, and NK cell detection; anti-CD43 PE (Biolegend 202812), anti-

CD161 AF647 (AbD Serotec MCA1427A647), and anti-ED9 FITC (AbD Serotec MCA620F) for monocytes detection; and anti-CD3 PerCP efluor (eBioscience 46-0030-80), anti-CD4 FITC (eBioscience 11-0040-85), anti-CD25 APC (eBioscience 17-0390-82), and anti-Fox P3 PE (eBioscience 12-4774-42) for Tregs detection. Cell membrane and nucleus permeabilization was needed for Tregs cytometric detection.

### 4.8. *Measurement of Serum Levels of Inflammatory Factors by Luminex Fluorescent Assay*

The determination of IFN$\gamma$, IL-2, IL-12/IL-23p40, MIP-1$\alpha$ (CCL3), RANTES (CCL5), IP-10 (CXCL10), and MCP-1 (CCL2) concentrations in serum was conducted using Luminex ProcartaPlex™ Multiplex Immunoassay (Thermo Fisher Scientific, Waltham, MA, USA) following the manufacturer's instructions. Results were calculated from the calibration curves and expressed in pg/mL.

### 4.9. *Quantification of Gene Expression in Kidneys from Warm Ischemia Model*

Snap-frozen rat kidneys from the ischemia-reperfusion study were stored at—80 °C. RNA samples with an A260/280 ratio of $\geq$1.8 were extracted using the PureLinkTM RNA MiniKit (Invitrogen, Madrid, Spain) following the manufacturer's instructions. For the reverse transcription, High-Capacity cDNA reverse Transcription Kit (Applied Biosystems, Madrid, Spain) was used following the manufacturer's instructions.

The tissue expression of immune-inflammatory mediators was quantified by Taqman Low Density Array microfluidic cards (ABI-PrismH-7700, Applied Biosystems, Madrid, Spain) using the comparative CT method: Emp1/Emp3/Lgals1/Lgals3/Reln/S100a6/S100a8/S100a9/Socs3/Socs5/Tnfrsf12a/Fcnb/CD4/CD40/CD80/CD86/Tnf/Nfkb1/Ctla4/Tlr2/Tlr4/Tlr6/Ccl2/Ccl3/Ccl5/Ccl7/Cxcr3/Cxcl10/Cxcl11/Ccr2/Ccr3/Ccr5/Ptprc/Junb/Igsf6/Ido2/Il2/Il9/Il10/Il15/Il17a/Tfcp2/Mapk9/Spp1/Bcl6 and eukaryotic 18S as an endogenous reference.

Moreover, the expression of genes validated in recent studies from our group [1] were quantified by TaqMan real-time PCR (Applied Biosystems, Madrid, Spain) using the comparative CT method: C1qa/C1qc/C1r/C1s/CD19/CD276/CD44/Cxcl3/Cxcr4/Fas/FoxP3/Hgf/Ifng/IL-10ra/IL-11/RORC/Socs1/Sox9/TLR8/TLR9/Tnfrsf1b/Vcam and GAPDH as endogenous reference. Controls, which were composed of distilled water, were negative for the target and reference genes.

A pathway analysis of single gene sets, it was set up using the online PathwaX.sbc.su.se web server, which applies the BinoX algorithm to KEGG pathways and FunCoup networks [65].

### 4.10. *Statistical Analysis*

For a statistical analysis, the Student's t-test compared two conditions, whereas the ANOVA was employed for the comparison of multiple conditions. Repeated measures ANOVAs were used to analyze differences in various parameters due to HYBRI treatment throughout the follow-up. Nonparametric analysis was used as needed. For the comparative CT method, the value shown is the one obtained by performing the Wilcoxon rank sum test when comparing the data of the study treatment with the data of the control treatment. The Kaplan-Meier method was performed and analyzed using the Mantel Cox test for a comparison of the survival distributions in the two groups. A value of $p < 0.05$ was considered significant. Data are given as a mean $\pm$ s.e.m.

**Supplementary Materials:** The following are available online at https://www.mdpi.com/1422-0067/22/3/1216/s1, Figure S1: PathwAX gene array results; Table S1: PathwAX list of the pathways related to gene array.

**Author Contributions:** Conceptualization, O.B., J.M.G. and J.T.; HYBRI design, J.M.G.; HYBRI recombinant synthesis, D.R.; methodology, J.G., L.D.R., E.C., N.B., S.B.-B., L.M.-V., P.F. and M.J.; formal analysis, J.G., J.M.G. and J.T.; writing—original draft preparation, J.G., L.D.R., J.M.G. and J.T.; writing—review and editing, J.G., J.M.G. and J.T.; visualization, J.G., A.T., O.B., J.M.G. and J.T.;

supervision, J.M.G. and J.T.; project administration, O.B., J.M.G. and O.B.; funding acquisition, J.G., O.B., J.M.G. and J.T. All authors have read and agreed to the published version of the manuscript.

**Funding:** This research was funded by grants from the Instituto de Salud Carlos III (Madrid, Spain) PI17/00277 and PI19/01710, co-funded by FEDER funds/European Regional Development Fund -a way to build Europe. The study was also supported by Fundación Renal Iñigo Alvarez de Toledo (20PSJ003).

**Institutional Review Board Statement:** The study was conducted according to the guidelines of the Declaration of Helsinki, and approved by "CEEA: Animal Experimentation Ethic Committee", the Institutional Ethics UB Committee for Animal Research (201/18, April 9th, 2018).

**Informed Consent Statement:** Not applicable.

**Data Availability Statement:** The data presented in this study are available on request from the corresponding author.

**Acknowledgments:** We thank Serveis Científico-Tècnics (UB, Campus Bellvitge) for technical support, Cristian Tebé from Unitat de Bioestadística of IDIBELL for the gene analyzing help and Josep Gardenyes (IDIBELL Scientific-Technical Services) for technical support with SPR experiments. We thank CERCA Programme/Generalitat de Catalunya for institutional support.

**Conflicts of Interest:** The authors declare no conflict of interest.

## References

1. De Ramon, L.; Ripoll, È.; Merino, A.; Lucia, M.; Aran, J.M.; Pérez-Rentero, S.; Lloberas, N.; Cruzado, J.M.; Grinyó, J.M.; Torras, J. CD154-CD40 T-cell co-stimulation pathway is a key mechanism in kidney ischemia-reperfusion injury. *Kidney Int.* **2015**, *88*, 538–549. [CrossRef]
2. Mannon, R.B. Delayed Graft Function: The AKI of Kidney Transplantation. *Nephron* **2018**, *140*, 94–98. [CrossRef] [PubMed]
3. Montagud-Marrahi, E.; Molina-Andújar, A.; Rovira, J.; Revuelta, I.; Ventura-Aguiar, P.; Piñeiro, G.; Ugalde-Altamirano, J.; Perna, F.; Torregrosa, J.; Oppenheimer, F.; et al. The impact of functional delayed graft function in the modern era of kidney transplantation—A retrospective study. *Transpl. Int.* **2021**, *34*, 175–184. [CrossRef] [PubMed]
4. Panisello-Roselló, A.; Roselló-Catafau, J. Molecular Mechanisms and Pathophysiology of Ischemia-Reperfusion Injury. *Int. J. Mol. Sci.* **2018**, *19*, 4093. [CrossRef] [PubMed]
5. Zhang, J.; Wei, X.; Tang, Z.; Miao, B.; Luo, Y.; Hu, X.; Luo, Y.; Zhou, Y.; Na, N. Elucidating the molecular pathways and immune system transcriptome during ischemia-reperfusion injury in renal transplantation. *Int. Immunopharmacol.* **2020**, *81*, 106246. [CrossRef]
6. Nieuwenhuijs-Moeke, G.J.; Pischke, S.E.; Berger, S.P.; Sanders, J.-S.F.; Pol, R.A.; Struys, M.M.; Ploeg, R.J.; Leuvenink, H.G.D. Ischemia and Reperfusion Injury in Kidney Transplantation: Relevant Mechanisms in Injury and Repair. *J. Clin. Med.* **2020**, *9*, 253. [CrossRef]
7. Eltzschig, M.H.K.; Eckle, T. Ischemia and reperfusion—from mechanism to translation. *Nat. Med.* **2011**, *17*, 1391–1401. [CrossRef]
8. Ogawa, S.; Gerlach, H.; Esposito, C.; Pasagian-Macaulay, A.; Brett, J.; Stern, D. Hypoxia modulates the barrier and coagulant function of cultured bovine endothelium. Increased monolayer permeability and induction of procoagulant properties. *J. Clin. Investig.* **1990**, *85*, 1090–1098. [CrossRef]
9. Bonventre, J.V.; Yang, L. Cellular pathophysiology of ischemic acute kidney injury. *J. Clin. Investig.* **2011**, *121*, 4210–4221. [CrossRef]
10. Lowenstein, C.J. Myocardial reperfusion injury. *N. Engl. J. Med.* **2007**, *357*, 2409.
11. Carroll, M.C.; Holers, V. Innate Autoimmunity. *Adv. Immunol.* **2005**, *86*, 137–157. [CrossRef] [PubMed]
12. Satpute, S.R.; Park, J.M.; Jang, H.R.; Agreda, P.; Liu, M.; Gandolfo, M.T.; Racusen, L.; Rabb, H. The Role for T Cell Repertoire/Antigen-Specific Interactions in Experimental Kidney Ischemia Reperfusion Injury. *J. Immunol.* **2009**, *183*, 984–992. [CrossRef] [PubMed]
13. Shen, X.; Wang, Y.; Gao, F.; Ren, F.; Busuttil, R.W.; Kupiec-Weglinski, J.W.; Zhai, Y. CD4 T cells promote tissue inflammation via CD40 signaling without de novo activation in a murine model of liver ischemia/reperfusion injury. *Hepatology* **2009**, *50*, 1537–1546. [CrossRef] [PubMed]
14. Ripoll, E.; Merino, A.; Gomà, M.; Aran, J.M.; Bolaños, N.; De Ramon, L.; Herrero-Fresneda, I.; Bestard, O.; Cruzado, J.M.; Grinyó, J.M.; et al. CD40 Gene Silencing Reduces the Progression of Experimental Lupus Nephritis Modulating Local Milieu and Systemic Mechanisms. *PLoS ONE* **2013**, *8*, e65068. [CrossRef]
15. Monteiro, R.M.; Camara, N.O.S.; Rodrigues, M.M.; Tzelepis, F.; Damião, M.J.; Cenedeze, M.A.; Teixeira, V.D.P.A.; Dos Reis, M.A.; Pacheco-Silva, Á. A role for regulatory T cells in renal acute kidney injury. *Transpl. Immunol.* **2009**, *21*, 50–55. [CrossRef]
16. De Greef, K.E.; Ysebaert, D.K.; Dauwe, S.; Persy, V.P.; Vercauteren, S.R.; Mey, D.; De Broe, M.E. Anti-B7-1 blocks mononuclear cell adherence in vasa recta after ischemia. *Kidney Int.* **2001**, *60*, 1415–1427. [CrossRef]

17. Bluestone, J.A.; Clair, E.W.S.; Turka, L.A. CTLA4Ig: Bridging the Basic Immunology with Clinical Application. *Immunity* **2006**, *24*, 233–238. [CrossRef]
18. Hathcock, K.S.; Laszlo, G.; Pucillo, C.; Linsley, P.; Hodes, R.J. Comparative analysis of B7-1 and B7-2 costimulatory ligands: Expression and function. *J. Exp. Med.* **1994**, *180*, 631–640. [CrossRef]
19. Takada, M.; Chandraker, A.; Nadeau, K.C.; Sayegh, M.H.; Tilney, N.L. The role of the B7 costimulatory pathway in experimental cold ischemia/reperfusion injury. *J. Clin. Investig.* **1997**, *100*, 1199–1203. [CrossRef]
20. Podojil, J.R.; Miller, S.D. Targeting the B7 family of co-stimulatory molecules: Successes and challenges. *BioDrugs* **2013**, *27*, 1–13. [CrossRef]
21. Wekerle, T.; Grinyó, J. Belatacept: From rational design to clinical application. *Transpl. Int.* **2011**, *25*, 139–150. [CrossRef] [PubMed]
22. Vincenti, F.; Rostaing, L.; Grinyo, J.; Rice, K.; Steinberg, S.; Gaite, L.; Moal, M.-C.; Mondragon-Ramirez, G.A.; Kothari, J.; Polinsky, M.S.; et al. Belatacept and Long-Term Outcomes in Kidney Transplantation. *N. Engl. J. Med.* **2016**, *374*, 333–343. [CrossRef] [PubMed]
23. Parsons, R.F.; Zahid, A.; Bumb, S.; Decker, H.; Sullivan, H.C.; Lee, F.E.; Badell, I.R.; Ford, M.L.; Larsen, C.P.; Pearson, T.C.; et al. The impact of belatacept on third-party HLA alloantibodies in highly sensitized kidney transplant recipients. *Am. J. Transplant.* **2020**, *20*, 573–581. [CrossRef] [PubMed]
24. Jaworska, K.; Ratajczak, J.; Huang, L.; Whalen, K.; Yang, M.; Stevens, B.K.; Kinsey, G.R. Both PD-1 Ligands Protect the Kidney from Ischemia Reperfusion Injury. *J. Immunol.* **2015**, *194*, 325–333. [CrossRef]
25. Sharpe, A.H.; Pauken, K.E. The diverse functions of the PD1 inhibitory pathway. *Nat. Rev. Immunol.* **2018**, *18*, 153–167. [CrossRef]
26. Francisco, L.M.; Salinas, V.H.; Brown, K.E.; Vanguri, V.K.; Freeman, G.J.; Kuchroo, V.K.; Sharpe, A.H. PD-L1 regulates the development, maintenance, and function of induced regulatory T cells. *J. Exp. Med.* **2009**, *206*, 3015–3029. [CrossRef]
27. Buermann, A.; Römermann, D.; Baars, W.; Hundrieser, J.; Klempnauer, J.; Schwinzer, R. Inhibition of B-cell activation and antibody production by triggering inhibitory signals via the PD-1/PD-ligand pathway. *Xenotransplantation* **2016**, *23*, 347–356. [CrossRef]
28. Hsu, J.; Hodgins, J.J.; Marathe, M.; Nicolai, C.J.; Bourgeois-Daigneault, M.-C.; Trevino, T.N.; Azimi, C.S.; Scheer, A.K.; Randolph, H.E.; Thompson, T.W.; et al. Contribution of NK cells to immunotherapy mediated by PD-1/PD-L1 blockade. *J. Clin. Investig.* **2018**, *128*, 4654–4668. [CrossRef]
29. Shim, Y.J.; Khedraki, R.; Dhar, J.; Fan, R.; Dvorina, N.; Valujskikh, A.; Fairchild, R.L.; Baldwin, W.M. Early T cell infiltration is modulated by programed cell death-1 protein and its ligand (PD-1/PD-L1) interactions in murine kidney transplants. *Kidney Int.* **2020**, *98*, 897–905. [CrossRef]
30. Lázár-Molnár, E.; Yan, Q.; Cao, E.; Ramagopal, U.; Nathenson, S.G.; Almo, S.C. Crystal structure of the complex between programmed death-1 (PD-1) and its ligand PD-L2. *Proc. Natl. Acad. Sci. USA* **2008**, *105*, 10483–10488. [CrossRef]
31. Cheng, X.; Veverka, V.; Radhakrishnan, A.; Waters, L.C.; Muskett, F.W.; Morgan, S.H.; Huo, J.; Yu, C.; Evans, E.J.; Leslie, A.J.; et al. Structure and Interactions of the Human Programmed Cell Death 1 Receptor. *J. Biol. Chem.* **2013**, *288*, 11771–11785. [CrossRef] [PubMed]
32. Tang, S.; Kim, P.S. A high-affinity human PD-1/PD-L2 complex informs avenues for small-molecule immune checkpoint drug discovery. *Proc. Natl. Acad. Sci. USA* **2019**, *116*, 24500–24506. [CrossRef] [PubMed]
33. Garo, L.P.; Ajay, A.K.; Fujiwara, M.; Beynon, V.; Kuhn, C.; Gabriely, G.; Sadhukan, S.; Raheja, R.; Rubino, S.; Weiner, H.L.; et al. Smad7 Controls Immunoregulatory PDL2/1-PD1 Signaling in Intestinal Inflammation and Autoimmunity. *Cell Rep.* **2019**, *28*, 3353–3366. [CrossRef] [PubMed]
34. Bardhan, K.; Anagnostou, T.; Boussiotis, V.A. The PD1: PD-L1/2 Pathway from Discovery to Clinical Implementation. *Front. Immunol.* **2016**, *7*, 550. [CrossRef] [PubMed]
35. Lim, W.C.; Olding, M.; Healy, E.; Millar, T.M. Human Endothelial Cells Modulate CD4+ T Cell Populations and Enhance Regulatory T Cell Suppressive Capacity. *Front. Immunol.* **2018**, *9*. [CrossRef]
36. Chun, N.; Fairchild, R.L.; Li, Y.; Liu, J.; Zhang, M.; Baldwin, W.M.; Heeger, P.S. Complement Dependence of Murine Costimulatory Blockade-Resistant Cellular Cardiac Allograft Rejection. *Am. J. Transplant.* **2017**, *11*, 2810–2819. [CrossRef]
37. Wieland, D.; Hofmann, M.; Thimme, R. Overcoming CD8+ T-Cell Exhaustion in Viral Hepatitis: Lessons from the Mouse Model and Clinical Perspectives. *Dig. Dis.* **2017**, *35*, 334–338. [CrossRef]
38. Nixon, B.G.; Li, M. Satb1: Restraining PD1 and T Cell Exhaustion. *Immunity* **2017**, *46*, 3–5. [CrossRef]
39. Sánchez-Fueyo, A.; Markmann, J.F. Immune Exhaustion and Transplantation. *Am. J. Transplant.* **2016**, *7*, 1953–1957. [CrossRef]
40. Barcelo-Batllori, S. *Analysis of Murine CD80 and PD-1 Proteins Competition to HYBRI Bindings Using the Surface Plasmon Resonance (SPR) Technique*; Molecular Interactions Unit, Institut d'Investigació Biomèdica de Bellvitge (IDIBELL) Scientific-Technical Services, L'Hospitalet de Llobregat: Barcelona, Spain, 2020.
41. Chen, L.; Flies, D.B. Molecular mechanisms of T cell co-stimulation and co-inhibtion. *Nat. Rev. Immunol.* **2013**, *13*, 227–242. [CrossRef]
42. Sharpe, A.H. Mechanisms of costimulation. *Immunol. Rev.* **2009**, *229*, 5–11. [CrossRef] [PubMed]
43. Alegre, M.-L.; Frauwirth, K.A.; Thompson, C.B. T-cell regulation by CD28 and CTLA-4. *Nat. Rev. Immunol.* **2001**, *1*, 220–228. [CrossRef] [PubMed]
44. Nurieva, R.I.; Liu, X.; Dong, C. Yin-Yang of costimulation: Crucial controls of immune tolerance and function. *Immunol. Rev.* **2009**, *229*, 88–100. [CrossRef] [PubMed]

45. Chen, L. Co-inhibitory molecules of the B7–CD28 family in the control of T-cell immunity. *Nat. Rev. Immunol.* **2004**, *4*, 336–347. [CrossRef]
46. Crespo, E. *In Vitro Activity Assessment of HYBRI Protein Using the Mixed Lymphocyte Reaction (MLR) Technique*; Experimental Nephrology Laboratory, University of Barcelona and Institut d'Investigació Biomèdica de Bellvitge (IDIBELL), L'Hospitalet de Llobregat: Barcelona, Spain, 2017.
47. Viricel, C.; Ahmed, M.; Barakat, K. Human PD-1 binds differently to its human ligands: A comprehensive modeling study. *J. Mol. Graph. Model.* **2015**, *57*, 131–142. [CrossRef]
48. UniProt. Available online: http://www.uniprot.org/ (accessed on 14 December 2020).
49. Lee, J.-R.; Bechstein, D.J.B.; Ooi, C.C.; Patel, A.; Gaster, R.S.; Ng, E.; Gonzalez, L.C.; Wang, S.X. Magneto-nanosensor platform for probing low-affinity protein–protein interactions and identification of a low-affinity PD-L1/PD-L2 interaction. *Nat. Commun.* **2016**, *7*, 12220. [CrossRef]
50. Li, K.; Cheng, X.; Tilevik, A.; Davis, S.J.; Zhu, C. In situ and in silico kinetic analyses of programmed cell death-1 (PD-1) receptor, programmed cell death ligands, and B7-1 protein interaction network. *J. Biol. Chem.* **2017**, *292*, 6799–6809. [CrossRef]
51. Philips, E.A.; Garcia-España, A.; Tocheva, A.S.; Ahearn, I.M.; Adam, K.R.; Pan, R.; Mor, A.; Kong, X.-P. The structural features that distinguish PD-L2 from PD-L1 emerged in placental mammals. *J. Biol. Chem.* **2020**, *295*, 4372–4380. [CrossRef]
52. Li, Y.; Liang, Z.; Tian, Y.; Cai, W.; Weng, Z.; Chen, L.; Zhang, H.; Bao, Y.; Zheng, H.; Zeng, S.; et al. High-affinity PD-1 molecules deliver improved interaction with PD-L1 and PD-L2. *Cancer Sci.* **2018**, *109*, 2435–2445. [CrossRef]
53. Zhang, T.; Song, N.; Fang, Y.; Teng, J.; Xu, X.; Hu, J.; Zhang, P.; Chen, R.; Lu, Z.; Yu, X.; et al. Delayed Ischemic Preconditioning Attenuated Renal Ischemia-Reperfusion Injury by Inhibiting Dendritic Cell Maturation. *Cell. Physiol. Biochem.* **2018**, *46*, 1807–1820. [CrossRef]
54. Suzuki, A.; Satoh, S.; Tsuchiya, N.; Kato, T.; Sato, M.; Senoo, H. Upregulation of Costimulatory Adhesion Molecule (Cd80) in Rat Kidney with Ischemia/Reperfusion Injury. *Jpn. J. Urol.* **2002**, *93*, 33–38. [CrossRef] [PubMed]
55. Costantini, A.; Viola, N.; Berretta, A.; Galeazzi, R.; Matacchione, G.; Sabbatinelli, J.; Storci, G.; De Matteis, S.; Butini, L.; Rippo, M.R.; et al. Age-related M1/M2 phenotype changes in circulating monocytes from healthy/unhealthy individuals. *Aging* **2018**, *10*, 1268–1280. [CrossRef]
56. Satoh, S.; Suzuki, A.; Asari, Y.; Sato, M.; Kojima, N.; Sato, T.; Tsuchiya, N.; Sato, K.; Senoo, H.; Kato, T. Glomerular Endothelium Exhibits Enhanced Expression of Costimulatory Adhesion Molecules, CD80 and CD86, by Warm Ischemia/Reperfusion Injury in Rats. *Lab. Investig.* **2002**, *82*, 1209–1217. [CrossRef] [PubMed]
57. Dowlatshahi, M.; Huang, V.; Gehad, A.E.; Jiang, Y.; Calarese, A.; Teague, J.E.; Dorosario, A.A.; Cheng, J.; Nghiem, P.; Schanbacher, C.F.; et al. Tumor-specific T cells in human Merkel cell carcinomas: A possible role for Tregs and T-cell exhaustion in reducing T-cell responses. *J. Investig. Dermatol.* **2013**, *133*, 1879–1889. [CrossRef] [PubMed]
58. Banu, N.; Meyers, C.M. IFN-γ and LPS differentially modulate class II MHC and B7-1 expression on murine renal tubular epithelial cells. *Kidney Int.* **1999**, *55*, 2250–2263. [CrossRef]
59. Salant, D.J. Podocyte Expression of B7-1/CD80: Is it a Reliable Biomarker for the Treatment of Proteinuric Kidney Diseases with Abatacept? *J. Am. Soc. Nephrol.* **2015**, *27*, 963–965. [CrossRef]
60. Zhang, Q.; Vignali, D.A.A. Co-stimulatory and Co-inhibitory Pathways in Autoimmunity. *Immunity* **2016**, *44*, 1034–1051. [CrossRef]
61. Wright, T.M. Cytokines in acute and chronic inflammation. *Front. Biosci.* **1997**, *2*. [CrossRef]
62. Coburn, L.A.; Singh, K.; Asim, M.; Barry, D.P.; Allaman, M.M.; Al-Greene, N.T.; Hardbower, D.M.; Polosukhina, D.; Williams, C.S.; Delgado, A.G.; et al. Loss of solute carrier family 7 member 2 exacerbates inflammation-associated colon tumorigenesis. *Oncogene* **2018**, *38*, 1067–1079. [CrossRef]
63. Lv, L.-L.; Hai-Feng, N.; Wen, Y.; Wu, W.-J.; Ni, H.-F.; Li, Z.-L.; Zhou, L.-T.; Wang, B.; Zhang, J.-D.; Crowley, S.D.; et al. Exosomal CCL2 from Tubular Epithelial Cells Is Critical for Albumin-Induced Tubulointerstitial Inflammation. *J. Am. Soc. Nephrol.* **2018**, *29*, 919–935. [CrossRef]
64. Zhang, Y.-Y.; Tang, P.M.-K.; Tang, P.C.-T.; Xiao, J.; Huang, X.-R.; Yu, C.; Ma, R.C.; Lan, H.-Y. LRNA9884, a Novel Smad3-Dependent Long Noncoding RNA, Promotes Diabetic Kidney Injury in db/db Mice via Enhancing MCP-1–Dependent Renal Inflammation. *Diabetes* **2019**, *68*, 1485–1498. [CrossRef] [PubMed]
65. Ogris, C.; Helleday, T.; Sonnhammer, E. PathwAX: A web server for network crosstalk based pathway annotation. *Nucleic Acids Res.* **2016**, *44*, W105–W109. [CrossRef] [PubMed]

International Journal of
*Molecular Sciences*

MDPI

*Review*

# Emerging Modes of Treatment of IgA Nephropathy

**Dita Maixnerova * and Vladimir Tesar**

1st Faculty of Medicine, General University Hospital, Department of Nephrology, Charles University, 128 08 Prague, Czech Republic; vladimir.tesar@vfn.cz

* Correspondence: ditama@centrum.cz; Tel.: +42-02-2496-6790

Received: 20 October 2020; Accepted: 19 November 2020; Published: 28 November 2020

check for updates

**Abstract:** IgA nephropathy is the most common primary glomerulonephritis with potentially serious outcome leading to end stage renal disease in 30 to 50% of patients within 20 to 30 years. Renal biopsy, which might be associated with risks of complications (bleeding and others), still remains the only reliable diagnostic tool for IgA nephropathy. Therefore, the search for non-invasive diagnostic and prognostic markers for detection of subclinical types of IgA nephropathy, evaluation of disease activity, and assessment of treatment effectiveness, is of utmost importance. In this review, we summarize treatment options for patients with IgA nephropathy including the drugs currently under evaluation in randomized control trials. An early initiation of immunosupressive regimens in patients with IgA nephropathy at risk of progression should result in the slowing down of the progression of renal function to end stage renal disease.

**Keywords:** IgAN; proteinuria; CKD; progression; ACEI; corticosteroids

---

## 1. Introduction, Diagnosis, Pathogenesis

IgA nephropathy (IgAN) is the most common primary glomerulonephritis worldwide with potentially serious renal outcome leading, in 30–50% of patients, to end stage renal disease (ESRD) within 20 to 30 years of follow-up [1,2].

Diagnosis of IgAN is currently based on evaluation of renal biopsy specimens with the demonstration of mesangial IgA1-dominant or co-dominant immunodeposits [3,4].

Clinical risk factors predicting poor renal outcome in patients with IgAN include time-averaged proteinuria, hypertension, decreased estimated glomerular filtration rate (eGFR) [2,5] at presentation or during follow up as well as histological findings evaluated using C-MEST classification [6,7].

IgAN is an autoimmune disease arising from a multi-hit pathophysiological process and is believed to be caused by the interaction of genetic and environmental contributing factors [2,8,9]. Genome-wide associated studies indicated a pathogenetic role of the intestinal immunity abnormalities in IgAN and confirmed a direct link of IgAN with the risk of inflammatory bowel disease or maintenance of the intestinal epithelial barrier [9].

A key role in the pathogenesis of IgAN is played by aberrantly glycosylated forms of IgA1 with galactose-deficient *O*-glycans (galactose-deficient IgA1; Gd-IgA1), which are recognized by antiglycan autoantibodies of IgG and/or IgA1 isotype, resulting in the formation of circulating immune complexes [10,11]. These complexes are deposited in the glomerular mesangium with subsequent mesangial-cell activation and local stimulation of the complement system, proliferation of mesangial cells, and production of extracellular matrix and cytokines, which could alter podocyte gene expression and glomerular permeability in clinical presentation of proteinuria and tubulointerstitial changes in IgAN [12–15]. If unabated, the damage progresses to glomerulosclerosis and interstitial fibrosis with impaired renal function with subsequent end-stage renal disease.

## 2. Treatment

Which goals do we have in treatment of patients with IgAN? We have to respect the possibility of induction of clinical remmission, reduction in proteinuria and hematuria, stabilization of renal parameters without further decline of GFR, a decrease in the rate of progression, prevention of the necessity of renal replacement therapy as well as the risk of adverse events in patients with corticosteroids and other immunosuppressive regimens. The balance of risks and benefits needs to be taken into account in all individual cases.

### *2.1. Low Risk Patients with IgAN*

Low risk patients with minor urinary abnormalities (proteinuria < 0.5 g/d and/or isolated microhematuria), normal glomerular filtration rate (GFR), no hypertension and without histological activity are at low risk of progression, do not require treatment and should be checked annually for at least 10 years according to KDIGO guidelines (Table 1) [16]. Supportive management such as diet modification, weight optimisation and smoking cessation should be taken into consideration. The ideal treatment of the initial phase of IgAN is focused on the decrease in or inhibition of production of Gd-IgA1 by means of a low cost drug with minimal adverse effects. Intestinal-associated lymphoid tissue and mucosal immunity show attractive targets [17,18]. Intestinal microbiota and/or diet regimens including gluten-free diet were suggested in an experimental mice model and human pilot studies [17,19].

Low protein diets were reported to decrease renal function decline [20]. The restriction of sodium was associated with sodium sensitivity of blood pressure and correlated with renal ultrastructural damage [21]. The decrease in proteinuria was shown even in normotensive patients with IgAN due to low-sodium diets [21]. The damaging effects of heightened sodium sensitivity are mediated due to the renin-angiotensin system and it was confirmed that sodium restriction improves the antiproteinuric effects of RAS inhibition in patients with IgAN [22]. Increased morbidity and mortality in patients with chronic kidney disease were associated with extreme body mass index [23]. The relation between body mass index and the probability of end stage renal disease was shown in patients with IgAN in a Chinese study [23]. Increased body mass index associated with lower remission of proteinuria subsequent to treatment was confirmed in a Japanese study [24]. It was assumed that obesity increased proteinuria in connection with hypertension and other parts of metabolic syndrome. Moreover, the advantages of losing weight in overweight patients with IgAN through protein/sodium restriction, and by attaining maximal control of hypertension using treatment with inhibitors of the renin-angiotension system, were confirmed [25].

In addition, the benefits of quitting smoking on slowing down the progression of renal function decline in patients with IgAN were assessed [26].

### *2.2. Intermediate Risk Patients with IgAN*

Intermediate risk IgAN patients with proteinuria > 0.5–1 g/d, and/or hypertension and a reduced GFR (without active histological findings in renal specimens) should obtain optimized supportive treatment with the inhibitors of the renin-angiotensin system (RAS) with up-titration of the drug depending on blood pressure to achieve proteinuria < 1 g/d, and should be thoroughly monitored [16]. The suggested therapeutic goals of blood pressure in patients with proteinuria < 1 g/d are <130/80 mmHg, and <125/75 mmHg in patients with initial proteinuria >1 g/d (Table 1) [16]. RAS inhibition was demonstrated to reduce proteinuria and may possibly also reduce the progression of chronic kidney disease in patients with IgAN; at least part of this effect is probably mediated by improved control of blood pressure. High risk of mortality of patients with IgAN might be caused by chronic kidney disease [27–29].

**Table 1.** KDIGO guidelines for the treatment of IgAN [16].

| Intervention | Recommendation | Grade |
|---|---|---|
| **Antiproteinuric and Antihypertensive Therapy** | Long-term treatment of ACE inhibitors or ARBs is recommended for patients with proteinuria > 1 g/day, with up-titration of the drug depending on blood pressure to achieve proteinuria < 1 g/day. | **1B** |
| | A target blood pressure of < 130/80 mmHg is recommended for patients with proteinuria < 1 g daily, and <125/75 for patients with proteinuria >1 g daily. | **Not graded** |
| **Corticosteroids** | A 6 month course of corticosteroids is recommended in patients with persistent proteinuria of >1 g/day despite 3–6 months of optimal supportive care and GFR > 50 mL/min per 1.73 $m^2$. | **2C** |
| **Other Immunosuppressive Agents** | Patients with crescentic IgAN involving over 50% of glomeruli and rapidly progressive course should be treated with steroids and cyclophosphamide. | **2D** |
| | Not treating with corticosteroids combined with cyclophosphamide or azathioprine (unless crescentic forms with rapidly progressive course). | **2D** |
| | Not using immunosuppressive regimen in patients with GFR < 30 mL/min per 1.73 $m^2$ (unless crescentic forms with rapidly progressive course). | **2C** |
| | Not using MMF. | **2C** |
| **Fish oils** | Fish oils may be potentially useful in patients with persistent proteinuria ≥ 1 g/day, despite 3–6 months of optimized supportive care. | **2D** |
| **Tonsilectomy, Antiplatelet Agents** | Not recommended. | **2C** |

It was suggested that patients with persistent proteinuria ≥ 1 g/d, despite 3–6 months of optimized supportive care (including RAS and blood pressure control), and GFR > 50 mL/min per 1.73 $m^2$, should receive a 6-month course of corticosteroid therapy (Table 1) [16]. The 10-year renal survival and median proteinuria were significantly better in patients who received a 6-month regimen of corticosteroids compared to patients with a symptomatic treatment (97% vs. 53%, $p = 0.0003$; median proteinuria 1.9 g/24 h at baseline, 1.1 g/24 h after six months and 0.6 g/24 h after a median of seven years) [30]. Other randomized and observational trials supported the potential effect of corticosteroids in IgAN [27,31]. The retrospective analysis of the VALIGA study showed, in patients treated with steroids and RAS blockers (RASB), significant reduction in proteinuria, renal function decline and increased renal survival, not only in patients with normal renal function but also in patients with eGFR < 50 mL/min per 1.73 $m^2$ (reaching proteinuria <1 g/day in 74% patients with corticosteroids and RASB vs. 37% in patients with RASB; slope of eGFR −0.3 ± 6.2 mL/min/1.73 $m^2$/year in patients with corticosteroids and RASB vs. −4.8 ± 7.4 mL/min/1.73 $m^2$/year in patients with RASB; $p = 0.001$) [32]. Nevertheless, little information is available about the doses, the duration of steroid treatment and the adverse events caused by corticosteroids [27].

The TESTING study, a randomized study by Lv et al., included 262 patients with persistent proteinuria 1 g/day and estimated GFR 20–120 mL/min/1.73 $m^2$, who were randomly assigned to receive 0.6–0.8 mg/kg/day of oral methylprednisolone or matching placebo [33]. The temporary results demonstrated a reduction in time-averaged proteinuria and a decreased rate of progression of CKD in the steroid-treated arm (1.37 vs. 2.36 g/day (42% lower), $p < 0.01$; −1.7 vs. −6.8 mL/min/1.73 $m^2$/year, $p = 0.031$) [33]. However, after a median follow-up of 1.5 years, serious adverse events occurred in patients with corticosteroids vs. placebo groups (14.7% vs. 3.2%, HR 4.95 (95% CI 1.87–17.0), $p = 0.03$) [33]. The additional long-term follow-up might reveal the balance of risks and benefits of steroid treatment [33]. Multiethnic trials such as the ongoing TESTING Low Dose trial (NCT01560052), should evaluate this issue further [34].

The recent STOP-IgAN Clinical Trial showed that the addition of immunosuppressive therapy (corticosteroids and cyclophosphamide followed by azathioprine) to intensive supportive care (ACEI-inhibitors or ARB) in patients with high-risk IgA nephropathy induced full remission of proteinuria (OR 4.82 (95% CI 1.43–16.30), $p = 0.01$) but did not significantly improve renal function (OR O.89 (95% CI 0.44–1.81), $p = 0.75$) and more adverse effects were observed among the patients with immunosuppressive regimens with no change in the rate of decrease in the eGFR (total number of infectious events in steroid treatment arm 182 vs. 111 in supportive care) [35]. However, of 309 patients who completed the 6-month supportive care run-in phase, 106 responded to supportive care (proteinuria level, <0.75 g of urinary protein excretion per day after the end of the run-in phase) and were not eligible for randomization. It needs to be highlighted that one third of patients were no longer suitable for randomization at the end of the run-in phase and the importance of RAS blockade was emphasized. The kidney function loss in the control group was 4 times slower in the STOP-IgAN trial than in the TESTING trial, suggesting a lower-risk population and/or differences in supportive therapy. Thus, it was assumed that low risk population of patients with IgAN with excellent prognosis with supportive care was selected in the STOP-IgAN trial. Nonetheless, detailed assessment of included patients with specific evaluation of histological renal findings and prolonged follow-up would be required for the elucidation of the results [35]. Included patients with inactive form of the disease might predominate in case of absent histological evaluation of renal specimens in the trials and the treatment of patients with inactive forms is useless. Recently, after ten years of follow-up from this study, the significant number of patients in both arms (supportive care plus immunosuppression and supportive care alone) reached the end-point with no benefits seen from the immunosuppression arm [36].

The enteric budesonide was evaluated for the treatment of IgAN in a European multicenter RCT [37]. In the NEFIGAN trial, a novel targeted-release formulation of budesonide was evaluated, designed to deliver the drug to the distal ileum with suspected suppression of B cells and inhibition of production of Gd-IgA1 moleculs transported to blood in patients with IgAN [37]. The results of the Nefigan study showed a significant reduction in proteinuria with full stabilization of eGFR without any serious side-effects [37]. A confirmatory phase 3 trial is currently underway (NCT 03643965). Other potential protease treatment with selective cleavage of IgA1 reverses mesangial deposits and hematuria in animal model and on human kidney biopsies [38,39].

Among patients with chronic kidney disease, regardless of the presence or absence of diabetes, the risk of a composite of a sustained decline in the estimated GFR of at least 50%, end-stage kidney disease, or death from renal or cardiovascular causes was significantly lower with dapagliflozin than with placebo. IgAN made up a significant proportion of the non-diabetic subgroup and the HR was an impressive 0.79 for IgAN. Unlike corticosteroid, the side effect profile is likely more favourable [40].

### 2.3. *High Risk Patients with IgAN*

Nevertheless, high risk patients with a rapid decrease in the GFR and crescentic glomerulonephritis should be treated in addition to supportive treatment with combined immunosuppression (corticosteroids and cyclophosphamide) in a regimen for induction treatment of ANCA vasculitides (Table 1) [16]. Extreme conditions with crescents involving >50% of glomeruli were considered by the KDIGO guidelines [16]. However, these cases are very rare. Just a few crescents are evaluated in majority of forms of crescentic IgAN, for which the need for aggressive treatment is doubtful. Moreover, a few glomeruli in biopsy specimens are sometimes detected with difficulties for calculation of a valid percentage of crescents. Furthermore, the percentage of glomeruli with crescents changes within a few days which makes comparison impossible among individual patients within cohort studies. Crescentic lesions were not found to have a prognostic value in the Oxford and VALIGA studies, but there was a bias in favour of using of corticosteroid/immunossupression treatment [4,41]. Another international study [7] demonstrated that C correlated with E1 and was associated with the use of CS/IS. The revised Oxford classification [42] suggested considering C1 (1–24% of glomeruli) and C2 (≥25% glomeruli with crescents). Crescents in 16% glomeruli increased the risk of renal function decline in untreated cases and crescents in 25% glomeruli predicted an unfavourable outcome independent of treatment.

Undoubtedly, crescents are a marker of histological activity but crescents can regress and do not require treatment in case of involvement of low percentages of glomeruli [43]. However in untreated patients, the negative effect of crescents on the renal function decline is well known [43]. Treatment with corticosteroids/immunossuppresion might to be initiated in case of involved crescents lesions >25% of the glomeruli (C2) and in patients with C1 involving >16% of glomeruli with other signs of disease activity such as endocapillary hypercellularity (E1 according to the Oxford classification) [43]. The importance of identifying patients at risk of progression was detailed mentioned and the task remains to avoid of exposure to immunosuppression regimen unnecessarily in patients with low risk of progression of renal function. The new international risk-prediction tool was recently developed in patients with IgAN [44,45].

Other immunosuppressive agents including calcineurin inhibitors, azathioprine, mycophenolate salts (MMF) or high-dose immunoglobulins failed to show an evident benefit or manifested with toxicity and therefore they were not recommended in clinical practice (Table 1) [46–49]. A Chinese trial randomized patients to 6 months of full dose steroids or lower dose steroid with MMF [50]. Complete proteinuria remission was similar between the two groups after one year but with fewer steroid-related adverse events in the arm with MMF [50]. Nevertheless, it was not a multiethnic study population, not all patients were treated by means of RAS-blockade and the time of follow-up was too short to evaluate the effect on renal parameters [50]. Although a possible positive effect of mycophenolate mofetil treatment in IgAN was noticed in a randomized controlled trial in China [51] with a significant reduction in the percentage of patients positive for histological change of E1 [50], the effect in Caucasian was not assessed [52] apart from the recent study on the effect of MMF therapy with a significant histological reduction in E1 score in repeated renal biopsies after 24 months ($p < 0.0001$) [53]. Further studies are needed for the assessment of treatment with mycophenolate mofetil in patients with IgAN. On the other hand several authors suggested potential benefits of rapamycin in animal and cell models of IgAN [54].

Moreover, Hydroxychloroquine in addition to optimized RAAS inhibition significantly reduced proteinuria in patients with IgAN over 6 months without evidence of adverse events. Undoubtadly, these findings require confirmation in larger treatment trials [55].

The question of the efficacy of fish oil in IgAN is uncertain (Table 1) [16]. Many randomizedclinical trials testing the efficacy of fish oil in patients with IgAN provided contrasting results [16]. It was reported that daily treatment with fish oil for 2 years may reduce the progression of renal function with few side effects in patients with IgAN [56]. Fish oil was also recommended by KDIGO guidelines if it was tolerated [16,34].

The role of adrenocorticotropic hormone (ACTH) was considered in the treatment of resistant glomerular diseases [57]. The potential involved mechanisms imagine stimulation of endogenous steroid production, activation of melanocortin receptors on inflammatory cells and direct binding to melanocortin receptors on the podocyte [57]. Administration of a 6-month course of ACTH gel in patients with IgAN at high risk of progression (proteinuria > 1 g per 24 h despite documented ACEI/ARB therapy and adequate blood pressure control for >3 months, 24-h creatinine clearance >30 mL/min/1.73 $m^2$) was prospectively investigated in an open-label pilot study (NCT 02282930). A significant decline in 24-h urinary protein (2.6 to 1.3 g; $p = 0.007$) with no significant changes in eGFR (65.5 to 61.1 mL/min, $p = 0.1$) was detected at 12-month follow-up in patients with IgAN treated with 6 months of ACTH [58].

A systematic review and meta-analysis of 14 studies indicated that tonsillectomy may induce clinical remission and decrease the rates of ESRD in IgAN patients [59]. Another multicenter controlled trial did not show a beneficial effect of tonsillectomy combined with steroid pulse therapy over steroid pulses alone to increase the incidence of clinical remission [60]. In the large VALIGA cohort (the European validation study of the Oxford classification of IgAN) of 1.147 European subjects with IgAN, no significant correlation was found between tonsillectomy and renal function decline [61].

A therapeutic option targeting B-cell pathway treatment against the production of Gd-IgA1 and its specific antibodies, such as rituximab, was involved [62,63]. A multicenter trial of 34 adult patients wih biopsy-proven IgA nephropathy and proteinuria > 1 g per day, maintained on ACEIs or ARBs with well-controlled blood pressure and eGFR < 90 mL/min/1.73 $m^2$, were randomized to receive supportive therapy either alone or with rituximab. Rituximab effectively depleted B cells (a monoclonal antiCD20 antibody) but neither serum levels of Gd-IgA1 nor its antibodies were reduced and the addition of rituximab failed to improve eGFR decline and proteinuria reduction [62]. CD20 positive B cells were targeted by rituximab but IgA positive plasma cells secreting antibodies were not affected therefore the treatment with rituximab was not efficient in patients with IgAN.

The activation of complement plays an important role in the pathogenesis of IgAN [64–70]. It was suggested that the process occurs both systemically on IgA-containing circulating immune complexes, and also locally in glomeruli, and is mediated through both the alternative and lectin pathways [13]. Pathway components were presented in the mesangial immunodeposits, including properdin and factor H (alternative pathway) and mannan-binding lectin, mannan-binding lectin-associated serine proteases 1 nad 2, and C4d (lectin pathway) [13]. Deletion of complement factor H-related genes 1 and 3 was identified as protective against the disease in GWAS [9,67].

C5a is a potent local inflammatory mediator and the presence of C5a in the kidney correlates with histological severity and proteinuria in IgAN [71]. Targeting C5a enables the suppression of local inflammation, contributing to progressive renal disease including the maintaining of the formation of C5b-9 (membrane attack complex), which plays a crucial role in the elimination of gram negative bacteria [71]. Avacopan (CCX 168), an inhibitor of the C5a receptor [72], was evaluated in an open-label Phase II trial in patients with IgAN. At the end of twelve weeks, proteinuria reduced in 6 of the 7 patients and a significant improvement of UPCR < 1 g/g was detected in 3 of the 7 patients. Undoubtedly, larger studies with longer follow up are needed in IgAN. Nevertheless, the efficacy of avacopan was confirmed in patients with ANCA-associated vasculitis where avacopan allowed the replacement of high-dose corticosteroids with respect of adverse effects of hepatic dysfunction and an increased risk of infection in a small amount of patients [73].

The alternative pathway forms an essential amplification mechanism for the activation of the classical and lectin pathways, resulting in enormous opsonisation and generation of the terminal lytic pathway [74]. The two proteases of Factor D and Factor B are elementary for this amplification process [74]. Selective reversible inhibitors of Factors B and D were developed to efficiently block the activation of alternative pathways [74]. A phase II trial of LNP023, a first in the class of oral inhibitor of Factor B, was recently recruited in patients with IgAN (Table 2). The key component of the lectin pathway demonstrates Mannose-binding lectin associated serine protease 2 (MASP-2), which elevates the production of C3 convertase and leads to further inflammatory consequences. Targeting MASP-2 seems to be promising in terms of reducing the activation of the glomerular lectin pathway and not affecting the formation of C3 convertase through the classical and alternative pathways. Presently, the MASP-2 inhibitor OMS 721 is being assessed in Phase II and Phase III studies in IgAN (Table 2).

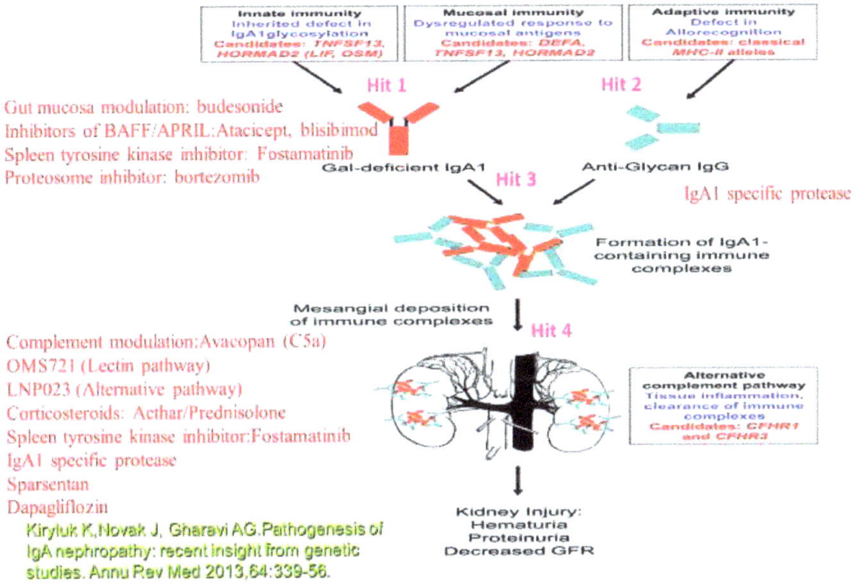


**Figure 1.** Therapeutic options related to the different targets. Target 1 **(Hit 1)**: B-lymphocyte activation results in the production of Gd-IgA1 (IgA1 poorly O-glycosylated at the hinge region). **Hit 2**: B-cell production of anti-Gd-IgA (IgG). Inhibitors of BAFF/APRIL:Atacicept, blisibimod; Spleen tyrosine kinase inhibitor: Fostamatinib;Gut mucosa modulation: budesonide; Proteosome inhibitor: bortezomib, microbiome modulation (may modulate B-lymphocyte activity with the reduction of Gd-IgA1). **Hit 3**: IgA1 specific protease. **Hit 4**:Spleen tyrosine kinase inhibitor:Fostamatinib; Corticosteroids: Acthar/Prednisolone, Complement mediation:Avacopan (C5a), OMS721 (Lectin pathway), LNP023 (Alternative pathway); IgA1 specific protease; Sparsentan; Dapagliflozin.

**Table 2.** Clinical trials in patients with IgA nephropathy—recruiting.

| | Phase | Target | Clinical Trials in Patients with IgA Nephropathy—Recruiting | Estimated Enrollment | | | | |
|---|---|---|---|---|---|---|---|---|
| | | | | Number of pts | Inclusion Criteria | Treatment—Both Arms | Primary Endpoint | Time of Follow Up |
| Therapeutic options related to different targets of the pathogenesis (See Figure 1) | | | | | | | | |
| NCT03633864 | 2 | 1 | Fecal microbiota transplantation | 30 | eGFR:20–120 mL/min/1.73 $m^2$, PU > 1 g/d | Exp:FMT arm/Biol.FMT | Change of urinary protein for 24 h | 8 wks |
| NCT04438603 | NA | 4 | The Role of T/B Cell Repertoire in Non-invasive Diagnosis and Disease Monitoring in pts with IgAN | 50 | eGFR ≥ 30 mL/min/1.73/$m^2$ | ACEI/ARB for non-progressive IgAN; Isu:CPA i.v./MMF p.o. for progressive IgAN | Urinary protein remission rate | 2 yrs |
| NCT03001947 | NA | others | Registration Initiative of High Quality (INSIGHT) | 10,000 | Biopsy proven IgAN | Observational/no intervention | Mortality, renal outcome (doubling of S-creat or ESRD) | 10 yrs |
| NCT04042623 | 2 | 4 | AVB-S6-500 (inhibitor of GAS6/AXL signaling pathway) | 24 | eGFR ≥ 45 mL/min/1.73 $m^2$, PU 1–3 g/d | Experimental: Treatment with AVB-S6-500 | Incidence od AE, UPE (g/d) | 14 wks |
| NCT03188887 | 3 | 4 | TIGER study (Treatment of IgA nEphropathy according to Renal lesions) | 122 | Biopsy proven IgAN < 45 days, PCR ratio > 0.75 g/g (within 30 days the renal biopsy) | RAS blockade treatment/Corticotherapy + RAS blockade treatment | Change of PCR, decline of eGFR | 2 yrs |
| NCT03945318 | 1 | 1 | BION-1301, a humanized IgG4 anti-a proliferation-inducing ligand (APRIL) monoclonal antibody | 92 | Biopsy proven IgAN within the past 10 years, PU ≥ 0.5 g/24 h, eGFR ≥4 5 mL/min/1.73 $m^2$ or 30–45 mL/min/1.73 $m^2$ with RB within 2 years before day 1 | Bion-1301/placebo | Incidence and severity of Treatment Emergent Adverse Events (TEAEs) | 2 yrs |
| NCT04014335 | 2 | 4 | IONIS-FB-LRx, an inhibitor of complement factor B | 10 | Biopsy proven IgAN | IONIS-FB-LRx | Percent reduction in 24-h urine protein excretion | 29 wks |
| NCT02954419 | NA | others | IgA nephropathy biomarkers evaluation study (INTEREST) | 2000 | Biopsy proven IgAN | no intervention | A doubling of serum creatinine level from baseline, progression to ESRD, death | 10 yrs |
| NCT03418779 | 2, 3 | 4 | Treatment effects of chinese medicine with immunosuppression therapies | 56 | Biopsy proven IgAN within 6 months before enrollment, PU > 1 g/24 h, eGFR 20–60 mL/min/1.73 $m^2$ | herbal compound/Isu (Prednisolon, CPA)/optimized supportive care | Increase in GFR from the baseline at the 24th week and 48th week, ESRD | 1 yr |
| NCT03373461 | 3 | 4 | LNP023 (complement-factor-B-inhibitor) | 146 | eGFR ≥ 30 mL/min/1.73/$m^2$, PU > 1 g/d, v accination against Neisseria meningitis | LNP023/Placebo | Change of UPCR at baseline and day 90 | 180 days |
| NCT03608033 | 3 | 4 | OMS 721 (mannan-binding lectin serine protease 2 (MASP2) protein inhibitor) | 450 | PU > 1 g/d within 6 months prior to screening, eGFR ≥ 30 mL/min/1.73/$m^2$ | OMS 721/Placebo | Change from baseline in 24-h UPE in g/day at 36 weeks from beginning of treatment | 3.5 yrs |
| NCT03643965 | 3 | 1 | NefIgArd (Nefecon-budesonide modified-release capsules) | 360 | eGFR ≥ 35 mL/min/1.73/$m^2$ and ≤90 mL/min/1.73/$m^2$, PU >1 g/24 h or UPCR ≥ 0.8 g/g | Nefecon/Placebo | Change of UPCR at baseline and 9 months | 25 mth |
| NCT03762850 | 3 | 4 | PROTECT (Sparsentan-a dual inhibitor of AT1 and ETA receptor) | 280 | eGFR ≥ 30 mL/min/1.73/$m^2$, PU > 1 g/24 h | Sparsentan/Irbesartan | Change of UPCR at baseline and week 36 | 110 wks |

Abbreviation: wks—weeks, yrs—years, mth—months.

The clinical effect of atacicept was investigated for treating systemic autoimmune diseases [75]. Studies in patients with IgA nephropathy investigate the contribution of dysregulation of IgA1 secretion in the intestinal epithelium to see if intestinal immunity or mucosal immunity inhibitors of overexpression of APRIL and B cell-activating factor would have a clinical effect [17,76,77]. Additional potential immunosuppressive regimens (such as blisibimod(NCT02062684)—A selective antagonist of the B-cell activating factor, atacicept (NCT02808429)—An inhibitor of B-cell activating factor (BLyS) and a proliferation-inducing ligand (APRIL), bortezomib—A proteasome inhibitor, fostamatinib–an inhibitor of spleen tyrosine kinase, leflunomide—A pyrimidine synthesis inhibitor) are currently being tested in ongoing trials (Table 2) [78–83].

BAFF (B-cell activating factor) and April (a proliferation inducing ligand) are members of the tumour necrosis factor family which mediate B-cell function and survival [84]. BAFF and April levels are elevated in the serum of patients with IgAN and correlate with the disease activity [85]. BAFF and April are bound by TACI (transmembrane activator and calcium-modulator and cyclophilin ligand interactor), which mediates their downflow effects through the NF-kB pathway. Blisibimod is a selective antagonist of BAFF and atacicept is a fusion protein containing the extracellular ligand binding domain of TACI and is able to block the downflow effects of BAFF and April.

The clinical effects of atacicept and blisibimod were investigated for treating systemic autoimmune diseases, including SLE and rheumatoid arthritis [75,86,87]. Studies in patients with IgAN investigate the contribution of dysregulation of IgA1 secretion in the intestinal epithelium to see if intestinal immunity or mucosal immunity inhibitors of overexpression of APRIL and B cell-activating factor would have a clinical effect [17,76,77].

Bortezomib, a plasma cell proteasome inhibitor, is applied in the treatment of multiple myeloma [88]. Proteasomes are indispensable intracellular protein complexes which destroy useless and impaired proteins by proteolysis [88]. Proteasomes are switched to immunoproteasomes but the dysregulation of the proteasome:immunoproteasome axis was confirmed in mononuclear cells in patients with IgAN with overexpression of the immunoproteasome, increased nuclear translocation of factors related to the NF-kB pathway, and more severe disease symptoms including higher proteinuria [89]. Nowadays, the treatment with bortezomib is more common in amyloidosis, lymphomas, tumours and antibody mediated allograft rejection [90]. A clinical trial to assess the safety and efficacy of bortezomib in patients with IgAN is currently underway (Table 2) but the use of bortezomib in mostly young asymptomatic patients with IgAN would probably be limited by the adverse effects of bortezomib (thrombocytopenia, rash, peripheral neuropathy, fatigue and anorexia) [90].

Tyrosine kinase pathways were asserted in the homeostasis of many diseases, and targeting of the tyrosine kinase signalling pathways was considered for treatment of immune-mediated glomerulonephritides [91]. Spleen tyrosine kinase is a non-receptor tyrosine kinase which might regulate the amount of key pathogenic pathways in IgAN [80]. Spleen tyrosine kinase is a signal transducer following B-cell receptor activation, arranging downflow signalling and promoting B-cell maturation and survival [80]. Spleen tyrosine kinase phosphorylation with the release of pro-inflammatory mediators was activated by stimulation of mesangial cells in vitro with IgA1 acquired from patients with IgAN [80].

Moreover, higher renal expression of spleen tyrosine kinase was confirmed in patients with endocapillary hypercellularity compared to patients without this sign in renal biopsy [92]. Fostamatinib, a selective inhibitor of spleen tyrosine kinase, was investigated in patients with rheumatoid artritis with a favourable effect on disease activity compared to placebo but with frequent adverse effects mostly involving diarrhoea and hypertension [93]. A Phase II trial of fostamatinib in patients with IgAN was recently completed.

Endothelin-1 (ET-1) is a growth factor for mesangial cells [94] and was shown to play a role in the progression of kidney disease in transgenic animals. In human subjects, urinary excretion of endothelin-1 correlates with the severity of kidney disease [95]. Expression of endothelin-1 and endothelin B receptor (mediating vasodilation and natriuresis), but not endothelin A receptor (mediating vasoconstriction and cell proliferation) was demonstrated in patients with IgAN and high-grade proteinuria [96] suggests that activation of the endothelin system in renal tubular cells may partly be a response to protein overload. We demonstrated association of the progresson of IgAN with polymorphisms of the ET-1 gene [97]. Association of ET-1 expression with the progression of IgAN was also confirmed using molecular profiling [98]. A specific ET-receptor antagonist (FR 139317) was shown to suppress the development of histologic lesions and proteinuria in ddY mice with IgAN [99]. Sparsentan, a dual inhibitor of the angiotensin II type 1 (AT1) and endothelin type A (ET-A) receptors was recently shown to significantly decrease proteinuria compared to irbesartan in patients with focal segmental glomerulosclerosis [100] and is currently tested in patients with FSGS in a phase 3 trial [101]. Recently, the PROTECT Study (Phase 3 NCT 03762850) evaluating the long-term nephroprotective potential of sparsentan for the treatment of IgAN was initiated. Activation of Nrf2/Keap 1 by bardoxolone methyl results in the suppression of the main proinflammatory transcription factor NFkappaB and activation of some antioxidative pathways [102]. In patients with type 2 diabetes and CKD4 bardoxolone, methyl was shown to increase the glomerular filtration rate by almost 50% [103]. Recently released data (PHOENIX–NCT03366337) demonstrated a significant increase in eGFR of 8 mL/min/1.73 $m^2$ in patients with IgAN treated with bardoxolone [104]. The increase in eGFR is, however, associated with a proportional increase in albuminuria with uncertain impact on the long-term outcome of the patients [105]. The updated KDIGO guideline will soon be released [34] and the current recommendation from KDIGO came from 2012 prior to STOP-IgAN, TESTING, Nefigan and DAPA-CKD. This is a rapidly evolving field and hence the importance of this review on currently recruiting trials was emphasized.

## 3. Conclusions

In conclusion, IgAN is a disease with variable clinical course. Validated urinary or serum biomarkers, able to provide information on the activity of the disease and the extent of fibrosis, are needed to stratify high risk patients with the necessity of use of immunossuppressive regimens with respect to possible adverse events. Nevertheless, IgAN patients with proteinuria $< 1$ g/d, and/or hypertension and a reduced GFR should obtain optimized supportive treatment with the inhibitors of the RAS. In IgAN patients with persistent proteinuria $\geq 1$ g/d, despite 3–6 months of optimized supportive care (including RAS and blood pressure control), and GFR $> 50$ mL/min per 1.73 $m^2$, a 6-month course of corticosteroid treatment is indicated. Combined immunosuppression with corticosteroids and cyclophosphamide is reserved for high risk patients with a rapid decrease in the GFR and crescentic glomerulonephritis. Nowadays, many specific biological regimens in RCT are evaluated with expected common use in the future (Table 2). The search for an effective and well tolerated treatment of IgAN, directly targeting its pathogenetic mechanisms, continues (Figure 1).

**Funding:** The authors received funding from grants PROGRES Q25/LF1 and DRO VFN 64165 from the Ministry of Health of the Czech Republic.

**Conflicts of Interest:** The authors declare no conflict of interest. The funders had no role in the design of the study; in the collection, analyses, or interpretation of data; in the writing of the manuscript, or in the decision to publish the result.

## References

1. Moriyama, T.; Tanaka, K.; Iwasaki, C.; Oshima, Y.; Ochi, A.; Kataoka, H.; Itabashi, M.; Takei, T.; Uchida, K.; Nitta, K. Prognosis in IgA nephropathy: 30-year analysis of 1012 patients at a single center in Japan. *PLoS ONE* **2014**, *9*, e91756. [CrossRef] [PubMed]
2. Wyatt, R.J.; Julian, B.A. IgA nephropathy. *N. Engl. J. Med.* **2013**, *368*, 2402–2414. [CrossRef] [PubMed]

3. Cattran, D.C.; Coppo, R.; Cook, H.T.; Feehally, J.; Roberts, I.S.; Troyanov, S.; Alpers, C.E.; Amore, A.; Barratt, J.; Berthoux, F.; et al. Working Group of the International IgA Nephropathy Network and the Renal Pathology Society, The Oxford classification of IgA nephropathy: Rationale, clinicopathological correlations, and classification. *Kidney Int.* **2009**, *76*, 534–545. [CrossRef] [PubMed]
4. Coppo, R.; Troyanov, S.; Camilla, R.; Hogg, R.J.; Cattran, D.C.; Cook, T.H.; Feehally, J.; Roberts, I.S.D.; Amore, A.; Alpers, C.E.; et al. Working Group of the International IgA Nephropathy Network and the Renal Pathology Society, The Oxford IgA nephropathy clinicopathological classification is valid for children as well as adults. *Kidney Int.* **2010**, *77*, 921–927. [CrossRef]
5. Reich, H.N.; Troyanov, S.; Scholey, J.W.; Cattran, D.C.; Toronto Glomerulonephritis Registry. Remission of proteinuria improves prognosis in IgA nephropathy. *J. Am. Soc. Nephrol.* **2007**, *18*, 3177–3183. [CrossRef]
6. Barbour, S.J.; Espino-Hernandez, G.; Reich, H.N.; Coppo, R.; Roberts, I.S.D.; Feehally, J.; Herzenberg, A.M.; Cattran, D.C. Oxford Derivation, North American Validation and VALIGA Consortia, The MEST score provides earlier risk prediction in lgA nephropathy. *Kidney Int.* **2016**, *89*, 167–175. [CrossRef]
7. Barbour, S.J.; Espino-Hernandez, G.; Reich, H.; Coppo, R.; Roberts, I.S.D.; Feehally, J.; Herzenberg, A.M.; Cattran, D.; Bavbek, N.; Cook, T.M.; et al. A multicenter study of the predictive value of crescents in IgA nephropathy. *J. Am. Soc. Nephrol.* **2017**, *28*, 691–701.
8. Haas, M.; Verhave, J.C.; Liu, Z.-H.; Alpers, C.E.; Barratt, J.; Becker, J.U.; Cattran, D.; Cook, H.T.; Coppo, R.; Feehally, J.; et al. Geographic differences in genetic susceptibility to IgA nephropathy: GWAS replication study and geospatial risk analysis. *PLoS Genet* **2012**, *8*, e1002765.
9. Kiryluk, K.; Li, Y.; Sanna-Cherchi, S.; Rohanizadegan, M.; Suzuki, H.; Eitner, F.; Snyder, H.J.; Choi, M.; Hou, P.; Scolari, F.; et al. Discovery of new risk loci for IgA nephropathy implicates genes involved in immunity against intestinal pathogens. *Nat. Genet* **2014**, *46*, 1187–1196. [CrossRef]
10. Tomana, M.; Matousovic, K.; Julian, B.A.; Radl, J.; Konecny, K.; Mestecky, J. Galactose-deficient IgA1 in sera of IgA nephropathy patients is present in complexes with IgG. *Kidney Int.* **1997**, *52*, 509–516. [CrossRef]
11. Tomana, M.; Novak, J.; Julian, B.A.; Matousovic, K.; Konecny, K.; Mestecky, J. Circulating immune complexes in IgA nephropathy consist of IgA1 with galactose-deficient hinge region and antiglycan antibodies. *J. Clin. Investig.* **1999**, *104*, 73–81. [CrossRef] [PubMed]
12. Novak, J.; Kafkova, L.R.; Suzuki, H.; Tomana, M.; Matousovic, K.; Brown, R.; Hall, S.; Sanders, J.T.; Eison, T.M.; Moldoveanu, Z.; et al. IgA1 immune complexes from pediatric patients with IgA nephropathy activate cultured human mesangial cells. *Nephrol. Dial Transpl.* **2011**, *26*, 3451–3457. [CrossRef] [PubMed]
13. Maillard, N.; Wyatt, R.J.; Julian, B.A.; Kiryluk, K.; Gharavi, A.; Fremeaux-Bacchi, V.; Novak, J. Current understanding of the role of complement in IgA nephropathy. *J. Am. Soc. Nephrol.* **2015**, *26*, 1503–1512. [CrossRef] [PubMed]
14. Schmitt, R.; Stahl, A.L.; Olin, A.; Kristoffersson, A.Ch.; Rebetz, J.; Novak, J.; Lindahl, G.; Karpman, D. The combined role of galactose-deficient IgA1 and streptococcal IgA-binding M protein in inducing IL-6 and C3 secretion from human mesangial cells: Implications for IgA nephropathy. *J. Immunol.* **2014**, *193*, 317–326. [CrossRef] [PubMed]
15. Lai, K.N.; Leung, J.C.K.; Chan, L.Y.Y.; Saleem, M.A.; Mathieson, P.W.; Lai, F.M.; Tang, S.C.W. Activation of podocytes by mesangial-derived TNF-alpha: Glomerulo-podocytic communication in IgA nephropathy. *Am. J. Physiol. Renal Physiol.* **2008**, *294*, F945–F955. [CrossRef]
16. KDIGO. KDIGO clinical practice guideline for glomerulonephritis. *Kidney Int.* **2012**, *2*, 139–274.
17. Coppo, R. The gut-kidney axis in IgA nephropathy: Role of microbiota and diet on genetic predisposition. *Pediatr. Nephrol.* **2018**, *33*, 53–61. [CrossRef]
18. Monteiro, R.C. Recent advances in the physiopathology of IgA nephropathy. *Nephrol. Ther.* **2018**, *14* (Suppl. 1), S1–S8. [CrossRef]
19. Papista, C.; Lechner, S.; Mkaddem, S.B.; LeStang, M.B.; Abbad, L.; Bex-Coudrat, J.; Pillebout, E.; Chemouny, J.M.; Jablonski, M.; Flamant, M.; et al. Gluten exacerbates IgA nephropathy in humanized mice through gliadin-CD89 interaction. *Kidney Int.* **2015**, *88*, 276–285. [CrossRef]
20. Koulouridis, E.; Koulouridis, I. Is the dietary protein restriction achievable in chronic kidney disease? The impact upon quality of life and the dialysis delay. *Hippokratia* **2011**, *15* (Suppl. 1), 3–7.
21. Konishi, Y.; Okada, N.; Okamura, M.; Morikawa, T.; Okumura, M.; Yoshioka, K.; Imanishi, M. Sodium sensitivity of blood pressure appearing before hypertension and related to histological damage in immunoglobulin a nephropathy. *Hypertension* **2001**, *38*, 81–85. [CrossRef] [PubMed]

22. Suzuki, T.; Miyazaki, Y.; Shimizu, A.; Ito, Y.; Okonogi, H.; Ogura, M. Sodium-sensitive variability of the antiproteinuric efficacy of RAS inhibitors in outpatients with IgA nephropathy. *Clin. Nephrol.* **2009**, *72*, 274–285. [CrossRef] [PubMed]
23. Ouyang, Y.; Xie, J.; Yang, M.; Zhang, X.; Ren, H.; Wang, W.; Chen, N. Underweight is an independent risk factor for renal function deterioration in patients with IgA nephropathy. *PLoS ONE* **2016**, *11*, e0162044. [CrossRef] [PubMed]
24. Shimamoto, M.; Ohsawa, I.; Suzuki, H.; Hisada, A.; Nagamachi, S.; Honda, D.; Inoshita, H.; Shimizu, Y. Impact of Body Mass Index on progression of IgA nephropathy among Japanese patients. *J. Clin. Lab. Anal.* **2015**, *29*, 353–360. [CrossRef] [PubMed]
25. Kittiskulnam, P.; Kanjanabuch, T.; Tangmanjitjaroen, K.; Chancharoenthana, W.; Praditpornsilpa, K.; Eiam-Ong, S. The beneficial effects of weight reduction in overweight patients with chronic proteinuric immunoglobulin a nephropathy: A randomized controlled trial. *J. Ren. Nutr.* **2014**, *24*, 200–207. [CrossRef] [PubMed]
26. Cha, Y.J.; Lim, B.J.; Kim, B.S.; Kim, Y.; Yoo, T.H.; Han, S.H.; Kang, S.W.; Choi, K.H. Smoking-related renal histologic injury in IgA nephropathy patients. *Yonsei Med. J* **2016**, *57*, 209–216. [CrossRef]
27. Ponticelli, C.; Glassock, R.J. IgA Nephritis with Declining Renal Function: Treatment with Corticosteroids May Be Worthwhile. *J. Am. Soc. Nephrol.* **2015**, *26*, 2071–2073. [CrossRef]
28. Sharma, P.; Blackburn, R.C.; Parke, C.L.; McCullough, K.; Marks, A.; Black, C. Angiotension-converting enzyme inhibitors and angiotensin receptor blockers for adults with early (stage 1 to 3)non-diabetic chronic kidney disease. *Cochrane Database Syst. Rev.* **2011**, *10*, CD007751.
29. Jarrick, S.; Lundberg, S.; Welander, A.; Carrero, J.J.; Höijer, J.; Bottai, M.; Ludvigsson, J.F. Mortality in IgA nephropathy: A nationwide population-based cohort study. *J. Am. Soc. Nephrol.* **2019**, *30*, 866–876. [CrossRef]
30. Pozzi, C.; Andrulli, S.; Del Vecchio, L.; Melis, P.; Fogazzi, G.B.; Altieri, P.; Ponticelli, C.; Locatelli, F. Corticosteroid effectiveness in IgA nephropathy: Long-term results of a randomized, controlled trial. *J. Am. Soc. Nephrol.* **2004**, *15*, 157–163. [CrossRef]
31. Lv, J.; Xu, D.; Perkovic, V.; Ma, X.; Johnson, D.W.; Woodward, M.; Levin, A.; Zhang, H. TESTING Study Group. Corticosteroid therapy in IgA nephropathy. *J. Am. Soc. Nephrol.* **2012**, *23*, 1108–1116. [CrossRef] [PubMed]
32. Tesar, V.; Troyanov, S.; Bellur, S.; Verhave, J.C.; Cook, H.T.; Feehally, J.; Roberts, I.S.D.; Cattran, D. VALIGA study of the ERA-EDTA Immunonephrology Working Group. Corticosteroids in IgA Nephropathy: A Retrospective Analysis from the VALIGA Study. *J. Am. Soc. Nephrol.* **2015**, *26*, 2248–2258. [CrossRef]
33. Lv, J.; Zhang, H.; Wong, M.G.; Jardine, M.J.; Hladunewich, M.; Jha, V.; Monaghan, H.; Zhao, M. TESTING Study Group. Effect of Oral Methylprednisolone on Clinical Outcomes in Patients With IgA Nephropathy: The TESTING Randomized Clinical Trial. *JAMA* **2017**, *318*, 432–442. [CrossRef]
34. Floege, J.; Barbour, S.J.; Cattran, D.C.; Hogan, J.J.; Nachman, P.H.; Tang, S.C.W.; Wetzels, J.F.M. Management and treatment of glomerular diseases (part 1): Conclusions from a Kidney Disease: Improving Global Outcomes (KDIGO) Controversies Conference. *Kidney Int.* **2019**, *95*, 268–280. [CrossRef] [PubMed]
35. Rauen, T.; Eitner, F.; Fitzner, C.; Sommerer, C.; Zeier, M.; Otte, B.; Panzer, U.; Peters, H. STOP-IgAN Investigators. Intensive Supportive Care plus Immunosuppression in IgA Nephropathy. *N. Engl. J. Med.* **2015**, *373*, 2225–2236. [CrossRef] [PubMed]
36. Rauen, T.; Wied, S.; Fitzner, C.; Eitner, F.; Sommerer, C.; Zeier, M.; Otte, B.; Panzer, U. After ten years of follow-up, no difference between supportive care plus immunosuppression and supportive care alone in IgA nephropathy. *Kidney Int.* **2020**, *98*, 1044–1052. [CrossRef] [PubMed]
37. Fellström, B.C.; Barratt, J.; Cook, H.; Coppo, R.; Feehally, J.; de Fijter, J.W.; Floege, J.; Hetzel, G. NEFIGAN Trial Investigators. Targeted-release budesonide versus placebo in patients with IgA nephropathy (NEFIGAN): A double-blind, randomised, placebo-controlled phase 2b trial. *Lancet* **2017**, *389*, 2117–2127. [CrossRef]
38. Lechner, S.M.; Abbad, L.; Boedec, E.; Papista, C.; LeStang, M.B.; Moal, C.; Maillard, J.; Jamin, A.; Bex-Coudrat, J.; Wang, Y.; et al. IgA1 Protease Treatment Reverses Mesangial Deposits and Hematuria in a Model of IgA Nephropathy. *J. Am. Soc. Nephrol.* **2016**, *27*, 2622–2629. [CrossRef]
39. Berthelot, L.; Papista, C.; Maciel, T.T.; Biarnes-Pelicot, M.; Tissandie, E.; Wang, P.H.M.; Tamouza, H.; Jamin, A.; Bex-Coudrat, J.; Gestin, A.; et al. Transglutaminase is essential for IgA nephropathy development acting through IgA receptors. *J. Exp. Med.* **2012**, *209*, 793–806. [CrossRef]

40. Heerspink, H.J.L.; Stefánsson, B.V.; Correa-Rotter, R.; Chertow, G.M.; Greene, T.; Hou, F.F.; Mann, J.F.E.; McMurray, J.J.V.; Lindberg, M.; Rossing, P.; et al. Dapagliflozin in Patients with Chronic Kidney Disease. *N. Engl. J. Med.* **2020**, *383*, 1436–1446. [CrossRef]
41. Roberts, I.S.; Cook, H.T.; Troyanov, S.; Alpers, C.E.; Amore, A.; Barratt, J.; Berthoux, F.; Bonsib, S.; Bruijn, J.A.; Cattran, D.C.; et al. The Oxford classification of IgA nephropathy: Pathology definitions, correlations, and reproducibility. *Kidney Int.* **2009**, *76*, 546–556. [CrossRef] [PubMed]
42. Trimarchi, H.; Barratt, J.; Cattran, D.C.; Cook, H.T.; Coppo, R.; Haas, M.; Liu, Z.H.; Roberts, I.S.; Yuzawa, Y.; Zhank, H.; et al. Oxford classification of IgA nephropathy 2016: An update from the IgA Nephropathy Classification Working Group. *Kidney Int.* **2017**, *91*, 1014–1021. [CrossRef] [PubMed]
43. Coppo, R. Towards a personalized treatment for IgA nephropathy considering pathology and pathogenesis. *Nephrol. Dial Transpl.* **2019**, *34*, 1832–1838. [CrossRef] [PubMed]
44. Barbour, S.J.; Coppo, R.; Zhang, H.; Liu, Z.H.; Suzuki, Y.; Matsuzaki, K.; Katafuchi, R.; Er, L.; Espino-Hernandez, G.; Kim, S.J.; et al. Evaluating a new international risk-prediction tool in IgA nephropathy. *JAMA Int. Med.* **2019**, *179*, 942–952. [CrossRef] [PubMed]
45. Barbour, S.J.; Canney, M.; Coppo, R.; Zhang, H.; Liu, Z.H.; Suzuki, Y.; Matsuzaki, K.; Katafuchi, R.; Induruwage, D.; Er, L.; et al. Improving treatment decisions using personalized risk assessment from the international IgA nephropathy prediction tool. *Kidney Int.* **2020**, *98*, 1009–1019. [CrossRef]
46. Sarcina, C.; Tinelli, C.; Ferrario, F.; Pani, A.; De Silvestri, A.; Scaini, P.; De Silvestri, A.; Scaini, P.; Del Vecchio, L.; Alberghini, E.; et al. Changes in Proteinuria and Side Effects of Corticosteroids Alone or in Combination with Azathioprine at Different Stages of IgA Nephropathy. *Clin. J. Am. Soc. Nephrol.* **2016**, *11*, 973–981. [CrossRef]
47. Pozzi, C.; Andrulli, S.; Pani, A.; Scaini, P.; Del Vecchio, L.; Fogazzi, G.; Vogt, B.; Cristofaro, V.D.; Allegri, L.; Cirami, L.; et al. Addition of azathioprine to corticosteroids does not benefit patients with IgA nephropathy. *J. Am. Soc. Nephrol.* **2010**, *21*, 1783–1790. [CrossRef]
48. Liu, H.; Xu, X.; Fang, Y.; Ji, J.; Zhang, X.; Yuan, M.; Liu, C.; Ding, X. Comparison of glucocorticoids alone and combined with cyclosporine a in patients with IgA nephropathy: A prospective randomized controlled trial. *Intern Med.* **2014**, *53*, 675–681. [CrossRef]
49. Xu, L.; Liu, Z.C.; Guan, G.J.; Lv, X.A.; Luo, Q. Cyclosporine A combined with medium/low dose prednisone in progressive IgA nephropathy. *Kaohsiung J. Med. Sci* **2014**, *30*, 390–395. [CrossRef]
50. Hou, J.H.; Le, W.B.; Chen, N.; Wang, W.M.; Liu, Z.S.; Liu, D.; Chen, J.H.; Tian, J.; Fu, P.; Hu, Z.X.; et al. Mycophenolate mofetil combined with prednisone versus full-dose prednisone in IgA nephropathy with active proliferative lesions: A randomized controlled trial. *Am. J. Kidney Dis.* **2017**, *69*, 788–795. [CrossRef]
51. Tang, S.C.; Tang, A.W.; Wong, S.S.; Leung, J.C.; Ho, Y.W.; Lai, K.N. Long-term study of mycophenolate mofetil treatment in IgA nephropathy. *Kidney Int.* **2010**, *77*, 543–549. [CrossRef] [PubMed]
52. Hogg, R.J.; Bay, R.C.; Jennette, J.C.; Sibley, R.; Kumar, S.; Fervenza, F.C.; Appel, G.; Cattran, D.; Fischer, D.; Hurley, R.M.; et al. Randomized controlled trial of mycophenolate mofetil in children, adolescents, and adults with IgA nephropathy. *Am. J. Kidney Dis.* **2015**, *66*, 783–791. [CrossRef] [PubMed]
53. Beckwith, H.; Medjeral-Thomas, N.; Galliford, J.; Griffith, M.; Levy, J.; Lightstone, L.; Palmer, A.; Roufosse, C.; Pusey, C.; Cook, H.T.; et al. Mycophenolate mofetil therapy in immunoglobulin a nephropathy: Histological changes after treatment. *Nephrol. Dial Transpl.* **2017**, *32*, 123–128. [CrossRef] [PubMed]
54. Liu, D.; Liu, Y.; Chen, G.; He, L.; Tang, C.; Wang, C.; Yang, D.; Li, H.; Dong, Z.; Liu, H. Rapamycin Enhances Repressed Autophagy and Attenuates Aggressive Progression in a Rat Model of IgA Nephropathy. *Am. J. Nephrol.* **2017**, *45*, 293–300. [CrossRef]
55. Liu, L.J.; Yang, Y.Z.; Shi, S.F.; Bao, Y.F.; Yang, C.; Zhu, S.N.; Sui, G.L.; Chen, Y.Q.; Lv, J.C.; Zhang, H. Effects of Hydroxychloroquine on Proteinuria in IgA Nephropathy: A Randomized Controlled Trial. *Am. J. Kidney Dis.* **2019**, *74*, 15–22. [CrossRef]
56. Donadio, J.V., Jr. Use of fish oil to treat patients with immunoglobulin a nephropathy. *Am. J. Clin. Nutr.* **2000**, *71*, 373S–375S. [CrossRef]
57. Bomback, A.S.; Canetta, P.A.; Beck, L.H., Jr.; Ayalon, R.; Radhakrhisnan, J.; Appel, G.B. Treatment of resistant glomerular diseases with adrenocorticotropic hormon gel: A prospective trial. *Am. J. Nephrol.* **2012**, *36*, 58–67. [CrossRef]
58. Zand, L.; Canetta, P.; Lafayette, R.; Aslam, N.; Novak, J.; Sethi, S.; Fervenza, C.F. An open-label pilot study of adrenocorticotrophic hormone in the treatment of IgA nephropathy at high risk of progression. *KI Rep.* **2020**, *5*, 58–65. [CrossRef]

59. Zand, L.; Canetta, P.; Lafayette, R.; Aslam, N.; Jan, N.; Sethi, S.; Fervenza, F.C. Tonsillectomy for IgA nephropathy: A meta-analysis. *Am. J. Kidney Dis.* **2015**, *65*, 80–87.
60. Kawamura, T.; Yoshimura, M.; Miyazaki, Y.; Okamoto, H.; Kimura, K.; Hirano, K.; Matsushima, M.; Utsunomiya, Y.; Ogura, M.; Yokoo, T.; et al. A multicenter randomized controlled trial of tonsillectomy combined with steroid pulse therapy in patients with immunoglobulin a nephropathy. *Nephrol. Dial Transpl.* **2014**, *29*, 1546–1553. [CrossRef]
61. Feehally, J.; Coppo, R.; Troyanov, S.; Bellur, S.S.; Cattran, D.; Cook, T.; Roberts, I.S.D.; Verhave, J.C.; Camilla, R.; Vergano, L.; et al. VALIGA study of ERA-EDTA Immunonephrology Working Group. Tonsillectomy in a European Cohort of 1,147 Patients with IgA Nephropathy. *Nephron* **2016**, *132*, 15–24. [CrossRef] [PubMed]
62. Lafayette, R.A.; Canetta, P.A.; Rovin, B.H.; Appel, G.B.; Novak, J.; Nath, K.A.; Sethi, S.; Tumlin, J.A.; Mehta, K.; Hogan, M.; et al. A Randomized, Controlled Trial of Rituximab in IgA Nephropathy with Proteinuria and Renal Dysfunction. *J. Am. Soc. Nephrol.* **2017**, *28*, 1306–1313. [CrossRef] [PubMed]
63. Sugiura, H.; Takei, T.; Itabashi, M.; Tsukada, M.; Moriyama, T.; Kojima, C.; Shiohira, T.; Shimizu, A.; Tsuruta, Y.; Amemiya, N.; et al. Effect of single-dose rituximab on primary glomerular diseases. *Nephron Clin. Pract* **2011**, *117*, 98–105. [CrossRef] [PubMed]
64. Coppo, R.; Peruzzi, L.; Loiacono, E.; Bergallo, M.; Krutova, A.; Russo, M.L.; Cocchi, E.; Amore, A.; Lundberg, S.; Maixnerova, D.; et al. Defective gene expression of the membrane complement inhibitor CD46 in patients with progressive immunoglobulin A nephropathy. *Nephrol. Dial Transpl.* **2018**, *34*, 587–596. [CrossRef] [PubMed]
65. Espinosa, M.; Ortega, R.; Sánchez, M.; Segarra, A.; Salcedo, M.T.; González, F.; Camacho, R.; Valdivia, M.A.; Cabrera, R.; López, K.; et al. Association of C4d deposition with clinical outcomes in IgA nephropathy. *Clin. J. Am. Soc. Nephrol.* **2014**, *9*, 897–904. [CrossRef]
66. Zhu, L.; Zhai, Y.L.; Wang, F.M.; Hou, P.; Lv, J.Ch.; Xu, D.M.; Shi, S.F.; Liu, L.J.; Yu, F.; Zhao, M.H.; et al. Variants in complement factor H and complement factor H-related protein genes, CFHR 3 and CFHR1, affect complement activation in IgA nephropathy. *J. Am. Soc. Nephrol.* **2015**, *26*, 1195–1204. [CrossRef]
67. Xie, J.; Kiryluk, K.; Li, Y.; Mladkova, N.; Zhu, L.; Hou, P.; Ren, H.; Wang, W.; Zhang, H.; Chen, N.; et al. Fine mapping implicates a deletion of CFHR1 nad CFHR3 in protection from IgA nephropathy in Han Chinese. *J. Am. Soc. Nephrol.* **2016**, *27*, 3187–3194. [CrossRef]
68. Jullien, P.; Laurent, B.; Claisse, G.; Masson, I.; Dinic, M.; Thibaudin, D.; Berthoux, F.; Alamartine, E.; Mariat, C.; Maillard, N.; et al. Deletion variants of CFHR1 and CFHR3 associate with mesangial immune deposits but not with progression of IgA nephropathy. *J. Am. Soc. Nephrol.* **2018**, *29*, 661–669. [CrossRef]
69. Daha, M.R.; van Kooten, C. Role of complement in IgA nephropathy. *J. Nephrol.* **2016**, *29*, 1–4. [CrossRef]
70. Block, G.A.; Whitaker, S. Maintenance of remission following completion of OMS721 treatment in patients with IgA nephropathy (IGAN). Abstract SA-PO278. *J. Am. Soc. Nephrol.* **2017**, *28*, 749–750.
71. Liu, L.; Zhan, Y.; Duan, X.; Peng, Q.; Liu, Q.; Zhou, Y.; Quan, S.; Xing, G. C3a, C5a renal expression and their receptors are correlated to severity of IgA nephropathy. *J. Clin. Immunol.* **2014**, *34*, 224–232. [CrossRef] [PubMed]
72. ChemoCentryx. Open-Label Study to Evaluate Safety and Efficacy of CCX168 in Subjects With Immunoglobulin A Nephropathy on Stable RAAS Blockade. In *ClinicalTrials.gov [Internet]*; National library of Medicine: Bethesda, MD, USA, 2015. Available online: https://www.clinicaltrials.gov/ct2/show/NCT02384317 (accessed on 20 December 2016).
73. Jayne, D.R.W.; Bruchfeld, A.N.; Harper, L.; Schaier, M.; Venning, M.C.; Hamilton, P.; Burst, V.; Grundmann, F.; Jadoul, M.; Szombati, I.; et al. Randomized trial of C5a receptor inhibitor Avacopan in ANCA-associated vasculitis. *J. Am. Soc. Nephrol.* **2017**, *28*, 2756–2767. [CrossRef] [PubMed]
74. Selvaskandan, H.; Cheung, C.K.; Muto, M.; Barratt, J. New strategies and perspectives on managing IgA nephropathy. *Clin. Exp. Nephrol.* **2019**, *23*, 577–588. [CrossRef]
75. Nakayamada, S.; Tanaka, Y. BAFF- and APRIL targeted therapy in systemic autoimmune diseases. *Inflamm Regen.* **2016**, *36*, 1–6. [CrossRef] [PubMed]
76. Lafayette, R.A.; Kelepouris, E. Immunoglobulin A nephropathy: Advances in understanding of pathogenesis and treatment. *Am. J. Nephrol.* **2018**, *47*, 43–53. [CrossRef] [PubMed]
77. Coppo, R. Biomarkers and targeted new therapies for IgA nephropathy. *Pediatr. Nephrol.* **2017**, *32*, 725–731. [CrossRef]
78. Coppo, R. Proteasome inhibitors in progressive renal diseases. *Nephrol. Dial Transpl.* **2014**, *29*, i25–i30. [CrossRef]

79. Xin, G.; Shi, W.; Xu, L.X.; Su, Y.; Yan, L.J.; Li, K.S. Serum BAFF is elevated in patients with IgA nephropathy and associated with clinical and histopathological features. *J. Nephrol.* **2013**, *26*, 683–690. [CrossRef]
80. Kim, M.J.; McDaid, J.P.; McAdoo, S.P.; Barratt, J.; Molyneux, K.; Masuda, E.S.; Pusey, C.D.; Tam, F.W. Spleen tyrosine kinase is important in the production of proinflammatory cytokines and cell proliferation in human mesangial cells following stimulation with IgA1 isolated from IgA nephropathy patients. *J. Immunol.* **2012**, *189*, 3751–3758. [CrossRef]
81. McAdoo, S.; Tam, F.W.K. Role of the Spleen Tyrosine Kinase Pathway in Driving Inflammation in IgA Nephropathy. *Semin. Nephrol.* **2018**, *38*, 496–503. [CrossRef]
82. Liu, X.W.; Li, D.M.; Xu, G.S.; Sun, S.R. Comparison of the therapeutic effects of leflunomide and mycophenolate mofetil in the treatment of immunoglobulin a nephropathy manifesting with nephrotic syndrome. *Int. J. Clin. Pharmacol. Ther.* **2010**, *48*, 509–513. [CrossRef] [PubMed]
83. Cheng, G.; Liu, D.; Margetts, P.; Liu, L.; Zhao, Z.; Liu, Z.; Tang, L.; Fang, Y.; Li, H.; Guo, Y.; et al. Valsartan combined with clopidogrel and/or leflunomide for the treatment of progressive immunoglobulin A nephropathy. *Nephrology* **2015**, *20*, 77–84. [CrossRef] [PubMed]
84. Samy, E.; Wax, S.; Huard, B.; Hess, H.; Schneider, P. Targeting BAFF and APRIL in systemic lupus erythematosus and oTher. antibody-associated diseases. *Int. Rev. Immunol.* **2017**, *36*, 3–19. [CrossRef] [PubMed]
85. Zhai, Y.; Zhu, L.; Shi, S.; Liu, L.; Lv, J.; Zhang, H. Increased APRIL expression induces IgA1 aberrant glycosylation in IgA nephropathy. *Medicine* **2016**, *95*, e3099. [CrossRef]
86. Isenberg, D.; Gordon, C.; Licu, D.; Copt, S.; Rossi, C.P.; Wofsy, D. Efficacy and safety of atacicept for prevention of flares in patients with moderate-to-severe systemic lupus erythematosus (SLE):52-week data (APRIL-SLE randomised trial). *Ann. Rheum. Dis.* **2015**, *74*, 2006–2015. [CrossRef]
87. Lenert, A.; Niewold, T.B.; Lenert, P. Spotlight on blisibimod and its potential in the treatment of systemic lupus erythematosus:evidenc to date. *Drug Des. Devel Ther.* **2017**, *11*, 747–757. [CrossRef]
88. Richardson, P.G.; Barlogie, B.; Berenson, J.; Singhal, S.; Jagannath, S.; Irwin, D.; Rajkumar, S.V.; Srkalovic, G.; Alsina, M.; Alexanian, R.; et al. A phase 2 study of bortezomib in relapsed, refractory myeloma. *N. Engl. J. Med.* **2003**, *26*, 2609–2617. [CrossRef]
89. Coppo, R.; Camilla, R.; Alfarano, A.; Balegno, S.; Mancuso, D.; Peruzzi, L.; Amore, A.; Canton, A.D.; Sepe, V.; Tovo, P.; et al. Upregulation of the immunoproteasome in peripheral blood mononuclear cells of patients with IgA nephropathy. *Kidney Int.* **2009**, *75*, 536–541. [CrossRef]
90. Bahleda, R.; Le Deley, M.; Bernard, A.; Chaturvedi, S.; Hanley, M.; Poterie, A.; Gazzah, A.; Varga, A.; Touat, M.; Deutsch, E.; et al. Phase I trial of bortezomib daily dose: Safety, pharmacokinetic profile, biological effects and early clinical evaluation in patients with advanced solid tumors. *Investig. New Drugs* **2017**, *5*, 66.
91. Ma, T.K.; McAdoo, S.P.; Tam, F.W.K. Targeting the tyrosine kinase signalling pathways for treatment of immune-mediated glomerulonephritis: From bench to bedside and beyond. *Nephrol. Dial Transpl.* **2017**, *32*, i138. [CrossRef]
92. McAdoo, S.P.; Bhangal, G.; Page, T.; Cook, H.T.; Pusey, C.D.; Tam, F.W.K. Correlation of disease activity in proliferative glomerulonephritis with glomerular spleen tyrosine kinase expression. *Kidney Int.* **2015**, *88*, 52–60. [CrossRef] [PubMed]
93. Taylor, P.C.; Genovese, M.C.; Greenwood, M.; Ho, M.; Nasonov, E.; Oemar, B.; Stoilov, R.; Vencovsky, J.; Weinblatt, M. OSKIRA-4: A phase IIb randomised, placebo-controlled study of the efficacy and safety of fostamatinib monotherapy. *Ann. Rheum. Dis.* **2015**, *74*, 2123–2129. [CrossRef] [PubMed]
94. Simonson, M.S.; Wann, S.; Mene, P.; Dubyak, G.R.; Kester, M.; Nakazato, Y.; Sedor, J.R.; Dunn, M.J. Endothelin stimulates phospholipase C, Na+/H+ exchange, c-Fos expression, and mitogenesis in rat mesangial cells. *J. Clin. Investig.* **1989**, *83*, 708–712. [CrossRef] [PubMed]
95. Ohta, K.; Hirata, Y.; Shichiri, M.; Kanno, K.; Emori, T.; Tomita, K.; Marumo, F. Urinary excretion of endothelin-1 in normal subjects and patients with renal disease. *Kidney Int.* **1991**, *39*, 307–311. [CrossRef] [PubMed]
96. Lehrke, I.; Waldherr, R.; Ritz, E.; Wagner, J. Renal endothelin-1 and endothelin receptor type B expression in glomerular diseases with proteinuria. *J. Am. Soc. Nephrol.* **2001**, *12*, 2321–2329. [PubMed]
97. Maixnerova, D.; Merta, M.; Reiterova, J.; Stekrova, J.; Rysava, R.; Obeidova, H.; Viklicky, O.; Potmesil, P.; Tesar, V. The influence of three endothelin-1 polymorphisms on the progression of IgA nephropathy. *Folia Biol.* **2007**, *53*, 27–32.

98. Tycova, I.; Hruba, P.; Maixnerova, D.; Girmanova, E.; Mrazova, P.; Straňavova, L.; Zachoval, R.; Merta, M.; Slatinska, J.; Kollar, M.; et al. Molecular Profiling in IgA Nephropathy and Focal and Segmental Glomerulosclerosis. *Physiol. Res.* **2018**, *67*, 93–105. [CrossRef]
99. Nakamura, T.; Ebihara, I.; Fukui, M.; Tomino, Y.; Koide, H. Effect of a specific endothelin receptor a antagonist on glomerulonephritis of ddY mice with IgA nephropathy. *Nephron* **1996**, *72*, 454–460. [CrossRef]
100. Trachtman, H.; Nelson, P.; Adler, S.; Campbell, K.N.; Chaudhuri, A.; Derebail, V.K.; Gambaro, G.; Gesualdo, L.; Gipson, D.S.; Hogan, J.; et al. DUET: A Phase 2 Study Evaluating the Efficacy and Safety of Sparsentan in Patients with FSGS. *J. Am. Soc. Nephrol.* **2018**, *29*, 2745–2754. [CrossRef]
101. Komers, R.; Diva, U.; Inrig, J.K.; Loewen, A.; Trachtman, H.; Rote, W.E. Study design of the phase 3 sparsentan versus irbesartan (DUPLEX) study in patients with focal segmental glomerulosclerosis. *Kidney Int. Rep.* **2020**, *5*, 494–502. [CrossRef]
102. Shelton, L.M.; Park, B.K.; Copple, I.M. Role of Nrf2 in protection against acute Kidney injury. *Kidney Int.* **2013**, *84*, 1090–1095. [CrossRef] [PubMed]
103. Pergola, P.E.; Raskin, P.; Toto, R.D.; Meyer, C.J.; Huff, J.W.; Grossman, E.B.; Krauth, M.; Ruiz, S.; Audhya, P.; Christ-Schmidt, H.; et al. Bardoxolone methyl and kidney function in CKD with type 2 diabetes. *N. Engl. J. Med.* **2011**, *365*, 327–336. [CrossRef] [PubMed]
104. Block, G.A. Primary Efficacy Analyses from a Phase 2 Trial of the Safety and Efficacy of Bardoxolone Methyl in Patients with IgA Nephropathy. *ASN Kidney Week* **2018**. poster TH-PO1039. [CrossRef]
105. Rossing, P.; Block, G.A.; Chin, M.P.; Goldsberry, A.; Heerspink, H.J.L.; McCullough, P.A.; Meyer, C.J.; Packham, D.; Pergola, P.E.; Spinowitz, B.; et al. Effect of bardoxolone methyl on the urine albumin-to-creatinine ratio in patients with type 2 diabetes and stage 4 chronic kidney disease. *Kidney Int.* **2019**, *96*, 1030–1036. [CrossRef] [PubMed]

International Journal of
*Molecular Sciences*

MDPI

*Article*

# Inhibition of Yes-Associated Protein by Verteporfin Ameliorates Unilateral Ureteral Obstruction-Induced Renal Tubulointerstitial Inflammation and Fibrosis

**Jixiu Jin [1], Tian Wang [1], Woong Park [1], Wenjia Li [1], Won Kim [1,2], Sung Kwang Park [1,2,*] and Kyung Pyo Kang [1,2,*]**

1 Department of Internal Medicine, Research Institute of Clinical Medicine, Jeonbuk National University Medical School, Jeonju 54907, Korea; gilsoo1215@gmail.com (J.J.); tianw0000@outlook.com (T.W.); mnipw@hanmail.net (W.P.); liwenjia1214@gmail.com (W.L.); kwon@jbnu.ac.kr (W.K.)
2 Biomedical Research Institute, Jeonbuk National University Hospital, Jeonju 54907, Korea
* Correspondence: parksk@jbnu.ac.kr (S.K.P.); kpkang@jbnu.ac.kr (K.P.K.); Tel.: +82-63-250-1683 (S.K.P.); +82-63-250-2361 (K.P.K.)

Received: 15 October 2020; Accepted: 31 October 2020; Published: 31 October 2020

check for updates

**Abstract:** Yes-associated protein (YAP) activation after acute ischemic kidney injury might be related to interstitial fibrosis and impaired renal tubular regeneration. Verteporfin (VP) is a photosensitizer used in photodynamic therapy to treat age-related macular degeneration. In cancer cells, VP inhibits TEA domain family member (TEAD)-YAP interactions without light stimulation. The protective role of VP in unilateral ureteral obstruction (UUO)-induced renal fibrosis and related mechanisms remains unclear. In this study, we investigate the protective effects of VP on UUO-induced renal tubulointerstitial inflammation and fibrosis and its regulation of the transforming growth factor-β1 (TGF-β1)/Smad signaling pathway. We find that VP decreased the UUO-induced increase in tubular injury, inflammation, and extracellular matrix deposition in mice. VP also decreased myofibroblast activation and proliferation in UUO kidneys and NRK-49F cells by modulating Smad2 and Smad3 phosphorylation. Therefore, YAP inhibition might have beneficial effects on UUO-induced tubulointerstitial inflammation and fibrosis by regulating the TGF-β1/Smad signaling pathway.

**Keywords:** kidney fibrosis; inflammation; myofibroblast activation; extracellular matrix; Hippo pathway; verteporfin

## 1. Introduction

Chronic kidney disease (CKD) is a heterogeneous condition characterized by reduced glomerular filtration rate, glomerular sclerosis, tubular atrophy, and interstitial fibrosis with inflammatory cell infiltration [1]. As human life expectancy has increased, CKD has become one of the most common non-communicable diseases [2,3]. End-stage renal disease that requires renal replacement therapy such as dialysis or kidney transplantation is associated with a decrease in residual life expectancy compared with healthy individuals [3]. Despite plenty of health resources in developed countries, CKD's global burden is steadily increasing, and CKD-related mortality is also increasing [4]. A nationwide cohort study in Korea found a higher mortality rate in patients with CKD than in healthy controls or even in patients with diabetes or hypertension but without CKD [5]. Therefore, strategies to enable the early recognition and prevention of CKD are needed to decrease the global health burden.

Organ fibrosis is characterized by a dynamic process of non-resolving inflammatory reactions [6] that cause the deterioration of organ function. After an ischemic or toxic injury to the kidneys causes damage to glomerular, vascular, and tubular cells, an inflammatory reaction can increase the deposition of the extracellular matrix (ECM) in the renal parenchyma [7]. Transforming growth factor-β1 (TGF-β1) is a multifunctional cytokine related to cell growth, differentiation, apoptosis, and wound repair [8]. Histologically, CKD is characterized by excessive ECM production from activated myofibroblasts, which causes renal tubulointerstitial fibrosis and organ dysfunction. TGF-β1 is a potent mediator in this fibrotic process [8,9]. Activated TGF-β1 binds to type I and type II cell surface receptors and phosphorylates the Smad2 and Smad3 proteins to activate the canonical (Smad-dependent) TGF-β signaling pathway [8,10]. TGF-β also activates other, non-canonical (Smad-independent) pathways, such as mitogen-activated protein kinase, phosphatidylinositol-3-kinase, and Rho-like GTPase [11]. Therefore, modulation of the TGF-β1 signaling pathway is an important therapeutic target for preventing progressive CKD.

The Hippo pathway is an evolutionarily conserved signaling pathway that regulates cell growth and fate decisions, organ size control, and regeneration [12]. The Hippo pathway consists of a kinase cascade (mammalian Ste20-like kinase 1/2, large tumor suppressor 1/2, and downstream effectors and transcriptional coactivators), the Yes-associated protein (YAP), and a transcriptional coactivator with a PDZ-binding motif (TAZ) [13]. Once the Hippo pathway has been activated, it limits tissue growth and cell proliferation through the phosphorylation and degradation of YAP/TAZ. In contrast, when the Hippo pathway is turned off, YAP/TAZ is dephosphorylated and translocated into the nucleus to induce target gene transcription [12,13]. During kidney development, *Yap* and *Taz* activation produce different phenotypes. YAP is related to nephron morphogenesis, and TAZ inactivation causes polycystic kidney disease [14]. YAP/TAZ function as physical sensors of cell structure, shape, and polarity, and YAP/TAZ activation is related to mechanical signaling in cells involved in tissue architecture and the surrounding ECM [14]. Therefore, modulating YAP/TAZ might reveal novel therapeutic targets for preventing renal fibrosis.

Verteporfin (VP) is a photosensitizer already used in photodynamic therapy to treat age-related macular degeneration [15]. Recently, Liu-Chittenden et al. showed that VP inhibits TEA domain family member (TEAD)–YAP interactions in cancer cells without light stimulation [16]. Notably, connective tissue growth factor (CTGF) and TGF-β, which regulate the extent of remodeling in the tissue architecture, are among the YAP transcription targets [17]. Recently, YAP and CTGF were found to be closely involved in determining blood vessel integrity and stability in the retina [18]. The constant activation of YAP after acute ischemic kidney injury might be related to interstitial fibrosis and impaired renal tubular regeneration [19]. Therefore, using VP to inhibit YAP might be a novel treatment strategy for renal tubulointerstitial inflammation and fibrosis. However, the protective role of VP in unilateral ureteral obstruction (UUO)-induced renal fibrosis and the related mechanisms remain unclear. Therefore, in this study, we investigate the protective effects of VP on UUO-induced renal tubulointerstitial inflammation and fibrosis and its regulatory role in the TGF-β signaling pathway.

## 2. Results

### 2.1. Verteporfin Decreases UUO-Induced Renal Tubular Injury and Fibrosis

To investigate the effect of VP on UUO-induced renal tubular injury and fibrosis, we examined kidney sections after periodic acid–Schiff (PAS) and Masson's trichrome staining. Histologically, Veh-treated UUO kidneys showed tubular dilation, epithelial desquamation, loss of brush border, inflammatory cell infiltration, and tubulointerstitial fibrosis. VP treatment decreased the UUO-induced increase in tubular dilation, inflammatory cell infiltration, and tubulointerstitial fibrosis compared with Veh-treated UUO kidneys (Figure 1A). Masson's trichrome staining revealed an increase in the fibrotic areas of the Veh-treated UUO kidneys compared with sham-operated kidneys treated with either Veh or VP. VP treatment, on the other hand, significantly decreased the UUO-induced increase in fibrotic areas (Figure 1B). Those data suggest that VP treatment has a protective effect against UUO-induced tubular injury and fibrosis.

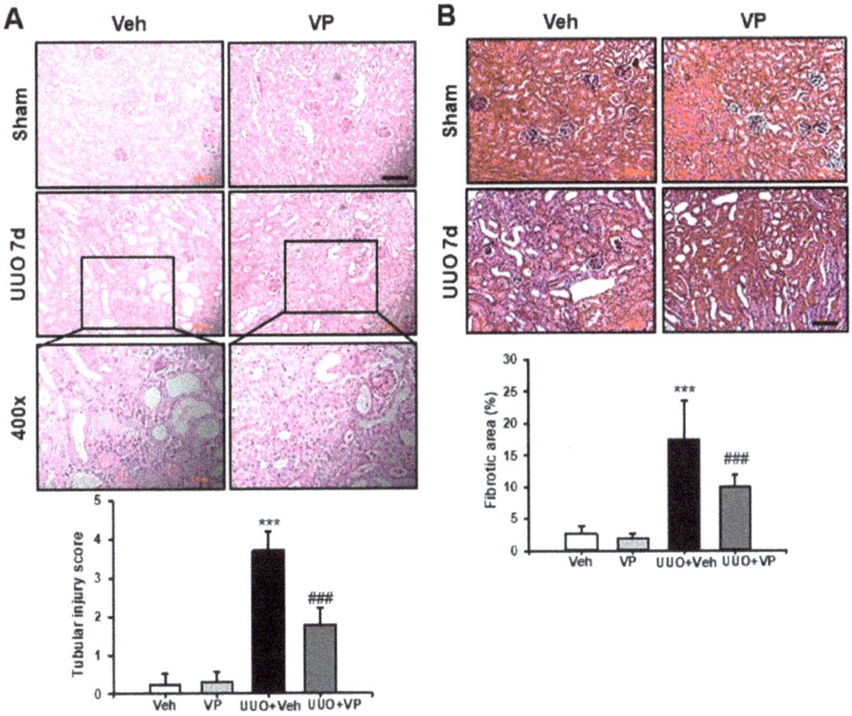


**Figure 1.** Effect of verteporfin on UUO-induced renal tubular injury and fibrosis. Representative PAS and MTC stains from the kidneys of sham- and UUO-operated mice treated with vehicle (Veh) or verteporfin (VP). Scale bar = 100 μm. Inlet shows a higher magnification view (400×) of UUO 7 d with Veh or VP treatment. The bar graphs show the semi-quantitative scoring of (**A**) tubular injury stained by PAS and (**B**) the area fraction (%) of tubulointerstitial fibrosis stained by MTC from ten randomly chosen, non-overlapping fields ($n = 10$) at a magnification of 200× ($n = 15$/group). Data are expressed as the mean ± SD. *** $p < 0.001$ versus Veh or VP; ### $p < 0.001$ versus UUO. Veh, vehicle; VP, verteporfin; Sham, sham-operated mice; UUO, unilateral ureteral obstruction operated mice.

### 2.2. *Verteporfin Decreases UUO-Induced Renal Fibroblast Activation and Excessive Extracellular Matrix Accumulation*

Renal fibrosis is characterized by renal fibroblast activation and excessive ECM accumulation that leads to tissue destruction, scarring, and kidney failure [6,20,21]. Therefore, we investigated renal fibroblast activation after UUO surgery by examining α-Smooth muscle actin (α-SMA) and fibroblast specific protein-1 (FSP-1) expression. Veh-treated UUO kidneys showed an increase in the α-SMA-positive area compared with sham-operated kidneys that received Veh or VP treatment, and VP treatment significantly attenuated that increase in UUO kidneys (Figure 2A). We also evaluated α-SMA expression in a Western blot analysis of UUO kidneys with or without VP treatment. Veh-treated UUO kidneys had significantly increased α-SMA expression compared with sham-operated kidneys treated with Veh or VP, and VP treatment significantly decreased the UUO-induced increase in α-SMA expression (Figure 2C). After UUO surgery, the number of FSP-1 (+) fibroblasts increased significantly compared with sham-operated kidneys treated with either Veh or VP, and VP treatment significantly decreased the number of FSP-1 (+) fibroblasts in UUO kidneys (Figure 2B). We also evaluated type I collagen expression using Western blotting of the UUO kidneys. Type I collagen expression was increased in Veh-treated UUO kidneys compared with sham-operated kidneys, and VP treatment significantly decreased the UUO-induced increase in type I collagen expression (Figure 2D). These data suggest that VP treatment reduces UUO-induced renal fibroblast activation and EMC accumulation in the kidney.

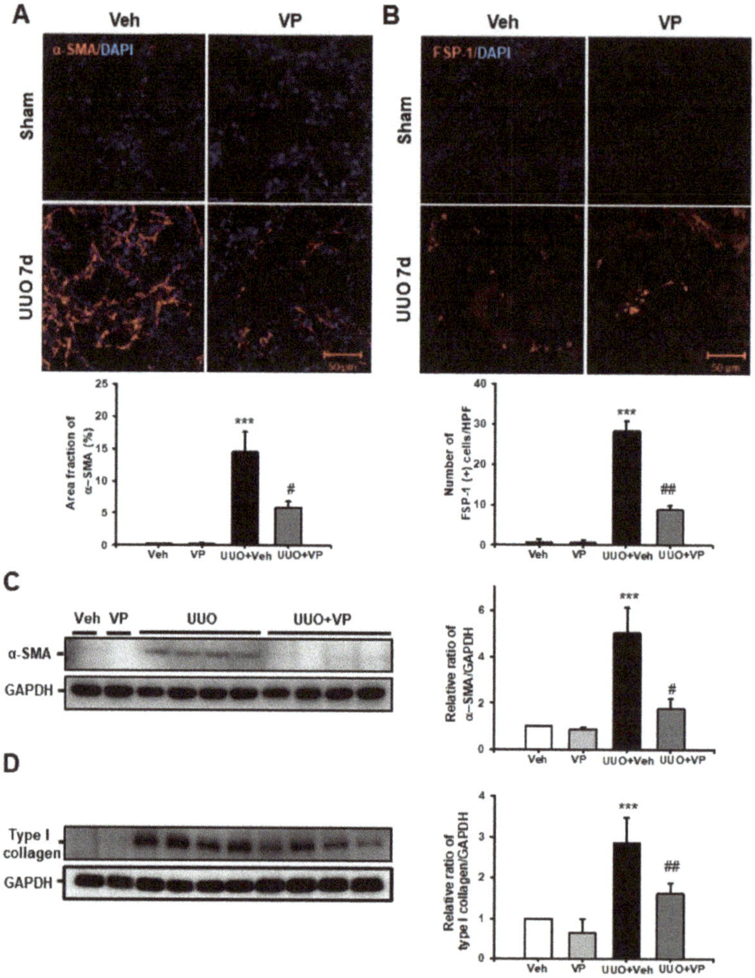


**Figure 2.** Effect of verteporfin on UUO-induced renal fibroblast activation. Representative immunofluorescence staining of α-SMA (**A**) and FPS-1 (**B**) from the kidneys of sham- and UUO-operated mice treated with vehicle (Veh) or verteporfin (VP). The nuclei were stained with DAPI. The bar graph shows the number of α-SMA and FPS-1 positive cells from ten randomly chosen, non-overlapping fields ($n$ = 10) at a magnification of x400 ($n$ = 15/group). Scale bar = 50 μm. Data are expressed as the mean ± SD. *** $p < 0.001$ versus Veh or VP; # $p < 0.05$, ## $p < 0.01$ versus UUO. α-SMA (**C**) and Type I collagen (**D**) expression in kidney tissue from sham and UUO-operated mice treated with Veh or VP was evaluated by Western blotting. Data from the densitometric analysis are presented as the relative ratio of each protein to GAPDH. The relative ratio measured in the kidneys from sham-operated mice treated with Veh is arbitrarily presented as 1. Data are expressed as the mean ± SD. # $p < 0.05$ versus UUO. Veh, vehicle; VP, verteporfin; UUO, unilateral ureteral obstruction operated mice; α-SMA, α-smooth muscle actin; FSP-1; fibroblast-specific protein-1; DAPI, 4′,6-diamidino-2-phenylindole; GAPDH, glyceraldehyde 3-phosphate dehydrogenase.

## 2.3. Verteporfin Decreases UUO-Induced Renal Inflammation

Renal inflammation, such as inflammatory cell infiltration and the increased expression of cell adhesion molecules, is an essential pathologic mechanism of UUO-induced renal tubulointerstitial fibrosis [21]. Therefore, we evaluated F4/80 (+) macrophage infiltration after UUO surgery and treatment with Veh or VP. Veh-treated UUO kidneys showed an increasing number of F4/80 (+) macrophages in the tubulointerstitial areas, and VP treatment significantly decreased the UUO-induced increase in F4/80 (+) macrophage infiltration (Figure 3A). We also used Western blot analysis to evaluate the expression of intercellular adhesion molecules (ICAM)-1 in UUO kidneys treated with Veh or VP. After UUO surgery, ICAM-1 expression increased, compared with sham-operated kidneys, and VP treatment significantly decreased the UUO-induced increase in ICAM-1 expression (Figure 3B). These data show that VP treatment reduces UUO-induced tubulointerstitial inflammation by regulating inflammatory cell infiltration and cell adhesion molecule expression.

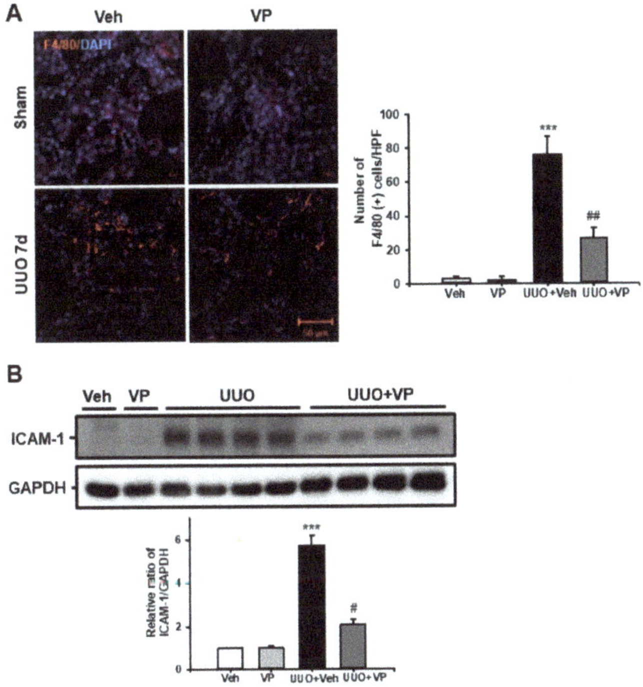


**Figure 3.** Effect of verteporfin on UUO-induced renal inflammation. (**A**) Representative immunofluorescence staining of F4/80 from the kidneys of sham- and UUO-operated mice treated with vehicle (Veh) or verteporfin (VP). The nuclei were stained with DAPI. The bar graph shows the number of F4/80 positive cells from ten randomly chosen, non-overlapping fields ($n$ = 10) at a magnification of ×400 ($n$ = 15/group). Scale bar = 50 μm. Data are expressed as the mean ± SD. *** $p < 0.001$ versus Veh or VP; ## $p < 0.01$ versus UUO. (**B**) ICAM-1 expression in kidney tissue from sham- and UUO-operated mice treated with Veh or VP was evaluated by Western blotting. Data from the densitometric analysis are presented as the relative ratio of each protein to GAPDH. The relative ratio measured in the kidneys of sham-operated mice treated with Veh is arbitrarily presented as 1. Data are expressed as the mean ± SD. *** $p < 0.001$ versus Veh or VP; # $p < 0.05$ versus UUO; Veh, vehicle; VP, verteporfin; Sham, sham-operated mice; UUO, unilateral ureteral obstruction operated mice; ICAM-1, intercellular adhesion molecule-1; DAPI, 4′,6-diamidino-2-phenylindole; GAPDH, glyceraldehyde 3-phosphate dehydrogenase.

### 2.4. *Verteporfin Decreases the UUO-Induced Increase in Connective Tissue Growth Factors by Regulating the Tgf-B1/Smad Signaling Pathway*

To address the protective mechanism of VP in UUO-induced renal fibrosis, we evaluated the TGF-β1/Smad signaling pathway. UUO kidneys showed an increase in Smad2 and Smad3 phosphorylation compared with sham-operated kidneys treated with Veh or VP, and VP treatment significantly decreased the UUO-induced increase in Smad2 and Smad3 phosphorylation (Figure 4A). CTGF is a matricellular protein that has been associated with wound healing and organ fibrosis [22]. CTGF is known to be a downstream mediator of the profibrotic TGF-β1 signaling pathway [23]. Therefore, we evaluated CTGF expression by Western blot analysis. After UUO surgery, CTGF expression increased compared with sham-operated kidneys treated with Veh or VP, and VP treatment significantly decreased the UUO-induced increase in CTGF expression (Figure 4B). These data suggest that VP modulates the UUO-induced activation of the TGF-β1/Smad signaling pathway and the expression of CTGF in UUO kidneys.

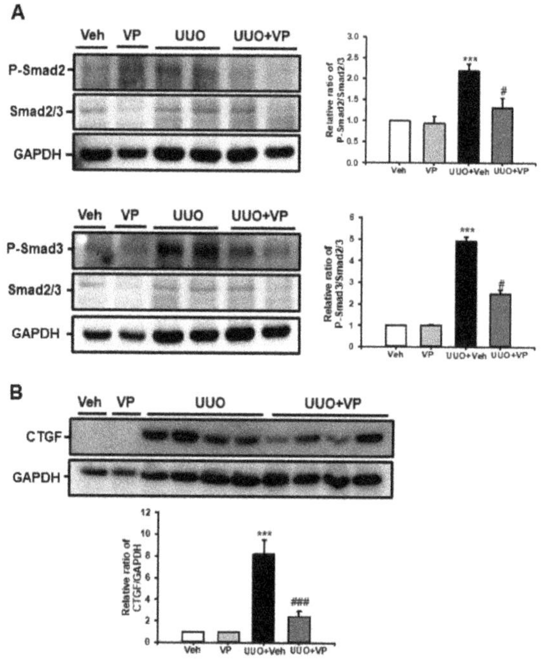


**Figure 4.** Effect of verteporfin on UUO-induced connective tissue growth factor expression through the regulation of Smad2 and Smad3 phosphorylation. (**A**) Phospho-Smad2 and phospho-Smad3 expression in kidney tissue from sham- and UUO-operated mice treated with vehicle (Veh) or verteporfin (VP) was evaluated by Western blotting. Data from the densitometric analysis of phospho-Smad2 and phospho-Smad3 are presented as the relative ratio of each protein to Smad2, Smad3, and GAPDH. The relative ratios measured in the kidneys of sham-operated mice treated with Veh are arbitrarily presented as 1. Data are expressed as the mean ± SD. *** $p < 0.001$ versus Veh or VP; # $p < 0.05$ versus UUO. (**B**) CTGF expression in kidney tissue from sham- and UUO-operated mice treated with Veh or VP was evaluated by Western blotting. Data from the densitometric analysis are presented as the relative ratio of each protein to GAPDH. The relative ratios measured in the kidneys of sham-operated mice treated with Veh are arbitrarily presented as 1. Data are expressed as the mean ± SD. *** $p < 0.001$ versus Veh or VP; ### $p < 0.001$ versus UUO; P-Smad, phospho-Smad; CTGF, connective tissue growth factor; Veh, vehicle; VP, verteporfin; UUO, unilateral ureteral obstruction operated mice, GAPDH, glyceraldehyde 3-phosphate dehydrogenase.

## 2.5. Verteporfin Decreases TGF-β1-Induced Renal Fibroblast Proliferation And Migration in NRK-49F Cells

We evaluated the effect of VP on TGF-β1-induced renal fibroblast proliferation and migration in normal rat fibroblasts (NRK-49F cells). Treatment with TGF-β1 increased renal fibroblast proliferation about 1.8-fold compared with Veh-treated NRK-49F cells. VP treatment significantly and dose-dependently decreased the TGF-β1-induced increase in renal fibroblast proliferation (Figure 5A). We also evaluated cell migration using a wound-healing assay. After TGF-β1 treatment, wound length was significantly decreased compared with baseline and Veh-treated NRK-49F cells. VP treatment decreased the TGF-β1-induced increase in NRK-49F cell migration (Figure 5B). These data suggest that VP treatment regulates TGF-β1-induced renal fibroblast proliferation and migration in NRK-49F cells.

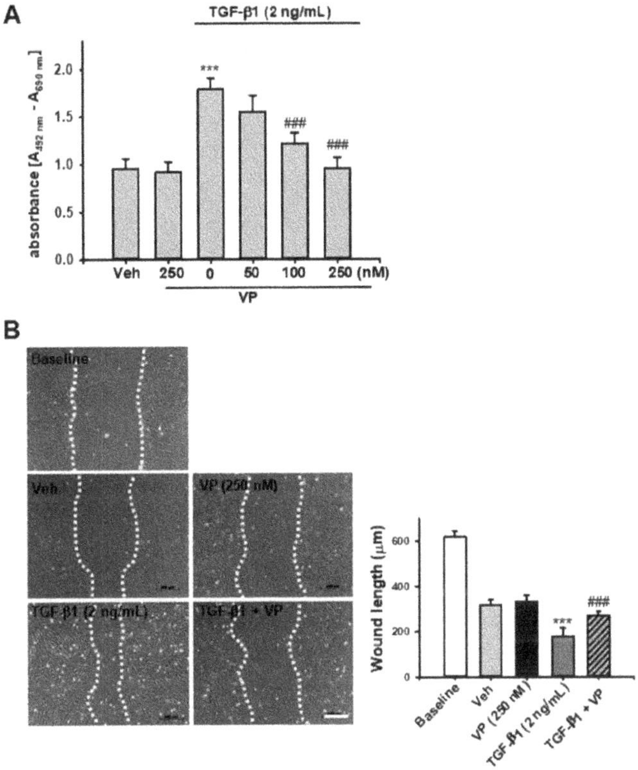


**Figure 5.** Effect of verteporfin on TGF-ß1-induced fibroblast proliferation and cell migration in NRK-49F cells. (**A**) NRK-49F cells were treated with vehicle (Veh) or TGF-β1 (2 ng/mL) with or without verteporfin (VP) at the indicated doses (50, 100, and 250 nM). After 24 h of treatment, cell proliferation was measured using the XTT assay. Data are expressed as the mean ± SD of three independent experiments performed in triplicate. *** $p < 0.001$ versus Veh or VP; ### $p < 0.001$ versus TGF-β1 (2 ng/mL). (**B**) Representative phase-contrast images of NRK-49F cells after the wound healing assay. The phase-contrast images of the migration of NRK-49F cells into the scratch area were obtained after treatment with either Veh or TGF-β1 (2 ng/mL) with or without VP (250 nM) at 0 h and 24 h after wounding. The bar graph shows the average length by which the gap between the NRK-49F cells closed at 0 h or 24 h after treatment with Veh, TGF-β1, and/or VP. *** $p < 0.001$ versus Veh or VP; ### $p < 0.001$ versus TGF-β1. Scale bar = 200 μm. Veh, vehicle; VP, verteporfin; TGF-β1, transforming growth factor-β1.

### 2.6. Verteporfin Decreases TGF-β1-Induced Renal Fibroblast Activation by Regulating the TGF-β1/Smad Signaling Pathway in NRK-49F Cells

We evaluated whether VP could modulate renal myofibroblast activation and matrix protein production in NFK49F cells. After 24 h of stimulation, TGF-β1 (2 ng/mL) significantly increased α-SMA and type I collagen expression in NRK-49F cells, and VP treatment significantly and dose-dependently decreased the TGF-β1-induced increase in α-SMA and type I collagen expression (Figure 6A). We further evaluated the effect of VP on the TGF-β1/Smad signaling pathway in NRK-49F cells. After 30 min of stimulation, TGF-β1 (2 ng/mL) increased Smad2 and Smad3 phosphorylation in NRK-49F cells, and VP treatment significantly and dose-dependently decreased the TGF-β1-induced increase in Smad2 and Smad3phosphorylation (Figure 6B). These data suggest that VP modulates TGF-β1-induced renal fibroblast activation through the TGF-β1/Smad signaling pathway.

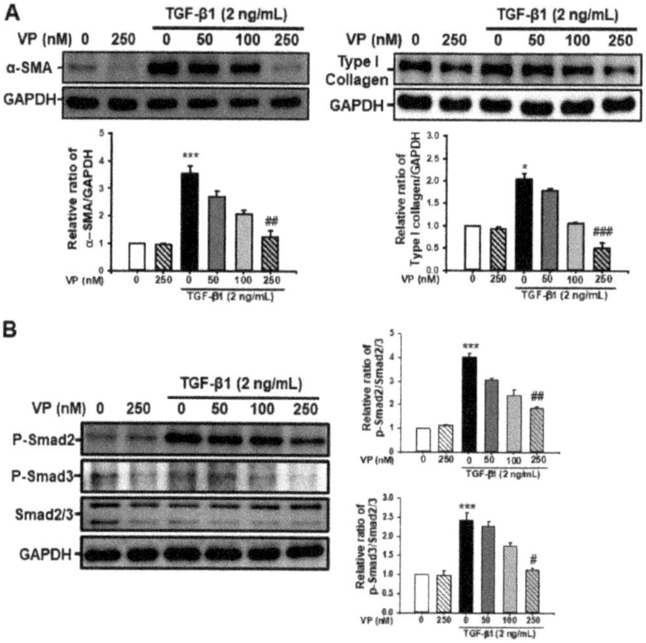


**Figure 6.** Effect of verteporfin on TGF-ß1-induced α-SMA and type I collagen through the regulation of the TGF-β1/Smad signaling pathway in NRK-49F cells. (**A**) Representative Western blot for α-SMA and type I collagen from NRK-49F cells treated with vehicle (Veh) or TGF-β1 (2 ng/mL) with or without verteporfin (VP) at the indicated doses (50, 100 and 250 nM). Treatment with TGF-β1 (2 ng/mL) for 24 h increased the expression of fibrotic markers. The expression of α-SMA and type I collagen decreased dose-dependently after VP treatment. The bar graph shows the densitometric quantification as the relative ratio of each protein to GAPDH. Data are presented as the mean ± SD. (**B**) Representative Western blot for phospho-Smad2 and phospho-Smad3 expression from NRK-49F cells treated with vehicle (Veh) or TGF-β1 (2 ng/mL), with or without VP at the indicated doses (50, 100, and 250 nM). TGF-β1 (2 ng/mL) treatment for 30 min increased the expression of phospho-Smad2 and phospho-Smad3, and VP treatment dose-dependently decreased that increase. The densitometric measurement of phospho-Smad2 and phospho-Smad3 protein expression is presented as the Smad2/3 protein expression ratio. The data are represented as the mean ± SD. *** $p < 0.001$ versus Veh or VP; # $p < 0.05$, ## $p < 0.01$ versus TGF-β1 treatment. Veh, vehicle; VP, verteporfin; TGF-β1, transforming growth factor-β1; α-SMA, α-smooth muscle actin; GAPDH, glyceraldehyde 3-phosphate dehydrogenase.

## 3. Discussion

Renal fibrosis is a common pathophysiologic endpoint of advanced CKD. The loss of the glomerular and peritubular capillary architecture, the proliferation of tubular cells and interstitial fibroblasts, the increases in proinflammatory cytokines and chemokines, the infiltration of inflammatory cells, and the diffuse accumulation of ECM are common histologic features in renal fibrosis [24]. Previously, we found that inhibiting the TGF/Smad signaling pathway by modulating estrogen receptor $\alpha$ and activating mitochondrial Sirt3 ameliorated UUO-induced renal inflammation and fibrosis [9,21]. In this study, we evaluated the protective effect of VP on UUO-induced renal fibrosis. Our results indicate that VP treatment decreases UUO-induced renal tubular injury, ECM deposition, and inflammatory processes. VP also inhibits TGF-β1-induced renal fibroblast activation. These results show that VP has a protective effect against kidney fibrosis by regulating the TGF-β1/Smad signaling pathway.

The excessive accumulation of ECM protein drives progressive organ fibrosis, which increases tissue stiffness and activates the mechanosensitive Hippo pathway effector YAP [25]. Active YAP upregulates ECM deposition and activates a positive-feedback loop that results in fibroblast activation [26]. Therefore, reducing ECM accumulation by modulating YAP activity is a critical target for preventing organ fibrosis and failure. In this study, we used a UUO model to induce renal fibrosis, which produced an increase in the number of FSP-1 (+) fibroblasts and α-SMA (+) myofibroblasts. VP treatment decreased the UUO-induced increase in fibroblast activation. VP treatment also decreased the UUO-induced increase in type I collagen and fibronectin expression. Therefore, using VP treatment to inhibit the Hippo pathway effector YAP might decrease UUO-induced ECM accumulation.

To initiate the wound healing process, the recruitment of inflammatory cells is a fundamental process [27]. The infiltration of polymorphonuclear neutrophils and monocytes is characteristic of the initial inflammatory response to injury [28,29]. An injured organ's parenchymal and endothelial cells and infiltrated inflammatory cells release many cytokines and chemokines that amplify the inflammatory response through complex interactions among the altered mesenchymal cells [27]. Dysregulation of the inflammatory and wound-healing processes leads to the formation of tissue fibrosis. In this study, VP treatment decreased the UUO-induced increase in F4/80 (+) macrophage infiltration and cell adhesion molecule expression. These data suggest that inhibiting the Hippo pathway might decrease the UUO-induced renal inflammatory response.

The TGF-β1/Smad signaling pathway is a crucial player in renal fibrosis [9,20]. The downstream target genes of the TGF-β1/Smad signaling pathway mediate myofibroblast activation and ECM deposition in injured tissues. Our in vitro data using NFR49F cells show that inhibiting the Hippo pathway decreases TGF-β1-induced renal fibroblast proliferation and migration by regulating Smad2 and Smad3 phosphorylation. Furthermore, VP treatment reduces TGF-β1-induced ECM production in NRK-49F cells. The action of TGF-β1 and YAP activity might by closely related at multiple levels of the fibrotic process, such as tissue stiffness by ECM accumulation, cell adhesion, and cell morphology [30]. In human lung fibrosis, increased TGF-β1 and aberrantly activated TAZ/YAP can contribute to fibroblast activation and survival and enhance the production of profibrogenic factors such as CTGF [30]. In diabetic nephropathy, EGF receptor-dependent upregulation of YAP increases the levels of downstream profibrotic factors such as CTGF and amphiregulin [31]. TGF-β1-dependent TAZ activation promotes maladaptive epithelial repair through Smad3-dependent CTGF up-regulation [32]. Xu et al. reported that constant YAP increases and activation are involved in regeneration and fibrogenesis after acute ischemic kidney injury [19]. In our in vivo experiment, the inhibition of YAP by VP decreased the UUO-induced increase in CTGF expression by regulating Smad2 and Smad3 phosphorylation.

The Hippo pathway plays an essential role in kidney and urinary tract development [33,34], cystic kidney disease [35,36], podocyte integrity [37], diabetic nephropathy [31], renal cell carcinoma [38], and tubulointerstitial fibrosis [39]. In the Hippo pathway, both YAP and TAZ can serve as central transcriptional coactivators after nuclear translocation. They associate with transcription factors such as the Runt-related transcription factor and TEAD to modulate transcription [40–43]. Recent research data have linked YAP and TAZ with fibrogenesis as critical regulators of fibroblast mechanoactivation and fibrogenic function [26]. Renal fibrosis that arises from numerous insults progresses to CKD, which is characterized by the deposition of ECM. The stiff ECM enhances TGF-β1-induced profibrotic Smad signaling in a process mediated by YAP and TAZ [44]. In addition to ECM deposition, YAP has an essential role in glomerular integrity. Podocyte-specific *Yap* deletion results in proteinuria between 5 and 6 weeks of age and leads to focal segmental glomerular sclerosis at 12 weeks [37]. Therefore, the modulation of the Hippo pathway might be a novel therapeutic target for kidney fibrosis.

In conclusion, YAP inhibition by means of VP treatment decreases UUO-induced renal fibroblast activation, inflammation, ECM deposition, and tubulointerstitial fibrosis by regulating the TGF-β1/Smad signaling pathway.

## 4. Materials and Methods

### 4.1. Animal Experiment

The animal experiment protocol was reviewed and approved by the Institutional Animal Care and Use Committee of Jeonbuk National University (CBNU 2018-040, 29 May 2018, Jeonju, Korea). Male C57BL/6 mice (7–8 weeks old; weight 20–25 g) were purchased from Orient Bio, Inc. (Seoul, Korea), maintained in a room with controlled temperature (23 ± 1 °C), humidity, and lighting (12-h light/12-h dark cycle), and given free access to food and water. For the experiment, we divided the mice into four groups: sham and UUO with Veh treatment, and sham and UUO with VP treatment ($n$ = 15/group). VP (Sigma-Aldrich; Merck KGaA, Darmstadt, Germany) was dissolved in dimethyl sulfoxide (DMSO, 0.05% *v*/*v*), and DMSO (0.05% *v*/*v*) was used as the vehicle. VP (100 mg/kg) was administered by daily intraperitoneal injection for 3 d before UUO surgery and continued for 7 d after surgery. Renal fibrosis was induced using a UUO operation described previously [21]. In brief, mice were anesthetized by intraperitoneal injection of ketamine (100 mg/kg, Huons, Seoul, Korea) and xylazine (10 mg/kg, Bayer Korea, Seoul, Korea) and placed on a temperature-controlled operating table to maintain body temperature at 37 °C. Through a midline incision in the abdomen, the right proximal ureter was exposed and ligated at two separated points using 3-0 black silk. We performed the sham operation using the same method without the ligation of the ureter. Seven days after the UUO operation, the obstructed kidney was harvested, prepared for histological examination, and stored at −80 °C for the Western blot analysis.

### 4.2. Renal Histologic Examination

Each kidney was fixed in 4% paraformaldehyde and embedded in paraffin. The block was cut into 5 μm sections and stained with PAS stain and Masson's trichrome. For immunofluorescence staining, freshly frozen renal tissues were fixed with 4% paraformaldehyde, permeabilized in 1% Triton X-100, and then incubated with a blocking buffer. The tissue samples were incubated with anti-α-smooth muscle actin (α-SMA; A2547 mouse; 1:1000; Sigma-Aldrich Merck KGaA, Darmstadt, Germany), anti-fibroblast specific protein (FSP)-1 (ab27957; 1:100; Abcam, Cambridge, UK) and F4/80 (14-4801-82; 1:200 eBioscience, San Diego, CA, USA) and then exposed to Cy3-labeled secondary antibody (Chemicon, Temecula, CA). Nuclear staining was performed using 300 nM 4′, 6-diamidino-2-phenylindole solution for 3 min (DAPI, Molecular Probes; Thermo Fisher Scientific, Inc.). For the morphometric analysis, two observers who were unaware of the origins of the samples used a Zeiss Z1 microscope or Zeiss LSM 510 confocal laser scanning microscope (Carl Zeiss, Göttingen, Germany) to evaluate all slides. Tubular injury was scored into six levels based on the percentage of tubular dilation, epithelial desquamation, and loss of brush border in 10 randomly chosen, non-overlapping fields at a magnification of 200× under a light microscope: 0, none; 0.5, <10%; 1, 10–25%; 2, 25–50%; 3, 50–75%; and 4, >75%. The fibrotic area was also measured in 10 randomly chosen, non-overlapping fields at a magnification of 200×. The area fraction of α-SMA was measured at a magnification of 400×. The numbers of FSP-1 positive fibroblasts and F4/80 positive macrophages were counted at a magnification of 400×. All images were analyzed using ImageJ software (http://rsb.info.nih.gov/ij).

### 4.3. Western Blotting

The Western blot analysis was performed as described previously [20]. Kidney tissue and cell lysates were separated by 10% SDS-PAGE. After electrophoresis, the samples were transferred to PVDF membranes (BIO-RAD, Hercules, CA, USA) and blocked with 5% skim milk (BIO-RAD, Hercules, CA, USA). Then we probed the blots with primary antibodies to α-SMA (A2547 mouse; 1:1000; Sigma-Aldrich Merck KGaA, Darmstadt, Germany), type I collagen (1310-01; goat; 1:1000; Southern Biotech, Birmingham, AL, USA), ICAM-1 (sc-1511; goat; 1:1000, Santa Cruz Biotechnology, Mississauga, CA, USA), CTGF (sc-365970; mouse; 1:1000; Santa Cruz Biotechnology, Inc., Dallas, TX, USA), phospho-Smad2 (3101; rabbit; 1:1000; Cell Signaling Technology Inc., Danvers, MA, USA), phospho-Smad3 (9520; rabbit; 1:1000; Cell Signaling Technology Inc.), Smad2/3 (07-408; rabbit; 1:1000; EMD Millipore, Billerica, MA, USA), and glyceraldehyde 3-phosphate dehydrogenase (GAPDH; AP0063; rabbit; 1:2000; Bioworld Technology, Inc., Danvers, MA, USA), which was used as an internal control. All signals were analyzed by a densitometric scanner (ImageQuant LAS 4000 Mini, GE Healthcare Life Sciences, Piscataway Township, NJ, USA).

### 4.4. Cell Culture Experiments

In vitro experiments were performed using a rat renal fibroblast cell line (NRK-49F, American Type Culture Collection, Manassas, VA). We cultured NRK-49F cells in Dulbecco's modified Eagle's medium with 4 mM L-glutamine adjusted to contain 1.5 g/L of sodium bicarbonate and 4.5 g/L of glucose supplemented with 5% (vol/vol) heat-inactivated fetal bovine serum and antibiotics (100 U/mL penicillin G and 100 μg/mL streptomycin) at 37 °C with 5% $CO_2$ in 95% air. To investigate the effect of VP on myofibroblast activation, ECM expression, and the activation of the TGF-β1/Smad signaling pathway, we incubated sub-confluent NRK-49F cells with VP (50, 100, and 250 nM) for 30 min and then stimulated them with TGF-β1 (2 ng/mL, Sigma Chemical Co.) for the indicated periods.

### 4.5. Cell proliferation Assay

After 24 h of treatment with VP (50, 100, and 250 nM) and TGF-β1 (2 ng/mL), the proliferation of NRK-49F cells was determined by a colorimetric assay (Cell Proliferation Kit II, Roche Diagnostics, Mannheim, Germany) according to the manufacturer's protocol. All experimental values were determined from triplicate wells.

### 4.6. Wound Healing Assay

Sub-confluent NRK-49F cells were cultured in 6-well dishes. Before treatment with VP and TGF-β1, we scratched the 6-well dishes using a sterile 200-μL pipette tip, causing three separate wounds. The cells were incubated with VP (250 nM) for 30 min and then stimulated with TGF-β1 (2 ng/mL) for 24 h. Wound lengths were measured using ImageJ. The wound length at 0 h after scratching was used as the control.

### 4.7. Statistical Analysis

The data are expressed as the mean ± standard deviation (SD). To confirm whether the dataset was normally distributed, we used the Shapiro-Wilk test. For normally distributed data, one-way analysis of variance (ANOVA) was used to evaluate differences within groups, followed by an individual comparison between groups with the Tukey post hoc test. For non-parametric data, the Kruskal-Wallis one-way ANOVA on ranks was used, followed by all multiple pairwise comparisons with the Dunn's method. $p < 0.05$ was considered statistically significant.

**Author Contributions:** Conceptualization, J.J. and K.P.K.; methodology, J.J., T.W., W.P., W.L., and K.P.K.; investigation, J.J., T.W., W.P., W.L., and K.P.K.; data curation, J.J. and K.P.K.; formal analysis, J.J. and K.P.K., writing—original draft preparation, J.J. and K.P.K.; writing—review and editing, K.P.K.; project administration, W.K., S.K.P., and K.P.K.; funding acquisition, S.K.P., and K.P.K. All authors have read and agreed to the published version of the manuscript.

**Funding:** This research was supported by the National Research Foundation of Korea (NRF) funded by the Korean government (NRF-2018R1D1A1B07045790 to K.P.K and NRF- 2017R1D1A3B03035494 to S.K.P) and by the Fund of Biomedical Research Institute, Jeonbuk National University Hospital (CUH2020-0014, to S.K.P).

**Acknowledgments:** We thank Kieu Thi Thu Trang for her excellent technical assistance.

**Conflicts of Interest:** The authors have no conflicts of interest to declare.

## Abbreviations

| | |
|---|---|
| α-SMA | α-smooth muscle actin |
| CKD | chronic kidney disease |
| CTGF | connective tissue growth factor |
| DAPI | 4′,6-diamidino-2-phenylindole |
| ECM, | extracellular matrix |
| FSP-1 | fibroblast-specific protein-1 |
| GAPDH | glyceraldehyde 3-phosphate dehydrogenase |
| ICAM-1 | intercellular adhesion molecule-1 |
| MTC | Masson's trichrome. |
| NRK | normal rat kidney |
| PAS | periodic acid–Schiff |
| Sham | sham-operated mice |
| TAZ | transcriptional coactivator with a PDZ-binding motif |
| TEAD | TEA domain family member |
| TGF-β1 | transforming growth factor-β1 |
| UUO | unilateral ureteral obstruction |
| YAP | Yes-associated protein |
| Veh | Vehicle |
| VP | Verteporfin |

## References

1. Chapter 1: Definition and classification of CKD. *Kidney Int. Suppl.* **2013**, *3*, 19–62. [CrossRef]
2. GBD 2015 Mortality and Causes of Death Collaborators. Global, regional, and national life expectancy, all-cause mortality, and cause-specific mortality for 249 causes of death, 1980–2015: A systematic analysis for the Global Burden of Disease Study 2015. *Lancet* **2016**, *388*, 1459–1544. [CrossRef]
3. Grams, M.E.; Chow, E.K.; Segev, D.L.; Coresh, J. Lifetime incidence of CKD stages 3-5 in the United States. *Am. J. Kidney Dis.* **2013**, *62*, 245–252. [CrossRef]
4. Li, P.K.; Garcia-Garcia, G.; Lui, S.F.; Andreoli, S.; Fung, W.W.; Hradsky, A.; Kumaraswami, L.; Liakopoulos, V.; Rakhimova, Z.; Saadi, G.; et al. World Kidney Day Steering, C. Kidney health for everyone everywhere-from prevention to detection and equitable access to care. *Kidney Int.* **2020**, *97*, 226–232. [CrossRef] [PubMed]
5. Kim, K.M.; Oh, H.J.; Choi, H.Y.; Lee, H.; Ryu, D.R. Impact of chronic kidney disease on mortality: A nationwide cohort study. *Kidney Res. Clin. Pract.* **2019**, *38*, 382–390. [CrossRef] [PubMed]
6. He, W.; Dai, C. Key Fibrogenic Signaling. *Curr. Pathobiol. Rep.* **2015**, *3*, 183–192. [CrossRef] [PubMed]
7. Boor, P.; Ostendorf, T.; Floege, J. Renal fibrosis: Novel insights into mechanisms and therapeutic targets. *Nat. Rev. Nephrol.* **2010**, *6*, 643–656. [CrossRef]
8. Sureshbabu, A.; Muhsin, S.A.; Choi, M.E. TGF-beta signaling in the kidney: Profibrotic and protective effects. *Am J Physiol Renal Physiol* **2016**, *310*, F596–F606. [CrossRef]
9. Kim, D.; Lee, A.S.; Jung, Y.J.; Yang, K.H.; Lee, S.; Park, S.K.; Kim, W.; Kang, K.P. Tamoxifen ameliorates renal tubulointerstitial fibrosis by modulation of estrogen receptor alpha-mediated transforming growth factor-beta1/Smad signaling pathway. *Nephrol Dial Transplant* **2014**, *29*, 2043–2053. [CrossRef]

10. Meng, X.M.; Nikolic-Paterson, D.J.; Lan, H.Y. TGF-beta: The master regulator of fibrosis. *Nat. Rev. Nephrol.* **2016**, *12*, 325–338. [CrossRef]
11. Finnson, K.W.; Almadani, Y.; Philip, A. Non-canonical (non-SMAD2/3) TGF-beta signaling in fibrosis: Mechanisms and targets. *Semin. Cell. Dev. Biol.* **2020**, *101*, 115–122. [CrossRef] [PubMed]
12. Ma, S.; Meng, Z.; Chen, R.; Guan, K.L. The Hippo Pathway: Biology and Pathophysiology. *Annu. Rev. Biochem.* **2019**, *88*, 577–604. [CrossRef] [PubMed]
13. Meng, Z.; Moroishi, T.; Guan, K.L. Mechanisms of Hippo pathway regulation. *Genes Dev.* **2016**, *30*, 1–17. [CrossRef]
14. Piccolo, S.; Dupont, S.; Cordenonsi, M. The biology of YAP/TAZ: Hippo signaling and beyond. *Physiol. Rev.* **2014**, *94*, 1287–1312. [CrossRef] [PubMed]
15. Chen, W.S.; Cao, Z.; Krishnan, C.; Panjwani, N. Verteporfin without light stimulation inhibits YAP activation in trabecular meshwork cells: Implications for glaucoma treatment. *Biochem. Biophys. Res. Commun.* **2015**, *466*, 221–225. [CrossRef] [PubMed]
16. Liu-Chittenden, Y.; Huang, B.; Shim, J.S.; Chen, Q.; Lee, S.J.; Anders, R.A.; Liu, J.O.; Pan, D. Genetic and pharmacological disruption of the TEAD-YAP complex suppresses the oncogenic activity of YAP. *Genes Dev.* **2012**, *26*, 1300–1305. [CrossRef]
17. Raghunathan, V.K.; Morgan, J.T.; Dreier, B.; Reilly, C.M.; Thomasy, S.M.; Wood, J.A.; Ly, I.; Tuyen, B.C.; Hughbanks, M.; Murphy, C.J.; et al. Role of substratum stiffness in modulating genes associated with extracellular matrix and mechanotransducers YAP and TAZ. *Invest. Ophthalmol. Vis. Sci.* **2013**, *54*, 378–386. [CrossRef]
18. Moon, S.; Lee, S.; Caesar, J.A.; Pruchenko, S.; Leask, A.; Knowles, J.A.; Sinon, J.; Chaqour, B. A CTGF-YAP Regulatory Pathway Is Essential for Angiogenesis and Barriergenesis in the Retina. *iScience* **2020**, *23*, 101184. [CrossRef]
19. Xu, J.; Li, P.X.; Wu, J.; Gao, Y.J.; Yin, M.X.; Lin, Y.; Yang, M.; Chen, D.P.; Sun, H.P.; Liu, Z.B.; et al. Involvement of the Hippo pathway in regeneration and fibrogenesis after ischaemic acute kidney injury: YAP is the key effector. *Clin. Sci. (Lond.)* **2016**, *130*, 349–363. [CrossRef]
20. Nguyen-Thanh, T.; Kim, D.; Lee, S.; Kim, W.; Park, S.K.; Kang, K.P. Inhibition of histone deacetylase 1 ameliorates renal tubulointerstitial fibrosis via modulation of inflammation and extracellular matrix gene transcription in mice. *Int. J. Mol. Med.* **2018**, *41*, 95–106. [CrossRef]
21. Quan, Y.; Park, W.; Jin, J.; Kim, W.; Park, S.K.; Kang, K.P. Sirtuin 3 Activation by Honokiol Decreases Unilateral Ureteral Obstruction-Induced Renal Inflammation and Fibrosis via Regulation of Mitochondrial Dynamics and the Renal NF-kappaBTGF-beta1/Smad Signaling Pathway. *Int. J. Mol. Sc.i* **2020**, *21*, 402. [CrossRef] [PubMed]
22. Brigstock, D.R. Connective tissue growth factor (CCN2, CTGF) and organ fibrosis: Lessons from transgenic animals. *J. Cell. Commun. Signal.* **2010**, *4*, 1–4. [CrossRef]
23. Grotendorst, G.R. Connective tissue growth factor: A mediator of TGF-beta action on fibroblasts. *Cytokine Growth Factor Rev.* **1997**, *8*, 171–179. [CrossRef]
24. Grande, M.T.; Lopez-Novoa, J.M. Fibroblast activation and myofibroblast generation in obstructive nephropathy. *Nat. Rev. Nephrol.* **2009**, *5*, 319–328. [CrossRef]
25. Herrera, J.; Henke, C.A.; Bitterman, P.B. Extracellular matrix as a driver of progressive fibrosis. *J. Clin. Investig.* **2018**, *128*, 45–53. [CrossRef] [PubMed]
26. Liu, F.; Lagares, D.; Choi, K.M.; Stopfer, L.; Marinkovic, A.; Vrbanac, V.; Probst, C.K.; Hiemer, S.E.; Sisson, T.H.; Horowitz, J.C.; et al. Mechanosignaling through YAP and TAZ drives fibroblast activation and fibrosis. *Am. J. Physiol. Lung Cell. Mol. Physiol.* **2015**, *308*, L344–L357. [CrossRef] [PubMed]
27. Sahin, H.; Wasmuth, H.E. Chemokines in tissue fibrosis. *Biochim. Biophys. Acta* **2013**, *1832*, 1041–1048. [CrossRef]
28. Wynn, T.A.; Ramalingam, T.R. Mechanisms of fibrosis: Therapeutic translation for fibrotic disease. *Nat. Med.* **2012**, *18*, 1028–1040. [CrossRef]
29. Serhan, C.N.; Chiang, N.; Van Dyke, T.E. Resolving inflammation: Dual anti-inflammatory and pro-resolution lipid mediators. *Nat. Rev. Immunol.* **2008**, *8*, 349–361. [CrossRef]
30. Saito, A.; Nagase, T. Hippo and TGF-beta interplay in the lung field. *Am. J. Physiol. Lung Cell. Mol. Physiol.* **2015**, *309*, L756–L767. [CrossRef]

31. Chen, J.; Harris, R.C. Interaction of the EGF Receptor and the Hippo Pathway in the Diabetic Kidney. *J. Am. Soc. Nephrol.* **2016**, *27*, 1689–1700. [CrossRef] [PubMed]
32. Anorga, S.; Overstreet, J.M.; Falke, L.L.; Tang, J.; Goldschmeding, R.G.; Higgins, P.J.; Samarakoon, R. Deregulation of Hippo-TAZ pathway during renal injury confers a fibrotic maladaptive phenotype. *FASEB J.* **2018**, *32*, 2644–2657. [CrossRef] [PubMed]
33. Morin-Kensicki, E.M.; Boone, B.N.; Howell, M.; Stonebraker, J.R.; Teed, J.; Alb, J.G.; Magnuson, T.R.; O'Neal, W.; Milgram, S.L. Defects in yolk sac vasculogenesis, chorioallantoic fusion, and embryonic axis elongation in mice with targeted disruption of Yap65. *Mol. Cell. Biol.* **2006**, *26*, 77–87. [CrossRef]
34. Reginensi, A.; Hoshi, M.; Boualia, S.K.; Bouchard, M.; Jain, S.; McNeill, H. Yap and Taz are required for Ret-dependent urinary tract morphogenesis. *Development* **2015**, *142*, 2696–2703. [CrossRef] [PubMed]
35. Hossain, Z.; Ali, S.M.; Ko, H.L.; Xu, J.; Ng, C.P.; Guo, K.; Qi, Z.; Ponniah, S.; Hong, W.; Hunziker, W. Glomerulocystic kidney disease in mice with a targeted inactivation of Wwtr1. *Proc. Natl. Acad. Sci. USA* **2007**, *104*, 1631–1636. [CrossRef]
36. Happe, H.; van der Wal, A.M.; Leonhard, W.N.; Kunnen, S.J.; Breuning, M.H.; de Heer, E.; Peters, D.J. Altered Hippo signalling in polycystic kidney disease. *J. Pathol.* **2011**, *224*, 133–142. [CrossRef]
37. Schwartzman, M.; Reginensi, A.; Wong, J.S.; Basgen, J.M.; Meliambro, K.; Nicholas, S.B.; D'Agati, V.; McNeill, H.; Campbell, K.N. Podocyte-Specific Deletion of Yes-Associated Protein Causes FSGS and Progressive Renal Failure. *J. Am. Soc. Nephrol.* **2016**, *27*, 216–226. [CrossRef]
38. Schutte, U.; Bisht, S.; Heukamp, L.C.; Kebschull, M.; Florin, A.; Haarmann, J.; Hoffmann, P.; Bendas, G.; Buettner, R.; Brossart, P.; et al. Hippo signaling mediates proliferation, invasiveness, and metastatic potential of clear cell renal cell carcinoma. *Transl. Oncol.* **2014**, *7*, 309–321. [CrossRef]
39. Szeto, S.G.; Narimatsu, M.; Lu, M.; He, X.; Sidiqi, A.M.; Tolosa, M.F.; Chan, L.; De Freitas, K.; Bialik, J.F.; Majumder, S.; et al. YAP/TAZ Are Mechanoregulators of TGF-beta-Smad Signaling and Renal Fibrogenesis. *J. Am. Soc. Nephrol.* **2016**, *27*, 3117–3128. [CrossRef]
40. Piersma, B.; Bank, R.A.; Boersema, M. Signaling in Fibrosis: TGF-beta, WNT, and YAP/TAZ Converge. *Front. Med. (Lausanne)* **2015**, *2*, 59. [CrossRef]
41. Zhao, B.; Li, L.; Lei, Q.; Guan, K.L. The Hippo-YAP pathway in organ size control and tumorigenesis: An updated version. *Genes Dev.* **2010**, *24*, 862–874. [CrossRef]
42. Yagi, R.; Chen, L.F.; Shigesada, K.; Murakami, Y.; Ito, Y. A WW domain-containing yes-associated protein (YAP) is a novel transcriptional co-activator. *EMBO J.* **1999**, *18*, 2551–2562. [CrossRef]
43. Kanai, F.; Marignani, P.A.; Sarbassova, D.; Yagi, R.; Hall, R.A.; Donowitz, M.; Hisaminato, A.; Fujiwara, T.; Ito, Y.; Cantley, L.C.; et al. TAZ: A novel transcriptional co-activator regulated by interactions with 14-3-3 and PDZ domain proteins. *EMBO J.* **2000**, *19*, 6778–6791. [CrossRef]
44. Wong, J.S.; Meliambro, K.; Ray, J.; Campbell, K.N. Hippo signaling in the kidney: The good and the bad. *Am. J. Physiol Renal. Physiol.* **2016**, *311*, F241–F248. [CrossRef]

International Journal of
*Molecular Sciences*

MDPI

*Article*

# B Cell Activating Factor (BAFF) Is Required for the Development of Intra-Renal Tertiary Lymphoid Organs in Experimental Kidney Transplantation in Rats

**Louisa Steines *, Helen Poth, Marlene Herrmann, Antonia Schuster, Bernhard Banas and Tobias Bergler**

Department of Nephrology, University Hospital Regensburg, 93042 Regensburg, Germany; helen_reinfrank@web.de (H.P.); marlene-herrmann@gmx.net (M.H.); antonia-margarete.schuster@ukr.de (A.S.); bernhard.banas@ukr.de (B.B.); tobias.bergler@ukr.de (T.B.)

* Correspondence: Louisa.Steines@ukr.de; Tel.: +49-941-9447301; Fax: +49-941-9447302

Received: 14 September 2020; Accepted: 25 October 2020; Published: 28 October 2020

check for updates

**Abstract:** Intra-renal tertiary lymphoid organs (TLOs) are associated with worsened outcome in kidney transplantation (Ktx). We used an anti-BAFF (B cell activating factor) intervention to investigate whether BAFF is required for TLO formation in a full MHC-mismatch Ktx model in rats. Rats received either therapeutic immunosuppression (no rejection, NR) or subtherapeutic immunosuppression (chronic rejection, CR) and were sacrificed on d56. One group additionally received an anti-BAFF antibody (CR + AB). Intra-renal T ($CD3^+$) and B ($CD20^+$) cells, their proliferation ($Ki67^+$), and $IgG^+$ plasma cells were analyzed by immunofluorescence microscopy. Formation of T and B cell zones and TLOs was assessed. Intra-renal expression of TLO-promoting factors, molecules of T:B crosstalk, and B cell differentiation was analyzed by qPCR. Intra-renal B and T cell zones and TLOs were detected in CR and were associated with elevated intra-renal mRNA expression of TLO-promoting factors, including CXCL13, CCL19, lymphotoxin-β, and BAFF. Intra-renal plasma cells were also elevated in CR. Anti-BAFF treatment significantly decreased intra-renal B cell zones and TLO, as well as intra-renal B cell-derived TLO-promoting factors and B cell differentiation markers. We conclude that BAFF-dependent intra-renal B cells promote TLO formation and advance local adaptive alloimmune responses in chronic rejection.

**Keywords:** tertiary lymphoid organs; kidney transplantation; B cells; BAFF

## 1. Introduction

Kidney transplantation is the best available treatment for many patients with end-stage kidney failure; however, kidney allograft survival is limited, with a 10-year graft survival rate of only 56% [1]. A shortage of organs for donation is therefore exacerbated by premature allograft failure. On top of this, patients with multiple consecutive transplants have a higher risk of graft failure due to rejection [2]. Improving allograft survival is therefore an important aim in renal and transplantation medicine.

Apart from antibody-mediated rejection (ABMR), which is a major cause of allograft failure [3], kidney allograft inflammation is an important predictor of reduced allograft survival [4]. Subclinical inflammation is associated with poorer outcomes [4,5] and may precede irreversible interstitial fibrosis [6]. Due to its prognostic relevance, inflammation in areas of fibrosis has recently been incorporated into Banff rejection grading as an independent score ("iIFTA", inflammation with interstitial fibrosis and tubular atrophy). The role of B cells in allograft inflammation has not been fully clarified. Intra-graft B cell clusters have been observed in animal and human transplant studies, and have been related to poorer outcomes [7,8]. Furthermore, overproportional amounts of B cells were found in allografts with subclinical rejection and fibrotic changes compared to grafts with subclinical rejection without fibrosis [9], suggesting a role of B cells in chronic rejection.

B cells can form organized follicular structures together with T cells and other immune cells [10,11]. Within these structures, termed tertiary lymphoid organs (TLOs), B cells can affect local immune activation [12]. TLOs resemble lymphoid follicles within secondary lymphoid organs and occur at sites of chronic inflammation. They have been detected in systemic lupus erythematodes (SLE), rheumatoid arthritis, multiple sclerosis, atherosclerosis, as well as heart and kidney transplantation, as reviewed by Pitzalis [13]. The formation of TLO is driven by local expression of factors required for formation of secondary lymphoid tissue, such as CCL19, CCL21, CXCL13, and lymphotoxin-$\alpha/\beta$ [14,15]. Furthermore, TLOs are sites of local activation of adaptive immunity, where locally antigen-activated B cells receive additional signals, clonally proliferate [16], and become a local source of donor-specific antibodies (DSAs) [12].

B cells are important mediators of TLO development due to their expression of lymphotoxin-$\alpha/\beta$ [17]. They can remain within allografts even after peripheral depletion of B cells using Rituximab [18]. B cell activating factor (BAFF) is an important survival factor for B cells and plasma cells [19]. In Ktx patients, elevated serum BAFF levels have also been associated with pre-sensitization, anti-HLA antibody formation, ABMR, and reduced graft survival [20,21]. We have previously demonstrated expression of BAFF in experimental rat kidney allografts [22], and also showed that anti-BAFF treatment interfered with humoral responses in Ktx using the same model [23]. However, a necessity of BAFF for TLO development has not previously been shown. Here, we tested the effects of an anti-BAFF antibody on intra-renal infiltrates of T and B cells, their microanatomical organization into TLOs, intra-renal expression of TLO-promoting factors and B cell differentiation factors, as part of local adaptive alloresponses in chronic rejection.

## 2. Results

### 2.1. Anti-BAFF Treatment Alters the T and B Cell Composition of Intra-Renal Infiltrates

We first examined the overall area of intra-renal infiltrates in the different experimental groups using immunohistochemistry. Infiltrates were significantly more expansive in CR and CR + AB compared to NR (CR vs. NR: 0.16 ± 0.05 vs. 0.01 ± 0.01 $mm^2$, $p = 0.0012$; CR + AB vs. NR: 0.10 ± 0.08 vs. 0.01 ± 0.01 $mm^2$, $p = 0.030$) (Figure 1A). The expansion of intra-renal infiltrates appeared to be reduced in CR + AB compared to CR, but the difference was not significant. Analysis of the microanatomical localization of infiltrates showed that the majority of infiltrates were localized in the vicinity of arterioles (perivascular), followed by localization surrounding glomeruli (periglomerular) and few were located interstitially without apparent contact to arterioles or glomeruli (Figure 1B). We then assessed the number of T ($CD3^+$) and B ($CD20^+$) cells within kidney sections, and found that there were significantly more T cells in CR and CR + AB compared to NR (CR vs. NR: 610 ± 204 vs. 30 ± 40 cells/$mm^2$, $p = 0.0032$; CR + AB vs. NR: 479 ± 338 vs. 30 ± 40 cells/$mm^2$, $p = 0.019$), but CR and CR + AB did not differ significantly in intra-renal T cell content (Figure 1C). The number of B cells was also significantly elevated in CR compared to NR (CR vs. NR: 431 ± 232 vs. 6 ± 13 cells/$mm^2$, $p = 0.0006$). Anti-BAFF treatment substantially reduced the number of intra-renal B cells (CR vs. CR + AB: 431 ± 232 vs. 60 ± 51 cells/$mm^2$, $p = 0.0013$) (Figure 1C). Since T cells were non-significantly reduced in CR + AB compared to CR, we also assessed the ratio of B:T cells and found that this was elevated in CR compared to NR (0.67 ± 0.29 vs. 0.12 ± 0.16, $p = 0.0067$), and significantly reduced after anti-BAFF treatment (CR vs. CR + AB: 0.67 ± 0.29 vs. 0.12 ± 0.05, $p = 0.0016$) (Figure 1D).

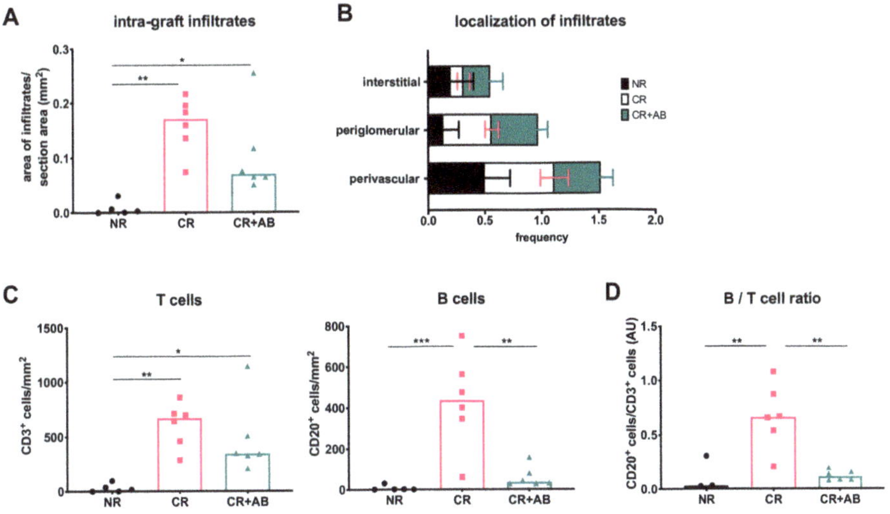


**Figure 1.** Intra-renal infiltrates, their microanatomical localization, and content of T and B lymphocytes. (**A**) shows intra-renal infiltrate expansion, which was measured using Histoquest software and was expressed as the cumulative area of infiltrates/area of the renal cortex. (**B**) shows the microanatomical localization of infiltrates, which was recorded as perivascular, periglomerular, or interstitial. (**C**) shows the intra-renal content of $CD3^+$ T cells and $CD20^+$ B cells, which was determined using Histoquest software after immunohistochemical staining and normalized to the area of renal cortex. (**D**) shows the ratio of intra-renal B/T cells in arbitrary units (AU). NR, no rejection (black); CR, chronic rejection (pink); CR + AB, chronic rejection and anti-BAFF antibody (green). Data is shown as individual data points per rat and group means. Statistical significance is shown as * $p < 0.05$, ** $p < 0.01$, and *** $p < 0.001$.

### 2.2. Anti-BAFF Treatment Interfered with TLO Formation

B cells and T cells can organize into distinct zones within infiltrates to form TLOs. We assessed the microanatomical organization of intra-renal T and B cells into T and B cell zones using immunofluorescence microscopy. Figure 2A shows representative images of staining of $CD3^+$ T cells (red), $CD20^+$ B cells (yellow), and $Ki67^+$ proliferating cells (green). In NR, infiltrates were rare and small compared to the other groups. In CR, large infiltrates containing distinct B and T cell zones were found as shown in Figure 2A. Infiltrates after anti-BAFF treatment showed dense T cell zones but a lack of B cell zones. We determined the presence of T and B cell zones per infiltrate, and found that T cell zones were similarly frequent in all groups (Figure 2B), but the frequency of B cell zones within infiltrates was significantly higher in CR compared to NR (CR vs. NR: 0.44 ± 0.20 vs. 0.00 ± 0.00, $p = 0.0001$) but substantially lower with anti-BAFF treatment (CR vs. CR + AB: 0.44 ± 0.20 vs. 0.05 ± 0.06, $p = 0.0002$) (Figure 2B). TLOs were defined by the presence of T and B cell zones, and were absent in NR but significantly elevated in CR (CR vs. NR: 0.44 ± 0.20 vs. 0.00 ± 0.00, $p = 0.0001$) (Figure 2C). However, the frequency of TLO was significantly diminished after anti-BAFF treatment (CR vs. CR + AB: 0.44 ± 0.20 vs. 0.048 ± 0.06, $p = 0.0002$) (Figure 2C).

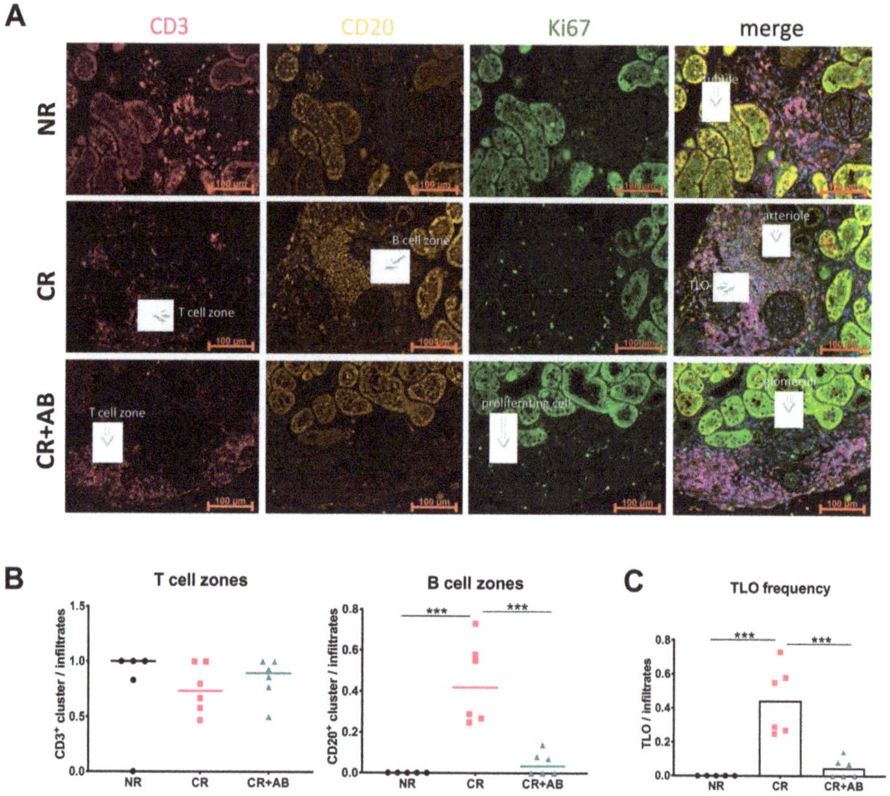


**Figure 2.** Effect of anti-BAFF treatment on intra-renal T and B cell zones and TLO formation. (**A**) shows representative allograft sections stained for CD3 (T cells, pink), CD20 (B cells, yellow), and Ki67 (proliferating cells, green) with distinct T and B cell zones. (**B**) shows the frequency of T cell ($CD3^+$) and B cell ($CD20^+$) zones, which were defined as dense clusters of predominantly one cell type. (**C**) shows the frequency of TLOs, which were defined as dense intra-renal infiltrates containing a T and a B cell zone. NR, no rejection (black); CR, chronic rejection (pink); CR + AB, chronic rejection and anti-BAFF antibody (green). Data is shown as group means and individual data points per rat. Statistical significance is shown as *** $p < 0.001$.

### 2.3. Proliferation of Intra-Renal T and B Cells Was Not Altered by Anti-BAFF Treatment

Since the number of B cells was significantly reduced within kidney allografts by anti-BAFF treatment, we were interested in whether anti-BAFF treatment had affected the local proliferation of intra-renal lymphocytes. We therefore analyzed the absolute numbers of proliferating T and B cells by co-staining for the proliferation marker $Ki67^+$. We found that proliferation of T cells was significantly increased in CR and CR + AB compared to NR (CR vs. NR: 31 ± 11 vs. 3 ± 3, $p = 0.0005$; CR + AB vs. NR: 25 ± 10 vs. 3 ± 3, $p = 0.0034$). In B cells, only CR + AB showed significantly increased proliferation compared to NR, while elevation of B cell proliferation in CR was not significant compared to NR (CR + AB vs. NR: 0.11 ± 0.04 vs. 0 ± 00, $p = 0.02$; CR vs. NR: 0.08 ± 0.03 vs. 0 ± 00, $p = 0.137$). However, anti-BAFF treatment did not change the number of proliferating T cells (Figure 3A) or B cells (Figure 3B).

Antigen-activated B cells may clonally proliferate in germinal centers (GCs) when given appropriate T helper cell signals. We analyzed infiltrates for the presence of GCs within TLOs and found that GCs were rare but could be detected in CR, as shown in Figure 3C.

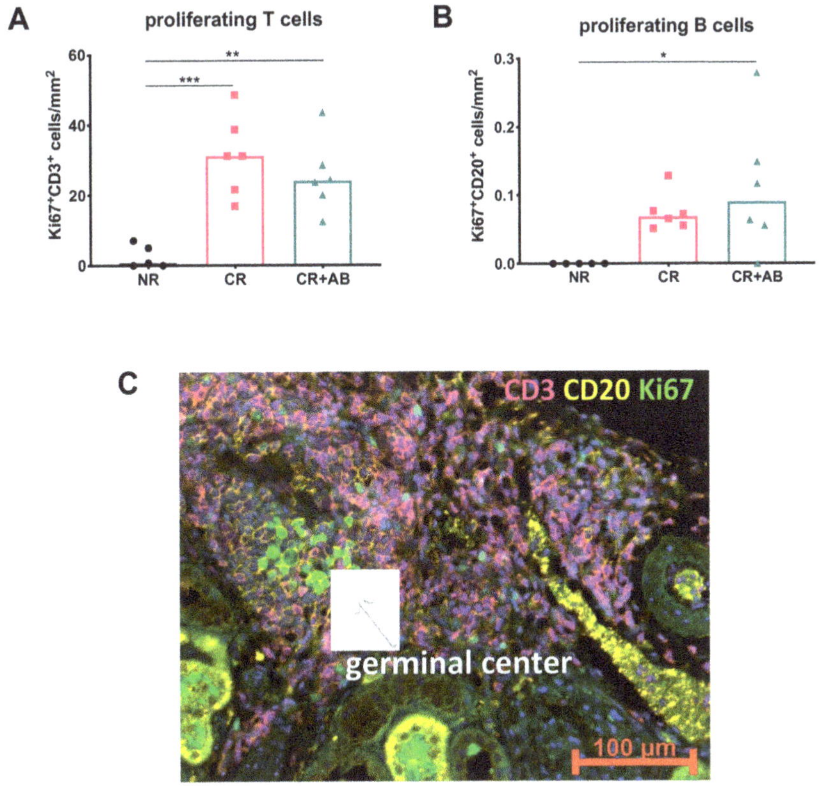


**Figure 3.** Intra-renal T and B cell proliferation and germinal center (GC) formation within TLOs. (**A**) shows the intra-renal content of proliferating Ki67$^+$CD3$^+$ T cells and (**B**) proliferating Ki67$^+$CD20$^+$ B cells, which were quantified using Histoquest software after immunohistochemical staining and normalized to the area of renal cortex. (**C**) shows a TLO with GC formation, which was defined as a dense cluster of Ki67$^+$ proliferating cells (green) within a CD20$^+$ B cell zone (yellow); the kidney section was from the CR group. NR, no rejection (black); CR, chronic rejection (pink); CR + AB, chronic rejection and anti-BAFF antibody (green). Data is shown as group means and individual data points per rat. Statistical significance is shown as * $p < 0.05$, ** $p < 0.01$, and *** $p < 0.001$.

### 2.4. *Effect of Anti-BAFF Treatment on Intra-Renal Plasma Cells*

Plasma cells are antibody-producing cells derived from B cells and have been found within kidney allograft infiltrates [24]. We therefore determined the amount of intra-renal plasma cells by staining for IgG$^+$ elliptical cells, as previously described [23]. Plasma cells were present in allografts from all groups and appeared increased in CR compared to NR and CR + AB, but the difference was not statistically significant (Figure 4).

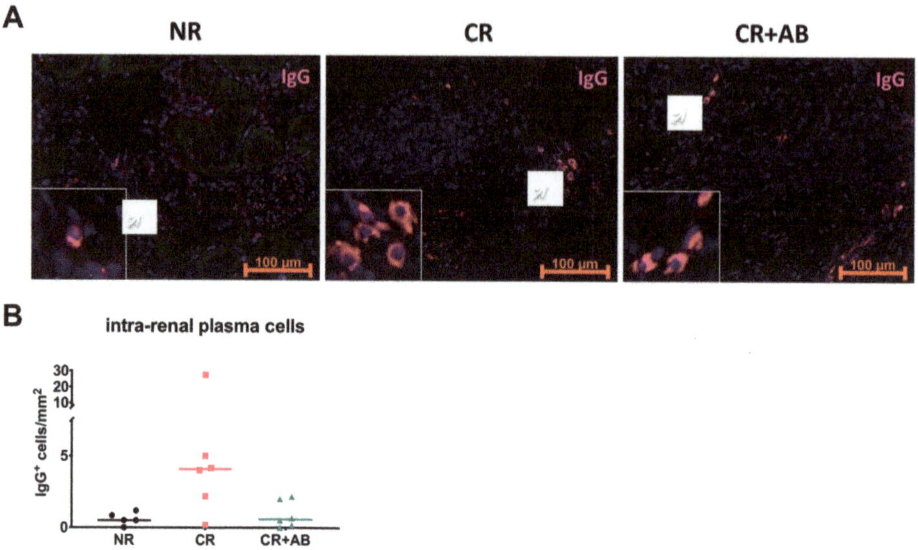


**Figure 4.** Effect of anti-BAFF treatment on intra-renal plasma cells. (**A**) shows immunofluorescence staining of IgG$^+$ plasma cells typically arranged in small nests within allografts. (**B**) shows the intra-renal content of IgG$^+$ plasma cells, which was determined by blinded manual counting of IgG$^+$ cells and normalized to the renal cortex area. NR, no rejection (black); CR, chronic rejection (pink); CR + AB, chronic rejection and anti-BAFF antibody (green). Data is shown as group means and individual data points per rat.

### *2.5. Anti-BAFF Treatment Regulated Expression of TLO-Promoting Factors and B Cell Differentiation Markers within Allografts*

Since BAFF was required for TLO formation, we were interested in the expression of TLO-promoting factors and B cell activation and differentiation molecules. To this end, we used a heat-map to visualize normalized gene expression (Figure 5). We analyzed the intra-renal mRNA expression of BAFF, its homolog APRIL (a proliferation-inducing ligand), and their receptors, BAFF-R (BAFF receptor), TACI (transmembrane activator and calcium modulator and cyclophilin ligand interactor), and BCMA (B cell maturation antigen). We found that BAFF and its receptors were more strongly expressed in CR than NR, but anti-BAFF treatment led to decreased expression of BAFF-R, TACI, and to a lesser degree BCMA (Figure 5A).

TLO formation is driven by lymphoid chemokines and cytokines. We therefore measured intra-renal mRNA expression of the B cell chemokine CXCL13 and its receptor CXCR5, as well as lymphotoxin-β and the T cell chemokine CCL19 and its receptor CCR7. We found that expression of B cell chemokine CXCL13 and its receptors CXCR5, as well as lymphotoxin-β, was elevated in CR but reduced after anti-BAFF, while expression of T cell chemokine CCL19 and its receptor CCR7 was increased in CR + AB (Figure 5B).

We found evidence of germinal center formation in CR, but anti-BAFF treatment did not affect the number of proliferating B cells within allografts. We therefore analyzed the expression of molecules, which drive B cell proliferation. We found that expression of interleukin (IL)-21, an important T cell cytokine, which stimulates B cell proliferation, was elevated in CR + AB compared to CR (Figure 5C). Similarly, the expression of T cell costimulatory molecules, CD40L (CD40 ligand) and ICOS (inducible T cell costimulator), was higher in CR + AB compared to CR, while expression of corresponding B cell ligands CD40 and ICOS ligand was lower in CR + AB compared to CR (Figure 5C).

Finally, BAFF is a survival factor for B cells at different differentiation stages. Therefore, we assessed the intra-renal expression of markers of B cell differentiation. Transmembrane IgD (transmemIgD) is expressed by immature and naïve B cells and its expression was elevated in CR and substantially reduced in CR + AB (Figure 5D). Pax5 (paired box protein 5), a pan-B cell lineage factor, was also elevated in CR and reduced in CR + AB (Figure 5D). Bcl-6 (B cell lymphoma 6) is expressed by germinal center B cells after activation in B cell follicles and was elevated in CR but lower in CR + AB (Figure 5D). Finally, XBP-1 (X-box binding protein 1) is a transcription factor for differentiating plasma cells and its intra-renal expression was elevated in CR compared to NR, and anti-BAFF treatment reduced its expression compared to CR (Figure 5D). Overall, early B cell differentiation markers appeared to be increased in CR and more strongly reduced by anti-BAFF treatment than markers of later differentiation stages (Figure 5D).

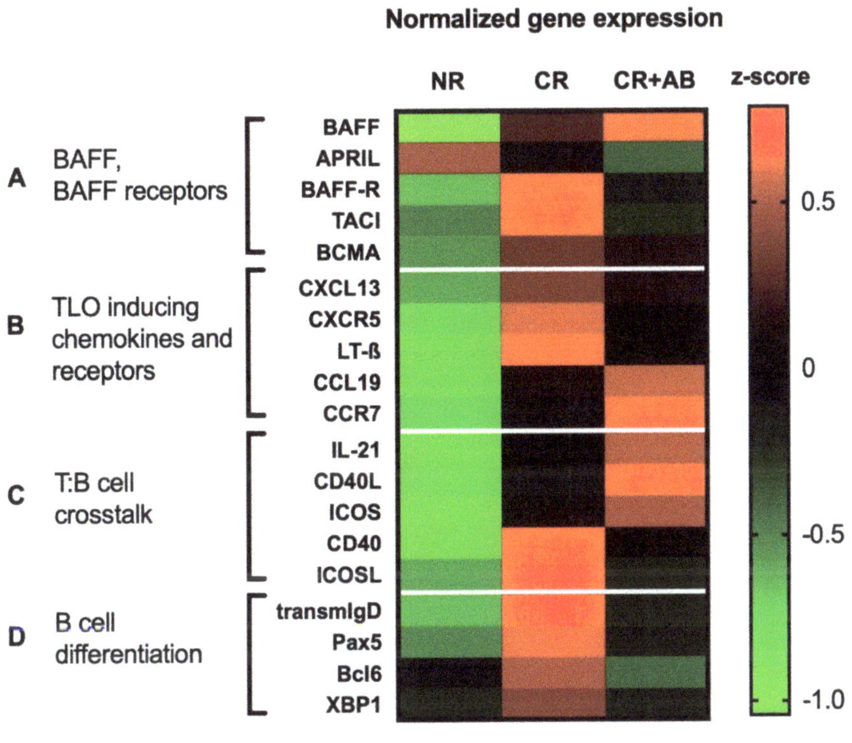


**Figure 5.** Effect of anti-BAFF treatment on intra-renal gene expression in chronic rejection. A heat-map was used to visualize relative mRNA expression of genes between groups. (**A**) BAFF, APRIL, and their receptors; (**B**) TLO-inducing chemokines and cytokines and receptors; (**C**) molecules of T:B cell crosstalk; (**D**) markers of B cell differentiation. MRNA expression of target genes was normalized to the house-keeper hypoxanthine-guanine-phosphoribosyl-transferase (HPRT,). The z-score was calculated from delta CT values per sample using the mean of all samples. Average z-scores from each group are shown using the indicated color scale for up- or downregulation.

Since we saw no significant difference in the amount of T cells present within allografts (Figure 1) or their proliferation rate (Figure 3) with or without anti-BAFF treatment, we analyzed the expression of molecules associated with T cell function by qPCR. We found no difference in the expression of interleukin-2, interferon-$\gamma$, interleukin-21, TGF-$\beta$, granzyme B, perforin, or foxp3 with or without anti-BAFF treatment (data not shown).

## 3. Discussion

TLOs are sites of adaptive alloimmune activation and have been detected in failed kidney allografts with chronic rejection [11]. We tested if BAFF is required for TLO formation in a model of chronic kidney allograft rejection in rats. Our results showed that intra-renal infiltrates were more frequent in chronic rejection than in non-rejecting allografts and included TLOs with distinct T and B cell zones. Furthermore, we observed B cell germinal center formation within TLOs. Anti-BAFF treatment diminished the number of intra-renal B cells and effectively blocked the formation of B cell zones and TLOs. Gene expression analysis showed that intra-renal expression of BAFF receptors and TLO-promoting factors was elevated in CR but diminished by anti-BAFF treatment. We found that B cells in early differentiation stages were particularly sensitive to anti-BAFF treatment. In summary, we showed that TLOs harbor local activation of alloresponses and that BAFF is required for TLO formation in chronic rejection.

In fully immunosuppressed non-rejecting allografts, intra-renal infiltrates were virtually absent; however, there was significant expansion of infiltrates within allografts in chronic rejection. Intra-renal infiltrates were most frequently found in the vicinity of arterioles, suggesting leukopedesis across existing blood vessels, rather than sprouting of high endothelial venules, which have been described in TLOs [14]. Anti-BAFF treatment did not affect the expansion of intra-renal infiltrates; it did, however, lead to a significant reduction in the number of intra-renal B cells and a lower B/T cell ratio.

Detailed analysis of the microanatomical organization of intra-renal T and B cells showed that a large portion of infiltrates consisted of distinct T and B cell zones forming lymphoid follicle-like structures or TLOs. Staining of the proliferation marker Ki67 revealed that germinal centers, or areas of clonal proliferation of antigen-specific B cells, could form within these TLOs in our model. Germinal centers are highly advanced structures, which arise from coordinated T:B cell crosstalk [25]. It is within germinal centers that B cells get fully activated, go through somatic hypermutation, get positively selected for the highest antibody affinity for alloantigens, and differentiate into antibody-secreting plasma cells and memory B cells [26]. Cheng et al. have previously shown that TLOs can harbor such diversification and clonal expansion of alloimmune responses in allografts [16]. Our results showed that anti-BAFF treatment can effectively prevent the formation of intra-renal TLOs, since B cell zones were mostly absent in anti-BAFF-treated rats. Although TLO formation has been observed in cardiac transplant models in mice [27], this is the first kidney transplant model showing TLO formation in chronic rejection. As such, the findings from our study may provide a basis for further investigation into the role of TLOs in kidney transplant rejection.

We were interested in the mechanism by which anti-BAFF treatment prevented TLO formation in allografts. There are three known receptors for BAFF and its homolog APRIL: BAFF-R, TACI, and BCMA, as reviewed by Parsons [28]. We found that the intra-renal expression of BAFF receptors was significantly lower after anti-BAFF treatment, which illustrated the dependency of BAFF receptor-expressing cells on the presence of BAFF as a survival factor. Whether there was a shortage of infiltrating B cells into allografts or intra-renal B cells locally succumbed to cell death in the absence of BAFF could not be determined by our experiments. CXCL13, a B cell chemokine that promotes TLO formation, was highly expressed during chronic rejection, but expression appeared lower after anti-BAFF treatment. The expression of CXCR5, the receptor for CXCL13, was also lower after anti-BAFF treatment. Furthermore, B cells are potent producers of lymphotoxin-β, an important factor for secondary and tertiary lymphoid organ formation [29,30]. The expression of lymphotoxin-β was elevated in chronic rejection but substantially diminished after anti-BAFF antibody. The regulation of these factors may have played in important role in preventing the development of TLO in anti-BAFF-treated rats in our model.

Intra-renal mRNA expression of B cell differentiation markers showed that anti-BAFF treatment strongly affected B cells at early differentiation stages and to a lesser extent reduced expression of advanced differentiation markers. Transmembrane IgD is expressed by immature transitional and naïve B cells. We found elevated transmembrane IgD expression in chronic rejection, reflecting the infiltration of these cells into allografts. Interestingly, expression of intra-renal transmembrane IgD was substantially reduced by anti-BAFF treatment. We also found increased expression of Pax5, a pan-B cell lineage transcription factor, within allografts with chronic rejection but a significant reduction of its expression after anti-BAFF treatment. Interestingly, the transcription factor Bcl-6 was also upregulated during chronic rejection but downregulated by anti-BAFF treatment. Bcl-6 is expressed in lymphoid follicles by germinal center B cells and T follicular helper cells, which provide essential activation signals to B cells, as reviewed by Vinuesa [31]. Bcl-6 is therefore a necessary factor for full activation of humoral alloresponses. Decreased Bcl-6 expression in rats treated with anti-BAFF antibody could reflect decreased humoral immune activation in allografts due to a lack of TLOs. Finally, expression of XBP-1, a transcription factor expressed during plasma cell differentiation [32], was elevated in chronic rejection. XBP-1 expression was also reduced in anti-BAFF, but the difference was much less pronounced compared with factors of early B cell differentiation. We investigated the presence of plasma cells within allografts in our model. Although the exact effector function of intra-renal plasma cells and their role in allograft rejection is not fully understood, intra-renal plasma cells have been associated with chronic allograft rejection and poor prognosis [24,33–36]. Although we have previously shown that anti-BAFF therapy reduced the number of splenic plasma cells [23], the difference in intra-renal plasma cells between groups was not statistically significant in this study. In summary, we found that intra-renal B cells during early differentiation stages were particularly sensitive to anti-BAFF treatment.

Signals required for B cell proliferation include antigen-activation, T cell help, and cytokines, but not BAFF, which was reflected by our data showing that B cell proliferation was not altered by anti-BAFF treatment. Analysis of B cell differentiation factors showed that early antigen-naïve B cells were particularly reduced by anti-BAFF treatment, suggesting that the remaining B cells were already antigen-activated. Proliferation of antigen-activated B cells depends on the expression of important signals by T helper cells, namely CD40L and IL-21. In line with this, we found that the relative expression of CD40L and IL-21 was not decreased by anti-BAFF treatment, demonstrating a potentially important gap in the mechanism of BAFF. This observation may point towards a shortcoming of BAFF-targeted therapy and raise interest in combining targets for therapy.

We demonstrated that TLOs are sites of humoral immune activation within allografts during chronic rejection, and that anti-BAFF treatment can hinder the formation of TLO in allografts. Belimumab®, a monoclonal anti-BAFF antibody, has been approved for treatment of lupus erythematodes and has been explored as an immunosuppressive agent in kidney transplant patients [37]. Our study shows that TLO formation may be prevented using an anti-BAFF antibody with a potential benefit to kidney transplant patients. We previously reported that anti-BAFF treatment interfered with systemic humoral responses and reduced formation of DSA of certain IgG subclasses in a Ktx model, but we found no direct evidence for any specific alteration in T cell function and it did not significantly affect allograft rejection according to Banff or allograft function [23]. A limitation of our study is the duration of our experiment. Extending experiments beyond d56 post-transplant may provide insight into the long-term effects of anti-BAFF treatment on cellular responses within allografts. To assess the long-term benefits of such an intervention, further investigation is needed.

## 4. Materials and Methods

### 4.1. Experimental Kidney Transplantation

Animal experiments were approved by the local inspecting authorities (Regierung von Unterfranken, No. 55.2-2532-2-47, 30-06-2015) and performed according to German animal protection laws and NIH's laboratory animal care principles. In brief, a previously described MHC-mismatched rat kidney transplantation model was used [22,23], in which male Brown Norway rats (BN) served as donors and male Lewis rats (LEW) as recipients (Charles River Laboratories, Sulzfeld, Germany, 200–250 g). Kidney transplantation was performed orthotopically as previously described [38].

Rats were either treated with daily cyclosporine A (CsA) at 10 mg/kg body weight (Neoral, Novartis, Basel, Switzerland), administered once daily by gavage (no rejection group, NR), or they received CsA 5 mg/kg daily until d6, then on every 2nd day to induce DSA and chronic rejection (CR). In addition, one group received CsA 5 mg/kg daily until d6, then on every 2nd day, and in addition a monoclonal anti-BAFF antibody (GSK, Hamburg, Germany) was injected in the peritoneal cavity on d3, d17, d31, and d45 after Ktx (CR + AB), as previously described [23]. Experimental groups are shown in Table 1 below. Rats were sacrificed on d56 after Ktx and allografts were harvested.

**Table 1.** Experimental groups.

| Group | Abbreviation | n= |
|---|---|---|
| Ktx CsA 10 mg/kg/d d56 (no rejection) | NR | 5 |
| Ktx CsA 5 mg/kg/2$^{nd}$ d d56 (chronic rejection) | CR | 6 |
| Ktx CsA 5 mg/kg/2nd d d56 + anti-BAFF antibody (chronic rejection + anti-BAFF antibody) | CR + AB | 6 |

### 4.2. Histology, Immunohistochemistry, and Immunofluorescence

Immunohistochemistry was performed on 3-μm formalin-fixed paraffin-embedded sections as previously described [39]. T cells were stained with rabbit anti-rat CD3 antibody (Abcam, ab5690, Cambridge, UK) and donkey anti-rabbit-Cy5 (Dianova, 711-175-152, Hamburg, Germany). B cells were stained with mouse anti-rat CD20 antibody (Santa Cruz, sc-393894, Heidelberg, Germany), goat anti-mouse-biotin (Thermofisher 31804), and Strep-Cy3 (Dianova, 016-160-084, Hamburg, Germany). Proliferation was stained using anti-Ki67-FITC (ebioscience, 11-5698), and plasma cells were stained using anti-rat-IgG-AlexaFluor647 (Thermofischer A21472, Waltham, MA, USA). Images were taken using a Zeiss observer Z.1 Fluorescence microscope at 20× magnification. Digital images from 10 high power fields (HPFs) per specimen were examined as previously described [39]. Using Histoquest® software (TissueGnostics GmbH, Vienna, Austria), the number of $CD20^+$, $CD3^+$, $Ki67^+CD20^+$, and $Ki67^+CD3^+$ cells were quantified within a defined section area. Intra-renal B cell ($CD20^+$) and T cell ($CD3^+$) zones were defined as dense clusters of predominantly one cell type (min. 20 cells/0.004 $mm^2$). TLO were defined as dense intra-renal infiltrates containing a T and B cell zone. Germinal centers (GCs) were defined as dense clusters of $Ki67^+$ proliferating cells within a B cell zone. The presence of T and B cell zones and GC was determined per infiltrate in a blinded manner. Intra-renal $IgG^+$ plasma cells, identified by strong intracellular IgG-positivity and typical cell shape, were counted manually in a blinded manner.

### 4.3. Real-Time PCR

Frozen tissue sections were homogenized using a RNeasy MiniKit® (cat. 74106, Qiagen, Hilden, Germany). Total RNA was extracted, and genomic DNA digested. Total RNA was reverse transcribed into cDNA. RT-PCR was performed on a ViiA7 detection system (Applied Biosystems, Darmstadt, Germany) using a QuantiTect SYBR Green PCR Kit (Qiagen, Hilden, Germany). The sequences of the primers are listed in Table S1). Copy numbers of target genes were normalized to the house-keeper gene hypoxanthine-guanine-phosphoribosyl-transferase (HPRT) and delta CT values were calculated. The z-score was calculated from delta CT values for each sample and target gene using the formula $z = (\chi-\mu)/\sigma$. Mean z-scores from each experimental group are shown in a heat map using a color scale for up- or downregulation of gene expression.

### 4.4. Statistical Analysis

Values are provided as individual data points and mean and SD. Statistical significance was calculated using Graphpad Prism software (Version 8.0, San Diego, CA, USA) using ANOVA; $p < 0.05$ was considered to be statistically significant.

**Supplementary Materials:** The following are available online at http://www.mdpi.com/1422-0067/21/21/8045/s1. Table S1: Primer sequences.

**Author Contributions:** L.S. designed experiments, performed data analysis and interpretation and prepared the manuscript. H.P. performed rat operations and treatments. M.H. analyzed intra-renal cell proliferation. A.S. assisted in data analysis and reviewed the manuscript. B.B. contributed to data interpretation and reviewed the manuscript. T.B. designed experiments, interpreted data and reviewed the manuscript. All authors have read and agreed to the published version of the manuscript.

**Funding:** This work was funded by the Deutsche Forschungsgemeinschaft (DFG, German Research Foundation), project number 387509280, SFB 1350 Project B6 to BT and BB. Anti-BAFF AB was provided by donation of GSK, Hamburg, Germany.

**Acknowledgments:** We thank Stefanie Ellmann and Alexandra Müller for their technical support.

**Conflicts of Interest:** The authors declare no conflict of interest. The funders had no role in the design of the study; in the collection, analyses, or interpretation of data; in the writing of the manuscript, or in the decision to publish the results.

## Abbreviations

| | |
|---|---|
| AB | antibody |
| ABMR | antibody-mediated rejection |
| APRIL | a proliferation inducing ligand |
| BAFF | B cell activating factor |
| BAFF-R | BAFF receptor |
| Bcl-6 | B cell lymphoma 6 |
| BCMA | B cell maturation antigen |
| BN | Brown Norway rat |
| CD | cluster of differentiation |
| CD40L | CD40 ligand |
| CR | chronic rejection |
| CR + AB | chronic rejection + anti-BAFF antibody |
| CsA | cyclosporine A |
| HPRT | hypoxanthine-guanine-phosphoribosyl-transferase |
| GC | germinal center |
| ICOS | inducible T cell costimulator |
| ICOSL | ICOS ligand |
| IFTA | interstitial fibrosis and tubular atrophy |
| Ig | immunoglobulin |
| IL | interleukin |
| Ktx | kidney transplantation |
| LEW | Lewis rat |
| MHC | major histocompatibility complex |
| NR | no rejection |
| Pax5 | paired box protein 5 |
| SLE | systemic lupus erythematosus |
| TACI | transmembrane activator and calcium modulator and cyclophilin ligand interactor |
| TLO | tertiary lymphoid organs |
| XBP-1 | X-box binding protein 1 |

## References

1. Gondos, A.; Dohler, B.; Brenner, H.; Opelz, G. Kidney graft survival in Europe and the United States: Strikingly different long-term outcomes. *Transplantation* **2013**, *95*, 267–274. [CrossRef] [PubMed]
2. Lefaucheur, C.; Loupy, A.; Hill, G.S.; Andrade, J.; Nochy, D.; Antoine, C.; Gautreau, C.; Charron, D.; Glotz, D.; Suberbielle-Boissel, C. Preexisting donor-specific HLA antibodies predict outcome in kidney transplantation. *J. Am. Soc. Nephrol.* **2010**, *21*, 1398–1406. [CrossRef] [PubMed]

3. Sellares, J.; Reeve, J.; Loupy, A.; Mengel, M.; Sis, B.; Skene, A.; de Freitas, D.G.; Kreepala, C.; Hidalgo, L.G.; Famulski, K.S.; et al. Molecular diagnosis of antibody-mediated rejection in human kidney transplants. *Am. J. Transplant.* **2013**, *13*, 971–983. [CrossRef] [PubMed]
4. Mannon, R.B.; Matas, A.J.; Grande, J.; Leduc, R.; Connett, J.; Kasiske, B.; Cecka, J.M.; Gaston, R.S.; Cosio, F.; Gourishankar, S.; et al. Inflammation in areas of tubular atrophy in kidney allograft biopsies: A potent predictor of allograft failure. *Am. J. Transplant.* **2010**, *10*, 2066–2073. [CrossRef] [PubMed]
5. Shishido, S.; Asanuma, H.; Nakai, H.; Mori, Y.; Satoh, H.; Kamimaki, I.; Hataya, H.; Ikeda, M.; Honda, M.; Hasegawa, A. The impact of repeated subclinical acute rejection on the progression of chronic allograft nephropathy. *J. Am. Soc. Nephrol.* **2003**, *14*, 1046–1052. [CrossRef] [PubMed]
6. Park, W.D.; Griffin, M.D.; Cornell, L.D.; Cosio, F.G.; Stegall, M.D. Fibrosis with inflammation at one year predicts transplant functional decline. *J. Am. Soc. Nephrol.* **2010**, *21*, 1987–1997. [CrossRef]
7. Tse, G.H.; Johnston, C.J.; Kluth, D.; Gray, M.; Gray, D.; Hughes, J.; Marson, L.P. Intrarenal B Cell Cytokines Promote Transplant Fibrosis and Tubular Atrophy. *Am. J. Transplant.* **2015**, *15*, 3067–3080. [CrossRef]
8. Sarwal, M.; Chua, M.S.; Kambham, N.; Hsieh, S.C.; Satterwhite, T.; Masek, M.; Salvatierra, O., Jr. Molecular heterogeneity in acute renal allograft rejection identified by DNA microarray profiling. *N. Engl. J. Med.* **2003**, *349*, 125–138. [CrossRef]
9. Hueso, M.; Navarro, E.; Moreso, F.; O'Valle, F.; Perez-Riba, M.; Del Moral, R.G.; Grinyo, J.M.; Seron, D. Intragraft expression of the IL-10 gene is up-regulated in renal protocol biopsies with early interstitial fibrosis, tubular atrophy, and subclinical rejection. *Am. J. Pathol.* **2010**, *176*, 1696–1704. [CrossRef]
10. Thaunat, O.; Field, A.C.; Dai, J.; Louedec, L.; Patey, N.; Bloch, M.F.; Mandet, C.; Belair, M.F.; Bruneval, P.; Meilhac, O.; et al. Lymphoid neogenesis in chronic rejection: Evidence for a local humoral alloimmune response. *Proc. Natl. Acad. Sci. USA* **2005**, *102*, 14723–14728. [CrossRef]
11. Thaunat, O.; Patey, N.; Caligiuri, G.; Gautreau, C.; Mamani-Matsuda, M.; Mekki, Y.; Dieu-Nosjean, M.C.; Eberl, G.; Ecochard, R.; Michel, J.B.; et al. Chronic rejection triggers the development of an aggressive intragraft immune response through recapitulation of lymphoid organogenesis. *J. Immunol.* **2010**, *185*, 717–728. [CrossRef] [PubMed]
12. Thaunat, O.; Graff-Dubois, S.; Brouard, S.; Gautreau, C.; Varthaman, A.; Fabien, N.; Field, A.C.; Louedec, L.; Dai, J.; Joly, E.; et al. Immune responses elicited in tertiary lymphoid tissues display distinctive features. *PLoS ONE* **2010**, *5*, e11398. [CrossRef]
13. Pitzalis, C.; Jones, G.W.; Bombardieri, M.; Jones, S.A. Ectopic lymphoid-like structures in infection, cancer and autoimmunity. *Nat. Rev. Immunol.* **2014**, *14*, 447–462. [CrossRef] [PubMed]
14. Luther, S.A.; Bidgol, A.; Hargreaves, D.C.; Schmidt, A.; Xu, Y.; Paniyadi, J.; Matloubian, M.; Cyster, J.G. Differing activities of homeostatic chemokines CCL19, CCL21, and CXCL12 in lymphocyte and dendritic cell recruitment and lymphoid neogenesis. *J. Immunol.* **2002**, *169*, 424–433. [CrossRef] [PubMed]
15. Ziegler, E.; Gueler, F.; Rong, S.; Mengel, M.; Witzke, O.; Kribben, A.; Haller, H.; Kunzendorf, U.; Krautwald, S. CCL19-IgG prevents allograft rejection by impairment of immune cell trafficking. *J. Am. Soc. Nephrol.* **2006**, *17*, 2521–2532. [CrossRef]
16. Cheng, J.; Torkamani, A.; Grover, R.K.; Jones, T.M.; Ruiz, D.I.; Schork, N.J.; Quigley, M.M.; Hall, F.W.; Salomon, D.R.; Lerner, R.A. Ectopic B-cell clusters that infiltrate transplanted human kidneys are clonal. *Proc. Natl. Acad. Sci. USA* **2011**, *108*, 5560–5565. [CrossRef] [PubMed]
17. Koenig, A.; Thaunat, O. Lymphoid Neogenesis and Tertiary Lymphoid Organs in Transplanted Organs. *Front. Immunol.* **2016**, *7*, 646. [CrossRef]
18. Thaunat, O.; Patey, N.; Gautreau, C.; Lechaton, S.; Fremeaux-Bacchi, V.; Dieu-Nosjean, M.C.; Cassuto-Viguier, E.; Legendre, C.; Delahousse, M.; Lang, P.; et al. B cell survival in intragraft tertiary lymphoid organs after rituximab therapy. *Transplantation* **2008**, *85*, 1648–1653. [CrossRef]
19. Mackay, F.; Figgett, W.A.; Saulep, D.; Lepage, M.; Hibbs, M.L. B-cell stage and context-dependent requirements for survival signals from BAFF and the B-cell receptor. *Immunol. Rev.* **2010**, *237*, 205–225. [CrossRef]
20. Irure-Ventura, J.; San Segundo, D.; Rodrigo, E.; Merino, D.; Belmar-Vega, L.; Ruiz San Millán, J.C.; Valero, R.; Benito, A.; López-Hoyos, M. High Pretransplant BAFF Levels and B-cell Subset Polarized towards a Memory Phenotype as Predictive Biomarkers for Antibody-Mediated Rejection. *Int. J. Mol. Sci.* **2020**, *21*, 779. [CrossRef]

21. Friebus-Kardash, J.; Wilde, B.; Keles, D.; Heinold, A.; Kribben, A.; Witzke, O.; Heinemann, F.M.; Eisenberger, U. Pretransplant serum BAFF levels are associated with pretransplant HLA immunization and renal allograft survival. *Transpl. Immunol.* **2018**, *47*, 10–17. [CrossRef] [PubMed]
22. Kuhne, L.; Jung, B.; Poth, H.; Schuster, A.; Wurm, S.; Ruemmele, P.; Banas, B.; Bergler, T. Renal allograft rejection, lymphocyte infiltration, and de novo donor-specific antibodies in a novel model of non-adherence to immunosuppressive therapy. *BMC Immunol.* **2017**, *18*, 52. [CrossRef] [PubMed]
23. Steines, L.; Poth, H.; Schuster, A.; Geissler, E.K.; Amann, K.; Banas, B.; Bergler, T. Anti-BAFF Treatment Interferes With Humoral Responses in a Model of Renal Transplantation in Rats. *Transplantation* **2020**, *104*, e16–e22. [CrossRef] [PubMed]
24. Hasegawa, J.; Honda, K.; Omoto, K.; Wakai, S.; Shirakawa, H.; Okumi, M.; Ishida, H.; Fuchinoue, S.; Hattori, M.; Tanabe, K. Clinical and Pathological Features of Plasma Cell-Rich Acute Rejection After Kidney Transplantation. *Transplantation* **2018**, *102*, 853–859. [CrossRef] [PubMed]
25. Kwun, J.; Manook, M.; Page, E.; Burghuber, C.; Hong, J.; Knechtle, S.J. Crosstalk Between T and B Cells in the Germinal Center After Transplantation. *Transplantation* **2017**, *101*, 704–712. [CrossRef]
26. Krautler, N.J.; Suan, D.; Butt, D.; Bourne, K.; Hermes, J.R.; Chan, T.D.; Sundling, C.; Kaplan, W.; Schofield, P.; Jackson, J.; et al. Differentiation of germinal center B cells into plasma cells is initiated by high-affinity antigen and completed by Tfh cells. *J. Exp. Med.* **2017**, *214*, 1259–1267. [CrossRef]
27. Baddoura, F.K.; Nasr, I.W.; Wrobel, B.; Li, Q.; Ruddle, N.H.; Lakkis, F.G. Lymphoid neogenesis in murine cardiac allografts undergoing chronic rejection. *Am. J. Transplant.* **2005**, *5*, 510–516. [CrossRef]
28. Parsons, R.F.; Vivek, K.; Redfield, R.R.; 3rd Migone, T.S.; Cancro, M.P.; Naji, A.; Noorchashm, H. B-lymphocyte homeostasis and BLyS-directed immunotherapy in transplantation. *Transplant. Rev.* **2010**, *24*, 207–221. [CrossRef]
29. Ngo, V.N.; Korner, H.; Gunn, M.D.; Schmidt, K.N.; Riminton, D.S.; Cooper, M.D.; Browning, J.L.; Sedgwick, J.D.; Cyster, J.G. Lymphotoxin alpha/beta and tumor necrosis factor are required for stromal cell expression of homing chemokines in B and T cell areas of the spleen. *J. Exp. Med.* **1999**, *189*, 403–412. [CrossRef]
30. Grabner, R.; Lotzer, K.; Dopping, S.; Hildner, M.; Radke, D.; Beer, M.; Spanbroek, R.; Lippert, B.; Reardon, C.A.; Getz, G.S.; et al. Lymphotoxin beta receptor signaling promotes tertiary lymphoid organogenesis in the aorta adventitia of aged ApoE-/- mice. *J. Exp. Med.* **2009**, *206*, 233–248. [CrossRef]
31. Vinuesa, C.G.; Linterman, M.A.; Yu, D.; MacLennan, I.C. Follicular Helper T Cells. *Annu. Rev. Immunol.* **2016**, *34*, 335–368. [CrossRef] [PubMed]
32. Reimold, A.M.; Iwakoshi, N.N.; Manis, J.; Vallabhajosyula, P.; Szomolanyi-Tsuda, E.; Gravallese, E.M.; Friend, D.; Grusby, M.J.; Alt, F.; Glimcher, L.H. Plasma cell differentiation requires the transcription factor XBP-1. *Nature* **2001**, *412*, 300–307. [CrossRef] [PubMed]
33. Wehner, J.R.; Fox-Talbot, K.; Halushka, M.K.; Ellis, C.; Zachary, A.A.; Baldwin, W.M., 3rd. B cells and plasma cells in coronaries of chronically rejected cardiac transplants. *Transplantation* **2010**, *89*, 1141–1148. [CrossRef] [PubMed]
34. Einecke, G.; Reeve, J.; Mengel, M.; Sis, B.; Bunnag, S.; Mueller, T.F.; Halloran, P.F. Expression of B cell and immunoglobulin transcripts is a feature of inflammation in late allografts. *Am. J. Transplant.* **2008**, *8*, 1434–1443. [CrossRef] [PubMed]
35. Desvaux, D.; Le Gouvello, S.; Pastural, M.; Abtahi, M.; Suberbielle, C.; Boeri, N.; Rémy, P.; Salomon, L.; Lang, P.; Baron, C. Acute renal allograft rejections with major interstitial oedema and plasma cell-rich infiltrates: High gamma-interferon expression and poor clinical outcome. *Nephrol. Dial. Transplant.* **2004**, *19*, 933–939. [CrossRef]
36. Hamada, A.M.; Yamamoto, I.; Kawabe, M.; Katsumata, H.; Yamakawa, T.; Katsuma, A.; Nakada, Y.; Kobayashi, A.; Koike, Y.; Miki, J.; et al. Clinicopathological features and outcomes of kidney allografts in plasma cell-rich acute rejection: A case series. *Nephrology* **2018**, *23*, 22–26. [CrossRef]
37. Banham, G.D.; Flint, S.M.; Torpey, N.; Lyons, P.A.; Shanahan, D.N.; Gibson, A.; Watson CJ, E.; O'Sullivan, A.M.; Chadwick, J.A.; Foster, K.E.; et al. Belimumab in kidney transplantation: An experimental medicine, randomised, placebo-controlled phase 2 trial. *Lancet* **2018**, *391*, 2619–2630. [CrossRef]
38. Bergler, T.; Hoffmann, U.; Bergler, E.; Jung, B.; Banas, M.C.; Reinhold, S.W.; Kramer, B.K.; Banas, B. Toll-like receptor 4 in experimental kidney transplantation: Early mediator of endogenous danger signals. *Nephron Exp. Nephrol.* **2012**, *121*, e59–e70. [CrossRef]

39. Hoffmann, U.; Bergler, T.; Jung, B.; Steege, A.; Pace, C.; Rummele, P.; Reinhold, S.; Kruger, B.; Kramer, B.K.; Banas, B. Comprehensive morphometric analysis of mononuclear cell infiltration during experimental renal allograft rejection. *Transpl. Immunol.* **2013**, *28*, 24–31. [CrossRef]

International Journal of
*Molecular Sciences*

MDPI

*Article*

# The Crucial Role of Xanthine Oxidase in CKD Progression Associated with Hypercholesterolemia

**You-Jin Kim [1,2], Se-Hyun Oh [1,2], Ji-Sun Ahn [1], Ju-Min Yook [1], Chan-Duck Kim [1,3], Sun-Hee Park [1,3], Jang-Hee Cho [1,3,*] and Yong-Lim Kim [1,2,3,*]**

1 Division of Nephrology, Kyungpook National University Hospital, Daegu 41944, Korea; pinkqic1004@naver.com (Y.-J.K.); ttily@nate.com (S.-H.O.); ggumsuni@hanmail.net (J.-S.A.); jumin18@hanmail.net (J.-M.Y.); drcdkim@mail.knu.ac.kr (C.-D.K.); sh-park@knu.ac.kr (S.-H.P.)
2 Cell and Matrix Research Institute, Kyungpook National University, Daegu 41944, Korea
3 Department of Internal Medicine, School of Medicine, Kyungpook National University, Daegu 41944, Korea
* Correspondence: jh-cho@knu.ac.kr (J.-H.C.); ylkim@knu.ac.kr (Y.-L.K.); Tel.: +82-10-6566-7551(J.-H.C.); +82-53-420-5553 (Y.-L.K.); Fax: +82-53-426-2046 (J.-H.C.); +82-53-423-7583 (Y.-L.K.)

Received: 28 August 2020; Accepted: 7 October 2020; Published: 9 October 2020

check for updates

**Abstract:** In the present study, we investigated the effects of xanthine oxidase (XO) inhibition on cholesterol-induced renal dysfunction in chronic kidney disease (CKD) mice, and in low-density lipoprotein (LDL)-treated human kidney proximal tubule epithelial (HK-2) cells. ApoE knockout (KO) mice underwent uninephrectomy to induce CKD, and were fed a normal diet or high-cholesterol (HC) diet along with the XO inhibitor topiroxostat (1 mg/kg/day). HK-2 cells were treated with LDL (200 μg/mL) and topiroxostat (5 μM) or small interfering RNA against xanthine dehydrogenase (siXDH; 20 nM). In uninephrectomized ApoE KO mice, the HC diet increased cholesterol accumulation, oxidative stress, XO activity, and kidney damage, while topiroxostat attenuated the hypercholesterolemia-associated renal dysfunction. The HC diet induced cholesterol accumulation by regulating the expressions of genes involved in cholesterol efflux (*Nr1h3* and *Abca1*) and synthesis (*Srebf2* and *Hmgcr*), which was reversed by topiroxostat. Topiroxostat suppressed the expressions of genes related to hypercholesterolemia-associated inflammation and fibrosis in the unilateral kidney. LDL stimulation evoked changes in the cholesterol metabolism, nicotinamide adenine dinucleotide phosphate (NADPH) oxidase, and NF-κB pathways in HK-2 cells, which were mitigated by XO inhibition with topiroxostat or siXDH. These findings suggest that XO inhibition exerts renoprotective effects against hypercholesterolemia-associated kidney injury. XO could be a novel therapeutic target for hypercholesterolemia-associated kidney injury in uninephrectomized patients.

**Keywords:** chronic kidney disease; hypercholesterolemia; xanthine oxidase; inflammation; fibrosis; NF-κB pathway

## 1. Introduction

Compared to people with normal cholesterol levels, those with high cholesterol levels are 1.5 times more likely to develop kidney dysfunction [1,2]. Individuals with metabolic syndrome who serve as kidney donors reportedly show a higher incidence of post-donation kidney disease due to dyslipidemia and obesity compared to normal donors [3,4]. These findings suggest that abnormal cholesterol metabolism independently increases the risk of chronic kidney disease.

Dyslipidemia may directly affect the kidney by causing deleterious renal lipid disturbances, and indirectly affect the kidney through systemic inflammation, oxidative stress and vascular injury [5,6]. We previously reported that high concentrations of uric acid synthesis metabolites lead to the generation of reactive oxygen species (ROS), which promotes hypercholesterolemia with cholesterol accumulation in hepatocytes and incites atherosclerosis in apolipoprotein E (ApoE)-deficient mice [7]. However, the effects of cholesterol on the kidneys have not been confirmed.

In a unilateral kidney, a high-fat diet alters the expressions of genes involved in the cytoskeletal remodeling, fibrosis, and oxidative stress pathways. This suggests that the high-fat diet has synergistic effects that promote gene expression changes related to kidney damage [8]. Additionally, in animal experiments, unilateral kidney dyslipidemia is associated with the exacerbation of kidney damage, characterized by decreased kidney function, vasodilation, fibrosis, oxidative stress, and ER stress, despite normal body weight [9]. These findings suggest that kidney lipid accumulation and lipid toxicity play important roles in the pathogenesis of kidney damage, and are associated with a higher risk of kidney damage in unilateral kidneys.

It has been postulated that oxidative stress—derived from nicotinamide adenine dinucleotide phosphate (NADPH) oxidase, mitochondrial oxidase, and xanthine oxidase (XO)—is involved in renal lipid disturbances [10]. Notably, high cholesterol levels activate XO and lead to excessive ROS formation, resulting in tissue damage, such as inflammation and atherosclerosis [11,12]. Consistently, XO inhibitors exhibit pronounced protective effects against vascular injuries, inflammatory diseases, and tissue damage [13,14]. XO inhibitors can also inhibit the expression of pro-inflammatory proteins. Therefore, XO inhibitors have potential for use as therapeutic drugs that reduce oxidative stress [15]. However, the XO inhibitor allopurinol does not inhibit renal dysfunction in patients with chronic kidney disease (CKD) and high risk of progression [16].Thus, the effect of XO inhibitors in terms of kidney protection remains controversial.

In the present study, we investigated the correlation between cell injury and non-oxidized LDL-induced ROS in vitro, as well as the effects of a high-cholesterol (HC) diet and hypercholesterolemia on lipid accumulation and renal tubule damage in vivo using a unilateral kidney model. We further aimed to identify potential signaling pathways that could be affected by lipid accumulation-induced xanthine oxidase and ROS under a CKD associated with hypercholesterolemia.

## 2. Results

### 2.1. Hypercholesterolemia Aggravates Renal Function Through Increased Kidney Lipid Accumulation, Xanthine Oxidase Activity, and Oxidative Stress

PAS staining confirmed that the high-cholesterol (HC) diet led to renal tubular damage in the unilateral kidney (Figure 1A). The HC diet yielded increased serum blood urea nitrogen (BUN) and creatinine, which were highest with HC+uninephrectomy (UN) group (Figure 1B,C). The XO inhibitor topiroxostat (TP) attenuated this kidney dysfunction (Figure 1A–C). Kidney weight was increased in uninephrectomized mice, whereas reduced by TP treatment (Figure 1D). In both sham-operated and UN mice, HC diet yielded increased serum total cholesterol (TC), low-density lipoprotein (LDL), and triglycerides (TG), and TP treatment restored these levels (Figure 1E–G).

Compared to normal control (NC), HC and HC+UN yielded increased lipid droplets in the kidney, showing higher levels with HC+UN versus HC (Figure 1H). Kidney TC was higher with HC and HC+UN versus NC, and was reduced by TP in the HC+UN+TP group (Figure 1I). Free cholesterol did not differ among groups. HC and HC+UN showed trends of increased kidney cholesterol esters (Figure 1J,K). TP decreased kidney cholesterol accumulation, consistent with decreased serum TC, LDL, and TG. The HC diet significantly elevated XO activity, dichlorodihydrofluorescein diacetate (DCFDA), and $H_2O_2$ excretion in kidney tissue, which were higher with HC+UN versus HC. TP decreased the increased XO activity and intracellular oxidative stress markers (Figure 1L–N).

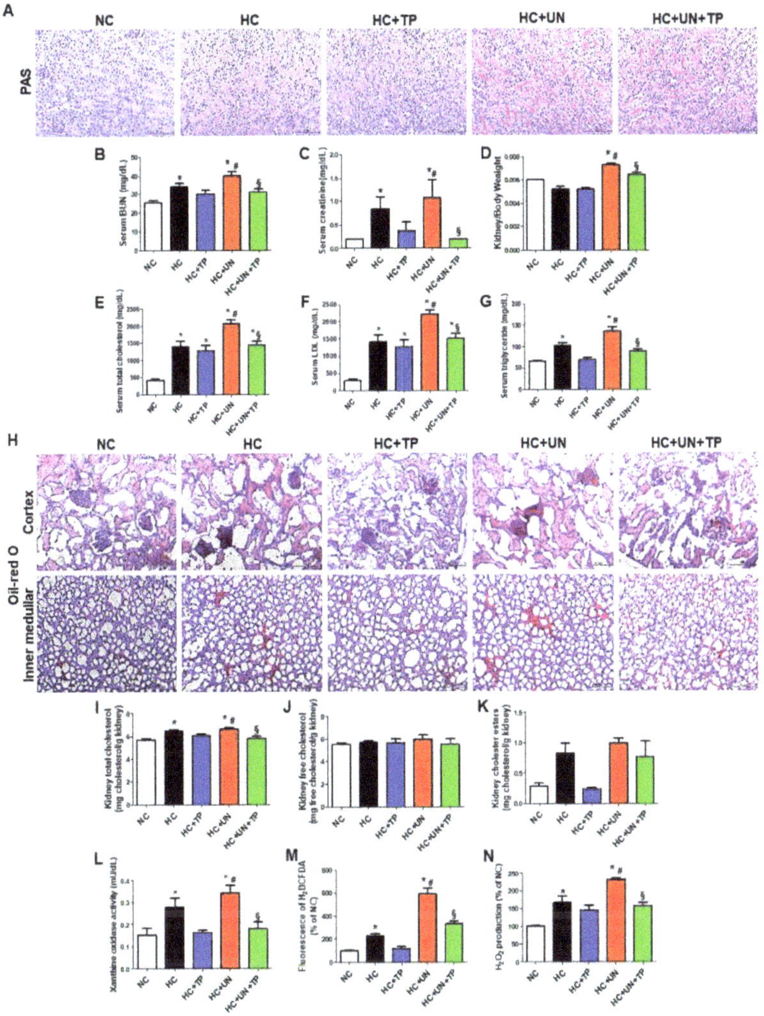


**Figure 1.** The effects of xanthine oxidase inhibition on high-cholesterol diet-induced cholesterol accumulation, oxidative stress, and damage in the kidney. (**A**) Representative images of periodic acid Schiff (PAS) staining of kidney tissue. Scale bars, 100 µm. (**B–D**) Levels of blood kidney injury factors (BUN and creatinine) and kidney/body weight in mice from different groups. (**E–G**) Serum cholesterol levels in mice from different groups. (**H**) Representative images of Oil red O staining of kidney tissue (upper: cortex, lower: inner-medullar). Scale bars, 100 µm. (**I–K**) Total cholesterol, free cholesterol, and cholesterol ester levels in the kidney. (**L–N**) Xanthine oxidase activity, DCFDA, and $H_2O_2$ production in kidney tissue. Differences among the groups were analyzed by a one-way non-parametric ANOVA, followed by Tukey's multiple comparison test. Data represent mean and SEM. * $p < 0.05$ vs. NC, # $p < 0.05$ vs. HC, § $p < 0.05$ vs. HC+UN. TP, topiroxostat; UN, uninephrectomy; NC, normal control; HC, high-cholesterol.

### 2.2. *Effects of Hypercholesterolemia on Genes Related to Cellular Cholesterol Transport and Synthesis in the Unilateral Kidney*

Compared to NC, the HC diet groups exhibited increased mRNA expression of genes related to cholesterol efflux (*Nr1h3* and *Abca1*), LDL and modified LDL uptake (*Ldlr*, *Msr1*, and *Scarb1*),

TG synthesis (*Srebf1*), and cholesterol synthesis (*Srebf2* and *Hmgcr*) (Figure 2A–I). HC+UN yielded decreased *Nr1h3* and *Abca1* (Figure 2A,B), increased *Msr1* and *Scarb1*, and decreased *Ldlr* expression (Figure 2C–E). *Lcat* expression was increased with the HC diet versus normal diet but did not differ between HC and HC+UN (Figure 2F). HC+UN yielded increased *Srebf1*, *Srebf2*, and *Hmgcr* expression (Figure 2G–I). TP treatment (HC+UN+TP) increased *Nr1h3* and *Abca1* expression, and decreased *Srebf1*, *Srebf2*, and *Hmgcr* expression (Figure 2A,B,G–I). The HC diet led to increased ABCA1 and HMGCR protein levels, which were higher with HC+UN versus HC. LXRα protein levels were not altered by HC diet (Figure 2J–L). Overall, TP treatment yielded increased cholesterol efflux gene expression and reduced cholesterol synthesis gene expression (Figure 2).

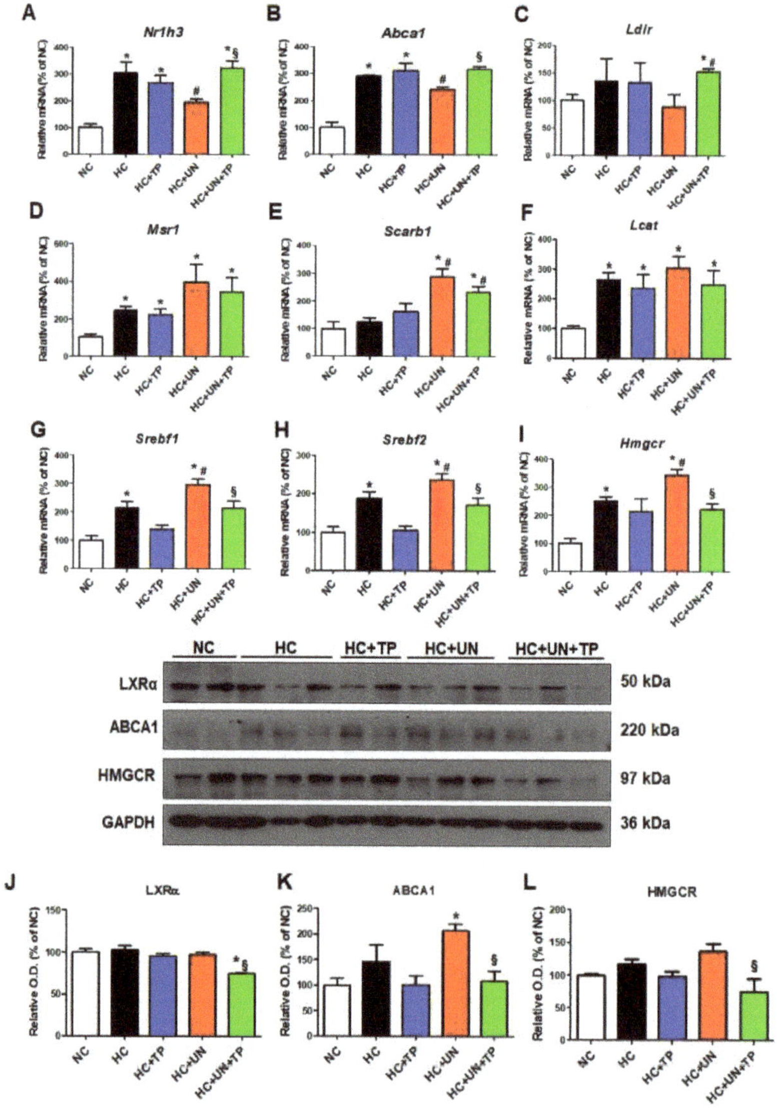


**Figure 2.** TP decreased cholesterol accumulation in the kidney through regulation of genes involved in cholesterol transport and synthesis. Real-time RT-PCR was performed to determine the expression

levels of genes involved in cholesterol efflux (**A**,**B**), LDL receptor (**C**), modified LDL influx transport (**D**,**E**), cholesterol esterase (**F**), triglyceride synthesis (**G**), and cholesterol synthesis (**H**,**I**). (**J**–**L**) Representative western blot for LXRα, ABCA1, HMGCR, and GAPDH. Relative protein expression was determined using densitometry. Differences among the groups were analyzed by one-way non-parametric ANOVA, followed by Tukey's multiple comparison test. Data represent mean and SEM. * $p < 0.05$ vs. NC, # $p < 0.05$ vs. HC, § $p < 0.05$ vs. HC+UN. LDL, low-density lipoprotein; TP, topiroxostat; UN, uninephrectomy; NC, normal control; HC, high-cholesterol.

### 2.3. Effects of LDL on Cholesterol Metabolism and Oxidative Stress in HK-2 Cells

LDL increased *NR1H3*, *ABCA1*, and *HMGCR* expression in human kidney proximal tubule epithelial (HK-2) cells, without affecting *LDLR*, *SREBF1*, or *SREBF2*. TP decreased only *HMGCR* expression (Figure 3A–F). LDL increased intracellular ROS over the basal level, which peaked at 30 min (Figure 3G), with elevated $H_2O_2$ level and ROS-dependent DCF fluorescence intensity. TP reduced cellular ROS, similar to the positive control NAC (Figure 3H–I).

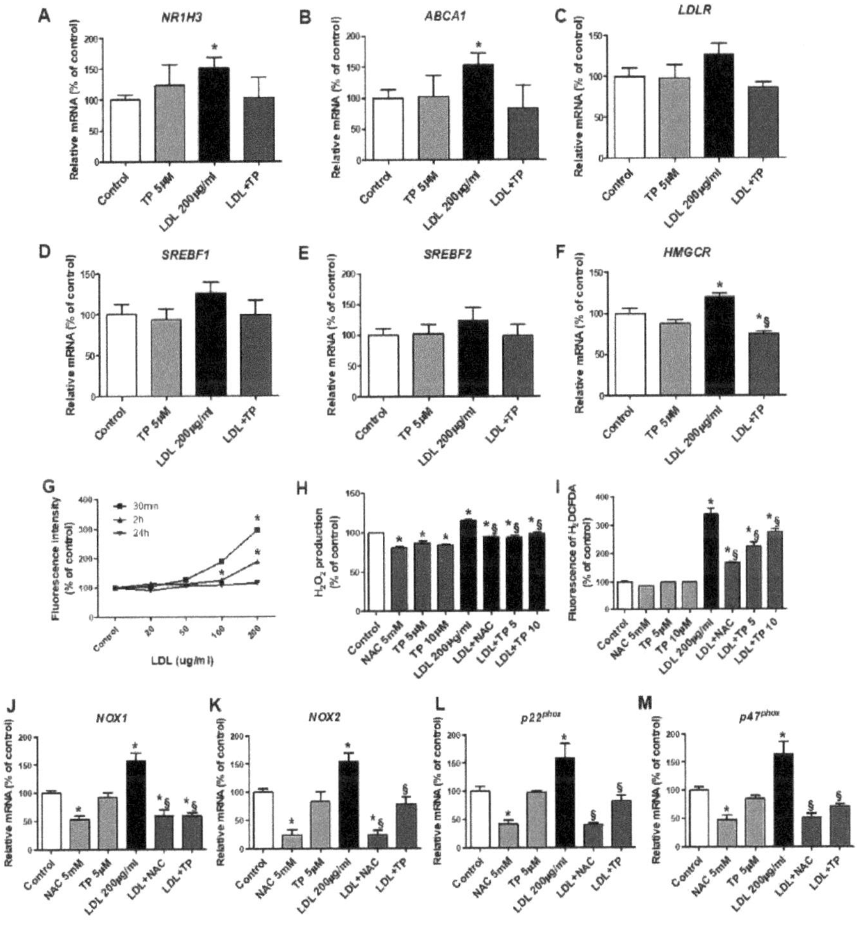


**Figure 3.** Effects of xanthine oxidase inhibitor on the expression of genes related to cholesterol transport and synthesis and ROS in LDL-stimulated HK-2 cells. Real-time RT-PCR was performed to determine the expression levels of genes related to cholesterol efflux (**A**,**B**), the LDL receptor (**C**), triglyceride synthesis (**D**), and cholesterol synthesis (**E**,**F**). (**G**) After pretreatment with TP (5 or 10 μM) for 1 h,

and stimulation with LDL (200 μg/mL) for 30 min, cellular ROS generation was measured based on the fluorescence intensity of DCF. (**H**,**I**) Measurement of $H_2O_2$ and DCFDA production. Quantitative PCR was performed to analyze the relative mRNA expression of *NOX1* (**J**), *NOX2* (**K**), and the NADPH oxidase subunits *p22*$^{phox}$ (**L**), *p47*$^{phox}$ (**M**). Differences among the groups were analyzed by one-way non-parametric ANOVA, followed by Tukey's multiple comparison test. NAC was used as a positive control. Data represent mean and SEM. * $p < 0.05$ vs. Control, § $p < 0.05$ vs. LDL. TP, topiroxostat; LDL, low-density lipoprotein; DCF, dichlorofluorescein.

Using siXDH, we evaluated how XO knock-down influenced cholesterol-related metabolism. LDL increased *XDH* expression in HK-2 cells (Figure 4G), and induced expression of the cholesterol transport genes *NR1H3* and *ABCA1*, but not *LDLR*. The siXDH reduced transport gene expression in LDL-treated HK-2 cells, to a greater extent than XO inhibitor (Figure 4A–C). XO deficiency regulated cholesterol synthesis genes upon LDL stimulation. LDL stimulation increased expressions of *SREBF1*, *SREBF2*, and *HMGCR*, while siXDH suppressed the increased expressions of *SREBF2* and *HMGCR* (Figure 4D–F).

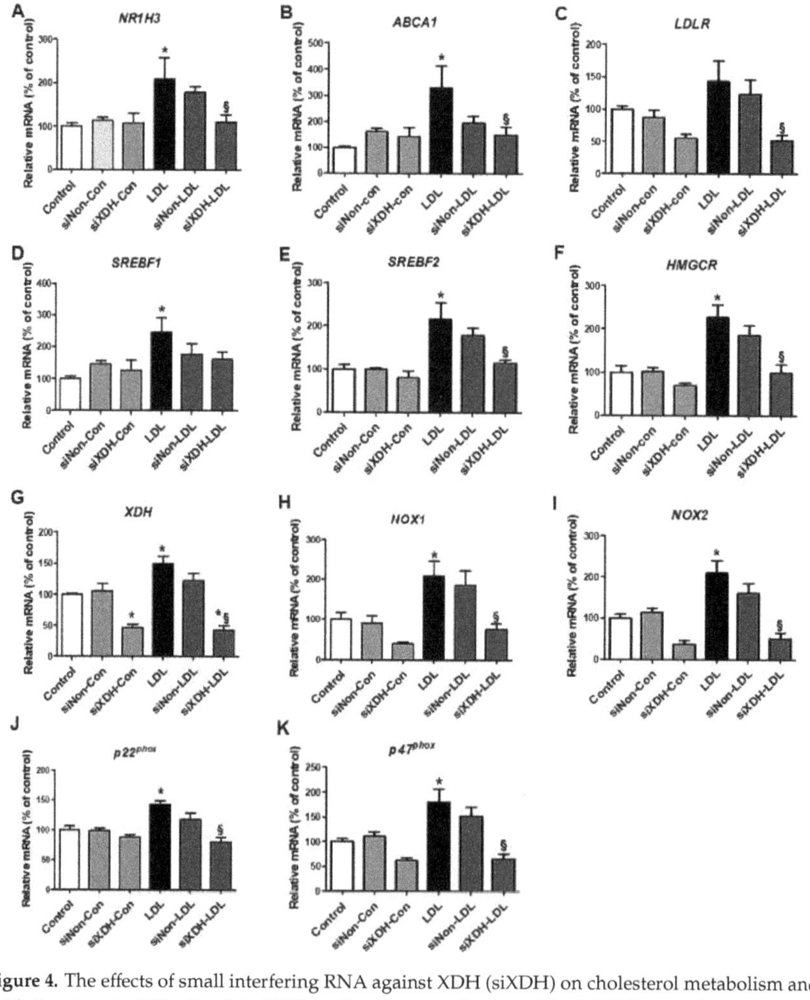


**Figure 4.** The effects of small interfering RNA against XDH (siXDH) on cholesterol metabolism and oxidative stress in LDL-stimulated HK-2 cells. After transfection with siXDH (20 μM) for 24 h, and

stimulation with LDL (200 μg/mL) for 30 min, real-time RT-PCR was performed to determine expression levels of cholesterol efflux genes (**A**,**B**), LDL receptor (**C**), triglyceride synthesis (**D**), cholesterol synthesis (**E**,**F**), *XDH* (**G**), *NOX1* (**H**), *NOX2* (**I**), and the NADPH oxidase subunits $p22^{phox}$ (**J**) and $p47^{phox}$ (**K**). Differences among the groups were analyzed by one-way non-parametric ANOVA, followed by Tukey's multiple comparison test. Data represent mean and SEM. * $p < 0.05$ vs. control, § $p < 0.05$ vs. LDL. LDL, low-density lipoprotein.

We examined mRNA expressions of subunits of the ROS generation enzyme NADPH oxidase. LDL-treated HK-2 cells exhibited increased mRNA expressions of *NOX1*, *NOX2*, $p22^{phox}$, and $p47^{phox}$. TP inhibited these increased expressions, similar to NAC (Figure 3J–M). siXDH transfection also reduced expression of *NOX1*, *NOX2*, $p22^{phox}$, and $p47^{phox}$ (Figure 4H–K).

### *2.4. XO Inhibition Reduces Hypercholesterolemia-Associated Kidney Inflammation and Fibrosis in CKD Mice*

We evaluated the inflammatory responses to high cholesterol and oxidative stress in the kidney of a CKD model. The HC diet increased inflammation cytokines (e.g., TNF-α) and the macrophage monocyte marker CD68, which were higher with HC+UN versus HC (Figure 5A). Expressions of the inflammation-related genes *Il-1β*, *Il-18*, and *Nlrp3* were also increased with HC+UN versus HC. TP reduced inflammation-related gene expression in uninephrectomized mice (Figure 5B–D). Compared to NC, HC groups showed progression in the fibrosis of glomeruli and interstitium, which was greatest with HC+UN, and was reduced by TP (Figure 5E). Compared to HC, HC+UN yielded increased *Acta2*, *Col1*, and *Fn1* expressions (Figure 5F–I). Fibronectin and α-SMA protein expressions were not significantly increased in the HC+UN group (Figure 5J,K).

Finally, we evaluated the effects of LDL on the NF-κB pathway [17], downstream of TNF-α. LDL-stimulated HK-2 cells showed increased NF-κB p50 and NF-κB p65 levels, which were decreased by TP (Figure 6A,B). We also investigated the NF-κB inhibitors JSH23 and BAY11-7082. In LDL-treated HK-2 cells, JSH23 treatment significantly decreased NF-κB p65, and IL-1β, but did not affect NLRP3 and NF-κB p50 (Figure 6C–F), while BAY11-7082 treatment reduced NF-κB p50, IL-1β, and NLRP3 levels, but did not affect NF-κB p65 (Figure 6G–J).

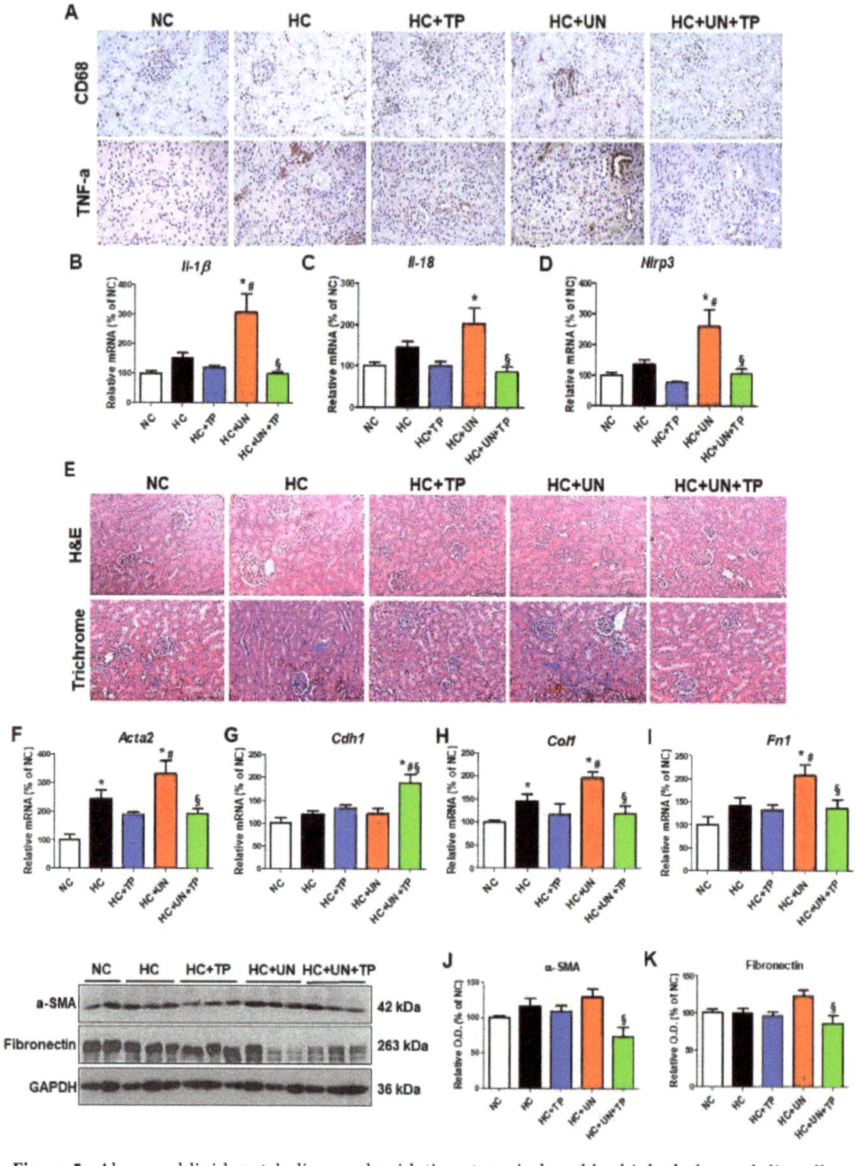


**Figure 5.** Abnormal lipid metabolism and oxidative stress induced by high-cholesterol diet affect inflammation and fibrosis progression in kidney tissue. (**A**) Representative images of TNF-α and CD68 staining of kidney tissue. Scale bars, 100 μm. (**B–D**) Real-time RT-PCR was performed to determine mRNA levels of *Il-1β*, *Il-18*, and *Nlrp3*. (**E**) Representative images of hematoxylin and eosin staining and trichrome staining of kidney tissue. Scale bars, 100 μm. (**F–I**) Real-time RT-PCR was performed to determine mRNA levels of *Acta2*, *Cdh1*, *ColI*, and *Fn1*. (**J**,**K**) Representative western blot for α-SMA, fibronectin, and GAPDH. Relative protein expression was determined using densitometry. Differences among the groups were analyzed by one-way non-parametric ANOVA, followed by Tukey's multiple comparison test. Data represent mean and SEM. * $p < 0.05$ vs. NC, # $p < 0.05$ vs. HC, § $p < 0.05$ vs. HC+UN. LDL, low-density lipoprotein; TP, topiroxostat; UN, uninephrectomy; NC, normal control; HC, high-cholesterol.

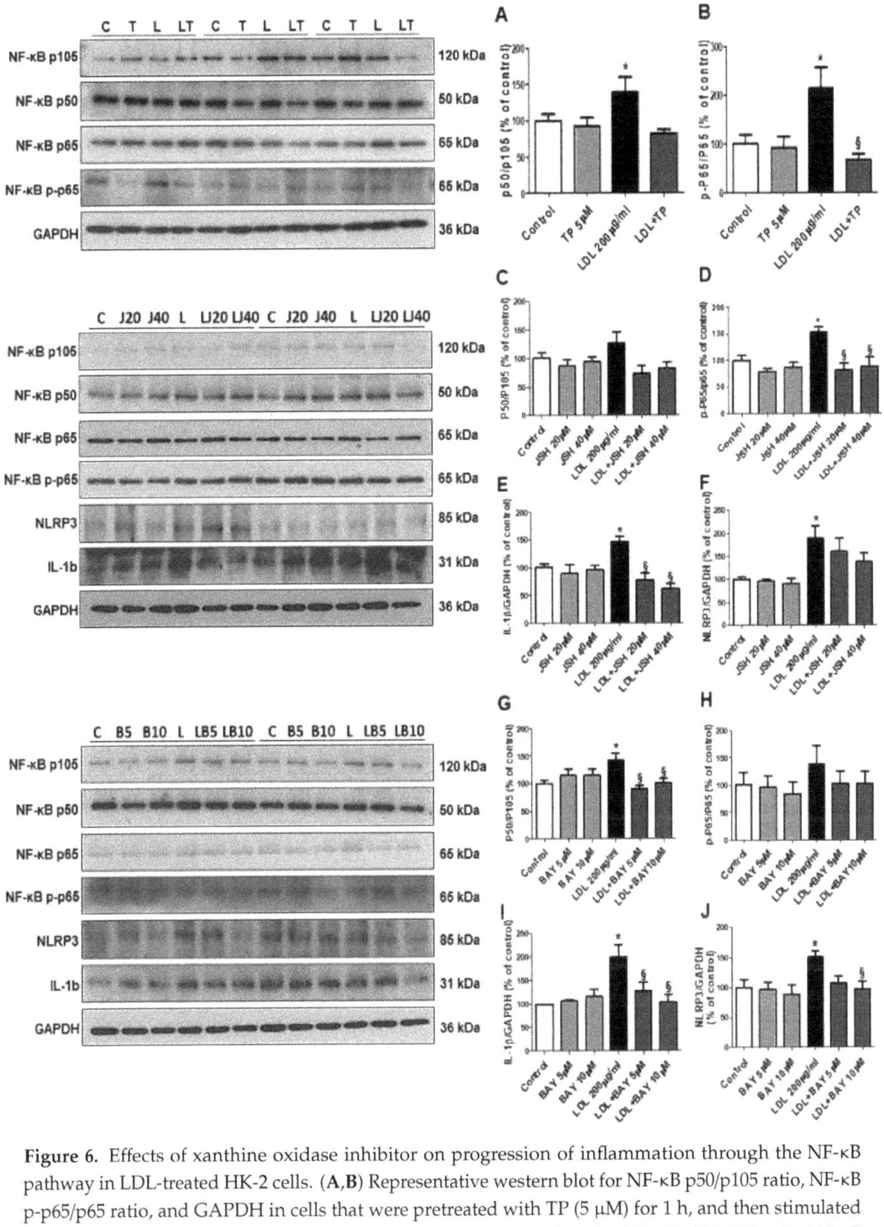


**Figure 6.** Effects of xanthine oxidase inhibitor on progression of inflammation through the NF-κB pathway in LDL-treated HK-2 cells. (**A**,**B**) Representative western blot for NF-κB p50/p105 ratio, NF-κB p-p65/p65 ratio, and GAPDH in cells that were pretreated with TP (5 μM) for 1 h, and then stimulated with LDL (200 μg/mL) for 30 min. (**C**–**F**) Representative western blot for NF-κB p50/p105 ratio, NF-κB p-p65/p65 ratio, IL-1b, NLRP3, and GAPDH in cells that were pretreated with NF-κB inhibitor (JSH23) for 1 h, and then stimulated with LDL (200 μg/mL) for 30 min. (**G**–**J**) Representative western blot for NF-κB p50/p105 ratio, NF-κB p-p65/p65 ratio, IL-1b, NLRP3, and GAPDH in cells that were pretreated with NF-κB inhibitor (BAY11-7028) for 2 h, and then stimulated with LDL (200 μg/mL) for 30 min. Relative protein expression was determined using densitometry. Differences among the groups were analyzed by a one-way non-parametric ANOVA, followed by Tukey's multiple comparison test. Data represent mean and SEM. * $p < 0.05$ vs. Control, § $p < 0.05$ vs. LDL. LDL, low-density lipoprotein; TP, topiroxostat.

## 3. Discussion

The present results demonstrated that XO inhibition significantly reduced hypercholesterolemia-associated kidney inflammation and fibrosis in uninephrectomized ApoE KO mice. In vitro experiments revealed that XO inhibition reduced LDL-induced oxidative stress and cholesterol synthesis. The HC diet induced cholesterol accumulation by regulating the expression of genes related to cholesterol efflux and synthesis. Additionally, hypercholesterolemia significantly increased XO activity and NADPH-dependent ROS generation, thus inducing kidney inflammation and fibrosis. LDL stimulation evoked changes in the cholesterol metabolism, NADPH oxidase, and NF-κB pathways in HK-2 cells. XO inhibition modulated the hypercholesterolemia-induced changes in the expression of genes related to cholesterol transport and synthesis. XO inhibition by topiroxostat attenuated inflammation and fibrosis in the unilateral kidney through inhibition of the NF-κB pathway.

Patients with CKD exhibit various lipid abnormalities [18], and abnormal lipid metabolism is associated with kidney disease progression [19,20]. However, the mechanism of lipid-induced kidney damage is not fully understood. In the present study, we used ApoE KO mice with unilateral nephrectomy as a model to evaluate the effects of hypercholesterolemia on CKD progression. Hypercholesterolemia aggravated renal function in the uninephrectomized ApoE KO mice by increasing kidney lipid accumulation. Moreover, these lipid abnormalities were associated with increases of factors mediating kidney injury, such as XO and oxidative stress.

Our results demonstrated that cholesterol accumulation in uninephrectomized mice was induced by upregulation of genes related to cholesterol synthesis, such as *Srebf2* and *Hmgcr*, and downregulation of efflux-related genes, such as *Abca1* and *Nr1h3*, upstream of ABCA1. Cholesterol homeostasis is regulated by multiple pathways, including intracellular cholesterol uptake, synthesis, and efflux actions [21]. Inflammatory stress promotes reduction of cholesterol efflux through the ABCA1 pathway, leading to lipid accumulation in the kidney [22]. ApoE promotes cholesterol efflux through the ABCA1 and ABCG1 cell surface transporters, which facilitate the efflux of phospholipids and cholesterol onto lipid-poor apolipoproteins [23]. The ABCA1 transporter facilitates the efflux of cellular phospholipids and cholesterol to acceptors, such as ApoA-I and ApoE [24]. Selective inactivation of macrophage ABCA1 yields substantially increased cholesterol accumulation in mice [25,26]. Our present results showed that the HC diet caused upregulated expression of both cholesterol synthesis and efflux genes. Furthermore, uninephrectomy plus hypercholesterolemia attenuated the increase of cholesterol efflux genes, while upregulating the increase of cholesterol synthesis genes. It is not yet known why uninephrectomy had different effects on the expression of genes related to cholesterol metabolism. However, our findings suggest that hypercholesterolemia-associated genes contributed to cholesterol accumulation in the kidney, and may potentially play a role in the dysfunction of the unilateral kidney.

The ABCA1 protein level differed from mRNA expression in the unilateral kidney with high cholesterol. The ABCA1 membrane protein rapidly responds to increased cholesterol, and the ABCA1 protein level is independent of its transcription [27]. Cholesterol accumulation inhibits ABCA1 degradation and ubiquitination by decreasing the proteasomal degradation [28]. In our study, the decrease of *Abca1* mRNA may have been associated with the reduced intracellular cholesterol efflux, and thus with the increased cholesterol accumulation in the kidney.

Abnormal lipid metabolism induces monocyte foam cells, and this change is more prominent in patients with kidney dysfunction [29]. Alterations in lipoprotein metabolism promote the production of ROS, such as hydrogen peroxide; however, the effect on intracellular cholesterol has not been clearly demonstrated. Since increased serum LDL level is a representative marker of dyslipidemia, we stimulated renal tubular cells with LDL to examine the molecular changes in cholesterol metabolism and inflammation. LDL stimulation increased the mRNA expression of *NR1H3*, *ABCA1*, *LDLR*, *SREBF2*, and *HMGCR* in HK-2 cells. These changes are consistent with our observations in the animal model, except for the expression of *SREBF1*, which is involved in TG synthesis. These findings suggest that the renal tubular cell damage is also mediated by the lipid accumulation associated with changes in the expression of genes related to cholesterol transport and synthesis.

XO is a key enzyme of the purine pathway, producing uric acid through various oxidized purines [30]. Recent studies demonstrate that XO plays a role as an ROS-producing enzyme, aggravating inflammation, atherosclerosis, and chronic disease [31]. XO activity is increased in obesity, and XO inhibitors regulate the inflammatory process by inhibiting production of ROS and uric acid [32,33]. We previously demonstrated that XO inhibition could decrease cancer cell migration and ROS generation [10]. In our present study, we found that XO activity and gene expression were increased in kidneys with hypercholesterolemia, and in LDL-treated HK-2 cells. This is the first report of cholesterol directly leading to increased XO enzyme activity in the kidney. We further found that XO inhibition improved hypercholesterolemia-associated kidney damage by modulating the expression of genes related to cholesterol metabolism and the progression of inflammation and fibrosis in a unilateral kidney. Overall, our findings suggest that XO is a promising treatment target for hypercholesterolemia-associated kidney injury in uninephrectomized patients.

Expression of NOX1, NOX2, and NOX4 in the kidney mediates oxidative stress and promotes vascular inflammation, dysfunction, and fibrosis in CKD [34]. NADPH oxidases of the kidney exhibit a distinct cellular localization and are activated by various stimuli, including LDL [35]. Our results demonstrated that hypercholesterolemia and LDL increased oxidative stress in kidney tissue and tubule cells, and that XO activity was associated with oxidative stress markers and increased expression of NADPH-related genes. XO inhibition reduced the expression of *NOX1* and *NOX2*, but not *NOX4* (data not shown), showing antioxidant effects similar to with NAC. Transfection with siXDH had the same effect as XO inhibitor in HK-2 cells. These results revealed that XO inhibition controlled NOX activity, thus suppressing oxidative stress and reducing renal damage.

The inflammatory process exacerbates lipid accumulation in the kidney by translocating plasma lipids to the kidney [36]. A high-fat diet activates the inflammatory response by increasing TNF-α expression in the kidney, thus causing kidney damage in obese humans and animal models [37,38]. XO activity is elevated in inflammation, and XO inhibition suppresses inflammation and oxidative stress in macrophages [14]. Treatment with XO inhibitors reportedly attenuates inflammation and fibrosis in animal models of atherosclerosis and nonalcoholic steatohepatitis [39]. Here we found that a HC diet led to increased TNF-α and CD68 in the unilateral kidney, which was downregulated after XO inhibition. These results showed that the mechanism of hypercholesterolemia-associated kidney damage is closely related to inflammation, and that the damage could be suppressed by XO inhibition.

Oxidative stress stimulates inflammatory cells to activate the NF-κB pathway through an intracellular signaling system, thus mediating inflammation [40]. In cells, oxidative stress induces NLRP3 activity, leading to inflammation and apoptosis, along with Caspase-1 activation. Obesity and metabolic syndrome induce NLRP3 inflammatory activation, which weakens phospholipid degradation, leading to kidney damage [41]. In this study, hypercholesterolemia increased NLRP3 and TNF-α, which is one of the most potent inducers of NF-κB. In vitro experiments demonstrated that the NF-κB pathway was an inflammatory mechanism of dyslipidemia-associated kidney damage. LDL stimulation increased the activity of the NF-κB pathway and NLRP3, whereas XO inhibition affected the NF-κB pathway by decreasing phosphorylated NF-κB p65 and NF-κB p50 in HK-2 cells. We further demonstrated that the NF-κB inhibitors JSH23 and BAY11-7028 had effects on NLRP3 similar to those of XO inhibition. This supports the theory that NF-κB is a main pathway of hypercholesterolemia-associated kidney damage.

In conclusion, our present data suggested that XO inhibition has renoprotective effects against hypercholesterolemia-associated kidney injury. This protection from XO inhibition was mediated by regulation of cholesterol metabolism, decreasing NADPH-dependent ROS generation, and reduction of inflammation through the NF-κB pathway. XO could be a novel therapeutic target for hypercholesterolemia-associated kidney disease in uninephrectomized patients.

## 4. Materials and Methods

### 4.1. Animals, Diets, and Specimen Collections

Male ApoE KO mice were purchased from Jackson Laboratory (Bar Harbor, ME, USA) at the age of 8 weeks. All animal experiments were approved and performed according to the regulations of the Kyungpook National University Animal Care and Use Committee (KNU-2018-0042, date; 08/03/2018). For 12 weeks, animals were fed normal control diet containing 20.3% protein, 5% fat, and 66% carbohydrate or a high-fat high-cholesterol diet (HC, diet D12336; Research Diets, New Brunswick, NJ, USA) containing 16.0% fat, 1.25% cholesterol, and 0.5% sodium cholic acid.

We randomized the eight-week-old ApoE KO mice into groups that did or did not receive topiroxostat (TP; 1 mg per kg body weight) treatment, and that did or did not undergo uninephrectomy (UN) surgery. There were a total of five groups: NC ($n$ = 5), fed a normal control diet; HC ($n$ = 6), fed a high-cholesterol diet; HC+TP ($n$ = 6), fed a high-cholesterol diet with TP; HC+UN ($n$ = 8), fed a high-cholesterol diet and received uninephrectomy surgery; and HC+UN+TP ($n$ = 8), fed a high-cholesterol diet with TP and received uninephrectomy surgery. All mice that did not undergo uninephrectomy were sham operated. TP was administered by oral gavage for 4 weeks before the end of the experiment.

Uninephrectomy was performed as described previously [42]. For uninephrectomy, after mice were anesthetized with 3–5% isoflurane, the left kidney was surgically removed via a left incision on the back. The adrenal gland was carefully freed from the upper pole of the renal capsule before removed the left kidney. The incision was closed with sutures. In sham surgery, the kidney was manipulated without ablation. At 12 weeks after surgery, all mice were anesthetized and then sacrifice, and kidneys were harvested for the analyses. Half of the kidneys were stored at −80 °C for molecular analysis and the other half was fixed with 4% paraformaldehyde for histological analysis.

### 4.2. Serum Chemistry

At the end of the experimental period, blood samples from each mouse were collected into tubes by cardiac puncture. The blood was sampled into ethylenediaminetetraacetic acid-free bottles for serum separation. The blood urea nitrogen (BUN), creatinine (Cr), uric acid, total cholesterol (TC), low-density lipoprotein (LDL) and triglycerides level in the serum were measured by GCLabs (Yongin, Korea) using the Cobas 8000 modular analyzer system (Roche, Basel, Switzerland).

### 4.3. Histopathology

To detect kidney injury, the fixed right kidney was dehydrated in ethanol and embedded in paraffin. Kidney tissue blocks were cut into 2-μm-thick sections and subjected to hematoxylin and eosin (H&E) staining, periodic acid Schiff (PAS) staining, and Masson's trichrome staining. For immunohistochemical analysis of kidney tissues, we used the following antibodies: mouse monoclonal against CD68 (ED1; 1:100; Abcam, Cambridge, MA, USA) and rabbit polyclonal against tumor necrosis factor-α (TNF-α; 1:200; Abcam). Next, secondary antibody was performed using HRP-conjugated polyclonal goat anti-rabbit IgG P0447 or goat anti-mouse IgG p0448 (Dako, Glostrup, Denmark) for 1 h. The sections were visualized using 3,3-diaminobenzidine (DAB; DAKO ChemMate Detection Kit) and counterstained with Mayer's hematoxylin.

### 4.4. Oil Red O Staining

Fixed frozen kidney tissue was cut into 6-μm-thick sections, and subjected to Oil Red O (Sigma-Aldrich, Saint Louis, MO, USA) staining following the manufacturer's protocol. After the sections were rinsed in distilled water and 60% isopropanol for 1 min, the sections were stained with Oil red O for 15 min. and then rinsed in 60% isopropanol and distilled water each for 1 min. Counterstaining was stained with hematoxylin for 1 min.

### 4.5. Cell Treatments

Human renal proximal tubule epithelial cells (HK-2 cells) were purchased from the Korean Cell Line Bank (KCLB, Seoul, South Korea). The cells were maintained in RPMI-1640 supplemented with 10% fetal bovine serum, and 100 units/mL penicillin and 100 μg/mL streptomycin antibiotic mixture at 37 °C in 5% $CO_2$ and 95% air. The Cells were pretreated with topiroxostat (TP), xanthine oxidase inhibitor (5 or 10 μM), and 5 mM N-acetylcysteine (NAC) (Sigma-Aldrich) for 1 h, and stimulated with LDL (200 μg/mL) for 30 min to induce lipotoxicity.

### 4.6. Hydrogen Peroxide Determination

$H_2O_2$ levels were measured using the Amplex Red Hydrogen Peroxide Assay Kit (Molecular Probes, Invitrogen, Eugene, OR, USA), following the manufacturer's protocol. To detect $H_2O_2$ released from kidney tissue and treated HK cells, cell lysate or culture media were reacted with the Amplex Red Reagent in the presence of horseradish peroxidase to produce the red-fluorescent oxidation product resorufin. The fluorescence of resorufin was determined at 530nm excitation and 590 nm emission using a fluorescence microplate reader (Molecular Devices, Sunnyvale, CA, USA). The concentrations of $H_2O_2$ were calculated using standard curves. The loading buffer was measured and subtracted from each value in order to exclude background fluorescence.

### 4.7. Intracellular ROS Measurement

Intracellular ROS generation was measured using 2′,7′-dichlorofluorescein diacetate (DCF-DA). HK-2 cells and kidney tissues were stained for 40 min with 10 μM 2′,7′-dichlorodihydrofluorescein diacetate ($H_2$DCFDA; Molecular Probes) in a black 96-well plate. DCF-DA is hydrolyzed by esterases to dichlorofluorescein (DCF), which is trapped within the cell. Then cellular oxidants oxidize this non-fluorescent molecule to fluorescent dichlorofluorescein (DCF). Fluorescence signal intensity was measured at 480 nm excitation and 520 nm emission using a fluorescence microplate reader (Molecular Devices). The value of the fluorescence signal was expressed as a percentage of the control.

### 4.8. Determination of Intracellular Total Cholesterol

From the kidney tissues of ApoE mice, we extracted cellular lipids by chloroform:methanol extraction (4:2:3, chloroform:methanol:water). Total cholesterol levels were determined using a commercially available kit (Cell Biolabs Inc., San Diego, CA, USA) following the manufacturer's protocol.

### 4.9. Transfection of HK-2 with XDH siRNA

ON-TARGETplus SMARTpool siRNAs used for silencing expression of human XDH genes (ID:7498) and non-targeting (negative control) siRNA were purchased from Dharmacon (Chicago, IL, USA). Four target sequences in human XDH are 5′- AGA GUG AGG UUG ACA AGU U -3′, 5′- GGA GUA ACA UAA CUG GAA U -3′, 5′- UAG AGG AGC UAC ACU AUU C -3′ and 5′- ACA CGG AGA UUG GCA UUG A -3′. siRNAs were used at a concentration of 20 nM. Transfection was performed using Opti-MEM™ transfection medium and Lipofectamine™ (both from Invitrogen, Paisley, UK). One day prior to transfection, HK-2 cells were seeded and cultured to reach 30–40% confluence on the following day. RNAi duplexes for XDH were mixed with Lipofectamine, forming a transfection complex that was added to the plated cells. After 24 h of incubation, the medium was replaced with RPMI, and cells were starved for 6 h. Transfected cells were used for quantitative real-time reverse transcription-polymerase chain reaction (qRT-PCR).

### 4.10. Quantitative Real-Time Polymerase Chain Reactions

Quantitative real-time RT-PCR analysis was performed as described previously [7]. Total RNA was extracted from cell lysates using TRIreagent (Thermo Fisher Scientific, Waltham, MA, USA) according to the provider's instructions. One microgram of total RNA was reverse transcribed to cDNA using the PrimeScript cDNA synthesis kit (TaKaRa, Otsu, Japan). Quantitative real-time RT-PCR was performed on the ABI PRISM 7700 Sequence Detection System (Applied Biosystems, Foster city, CA, USA) using the SYBR green PCR Master Mix (Applied Biosystems, Foster City, CA, USA). The results were analyzed using the comparative Ct method for relative quantification of gene expression. The primer sets used in this study are listed in Table 1.

**Table 1.** Oligonucleotide primer sequences.

| Gene | Forward Primer (5′–3′) | Reverse Primer (5′–3′) |
|---|---|---|
| Mouse *Msr1* | CAC GGG ACG CTT CCA GAA T | TGG ACT GAC GAA ATC AAG GAA TT |
| Mouse *Scarb1* | GGC CTG TTT GTT GGG ATG AA | CGT TCC ATT TGT CCA CCA GAT |
| Mouse *Lcat* | AGC CTT GGC TGT CTG CAT GT | CCCGAGAGAGATAAAACCATCAA |
| Mouse *Srebf1* | GGC TAT TCC GTG AAC ATC TCC TA | ATC CAA GGG CAT CTG AGA ACT C |
| Mouse *Srebf2* | GGT CCT CCA TCA ACG ACA AAA T | TAA TCA ATG GCC TTC CTC AGA AC |
| Mouse *Nr1h3* | GAG TGT CGA CTT CGC AAA TGC | CCT CTT CTT GCC GCT TCA GT |
| Mouse *Abca1* | GGC AAT GAG TGT GCC AGA GTT A | TAG TCA CAT GTG GCA CCG TTT T |
| Mouse *Ldlr* | CCAAATGGCATCACACTAGATCTT | CCGATTGCCCCCATTG |
| Mouse *Hmgcr* | GGG CCC CAC ATT CAC TCT T | GCC GAA GCA GCA CAT GAT CT |
| Mouse *Il-1β* | TCG TGC TGT CGG ACC CAT AT | GGTTCTCCTTGTACAAAGCTCATG |
| Mouse *Nlrp3* | TCTCCCGCATCTCCATTTGTA | CGC GCG TTC CTG TCC TT |
| Mous *Il-18* | GACAACTTTGGCCGACTTCAC | TCCTCGAACACAGGCTGTCTT |
| Mouse *Acta2* | CTGACAGAGGCACCACTG | CATCTCCAGAGTCCAGCA |
| Mouse *Cdh* | GCAGTTCTGCCAGAGAAACC | TGGATCCAAGATGGTGATGA |
| Mouse *Fn1* | CCA TTC TCC TTC TTC AAG TTT GC | AGG AAT GGC TGT CAG GAT GGT |
| Mouse *Col1* | ACA ACC GCT TTG CCA CTT CT | CGT AAG TCA CGG GCA CGT T |
| Mouse *Gapdh* | TAA AGG GCA TCC TGG GCT ACA CT | TTA CTC CTT GGA GGC CAT GTA GG |
| Human *LDLR* | AGT TGG CTG CGT TAA TGT GAC A | TCT CTA GCC ATG TTG CAG ACT TTG |
| Human *SREBF1* | GCT CCT CCA TCA ATG ACA AAA TC | TGC AGA AAG CGA ATG TAG TCG AT |
| Human *SREBF2* | AGG CGG ACA ACC CAT AAT ATC A | CTT GTG CAT CTT GGC GTC TGT |
| Human *ABCA1* | GAC ATC GTG GCG TTT TTG G | CGA GAT ATG GTC CGG ATT GC |
| Human *HMGCR* | GGA CAG GAT GCA GCA CAG AA | GCATGGTGCAGCTGATATATAAATCT |
| Human *NR1H3* | CAC CTA CAT GCG TCG CAA GT | CAG GCG GAT CTG TTC TTC TGA |
| Human *NOX1* | TGCCTAGAAGGGCTCCAAAC | ACATTCAGCCCTAACCAAACAAC |
| Human *NOX2* | AGGGTCAAGAACAGGCTAAGGA | TTCTCCACCTCCAACCCTCTTT |
| Human $p47^{phox}$ | GGCAGGACCTGTCGGAGAA | ATCGCCCCTGCCTCAATAG |
| Human $p22^{phox}$ | ACTTTGGTGCCTACTCCATTGTG | TGTCCCCAGCGCTCCAT |
| Human *XDH* | GAAGGCCATCTATGCATCGAA | GAAGGCCATCTATGCATCGAA |
| Human *GAPDH* | TTCACCACCATGGAGAAGGCT | TGGTTCACACCCATGACGAAC |

### 4.11. Immunoblot Analysis

Protein concentration was measured using Bradford's method in lysates of treated HK2 cells and tissues. Total protein (20 μg) was separated by 10% SDS-polyacrylamide gel electrophoresis and transferred to a nitrocellulose membrane. The membrane was blocked with 10% skim milk for 1 h at room temperature, and incubated overnight at 4 °C with primary antibodies. The membrane was incubated with HRP-conjugated polyclonal goat anti-rabbit IgG P0447 or goat anti-mouse IgG p0448 (Dako, Glostrup, Denmark) as the secondary antibody for 1 h and detected using advanced ECL reagents (Amersham Bioscience, Piscataway, NJ, USA). The target protein bands were normalized to that of GAPDH. Expression levels were estimated using Scion Image software (Scion, Frederick, MD, USA). The primary antibodies that detect proteins are listed in Table 2.

**Table 2.** List of antibodies used in immunohistochemistry and immunoblotting.

| Antibodies | Cat. No. | Company |
|---|---|---|
| **LXRα** | Ab176323 | abcam |
| **HMGCR** | Ab174830 | abcam |
| **ABCA1** | Ab18180 | abcam |
| **α-SMA** | Ab5694 | abcam |
| **Fibronectin** | Ab2413 | abcam |
| **IL-1β** | 12242 | Cell signaling |
| **NLRP3** | 13158 | Cell signaling |
| **NF-kappaB p65** | 8242S | Cell signaling |
| **NF-kappaBphos-p65** | 3036S | Cell signaling |
| **NF-kappaBp105/p50** | 3035S | Cell signaling |
| **GAPDH** | 2118S | Cell signaling |

### 4.12. Statistical Analysis

Data are presented as mean ± SEM. Statistical analyses were performed using GraphPad Prism 5.01 (GraphPad Software Inc., La Jolla, CA, USA). The difference among the groups was analyzed using a one-way nonparametric ANOVA followed by Tukey's multiple comparison test. A $p$ value of <0.05 was considered statistically significant.

**Author Contributions:** Conceptualization, Y.-J.K., J.-H.C. and Y.-L.K.; Formal analysis, Y.-J.K., S.-H.O., C.-D.K., S.-H.P., J.-H.C. and Y.-L.K.; Funding acquisition, Y.-J.K. and Y.-L.K.; Investigation, Y.-J.K., S.-H.O., J.-S.A. and J.-M.Y.; Methodology, Y.-J.K.; Visualization, Y.-J.K. and S.-H.O.; Writing—original draft, Y.-J.K.; Writing—review & editing, J.-H.C. and Y.-L.K. All authors have read and agreed to the published version of the manuscript.

**Funding:** This research was supported by Basic Science Research Program through the National Research Foundation of Korea (NRF) funded by the Ministry of Education (2017R1A6A3A01008277, 2020R1I1A1A01055554, 2020R1I1A3068253).

**Conflicts of Interest:** The authors declare no conflict of interest.

## Abbreviations

| | |
|---|---|
| ABCA1 | ATP Binding Cassette Subfamily A Member 1 |
| ABCG1 | ATP-binding cassette super-family G Member 1 |
| ApoE KO | Apolipoprotein E Knockout |
| BUN | Blood urea nitrogen |
| CD68 | Cluster of Differentiation 68 |
| CKD | Chronic kidney disease |
| DCFDA | Dichlorodihydrofluorescein diacetate |
| HC | High-cholesterol |
| HMGCR | 3-Hydroxy-3-Methylglutaryl-CoA Reductase |
| Il-1 | Interleukin-1 |
| LCAT | Lecithin-cholesterol acyltransferase |
| LDL | Low-density lipoprotein |
| LDLR | Low density lipoprotein receptor |
| LXRα | Liver X receptor α |
| MSR1 | Macrophage scavenger receptor types I |
| NR1H3 | Nuclear receptor subfamily 1 group H member 3 |
| NADPH | Nicotinamide adenine dinucleotide phosphate |
| NF-κB | Nuclear Factor-kappaB |
| NLRP3 | NOD-, LRR- and pyrin domain-containing protein 3 |

| | |
|---|---|
| NOX | NADPH oxidase |
| PAS | Periodic acid-Schiff |
| ROS | Reactive oxygen species |
| siXDH | Small interfering RNA against XDH |
| SCARB1 | Scavenger receptor class B type 1 |
| SREBF | Sterol regulatory element binding transcription factor |
| TC | Total cholesterol |
| TG | Triglyceride |
| TNF-α | Tumor necrosis factor α |
| TP | Topiroxostat |
| XO | Xanthine oxidase |
| α-SMA | Alpha-smooth muscle actin |

## References


1. Gelber, R.P.; Kurth, T.; Kausz, A.T.; Manson, J.E.; Buring, J.E.; Levey, A.S.; Gaziano, J.M. Association between body mass index and CKD in apparently healthy men. *Am. J. Kidney Dis.* **2005**, *46*, 871–880. [CrossRef] [PubMed]
2. Reiss, A.B.; Voloshyna, I.; De Leon, J.; Miyawaki, N.; Mattana, J. Cholesterol Metabolism in CKD. *Am. J. Kidney Dis.* **2015**, *66*, 1071–1082. [CrossRef] [PubMed]
3. Locke, J.E.; Reed, R.D.; Massie, A.; MacLennan, P.A.; Sawinski, D.; Kumar, V.; Mehta, S.; Mannon, R.B.; Gaston, R.; Lewis, C.E.; et al. Obesity increases the risk of end-stage renal disease among living kidney donors. *Kidney Int.* **2017**, *91*, 699–703. [CrossRef] [PubMed]
4. Muzaale, A.D.; Massie, A.B.; Wang, M.C.; Montgomery, R.A.; McBride, M.A.; Wainright, J.L.; Segev, D.L. Risk of end-stage renal disease following live kidney donation. *JAMA* **2014**, *311*, 579–586. [CrossRef] [PubMed]
5. Amiya, E. Interaction of hyperlipidemia and reactive oxygen species: Insights from the lipid-raft platform. *World J. Cardiol.* **2016**, *8*, 689–694. [CrossRef] [PubMed]
6. Bobulescu, I.A. Renal lipid metabolism and lipotoxicity. *Curr. Opin. Nephrol. Hypertens.* **2010**, *19*, 393–402. [CrossRef] [PubMed]
7. Ryu, H.M.; Kim, Y.J.; Oh, E.J.; Oh, S.H.; Choi, J.Y.; Cho, J.H.; Kim, C.D.; Park, S.H.; Kim, Y.L. Hypoxanthine induces cholesterol accumulation and incites atherosclerosis in apolipoprotein E-deficient mice and cells. *J. Cell Mol. Med.* **2016**, *20*, 2160–2172. [CrossRef]
8. Gai, Z.; Hiller, C.; Chin, S.H.; Hofstetter, L.; Stieger, B.; Konrad, D.; Kullak-Ublick, G.A. Uninephrectomy augments the effects of high fat diet induced obesity on gene expression in mouse kidney. *Biochim. Biophys. Acta* **2014**, *1842*, 1870–1878. [CrossRef]
9. Bro, S.; Bentzon, J.F.; Falk, E.; Andersen, C.B.; Olgaard, K.; Nielsen, L.B. Chronic renal failure accelerates atherogenesis in apolipoprotein E-deficient mice. *J. Am. Soc. Nephrol.* **2003**, *14*, 2466–2474. [CrossRef]
10. Oh, S.H.; Choi, S.Y.; Choi, H.J.; Ryu, H.M.; Kim, Y.J.; Jung, H.Y.; Cho, J.H.; Kim, C.D.; Park, S.H.; Kwon, T.H.; et al. The emerging role of xanthine oxidase inhibition for suppression of breast cancer cell migration and metastasis associated with hypercholesterolemia. *FASEB J.* **2019**, *33*, 7301–7314. [CrossRef]
11. Gwinner, W.; Scheuer, H.; Haller, H.; Brandes, R.P.; Groene, H.J. Pivotal role of xanthine oxidase in the initiation of tubulointerstitial renal injury in rats with hyperlipidemia. *Kidney Int.* **2006**, *69*, 481–487. [CrossRef] [PubMed]
12. Kataoka, H.; Yang, K.; Rock, K.L. The xanthine oxidase inhibitor Febuxostat reduces tissue uric acid content and inhibits injury-induced inflammation in the liver and lung. *Eur. J. Pharmacol.* **2015**, *746*, 174–179. [CrossRef] [PubMed]
13. Pacher, P.; Nivorozhkin, A.; Szabó, C. Therapeutic effects of xanthine oxidase inhibitors: Renaissance half a century after the discovery of allopurinol. *Pharmacol. Rev.* **2006**, *58*, 87–114. [CrossRef]
14. Nomura, J.; Busso, N.; Ives, A.; Matsui, C.; Tsujimoto, S.; Shirakura, T.; Tamura, M.; Kobayashi, T.; So, A.; Yamanaka, Y. Xanthine oxidase inhibition by febuxostat attenuates experimental atherosclerosis in mice. *Sci. Rep.* **2014**, *4*, 1–9. [CrossRef] [PubMed]
15. Dandona, P.; Ghanim, H.; Brooks, D.P. Antioxidant activity of carvedilol in cardiovascular disease. *J. Hypertens.* **2007**, *25*, 731–741. [CrossRef] [PubMed]

16. Badve, S.V.; Pascoe, E.M.; Tiku, A.; Boudville, N.; Brown, F.G.; Cass, A.; Clarke, P.; Dalbeth, N.; Day, R.O.; de Zoysa, J.R.; et al. Effects of Allopurinol on the Progression of Chronic Kidney Disease. *N. Engl. J. Med.* **2020**, *382*, 2504–2513. [CrossRef] [PubMed]
17. Janabi, M.; Yamashita, S.; Hirano, K.; Sakai, N.; Hiraoka, H.; Matsumoto, K.; Zhang, Z.; Nozaki, S.; Matsuzawa, Y. Oxidized LDL-induced NF-kappa B activation and subsequent expression of proinflammatory genes are defective in monocyte-derived macrophages from CD36-deficient patients. *Arterioscler Thromb Vasc Biol.* **2000**, *20*, 1953–1960. [CrossRef]
18. Cases, A.; Coll, E. Dyslipidemia and the progression of renal disease in chronic renal failure patients. *Kidney Int. Suppl.* **2005**, *68*, S87–S93. [CrossRef]
19. Moorhead, J.; El-Nahas, M.; Chan, M.; Varghese, Z. Lipid nephrotoxicity in chronic progressive glomerular and tubulo-interstitial disease. *Lancet* **1982**, *320*, 1309–1311. [CrossRef]
20. Scarpioni, R.; Ricardi, M.; Albertazzi, V.; Melfa, L. Treatment of dyslipidemia in chronic kidney disease: Effectiveness and safety of statins. *World J. Nephrol.* **2012**, *1*, 184–194. [CrossRef]
21. Afonso, M.S.; Machado, R.M.; Lavrador, M.S.; Quintao, E.C.R.; Moore, K.J.; Lottenberg, A.M. Molecular Pathways Underlying Cholesterol Homeostasis. *Nutrients* **2018**, *10*, 760. [CrossRef] [PubMed]
22. Ruan, X.Z.; Moorhead, J.F.; Fernando, R.Y.; Wheeler, D.C.; Powis, S.H. PPAR agonists protect mesangial cells from interleukin 1β-induced intracellular lipid accumulation by activating the ABCA1 cholesterol efflux pathway. *J. Am. Soc. Nephrol.* **2003**, *14*, 593–600. [CrossRef] [PubMed]
23. Gelissen, I.C.; Harris, M.; Rye, K.A.; Quinn, C.; Brown, A.J.; Kockx, M.; Cartland, S.; Packianathan, M.; Kritharides, L.; Jessup, W. ABCA1 and ABCG1 synergize to mediate cholesterol export to apoA-I. *Arter. Thromb. Vasc. Biol.* **2006**, *26*, 534–540. [CrossRef] [PubMed]
24. Brooks-Wilson, A.; Marcil, M.; Clee, S.M.; Zhang, L.-H.; Roomp, K.; van Dam, M.; Yu, L.; Brewer, C.; Collins, J.A.; Molhuizen, H.O. Mutations in ABC1 in Tangier disease and familial high-density lipoprotein deficiency. *Nat. Genet.* **1999**, *22*, 337. [CrossRef] [PubMed]
25. Zuo, Y.; Yancey, P.; Castro, I.; Khan, W.N.; Motojima, M.; Ichikawa, I.; Fogo, A.B.; Linton, M.F.; Fazio, S.; Kon, V. Renal dysfunction potentiates foam cell formation by repressing ABCA1. *Arter. Thromb. Vasc. Biol.* **2009**, *29*, 1277–1282. [CrossRef]
26. Joyce, C.; Freeman, L.; Brewer, H.B., Jr.; Santamarina-Fojo, S. Study of ABCA1 function in transgenic mice. *Arter. Thromb. Vasc. Biol.* **2003**, *23*, 965–971. [CrossRef]
27. Hsieh, V.; Kim, M.J.; Gelissen, I.C.; Brown, A.J.; Sandoval, C.; Hallab, J.C.; Kockx, M.; Traini, M.; Jessup, W.; Kritharides, L. Cellular cholesterol regulates ubiquitination and degradation of the cholesterol export proteins ABCA1 and ABCG1. *J. Biol. Chem.* **2014**, *289*, 7524–7536. [CrossRef]
28. Wellington, C.L.; Walker, E.K.; Suarez, A.; Kwok, A.; Bissada, N.; Singaraja, R.; Yang, Y.-Z.; Zhang, L.-H.; James, E.; Wilson, J.E. ABCA1 mRNA and Protein Distribution Patterns Predict Multiple Different Roles and Levels of Regulation. *Regulation* **2002**, *82*, 273–283. [CrossRef]
29. Eom, M.; Hudkins, K.L.; Alpers, C.E. Foam cells and the pathogenesis of kidney disease. *Curr. Opin. Nephrol. Hypertens.* **2015**, *24*, 245–251. [CrossRef]
30. Kushiyama, A.; Tanaka, K.; Hara, S.; Kawazu, S. Linking uric acid metabolism to diabetic complications. *World J. Diabetes* **2014**, *5*, 787–795. [CrossRef]
31. Nomura, J.; Busso, N.; Ives, A.; Tsujimoto, S.; Tamura, M.; So, A.; Yamanaka, Y. Febuxostat, an inhibitor of xanthine oxidase, suppresses lipopolysaccharide-induced MCP-1 production via MAPK phosphatase-1-mediated inactivation of JNK. *PLoS ONE* **2013**, *8*, e75527. [CrossRef] [PubMed]
32. Klisic, A.; Kocic, G.; Kavaric, N.; Jovanovic, M.; Stanisic, V.; Ninic, A. Body mass index is independently associated with xanthine oxidase activity in overweight/obese population. *Eat. Weight Disord.* **2020**, *25*, 9–15. [CrossRef] [PubMed]
33. Ives, A.; Nomura, J.; Martinon, F.; Roger, T.; LeRoy, D.; Miner, J.N.; Simon, G.; Busso, N.; So, A. Xanthine oxidoreductase regulates macrophage IL1beta secretion upon NLRP3 inflammasome activation. *Nat. Commun.* **2015**, *6*, 6555. [CrossRef] [PubMed]
34. Honda, T.; Hirakawa, Y.; Nangaku, M. The role of oxidative stress and hypoxia in renal disease. *Kidney Res Clin Pract.* **2019**, *38*, 414–426. [CrossRef]
35. Ratliff, B.B.; Abdulmahdi, W.; Pawar, R.; Wolin, M.S. Oxidant Mechanisms in Renal Injury and Disease. *Antioxid. Redox Signal.* **2016**, *25*, 119–146. [CrossRef]

36. Ruan, X.Z.; Moorhead, J.F.; Varghese, Z. Lipid redistribution in renal dysfunction. *Kidney Int.* **2008**, *74*, 407–409. [CrossRef]
37. Laurencikiene, J.; van Harmelen, V.; Arvidsson Nordstrom, E.; Dicker, A.; Blomqvist, L.; Naslund, E.; Langin, D.; Arner, P.; Ryden, M. NF-kappaB is important for TNF-alpha-induced lipolysis in human adipocytes. *J. Lipid Res.* **2007**, *48*, 1069–1077. [CrossRef]
38. Wang, Z.; Huang, W.; Li, H.; Tang, L.; Sun, H.; Liu, Q.; Zhang, L. Synergistic action of inflammation and lipid dysmetabolism on kidney damage in rats. *Ren. Fail.* **2018**, *40*, 175–182. [CrossRef]
39. Mizuno, Y.; Yamamotoya, T.; Nakatsu, Y.; Ueda, K.; Matsunaga, Y.; Inoue, M.K.; Sakoda, H.; Fujishiro, M.; Ono, H.; Kikuchi, T.; et al. Xanthine Oxidase Inhibitor Febuxostat Exerts an Anti-Inflammatory Action and Protects against Diabetic Nephropathy Development in KK-Ay Obese Diabetic Mice. *Int. J. Mol. Sci.* **2019**, *20*, 4680. [CrossRef]
40. Kim, J.Y. Antioxidants in Sepsis. *Korean J. Crit. Care Med.* **2010**, *25*, 57–60. [CrossRef]
41. Fu, H.; Hu, Z.; Di, X.; Zhang, Q.; Zhou, R.; Du, H. Tenuigenin exhibits protective effects against LPS-induced acute kidney injury via inhibiting TLR4/NF-κB signaling pathway. *Eur. J. Pharmacol.* **2016**, *791*, 229–234. [CrossRef] [PubMed]
42. Arsenijevic, D.; Cajot, J.-F.; Dulloo, A.G.; Montani, J.-P. Uninephrectomy in rats on a fixed food intake results in adipose tissue lipolysis implicating spleen cytokines. *Front. Physiol.* **2015**, *6*, 195. [CrossRef] [PubMed]

International Journal of
*Molecular Sciences*

MDPI

*Article*

# Protective Effects of Simvastatin on Endotoxin-Induced Acute Kidney Injury through Activation of Tubular Epithelial Cells' Survival and Hindering Cytochrome C-Mediated Apoptosis

**Lana Nežić [1,*,†], Ranko Škrbić [1], Ljiljana Amidžić [2], Radoslav Gajanin [3], Zoran Milovanović [4], Eugenie Nepovimova [5], Kamil Kuča [5,6,*] and Vesna Jaćević [5,7,8,†]**

1 Department of Pharmacology, Toxicology and Clinical Pharmacology, School of Medicine, University of Banja Luka, 14 Save Mrkalja St, 78000 Banja Luka, Bosnia and Herzegovina; ranko.skrbic@med.unibl.org

2 Center for Biomedical Research, School of Medicine, University of Banja Luka, 14 Save Mrkalja St, 78000 Banja Luka, Bosnia and Herzegovina; ljiljana.amidzic@med.unibl.org

3 Institute of Pathology, University Clinical Center of Republic of Srpska, School of Medicine, University of Banja Luka, 12 Beba St, 78000 Banja Luka, Bosnia and Herzegovina; radoslav.gajanin@med.unibl.org

4 Special Police Unit, Police Department of the City of Belgrade, Ministry of Interior, Trebevićka 12/A, 11030 Belgrade, Serbia; tinahoks41@gmail.com

5 Department of Chemistry, Faculty of Science, University of Hradec Kralove, Rokitanského 62, 500 03 Hradec Králové, Czech Republic; evzenie.n@seznam.cz (E.N.); v_jacevic@yahoo.com (V.J.)

6 Biomedical Research Center, University Hospital Hradec Kralove, 500 02 Hradec Kralove, Czech Republic

7 Department for Experimental Toxicology and Pharmacology, National Poison Control Centre, Military Medical Academy, 11 Crnotravska St, 11000 Belgrade, Serbia

8 Department of Pharmacological Sciences, Medical Faculty of the Military Medical Academy, the University of Defence in Belgrade, 17 Crnotravska St, 11000 Belgrade, Serbia

* Correspondence: lana.nezic@med.unibl.org (L.N.); kamil.kuca@uhk.cz (K.K.); Tel.: +387-66-125222 (L.N.); +420-603289 (K.K.)

† These authors contributed equally to this work.

Received: 6 September 2020; Accepted: 28 September 2020; Published: 30 September 2020

check for updates

**Abstract:** Increasing evidence suggests that apoptosis of tubular cells and renal inflammation mainly determine the outcome of sepsis-associated acute kidney injury (AKI). The study aim was to investigate the molecular mechanism involved in the renoprotective effects of simvastatin in endotoxin (lipopolysaccharide, LSP)-induced AKI. A sepsis model was established by intraperitoneal injection of a single non-lethal LPS dose after short-term simvastatin pretreatment. The severity of the inflammatory injury was expressed as renal damage scores (RDS). Apoptosis of tubular cells was detected by Terminal deoxynucleotidyl transferase-mediated dUTP Nick End Labeling (TUNEL assay) (apoptotic DNA fragmentation, expressed as an apoptotic index, AI) and immunohistochemical staining for cleaved caspase-3, cytochrome C, and anti-apoptotic Bcl-xL and survivin. We found that endotoxin induced severe renal inflammatory injury (RDS = 3.58 ± 0.50), whereas simvastatin dose-dependently prevented structural changes induced by LPS. Furthermore, simvastatin 40 mg/kg most profoundly attenuated tubular apoptosis, determined as a decrease of cytochrome C, caspase-3 expression, and AIs ($p < 0.01$ vs. LPS). Conversely, simvastatin induced a significant increase of Bcl-XL and survivin, both in the strong inverse correlations with cleaved caspase-3 and cytochrome C. Our study indicates that simvastatin has cytoprotective effects against LPS-induced tubular apoptosis, seemingly mediated by upregulation of cell-survival molecules, such as Bcl-XL and survivin, and inhibition of the mitochondrial cytochrome C and downstream caspase-3 activation.

**Keywords:** simvastatin; endotoxin; tubular apoptosis; cytochrome C; Bcl-XL; survivin

## 1. Introduction

Acute kidney injury (AKI) is one of the major complications of sepsis-induced multiple organ failure and is accompanied by high mortality [1]. During sepsis, a major mechanism of AKI includes severe inflammation in the renal parenchyma, heterogeneous distortion of microvascular flow at the peritubular and glomerular levels, and severe tubular epithelial injury and apoptosis [1,2].

Lipopolysaccharide (LPS), an endotoxin from the Gram-negative bacteria, has been identified as the major factor associated with the development of sepsis-associated AKI [3]. Proinflammatory cytokine, tumor necrosis factor-$\alpha$ (TNF-$\alpha$), has a crucial role in the pathogenesis of the AKI caused by endotoxemia, leading to renal inflammatory injury, and acute tubular cell apoptosis presumably by activation of the extrinsic apoptotic pathway [1,4]. The pleiotropic cytokine TNF-$\alpha$ has a particular role in the initiation of cell-survival signaling molecules such as upregulation of anti-apoptotic molecules Bcl-2, and survivin (an inhibitor of apoptosis—IAP) through activation of nuclear factor-kappa (NF-κB) [5]. In addition to the severe inflammatory syndrome, LPS activates Toll-like receptor 4 (TLR4) that is present in the membrane of immune cells and renal tubular epithelial cells, triggering the excessive release of proinflammatory cytokines, oxidative stress, and tubular cell apoptosis [3,6]. Severe tubular cell apoptosis plays an important role in LPS-induced AKI, showing caspase-3-positivity in tubular epithelial cells even at the early phase of AKI [3,7].

Mitochondrial dysfunction and damage are confirmed in the LPS and cecal ligation puncture (CLP) model of septic AKI. Oxidative stress has also been known to contribute to the overproduction of mitochondrial reactive oxygen species (ROS) and early mitochondrial dysfunction after the LPS challenge, which triggers intrinsic apoptosis through the release of pro-apoptotic cytochrome C into the cytosol and activating the caspase cascade. Importantly, antiapoptotic Bcl-2 members, such as Bcl-XL, inhibit cell death by blocking of the cytochrome C release from mitochondria and thereby prevent downstream caspases' (caspase-9, -3, -7) activation [1,2,8,9].

Consistent with these results, LPS-induced AKI and renal tubular cells apoptosis were ameliorated by novel potential agents, such as a pluripotent autocrine growth factor progranulin, an anion transporter uncoupling protein 2 [10], the bee venom [11], and peroxiredoxin protein DJ-1 (Parkinson disease protein 7, Park7) [12], as well as by vitamin D that suppressed p53-upregulated modulator of apoptosis (PUMA) and upregulated expression of a Bcl-2 family antiapoptotic protein [13]. Thus, an LPS-induced AKI model has been commonly recognized to study the pathophysiology of renal tissue injury and tubular cell apoptosis and to evaluate potential new therapeutic agents for this medical condition [2,3].

Numerous experimental studies demonstrated that statins, well-known lipid-lowering drugs, improved survival, and prevent tissue and organ injuries in local inflammation [14] or sepsis induced by LPS or CLP [15,16]. By inhibition of hydroxy-3-methylglutaryl-CoA (HMG-CoA), reductase statins block the mevalonate pathway and activation of intermediate products involved in cell signaling pathways, such as apoptosis or cell survival. One previous study showed that atorvastatin ameliorated contrast-induced nephropathy and reduced the extent of renal tubular cell apoptosis that is associated with the decreased expression of proapoptotic Bax/caspase-3 and increased Bcl-2 [17]. Another study that demonstrated the renoprotective effects of pitavastatin on cisplatin-induced AKI pointed to suppression of the mitogen-activated protein kinase (MAPK)/NF-kB/inflammation axis and intrinsic apoptotic pathway [18].

In the context of the experimental sepsis, we have previously shown that simvastatin improved survival rate and significantly suppressed LPS-induced over-production of proinflammatory cytokines, TNF$\alpha$ and interleukin (IL)-1$\beta$ [19]. Furthermore, the cell-protective effect of simvastatin pretreatment against LPS has been confirmed on cardiomyocytes [20], hepatocytes, and spleen lymphocytes [21]. These results showed that pretreatment with simvastatin mitigated myocardial, liver, and spleen tissue injuries, and decreased activation of the cleaved caspase-3 along to the reduced apoptotic-cell death in the parenchyma. Simvastatin targets the cell-survival signaling pathway survivin/NF-κB/p65 and anti-apoptotic Bcl-XL in these cells, which appears a protective mechanism in response to LPS-induced tissue injury and programmed cell death [20,21].

Therefore, the present study was designed to determine whether pretreatment with simvastatin (1) ameliorates LPS-induced AKI, and, if it does, (2) to elucidate its role in hindering apoptotic death-inducing pathways in the tubular epithelial cells, and (3) subsequent upregulation of cell-survival mechanisms like survivin and Bcl-XL.

## 2. Results

### 2.1. Protective Effects of Simvastatin on the LPS-Induced Acute Renal Injury

Renal specimens taken from the control rats revealed the normal histological structure of the glomeruli and renal tubules (Figure 1A). Treatment with LPS only (Figure 1B) induced congestion and small multifocal hemorrhages in the cortical and interstitial blood vessels with the presence of polymorphonuclear leukocytes (PMNL) infiltrate. Glomerular lesions were characterized by increased numbers of epithelial cells and pericapilar infiltration by PMNL and erythrocytes, predominantly. Both proximal and distal convoluted tubules showed diffuse epithelial cell swelling, loss of brush border, vacuolar degeneration, and focal necrosis. These changes were correlated with the RDS of 3.58 ± 0.50 confirming the LPS-induced severe renal damage (Table 1). Pretreatment with simvastatin 10 mg/kg reduced histopathological changes (RDS = 2.67 ± 0.48, not significantly vs. LPS group). Renal histopathological examination in the simvastatin 20 group (Figure 1C) showed the decreased intensity of tissue damage with the distinct renal tubular epithelial cell swelling and degeneration. Only individual glomeruli showed hypercellularity, with increased numbers of both resident cells and infiltrating leukocytes, indicative of the significantly lower RDS of 2.33 ± 0.47 ($p < 0.05$ vs. control and vs. LPS group, respectively). Renal histology in the simvastatin 40 group was mostly unchanged and showed mild edema and hyperemia, rare small hemorrhages, and a single PNML infiltration throughout the cortex with irregular swelling of renal tubular cells. A mean RDS was minimal, 1.42 ± 0.50, in comparison to the LPS ($p < 0.01$). Semiquantitative assessment of renal tissue lesions reveals that simvastatin ameliorated LPS-induced histopathological changes in a dose-dependent manner (Figure 1C,D).

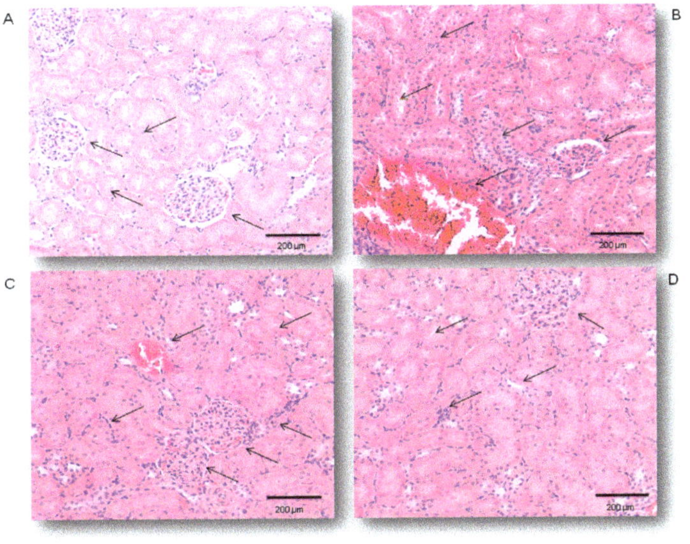


**Figure 1.** Protective effects of simvastatin pretreatment against LPS-induced acute renal damages, Hematoxylin and Eosin (H&E) method, 200× magnified images, black arrows indicates the gromeruls

and tubules. (**A**) Appearance of renal tissue of control animals, (**B**) renal tissue challenged with LPS, (**C**) renal tissue from simvastatin 20 group, (**D**) renal tissue from simvastatin 40 group. Histopathological analysis revealed decreased renal inflammatory damages in both simvastatin-treated groups, while severe alterations persisted only in the LPS-treated group.

**Table 1.** The effects of different treatments on the degree of renal alterations—Renal Damage Score (RDS)

| Treatment (mg/kg) | Renal Damage Score (6 Kidneys/Group × 6 Slices/Kidney) | | | | | $\overline{X} \pm$ S.D. |
|---|---|---|---|---|---|---|
| | 0 | 1 | 2 | 3 | 4 | |
| Control | 30 | 6 | 0 | 0 | 0 | 0.67 ± 0.48 |
| LPS | 0 | 0 | 0 | 15 | 21 | 3.58 ± 0.50 $a^3$ |
| Simvastatin 10 group | 0 | 0 | 12 | 24 | 0 | 2.67 ± 0.48 $a^1$ |
| Simvastatin 20 group | 0 | 0 | 24 | 12 | 0 | 2.33 ± 0.47 $a^1$ |
| Simvastatin 40 group | 0 | 21 | 15 | 0 | 0 | 1.42 ± 0.50 $b^2$ |

Statistical analysis was performed using the Kruskal–Wallis test. $a^1$, $a^3$—$p < 0.05$, 0.001 in comparison to the control group, $b^2$—$p < 0.01$ in comparison to the LPS-only treated group. ($\overline{X}$—mean value, S.D—standard deviation).

## 2.2. *Simvastatin Inhibited Cleaved Caspase-3 Expression and Apoptotic Cell Death of Renal Tubular Epithelial Cells Induced by LPS*

Occurrence and the extent of apoptosis of the renal tubular epithelium was assessed based on the expression of cleaved caspase-3 and confirmed by the TUNEL assay with quantification of apoptotic index (AIs, see Methods and Materials Section) (Figure 2A–D and Figure 3A–D). We analyzed tissue sections challenged with simvastatin of 20 and 40 mg/kg, as the dose of 10 mg/kg did not show a significant protective effect on RDS. LPS induced cleavage of caspase-3 (active molecule) predominantly in the renal tubular epithelial cells, characteristically localized in the cytoplasm and perinuclear region of apoptotic cells. As shown in Figure 2, a substantial increase of cleaved caspase-3 expression in the LPS group (43.6% ± 4.4%, $p < 0.01$ vs. control group), was the most profoundly reduced with simvastatin 40 mg/kg (17.2% ± 2.9%, $p < 0.01$ vs. LPS group, and $p < 0.05$ vs. simvastatin 20 group), showing also and dose-dependent efficacy (Figures 2 and 3E).

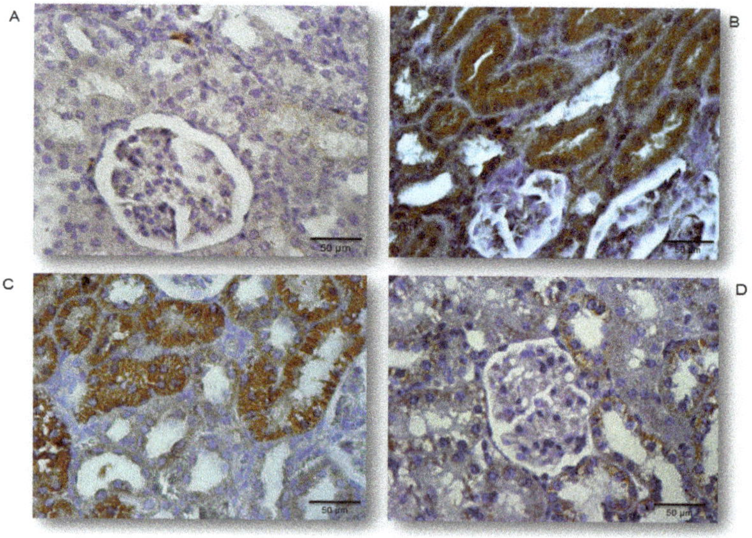


**Figure 2.** Representative images of apoptotic renal tubular epithelial cells that were challenged with

LPS or pretreated with simvastatin prior to LPS, simvastatin 20 mg/kg or 40 mg/kg, respectively. Attenuation of the renal apoptosis induced by LPS shown as decreased cleaved caspase-3 expression in the tubular epithelial cells, assessed by immunohistochemistry, magnification 400×. (**A**) The control group, (**B**) intense cytoplasmic staining of cleaved caspase 3 in the tubular epithelium in the LPS group, as one of the feature of apoptotic cell, significant reduction of apoptotic cells in the groups treated with simvastatin 20 mg/kg (**C**) and 40 mg/kg, respectively (**D**).

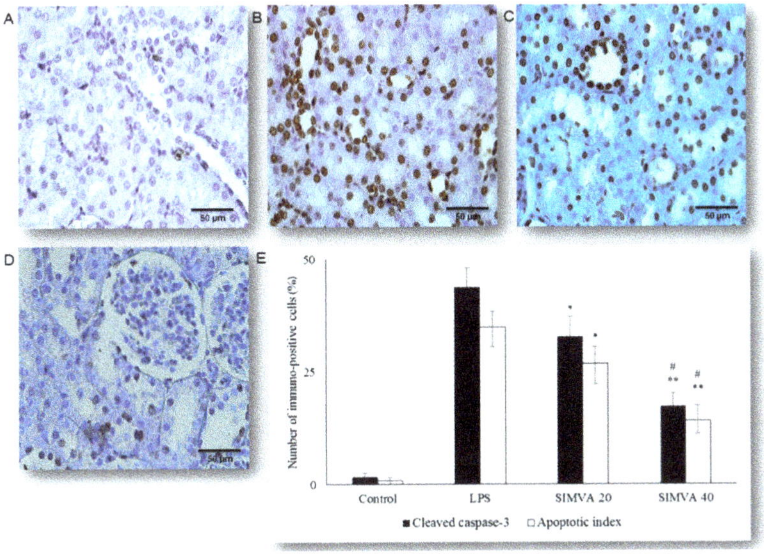


**Figure 3.** Simvastatin inhibited apoptosis of renal tubular epithelial cells in inflammatory injury induced by LPS, confirmed by TUNEL assay, magnification 400×. The apoptotic indices (AI) are based on the relative number of brown stained nuclei (TUNEL-positive renal tubular epithelial cells) and showed significant increase in the LPS group (**B**), simvastatin 20 mg/kg (**C**), and 40 mg/kg group (**D**) respectively, compared with the control group (**A**). LPS challenge led to a marked increase of TUNEL-positive tubular epithelial cells (shown as AIs in white columns AIs) while the AIs were significantly decreased in the simvastatin groups. Quantitative comparison of the immunohistochemically stained renal tissue for cleaved caspase 3 and the TUNEL positive tubular epithelial cells expressed as AIs (* $p < 0.05$ vs. LPS group, ** $p < 0.05$ vs. simvastatin 20 group, # $p < 0.01$ vs. LPS group) (**E**).

Definite apoptosis was confirmed with the TUNEL assay that detected chromatin condensation and DNA fragmentation, with the main features of apoptosis shown as dark brown nuclei (Figure 3). The apoptotic indices, as the degrees of apoptosis in renal tissue, significantly increased after LPS administration (in all experimental treated groups) compared with the control ($p < 0.01$), but they were markedly decreased in the group with simvastatin 20 (AI = 26.7% ± 3.7%, $p < 0.05$) and simvastatin 40 group (AI = 14.0% ± 3.3%, $p < 0.01$) in respect to the LPS group (AI = 34.8% ± 3.6%) (Figure 3). Immunohistochemical staining and TUNEL assay revealed insignificant differences in the cleaved caspase-3 expression (total number of immuno-positive cells) compared to the AIs, that were strongly positively correlated across the experimental groups ($p < 0.05$) (Figure 3E). This could be explained by the fact that cytoplasmic immune-positivity of cleaved caspase-3 represents both apoptotic and the cells in pre-apoptosis without condensation of chromatin (TUNEL-positive cells) and with preserved cellular morphology.

## 2.3. Simvastatin Attenuated Expression of Pro-Apoptotic Cytochrome C in Renal Tubular Epithelial Cells after LPS Administration

To further investigate an apoptotic pathway targeted by simvastatin in LPS-induced AKI, we assessed mitochondrial pro-apoptotic marker, cytochrome C. The control group showed minimal immunostaining in the sporadic tubular epithelial cells. LPS administration increased expression of cytochrome C, quantified as the intense brown cytoplasmic staining in the affected tubular cells (45.11% ± 4.14%). Conversely, simvastatin markedly mitigated LPS-induced cytochrome C expression in comparison to the LPS group (Figure 4A–D). Consistently, quantitative analysis of cytochrome C immunopositivity showed a significant difference among groups ($p < 0.05$ in simvastatin 20 group and $p < 0.01$ in simvastatin 40 group vs. LPS, respectively), while very strong positive correlations between apoptotic markers, cleaved caspase-3, and cytochrome C were determined across the groups ($p = 0.01$).

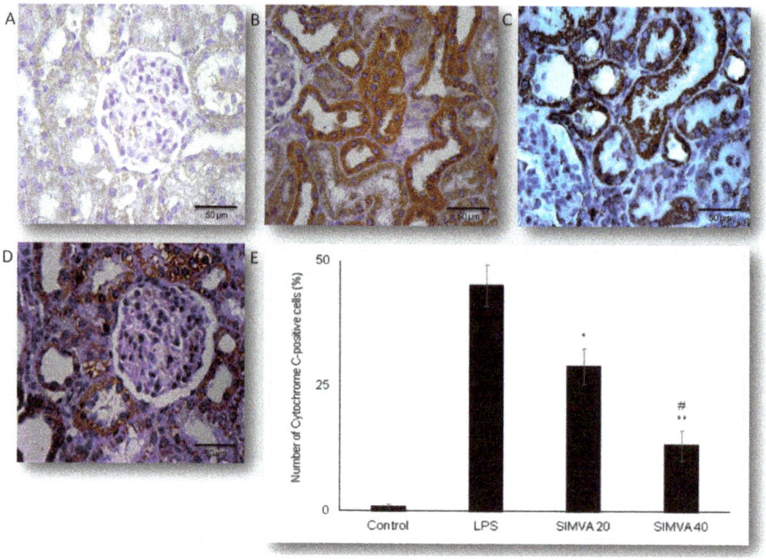


**Figure 4.** Simvastatin attenuated cytochrome C expression in renal tubular epithelial cells after LPS-administration. The expression of cytochrome C in rat renal tissue examined by immunohistochemical staining, magnification 400×, (**A**) negative immunostaining in the control group, (**B**) intense brown cytoplasmic staining in the tubular epithelium in the LPS group indicates increased expression of the pro-apoptotic protein cytochrome C. A significant decrease of cytochrome C-positive cells in the groups pretreated with simvastatin 20 mg/kg (**C**) and 40 mg/kg group (**D**), respectively. A quantitative analysis of cytochrome C-positive renal tubular epithelial cells assessed in the immunohistochemically stained sections in the renal tissue (* $p < 0.05$ vs. LPS group, ** $p < 0.01$ vs. simvastatin 20 group, # $p < 0.01$ vs. LPS group) (**E**).

## 2.4. Expression of Anti-Apoptotic Bcl-XL in Renal Tubular Epithelial Cells after Simvastatin and LPS Administration

Expression of anti-apoptotic Bcl-xL in renal tubular epithelial cells significantly differed among LPS and simvastatin groups (Figure 5). Immuno-positive Bcl-XL renal tubular cells were sporadically determined in the control, and significantly in the LPS groups (36.4%, $p < 0.05$ vs. control) (Figure 5A,B). Upregulation of Bcl-XL implied that LPS might trigger a potential cell self-protective mechanism against the intrinsic apoptotic pathway. Pretreatment with simvastatin 20 mg/kg and simvastatin 40 mg/kg produced a gradual and significant increase in Bcl-xL expression in the tubular cells compared to the LPS group (56.4% ± 4.8%, $p < 0.05$ and 71.6% ;± 4.9%, $p < 0.01$, respectively), showing intensive brown cytoplasmic staining (Figure 5A–E). To compare the expression of key apoptotic proteins and Bcl-XL in tubular cells in the treated groups, we analyzed their correlations (Figure 6). The result showed the strong inverse correlation between Bcl-XL and cleaved caspase-3-positive cells in the simvastatin 20 group ($R^2 = 0.61$, $p < 0.05$) and simvastatin 40 group ($R^2 = 0.78$, $p < 0.05$) group. As it is shown (Figure 7), Bcl-XL expression is in a very strong negative correlation with cytochrome C in the simvastatin 40 group ($R^2 = 0.81$, $p < 0.05$), similarly as in the simvastatin 20 group, suggesting that through induction of anti-apoptotic Bcl-XL, simvastatin might express a cell-protective mechanism.

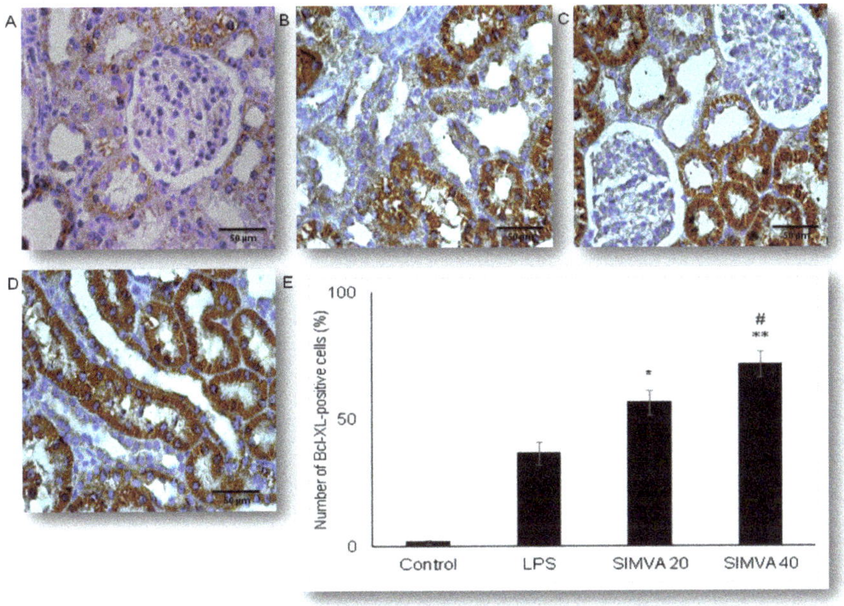


**Figure 5.** Simvastatin increased Bcl-XL expression in renal tubular epithelial cells after LPS administration. The expression of Bcl-XL in renal tissue was examined by immunohistochemical staining, magnification 400×, (**A**) the control group showed rare immuno-positive cells, (**B**) note Bcl-XL-expression in the tubular epithelial cells in the LPS group, in simvastatin 20 mg/kg (**C**) and 40 mg/kg group (**D**), respectively. Bcl-XL expression significantly increased, and it is determined as intensive brown cytoplasmic staining widely distributed in renal tubular epithelial cells. (**E**) A quantitative analysis of Bcl-XL-positive renal tubular epithelial cells assessed in immunohistochemically stained sections of the renal tissue (* $p < 0.05$ vs. LPS group, ** $p < 0.05$ vs. simvastatin 20 group, # $p < 0.01$ vs. LPS group).

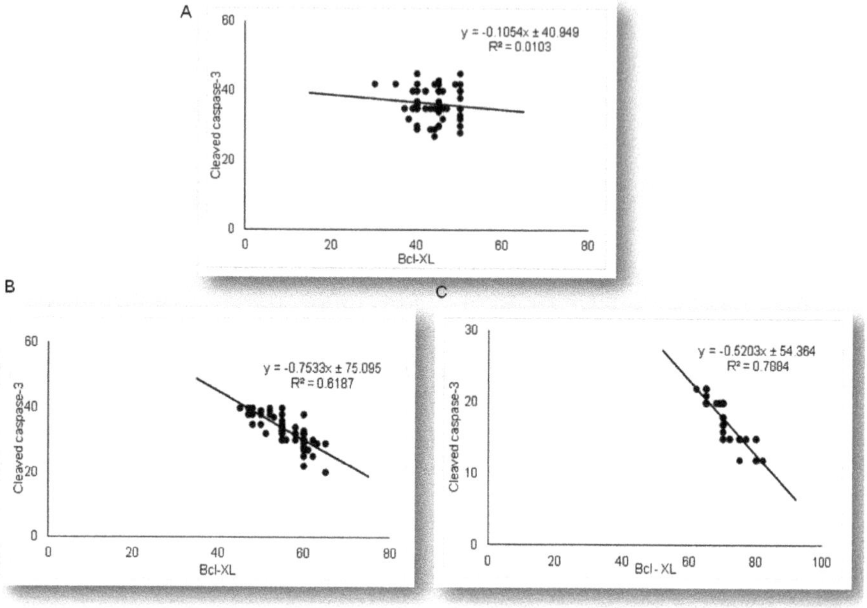


**Figure 6.** The correlations are shown for Bcl-XL and cleaved-caspase-3 in the renal tubular epithelial cells: (**A**) LPS group only, (**B**) simvastatin 20 mg/kg group, (**C**) simvastatin 40 mg/kg group.

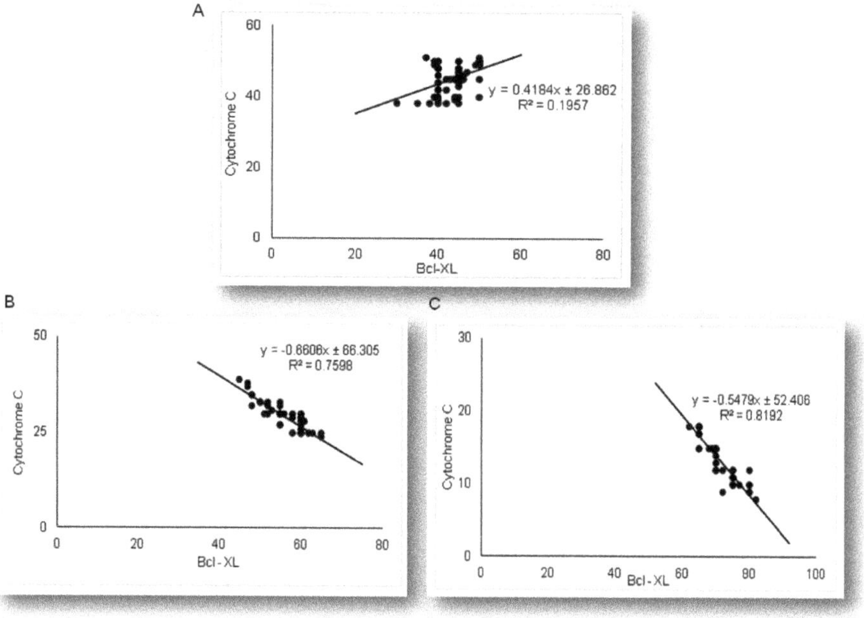


**Figure 7.** The correlations are shown for Bcl-XL and cytochrome C in the renal tubular epithelial cells: (**A**) LPS group only, (**B**) simvastatin 20 mg/kg group, (**C**) simvastatin 40 mg/kg group.

### 2.5. Simvastatin Enhanced Survivin Expression in Renal Tubular Epithelial Cells after LPS Administration

As the results demonstrated that simvastatin enhanced Bcl-XL expression in renal tubular epithelial cells after LPS administration, we further analyzed if simvastatin upregulates expression of a downstream inhibitor of apoptosis, survivin (Figure 8). Weak cytoplasmic staining assessed as positive survivin expression in the control was considered as its basal expression (Figure 8A). The LPS challenge resulted in a marked increase of survivin expression in tubular cells ($p < 0.05$ vs. control group), suggesting that survivin itself presents a cell-protective mechanism in LPS injury (Figure 8B). Further results demonstrated that simvastatin induced cell survival pathways, showing a dose-dependent increase in strong cytoplasmic expression of survivin (Figure 8C,D). Quantitative analysis revealed that pretreatment in simvastatin 20 and 40 groups led to a striking increase of survivin expression (49.5% ± 4.7% and 73.3% ± 5.3% vs. LPS group, $p < 0.01$, respectively) (Figure 8E). As survivin is one of the IAPs, we tested its correlation with cleaved caspase-3 and cytochrome C. As illustrated in Figure 9, strong inverse correlations were determined between survivin and cleaved caspase-3 in simvastatin 20 and 40 groups ($R^2 = 0.71$ and $R^2 = 0.83$, $p < 0.01$, respectively). Consistently, Pearson's correlation analysis revealed a strong inverse correlation of survivin with cytochrome C-positive tubular cells in simvastatin 20 and 40 groups ($R^2 = 0.69$ and $R^2 = 0.85$, $p < 0.01$, respectively) (Figure 10), suggesting that simvastatin protects tubular cells in LPS-induced AKI by inhibiting key apoptotic proteins of the intrinsic pathway and activates cell-survival mechanisms.

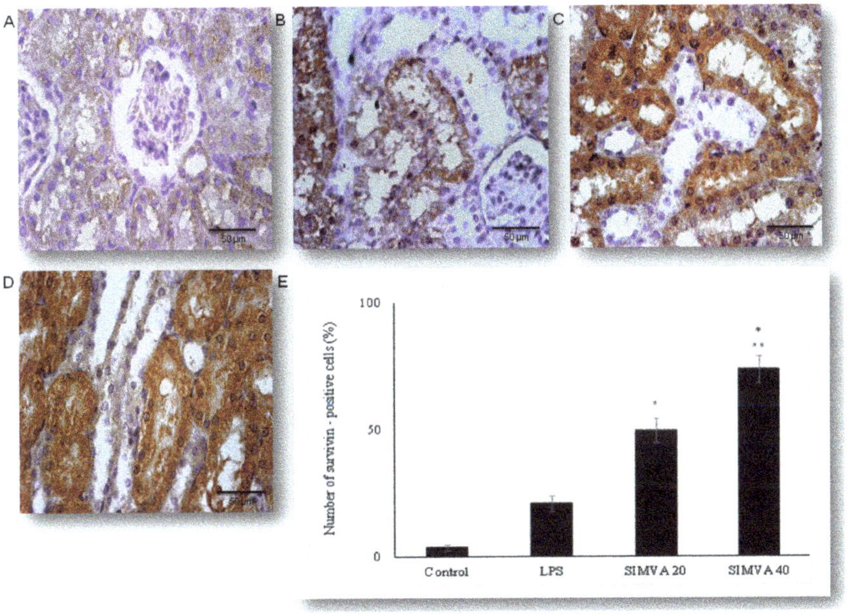


**Figure 8.** Simvastatin increased survivin expression in renal tubular epithelial cells after LPS administration. The expression of survivin in renal tissue examined by immunohistochemical staining, magnification 400×, (**A**) the control group showed rare immuno-positive cell, (**B**) note immuno-positive survivin cells in the LPS group, in simvastatin 20 group (**C**), and simvastatin 40 group (**D**), survivin expression significantly increased, and it is determined as intensive brown cytoplasmic staining widely distributed in renal tubular epithelial cells. (**E**) A quantitative analysis of survivin-positive renal tubular epithelial cells assessed in immunohistochemically stained sections of the renal tissue (* $p < 0.01$ vs. LPS group, ** $p < 0.05$ vs. simvastatin 20 group).

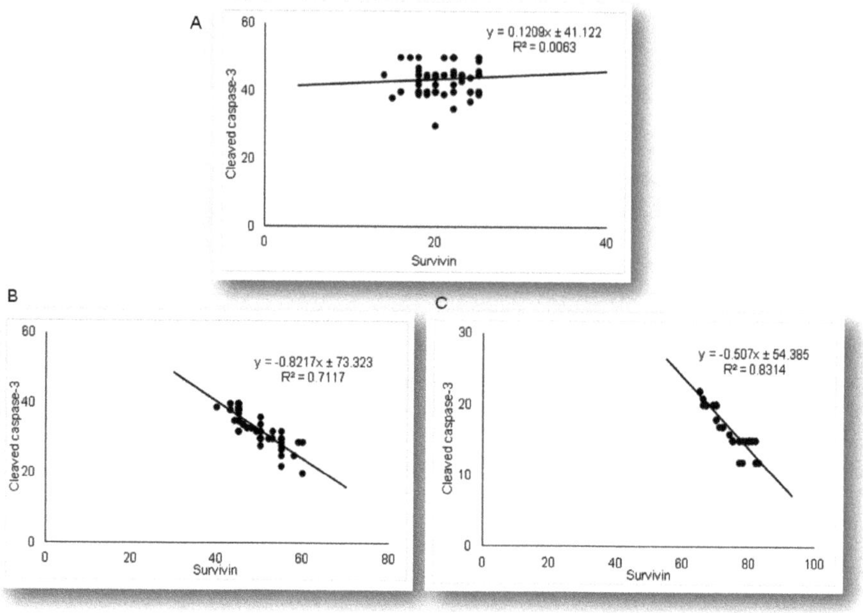


**Figure 9.** The correlations are shown for survivin and cleaved-caspase-3 in the renal tubular epithelial cells: (**A**) LPS group only, (**B**) simvastatin 20 mg/kg group, (**C**) simvastatin 40 mg/kg group.

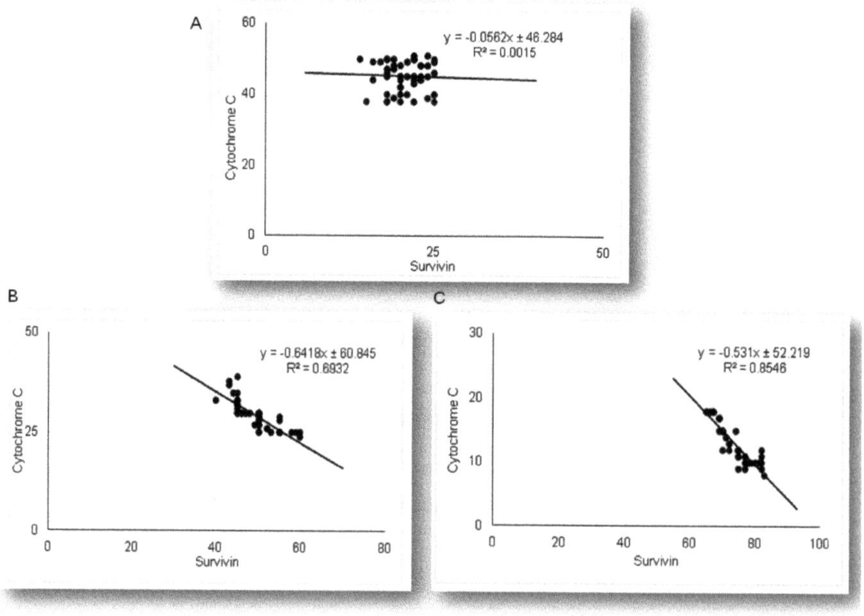


**Figure 10.** The correlations are shown for survivin and cytochrome C in the renal tubular epithelial cells: (**A**) LPS, (**B**) simvastatin 20 mg/kg group, (**C**) simvastatin 40 mg/kg group.

## 3. Discussion

In the present study, a standard model of AKI induced by LPS was used to investigate the renoprotective effects of simvastatin on apoptotic signaling molecules in the development of AKI. The main findings indicate that without simvastatin, LPS severely damaged renal tissue, mainly due to induction of glomerular cell proliferation and tubular epithelial cell apoptosis mediated by a mitochondrial apoptotic pathway leading to caspase-3 cleavage. In contrast, with simvastatin pretreatment, the rats were protected against LPS-induced renal inflammatory injury, that is confirmed by attenuated apoptosis of tubular epithelial cells, and significantly increased expression of anti-apoptotic molecules, Bcl-XL and survivin. These results demonstrate that inhibition of cytochrome C apoptotic cascade and activation of IAP might be a mechanism of simvastatin cell-protective effects against bacterial toxin-associated AKI.

Growing experimental evidence has shown that pretreatment with statins prevents tissue injuries induced by bacterial toxins [20–24]. Consistently, our work and the studies by Apaya et al. [25] and Ozkok et al. [26] demonstrated that simvastatin attenuated LPS-induced renal injury, seen as a significantly reduced amount of infiltrating leukocytes associated with minimal histopathological features. It has been known that LPS/TLR4 signaling triggers systemic inflammation but also local renal inflammatory injury and apoptosis through the proinflammatory cytokines TNF-$\alpha$ release, to induce AKI [13]. Our previous results showed that simvastatin dose-dependently decreased overproduction of TNF-$\alpha$ and IL-1$\beta$ in endotoxemia [19], therefore it is conceivable that in this study, simvastatin targets both inflammatory pathways to protect renal tubules against LPS.

Statins are known to have potent renoprotective effects in gentamicin-, cisplatin-, and cyclosporine-induced nephrotoxicity by a variety of mechanisms, ranging from antioxidant, anti-inflammatory, and anti-apoptotic effects [27]. However, to our knowledge, simvastatin suppression of tubular cell apoptosis in AKI associated with a septic condition has not been reported. Here, we showed that one of the potential protective mechanisms of simvastatin against AKI is blockade of renal tubular cell apoptosis, confirmed by reduced cytochrome C and cleaved caspase-3 expression and corresponding DNA fragmentation. Interestingly, results of antiapoptotic actions of simvastatin through inhibition of pro-apoptotic Bim/Bax and effectors caspases have been well documented in hepatocytes and lymphocytes, and cardiomyocyte in other's and our previous studies [20,21,28,29].

Ultrastructural changes and dysfunctions of renal epithelial mitochondria appear to be an underlying mechanism in septic AKI, similarly to other sepsis-induced multi-organ failure [1,8]. A recent study by Liu et al. [9] showed dominant mitochondrial-mediated apoptosis in CLP-induced AKI with notable leakage of cytochrome C, followed by activation of downstream caspase-9 and -3, and disturbance of mitochondrial dynamics. In the present study, we observed that simvastatin abolished an LPS-induced significant increase of cytochrome C in renal tubular cells. This observation tightly correlates with a marked inhibition of cleaved caspase-3 in simvastatin groups, indicating its cell-protective mechanism against LPS.

Importantly, Bcl-2-related antiapoptotic protein such as Bcl-XL, control outer mitochondrial membrane integrity, bind to proapoptotic Bim/Bax proteins, and inhibit cell-death by preventing the release of pro-apoptotic factors such as cytochrome C or apoptosis-inducing factor [8,30]. Our results showed overexpression of Bcl-XL in tubular cells in simvastatin groups, accompanied by significantly decreased cytochrome C.

Consistently, our previous studies demonstrated that simvastatin upregulated Bcl-XL expression in LPS-challenged organs [20,21], while vitamin D or glycyrrhizin acid, an active ingredient of licorice, by targeting Bcl-2, suppressed tubular apoptosis, and markedly prevented LPS-induced AKI [13,31]. As Bcl-XL is one of the key anti-apoptotic proteins in renal tubular cells, our findings strongly suggest that simvastatin controls apoptosis by targeting Bcl-2 proteins and inhibiting cytochrome C.

Survivin, the unique member of the IAPs family, has a dual cellular role in the regulation of mitosis and inhibition of apoptosis. Biological functions of survivin depend on localization, so that in the cytosol (mitochondrial survivin), it initiates anti-apoptotic activity by blockade caspase cascade, while nuclear localization enables cell division. Cytoprotection by survivin is more selective and appears to target the cascade of mitochondrial cytochrome C-mediated apoptosis in order to prevent caspase-9 and downstream caspase-3 activation [5,32,33]. Previous studies have demonstrated that survivin, expressed dominantly in the proximal tubular cells, prevents development of AKI and renal apoptosis induced by various nephrotoxins (such as folic acid, cisplatin) by suppression of expression of the p53 gene [34,35] and in ischemia/reperfusion (I/R) injury through activation of the Notch-2 intracellular signaling pathway [36]. Our results have demonstrated increased cytoplasmic survivin expression in renal tubular cells in response to LPS that we assumed as induction of a cell-protection mechanism. Further, simvastatin induced intense and dose-dependent expression of survivin in the tubular epithelium that is inversely correlated with cytochrome C and cleaved caspase-3 respectively, and indicates its evident anti-apoptotic effects. Because our previous studies indicated an important role of survivin/NF-κB/p65 pathway activation in cytoprotection against LPS-injury [20,21], similar to Wilson et al. [37], in CLP-induced cardiomyopathy, we hypothesized that simvastatin has significant cell-protective effects in septic AKI but not only by inhibiting of apoptotic cell death but through induction of the important intracellular survival pathways in renal tubular epithelium.

## 4. Materials and Methods

### 4.1. Experimental Animals

Adult Wistar rats, 6–8 weeks old (200–220 g), raised at the Institute for Biomedical Researches, Military Medical Academy, Belgrade, Republic of Serbia, were used in this trial.

A typical macrolon plastic cage (Bioscape, Castrop-Rauxel, Germany) filled with clear sawdust (Versele-Laga, Deinze, Belgium) was used for experimental animals' housing. Ambient conditions, the temperature of 22 ± 2 °C, the humidity of 55% ± 15%, air changes/h of 15–20, and the light/dark cycle of 12/12 h, in the animal housing room were centrally regulated. A commercial diet mixture for rats (Veterinary Institute Subotica, Subotica, Republic of Serbia) and tap water ad libitum were applied for animals' feeding.

Before the start of the study, the experimental design, laboratory protocol, and welfare of the experimental animals were approved by the Ethics Committee of Experimental Animals of the Military Medical Academy, Belgrade, Serbia (No. 282-12/2002). This decision confirmed that in the complete experimental study, animal care and all treatments throughout the research are in compliance with Directive 2010/63/EU on the protection of animals used for scientific purposes and the Guidelines for Animal Welfare adopted by the Republic of Serbia (No. 323-07-04943/2014-05/1).

### 4.2. Drugs

The drug used in the experiment, simvastatin (donation for research purposes only, from pharmaceutical company Krka, Novo Mesto, Slovenia), was prepared in 0.5% methylcellulose as 10 or 20 mg/mL stocks.

Lipopolysaccharide (LPS, endotoxin, producer Sigma Aldrich, Munich, Germany), serotype 0127:B8 *Escherichia coli* was dissolved with sterile pyrogen-free physiologic saline and administered intraperitoneally (i.p.) immediately after dilution.

Each invasive procedure in animals was operated under aseptic conditions.

### 4.3. Experimental Design

In the model of experimental sepsis, we used endotoxin, and challenged the experimental animals with a non-lethal single dose of LPS i.p. (0.25 $LD_{50}$/kg). This experimental sepsis is a widely accepted model that is featured with high-grade acute systemic inflammation, inflammatory infiltration, increased oxidative stress, and apoptosis of organ tissues [14,38,39]. Simvastatin was administered in the three different dose regimens (10, 20, and 40 mg/kg p.o.), that was confirmed in our previous experiments as the doses that completely protect the animals against the single median lethal dose

($LD_{50}$) of 22.15 mg/kg i.p. of LPS in rats (95% CI 16.5–29.1) [19]. The dose selection of simvastatin was based on the previous rat/murine in vivo studies where the dose range was 10–100 mg/kg/day, considering a rapid upregulation (3- to 10-fold) of HMG-CoA reductase's activity induced by statin treatment or other inhibitors in rodents. Therefore, the simvastatin doses in this experiment were higher compared to those recommended in clinical medicines [14,40,41].

A total of 30 animals were divided into five experimental groups and received the following treatments: (1) Control group (0.5% methylcellulose 1 mL/kg i.p.), (2) LPS group (non-lethal dose as 0.25 $LD_{50}$/kg i.p., that is equal to 5.5 mg/kg of LPS i.p.), (3) Simvastatin 10 group (simvastatin 10 mg/kg p.o. + 0.25 $LD_{50}$/kg LPS i.p.), (4) Simvastatin 20 group (simvastatin 20 mg/kg p.o. + 0.25 $LD_{50}$/kg LPS i.p.), and (5) Simvastatin 40 group (simvastatin 40 mg/kg p.o. + 0.25 $LD_{50}$/kg LPS i.p.).

After dissolution, simvastatin was given per os via oral gavage in the short-term treatment of 5 days, and the single non-lethal dose of LPS was administered 1.5 h after the simvastatin pretreatment. In the LPS group, animals received the same vehicle (1 mL/kg) of 0.5% methylcellulose for the same period as the simvastatin treatment, prior to LPS injection. The control group received an identical volume of vehicle only. After LPS administration, the animals were monitored continuously for 48 h and then sacrificed.

### 4.4. Histopathological Examination and Semiquantitative Analysis of Renal Damage Score

The renal protective effect of simvastatin was evaluated after receiving the last treatment. Before sacrification, all animals were immobilized in a dorsal position and euthanized by using sodium pentobarbital in a single dose of 30 mg/kg i.p. (Hemofarm AD, Vršac, Republic of Serbia). Shortly after the autopsy, a renal tissue sample from each animal was fixed in 10% neutral solution during the one-week period. Then, fixed renal tissue samples were divided into six equal sections, which were dehydrated in a series of alcohol (70%, 96%, and 100%) and xylene. After fitting into paraffin blocks, each 2 μm thick renal tissue section was stained using the hematoxylin and eosin (H&E) method.

The whole visual field from each renal slice was analyzed and photographed at magnification 200×, by using a light microscope connected with a digital camera (BX-45, Olympus, Tokyo, Japan) for histopathological examination, as per our method previously published in the literature [42–48]. To assess the degree of renal damages, which consists of edema, hyperemia, neutrophils infiltration, glomerular cells' proliferation, and renal hemorrhages, a semi-quantitative 5-point scale was applied as previously described [43]. The severity of renal impairment expressed as Renal Damage Score (RDS) is shown in Table 2. The exact method for RDS calculation is presented in Table 1.

**Table 2.** Tissue scoring scale for renal alterations—Renal Damage Score (RDS).

| Degree | Description |
|---|---|
| 0 | Normal finding. |
| 1 | Mild damage: Single glomerular cells slightly enlarged. Mild dilatation of small blood vessels. A few foci of inflammatory cell infiltrates. |
| 2 | Moderate damage: < 50% glomerular cells with proliferation. Severe vasodilatation associated with hyperemia and edema. Various numbers of inflammatory cells infiltrates. |
| 3 | Severe and focal damage: > 50% glomerular cells with proliferation. Transmural rupture of the blood vessels (up to 50%) associated with an accumulation of inflammatory cells. |
| 4 | Severe and diffuse damage: Complete loss of the normal glomerular architecture, and the basal membrane and endothelial cells of the blood vessels (>50%). High-intensity hemorrhages and diffuse accumulation of inflammatory cells. |

### *4.5. Detection and Quantification of Tubular Cell Apoptosis in Situ by TUNEL Method*

The TUNEL (Terminal deoxynucleotidyl transferase-mediated dUTP Nick End Labeling) assay was used to assess the apoptosis of renal tubular cells. To perform TUNEL staining on paraffin-embedded sections (4–6 μm thickness), we used the In-Situ Cell Death Detection Kit POD (Roche Molecular Biochemicals, Basel, Switzerland, Cat. No 11 684 817 910) according to the manufacturer's instructions. Renal tissue slides were incubated with anti-fluorescein antibody conjugated with horseradish peroxidase (POD), and then color development was performed using diaminobenzidine (DAB) substrate. According to these instructions, negative (incubation with Label Solution, instead of TUNEL reaction) and positive controls (incubation with DNase I recombinant, grade I) were performed.

Two blinded pathologists assessed TUNEL cells (immuno-positive reaction). The slides were examined under a light microscope (Olympus Plaza, Tokyo, Japan) at 400× magnifications. Twenty non-successive fields per sample were counted for the number of TUNEL-positive tubular cells. Apoptotic index (AI) defined as the percentage (%) of apoptotic tubular cells was calculated according to the formula (1):

$$\text{AI } (\% \text{ of apoptotic cells}) = \frac{\text{the number of TUNEL} - \text{positive tubular cells} \times 100}{\text{total number of tubular cells}} \quad (1)$$

### *4.6. Detection and Quantification of Apoptosis Regulating Molecules by Immunohistochemistry*

Paraffin-embedded sections of kidney tissues were stained with polyclonal rabbit antibodies for cleaved caspase-3 (Asp 175, Cat. 9661, Cell Signaling Technology, Frankfurt, Germany), monoclonal mouse antibody for Cytochrome C, clone 7H8.2C12 (Cat. MA5-11674, Invitrogen, Thermo Fisher Scientific, Walthman, MA, United States), polyclonal rabbit antibody for anti-apoptotic Bcl-XL (Cat. PA1-37161, Invitrogen, Thermo Fisher Scientific, Walthman, MA, United States), and monoclonal mouse antibody for survivin, clone 8E2 (Cat. MS-1201-P1 NeoMarkers Inc., Fremont, CA, The United States), according to the manufacturer's instructions.

The standard protocol was followed for the immunohistochemistry staining on 3–4 μm deparaffinized and rehydrated tissue sections. Slides were then boiled for 20 min in a microwave oven with a citric acid buffer solution (0.01 mol/L citrate buffer, pH 6.0.). To reduce nonspecific background staining, slides were incubated in 3% hydrogen peroxide for 10 min. Primary antibodies for cleaved caspase-3 (1:300), Cytochrome C (1:100), Bcl-XL (RTU), and survivin (1:50) were applied according to the manufacturer's recommended protocol. The slides were washed thoroughly with phosphate-buffered saline, pH 7.4, between the steps. 3,3′-Diaminobenzidine (DAB) (TL-015-HDJ, Thermo Scientific Lab Vision UltraVision ONE Detection System) was used as chromogen, to develop the antigen-antibody complex, and all slides were then counterstained with H&E, dehydrated, and mounted. Appropriate positive and negative controls were processed in parallel.

The slides were analyzed with a microscope (Olympus, Tokyo, Japan) at 400× magnification. For these sections, the average number of immune-positive cells (tubular cells with intensive optical density expression of cleaved caspase-3, Cytochrome C, BCL-XL, and survivin) across twenty non-successive fields was calculated by two independent pathologists in a blinded manner, using ImageJ software 1.50 (National Institute of Health, Bethesda, Rockville, MD, United States).

Quantitative measurement of the immuno-positive tubular cells was expressed according to this formula (2):

$$\% \text{ of positively stained cells } = \frac{\text{the number of positively stained tubular cells} \times 100}{\text{total number of tubular cells}} \quad (2)$$

Survivin expression was evaluated qualitatively, where tubular cells positive for cytoplasmic staining were considered immuno-positive and taken into account [33,49,50].

### 4.7. Statistical Analysis

The statistical software package SPSS 19.0. (IBM Corporation, New York, NY, The United States) was used to analyze the results which were presented as mean value ($\overline{\mathbf{X}}$) ± standard deviation (SD). To differentiate the renal damage score (RDS) as well as the expression of biomarkers among the groups, we used the Kruskal–Wallis rank test and analysis of variance (one-way ANOVA) followed by the Tamhane's T2 post hoc test, respectively. Correlation analysis was presented as Pearson's correlation coefficient. $p < 0.05$ was considered statistically significant.

## 5. Conclusions

This study broadened the current understanding of simvastatin anti-apoptotic and cytoprotective effects against LPS-induced AKI. Mechanistically, it seems that simvastatin inhibits the mitochondrial release of cytochrome C and consequent cleavage of the effector caspase-3, resulting in the blockade of tubular cells' apoptosis. Moreover, simvastatin promotes cell-survival by enhancing Bcl-XL and survivin expression, signaling molecules are known that inhibit the intrinsic apoptotic pathway mediated by cytochrome C and directly block caspase-3 respectively, and in turn, inhibits apoptosis in tubular epithelium. Based on our findings in the AKI model reported here, we suggest that using simvastatin for the prevention of AKI in septic conditions is a promising therapeutic option in targeting apoptosis, and more preclinical and clinical studies should be encouraged in this regard.

**Author Contributions:** Conceptualization, L.N., R.Š., L.A., and V.J.; methodology, L.N., L.A., Z.M., and V.J.; software, L.N., L.A., and V.J.; validation, L.N., R.Š., E.N., and V.J.; formal analysis, L.N., L.A., and V.J.; investigation, L.N., Z.M., and V.J.; resources, L.N., R.Š., R.G., E.N., K.K., and V.J.; writing—original draft preparation, L.N. and V.J.; writing—review and editing, L.N., E.N., K.K., and V.J.; visualization, L.N., L.A., and V.J.; supervision, K.K.; project administration, E.N.; funding acquisition, L.N., R.Š., E.N., K.K., and V.J. All authors have read and agreed to the published version of the manuscript.

**Funding:** This research received no external funding.

**Acknowledgments:** The research was conducted by the support given from the Ministry of Science and Technology, Republic of Srpska, Bosnia and Herzegovina. This work also supported by the University of Hradec Kralove (Faculty of Science VT2019-2021) and FNHK (UHHK, 00179906), Hradec Kralove, Czech Republic. The Medical Faculty of the Military Medical Academy, the University of Defence in Belgrade, Republic of Serbia (MFVMA/04/20-22) also took part in support of this work.

**Conflicts of Interest:** The authors declare no conflict of interest.

## References

1. Gomez, H.; Kellum, J.A. Sepsis-induced acute kidney injury. *Curr. Opin. Crit. Care.* **2016**, *22*, 546–553. [CrossRef]
2. Plotnikov, E.Y.; Brezgunova, A.A.; Pevzner, I.B.; Zorova, L.D.; Manskikh, V.N.; Popkov, V.A.; Silachev, D.N.; Zorov, D.B. Mechanisms of LPS-Induced acute kidney injury in neonatal and adult rats. *Antioxidants* **2018**, *7*, 105. [CrossRef] [PubMed]
3. Stasi, A.; Intini, A.; Divella, C.; Franzin, R.; Montemurno, E.; Grandaliano, G.; Ronco, C.; Fiaccadori, E.; Pertosa, G.B.; Gesualdo, L.; et al. Emerging role of Lipopolysaccharide binding protein in sepsis-induced acute kidney injury. *Nephrol. Dial. Transpl.* **2017**, *32*, 24–31. [CrossRef] [PubMed]
4. Jo, S.K.; Cha, D.R.; Cho, W.Y.; Kim, H.K.; Chang, K.H.; Yun, S.Y.; Won, N.H. Inflammatory cytokines and lipopolysaccharide induce Fas-mediated apoptosis in renal tubular cells. *Nephron* **2002**, *91*, 406–415. [CrossRef]
5. Flusberg, D.A.; Sorger, P.K. Surviving apoptosis: Life-death signalling in single cells. *Trends Cell. Biol.* **2015**, *25*, 446–458. [CrossRef] [PubMed]
6. Zhang, S.; Li, R.; Dong, W.; Yang, H.; Zhang, L.; Chen, Y.; Wang, W.; Li, C.; Wu, Y.; Ye, Z.; et al. RIPK3 mediates renal tubular epithelial cell apoptosis in endotoxin-induced acute kidney injury. *Mol. Med. Rep.* **2019**, *20*, 1613–1620. [CrossRef]

7. Jacobs, R.; Honore, P.M.; Joannes-Boyau, O.; Boer, W.; De Regt, J.; De Waele, E.; Collin, V.; Spapen, H.D. Septic acute kidney injury: The culprit is inflammatory apoptosis rather than ischemic necrosis. *Blood Purif.* **2011**, *32*, 262–265. [CrossRef]
8. Parikh, S.M.; Yang, Y.; He, L.; Tang, C.; Zhan, M.; Dong, Z. Mitochondrial function and disturbances in the septic kidney. *Semin. Nephrol.* **2015**, *35*, 108–119. [CrossRef]
9. Liu, J.X.; Yang, C.; Zhang, W.H.; Su, H.Y.; Liu, Z.J.; Pan, Q.; Liu, H.F. Disturbance of mitochondrial dynamics and mitophagy in sepsis-induced acute kidney injury. *Life Sci.* **2019**, *235*, 116828. [CrossRef]
10. Zhong, X.; He, J.; Zhang, X.; Li, C.; Tian, X.; Xia, W.; Gan, H.; Xia, Y. UCP2 alleviates tubular epithelial cell apoptosis in lipopolysaccharide-induced acute kidney injury by decreasing ROS production. *Biomed. Pharm.* **2019**, *115*, 108914. [CrossRef]
11. Kim, J.Y.; Lee, S.J.; Maeng, Y.I.; Leem, J.; Park, K.K. Protective Effects of Bee Venom against Endotoxemia-Related Acute Kidney Injury in Mice. *Biology* **2020**, *9*, 154. [CrossRef] [PubMed]
12. Leeds, J.; Scindia, Y.; Loi, V.; Wlazlo, E.; Ghias, E.; Cechova, S.; Portilla, D.; Ledesma, J.; Swaminathan, S. Protective Role of DJ-1 in Endotoxin-induced Acute Kidney Injury. *Am. J. Physiol. Renal. Physiol* **2020**. [CrossRef] [PubMed]
13. Du., J.; Jiang, S.; Hu, Z.; Tang, S.; Sun, Y.; He, J.; Li, Z.; Yi, B.; Wang, I.; Zhang, H.; et al. Vitamin D receptor activation protects against lipopolysaccharide-induced acute kidney injury through suppression of tubular cell apoptosis. *Am. J. Physiol. Ren. Physiol.* **2019**, *316*, F1068–F1077. [CrossRef] [PubMed]
14. Nežić, L.; Škrbić, R.; Dobrić, S.; Stojiljković, M.P.; jaćevič, V.; Stoisavljević, S.; Milovanović, Z.A.; Stojaković, N. Simvastatin and indomethacin have similar anti-inflammatory activity in a rat model of acute local inflammation. *Basic Clin. Pharm. Toxicol.* **2009**, *104*, 185–191. [CrossRef]
15. Zhao, G.; Yu, Y.M.; Kaneki, M.; Bonab, A.A.; Tompkins, R.G.; Fischman, A.J. Simvastatin reduces burn injury-induced splenic apoptosis via down-regulation of the TNF-α/ NF-κB pathway. *Ann. Surg.* **2015**, *261*, 1006–1012. [CrossRef]
16. Wang, Y.; Yang, W.; Zhao, X.; Zhang, R. Experimental study of the protective effect of simvastatin on lung injury in rats with sepsis. *Inflammation* **2018**, *41*, 104–113. [CrossRef]
17. He, X.; Yang, J.; Li, L.; Tan, H.; Wu, Y.; Ran, P.; Sun, S.; Chen, J.; Zhou, Y. Atorvastatin protects against contrast-induced nephropathy via anti-apoptosis by the upregulation of Hsp27 in vivo and in vitro. *Mol. Med. Rep.* **2017**, *15*, 1963–1972. [CrossRef] [PubMed]
18. Kaushik, S.; Tomar, A.; Puthanmadhom Narayanan, S.; Nag, T.C.; Arya, D.C.; Bhatia, J. Pitavastatin attenuates cisplatin–induced renal injury by targeting MAPK and apoptotic pathways. *J. Pharm. Pharm.* **2019**, *71*, 1072–1081. [CrossRef]
19. Nežić, L.; Škrbić, R.; Dobrić, S.; Stojiljković, M.P.; Šatara, S.S.; Milovanović, Z.A.; Stojaković, N. Effect of simvastatin on proinflammatory cytokines production during lipopolysaccharide-induced inflammation in rats. *Gen. Physiol. Biophys.* **2009**, *28*, 119–126.
20. Nežić, L.; Škrbić, R.; Amidžić, L.j.; Gajanin, R.; Kuča, K.; Jaćević, V. Simvastatin protects cardiomyocytes against endotoxin-induced apoptosis and up-regulates survivin/NF-κB/p65 expression. *Sci. Rep.* **2018**, *8*, 14652. [CrossRef]
21. Nežić, L.; Amidžić, L.j.; Škrbić, R.; Gajanin, R.; Nepovimova, E.; Vališ, M.; Kuča, K.; Jaćević, V. Simvastatin inhibits endotoxin-induced apoptosis in liver and spleen through up-regulation of survivin/NF-kB/p65 expression. *Front. Pharm.* **2019**, *10*, 54. [CrossRef] [PubMed]
22. Yasuda, H.; Yuen, P.S.; Hu, X.; Zhou, H.; Star, R.A. Simvastatin improves sepsis-induced mortality and acute kidney injury via renal vascular effects. *Kidn. Int.* **2006**, *69*, 1535–1542. [CrossRef]
23. Chen, C.H.; Lee, R.P.; Wu, W.T.; Liao, K.W.; Hsu, N.; Hsu, B.G. Fluvastatin ameliorates endotoxin-induced multiple organ failure in conscious rats. *Resuscitation* **2007**, *74*, 166–174. [CrossRef]
24. Wang, Y.; Zhang, L.; Zhao, X.; Yang, W.; Zhang, R. An experimental study of the protective effect of simvastatin on sepsis-induced myocardial depression in rats. *Biomed. Pharm.* **2017**, *94*, 705–711. [CrossRef]
25. Apaya, M.K.; Lin, C.Y.; Chiou, C.Y.; Yang, C.C.; Ting, C.Y.; Shyur, L.F. Simvastatin and a plant galactolipid protect animals from septic shock by regulating oxylipin mediator dynamics through the MAPK-cPLA2 signalling pathway. *Mol. Med.* **2016**, *21*, 988–1001. [CrossRef]
26. Özkök, E.; Yorulmaz, H.; Ateş, G.; Aydın, I.; Ergüven, M.; Tamer, Ş. The impact of pretreatment with simvastatin on kidney tissue of rats with acute sepsis. *Physiol. Int.* **2017**, *104*, 158–170. [CrossRef] [PubMed]

27. Yang, Y.; Song, M.; Liu, Y.; Liu, H.; Sun, L.; Peng, Y.; Liu, F.; Venkatachalam, M.A.; Dong, Z. Renoprotective approaches and strategies in acute kidney injury. *Pharm. Ther.* **2016**, *163*, 58–73. [CrossRef] [PubMed]
28. Shinozaki, S.; Inoue, Y.; Yang, W.; Fukaya, M.; Carter, E.A.; Yu, Y.; Fishman, A.; Tompkins, R.; Kanrki, M. Farnesyltransferase inhibitor improved survival following endotoxin challenge in mice. *Biochem. Biophys. Res. Commun.* **2010**, *391*, 1459–1464. [CrossRef]
29. Slotta, J.E.; Laschke, M.W.; Schilling, M.K.; Menger, M.D.; Jeppsson, B.; Thorlacius, H. Simvastatin attenuate hepatic sensitization to lipopolysaccharide after partial hepatectomy. *J. Surg. Res.* **2010**, *162*, 184–192. [CrossRef]
30. Lee, E.F.; Fairlie, W.D. The Structural Biology of Bcl-xL. *Int. J. Mol. Sci.* **2019**, *20*, 2234. [CrossRef]
31. Zhao, H.; Liu, Z.; Shen, H.; Jin, S.; Zhang, S. Glycyrrhizic acid pretreatment prevents sepsis-induced acute kidney injury via suppressing inflammation, apoptosis and oxidative stress. *Eur. J. Pharm.* **2016**, *781*, 92–99. [CrossRef]
32. Dohi, T.; Beltrami, E.; Wall, N.R.; Plescia, J.; Altieri, D.C. Mitochondrial survivin inhibits apoptosis and promotes tumorigenesis. *J. Clin. Inv.* **2004**, *114*, 1117–1127. [CrossRef]
33. Tsang, T.J.; Hsueh, Y.C.; Wei, E.I.; Lundy, D.J.; Cheng, B.; Chen, Y.T.; Wang, S.S.; Hsieh, P.C.H. Subcellular localization of survivin determines its function in cardiomyocytes. *Theranostics* **2017**, *7*, 4577–4590. [CrossRef] [PubMed]
34. Kindt, N.; Menzebach, A.; Van de Wouwer, M.; Betz, I.; De Vriese, A.; Conway, E.M. Protective role of the inhibitor of apoptosis protein, survivin, in toxin-induced acute renal failure. *Faseb. J.* **2008**, *22*, 510–521. [CrossRef] [PubMed]
35. Yang, C.; Guo, Y.; Huang, T.S.; Zhao, J.; Huang, X.J.; Tang, H.X.; An, N.; Pan, Q.; Xu, Y.-Z.; Liu, H.-F. Asiatic acid protects against cisplatin-induced acute kidney injury via anti-apoptosis and anti-inflammation. *Biomed. Pharmacother.* **2018**, *107*, 1354–1362. [CrossRef]
36. Chen, J.; Chen, J.K.; Conway, E.M.; Harris, R.S. Survivin mediates renal proximal tubule recovery from AKI. J. *Am. Soc. Nephrol.* **2013**, *24*, 2023–2033. [CrossRef]
37. Wilson, R.L.; Selvaraju, V.; Lakshmanan, R.; Thirunavukkarasu, M.; Campbell, J.; McFadden, D.W.; Maulik, D.W. Thioredoxin-1 attenuates sepsis-induced cardiomyopathy after cecal ligation and puncture in mice. *J. Surg. Res.* **2017**, *220*, 68–78. [CrossRef]
38. Seemann, S.; Zohles, F.; Lupp, A. Comprehensive comparison of three different animal models for systemic inflammation. *J. Biomed. Sci.* **2017**, *24*, 60. [CrossRef]
39. Kosaka, J.; Lankadeva, Y.R.; May, C.N.; Bellomo, R. Histopathology of septic acute kidney injury: A systematic review of experimental data. *Crit. Care Med.* **2016**, *44*, e897–e903. [CrossRef]
40. Kita, T.; Brown, M.S.; Goldstein, J.L. Feedback regulation of 3-hydroxy-3-methylglutaryl coenzyme A reductase in livers of mice treated with mevinolin, a competitive inhibitor of the reductase. *J. Clin. Inv.* **1980**, *66*, 1094–1100. [CrossRef]
41. Morel, J.; Hargreaves, I.; Brealey, D.; Neergheen, V.; Backman, J.T.; Lindig, S.; Bläss, M.; Bauer, M.; McAuley, D.F.; Singer, M. Simvastatin pre-treatment improves survival and mitochondrial function in a 3-day fluid-resuscitated rat model of sepsis. *Clin. Sci.* **2017**, *131*, 747–758. [CrossRef] [PubMed]
42. Jaćević, V.; Jovic, D.; Kuča, K.; Dragojevic-Simic, V.; Dobric, S.; Trajkovic, S.; Borisev, I.; Segrt, Z.; Milovanovic, Z.; Bokonjic, D.; et al. Effects of Fullerenol nanoparticles and Amifostine on radiation-induced tissue damages: Histopathological analysis. *J. Appl. Biomed.* **2016**, *14*, 285–297. [CrossRef]
43. Jaćević, V.; Djordjevic, A.; Srdjenovic, B.; Milic-Tores, V.; Segrt, Z.; Dragojevic-Simic, V.; Kuca, K. Fullerenol nanoparticles prevent doxorubicin-induced acute hepatotoxicity in rats. *Exp. Mol. Pathol.* **2017**, *102*, 360–369. [CrossRef]
44. Jaćević, V.; Dragojević-Simić, V.; Tatomirović, Ž.; Dobrić, S.; Bokonjić, D.; Kovačević, A.; Nepovimova, E.; Vališ, M.; Kuča, K. The efficacy of amifostine against multiple-dose doxorubicin-induced toxicity in rats. *Int. J. Mol. Sci.* **2018**, *19*, 2370. [CrossRef] [PubMed]
45. Jaćević, V.; Nepovimova, E.; Kuča, K. Toxic injury to the muscle tissue of rats following acute oximes exposure. *Sci. Rep.* **2019**, *9*, 1457. [CrossRef]
46. Jaćević, V.; Nepovimova, E.; Kuča, K. Acute toxic injuries of rat's visceral tissues induced by different oximes. *Sci. Rep.* **2019**, *9*, 16425. [CrossRef]
47. Jaćević, V.; Wu, Q.; Nepovimova, E.; Kuča, K. Efficacy of methylprednisolone on T-2 toxin-induced cardiotoxicity in vivo: A pathohistological study. *Environ. Toxicol. Pharm.* **2019**, *71*, 103221. [CrossRef]

48. Jaćević, V.; Wu, Q.; Nepovimova, E.; Kuča, K. Cardiomiopythy induced by T-2 toxin. *Food Chem. Toxicol.* **2020**, *137*, 111138. [CrossRef]
49. Wang, K.; Brems, J.J.; Gamelli, R.L.; Holterman, X.A. Survivin signalling is regulated through the nuclear factor-kappa B pathway during glycochenodeoxycholate-induced hepatocyte apoptosis. *Biochim. Biophys. Acta* **2010**, *1803*, 1368–1375. [CrossRef]
50. Scheer, A.; Knauer, S.K.; Verhaegh, R. Survivin expression pattern in the intestine of normoxic and ischemic rats. *BMC Gastroenterol.* **2017**, *17*, 76. [CrossRef]

International Journal of
*Molecular Sciences*

MDPI

*Article*

# Autophagy Dynamics and Modulation in a Rat Model of Renal Ischemia-Reperfusion Injury

**Jean-Paul Decuypere [1,2], Shawn Hutchinson [1,2], Diethard Monbaliu [1,2], Wim Martinet [3], Jacques Pirenne [1,2] and Ina Jochmans [1,2,*]**

1 Laboratory of Abdominal Transplantation, Transplantation Research Group, Department of Microbiology and Immunology, KU Leuven, B-3000 Leuven, Belgium; jeanpaul.decuypere@kuleuven.be (J.-P.D.); shawn.hutchinson@uhn.ca (S.H.); diethard.monbaliu@uzleuven.be (D.M.); jacques.pirenne@uzleuven.be (J.P.)

2 Department of Abdominal Transplant Surgery, University Hospitals Leuven, B-3000 Leuven, Belgium

3 Department of Pharmaceutical Sciences, University of Antwerp, B-2610 Antwerp, Belgium; wim.martinet@uantwerpen.be

* Correspondence: ina.jochmans@uzleuven.be; Tel.: +32-16-348727

Received: 20 August 2020; Accepted: 25 September 2020; Published: 29 September 2020

check for updates

**Abstract:** Renal ischemia-reperfusion (IR) injury leading to cell death is a major cause of acute kidney injury, contributing to morbidity and mortality. Autophagy counteracts cell death by removing damaged macromolecules and organelles, making it an interesting anchor point for treatment strategies. However, autophagy is also suggested to enhance cell death when the ischemic burden is too strong. To investigate whether the role of autophagy depends on the severity of ischemic stress, we analyzed the dynamics of autophagy and apoptosis in an IR rat model with mild (45 min) or severe (60 min) renal ischemia. Following mild IR, renal injury was associated with reduced autophagy, enhanced mammalian target of rapamycin (mTOR) activity, and apoptosis. Severe IR, on the other hand, was associated with a higher autophagic activity, independent of mTOR, and without affecting apoptosis. Autophagy stimulation by trehalose injected 24 and 48 h prior to onset of severe ischemia did not reduce renal injury markers nor function, but reduced apoptosis and restored tubular dilation 7 days post reperfusion. This suggests that trehalose-dependent autophagy stimulation enhances tissue repair following an IR injury. Our data show that autophagy dynamics are strongly dependent on the severity of IR and that trehalose shows the potential to trigger autophagy-dependent repair processes following renal IR injury.

**Keywords:** ischemia-reperfusion injury; acute kidney injury; autophagy; apoptosis; trehalose

## 1. Introduction

Renal ischemia-reperfusion (IR) injury is a major contributor to acute kidney injury (AKI), leading to acute tubular necrosis [1,2]. AKI is a very common condition, affecting 3–18% of hospitalized patients and 33–66% of those admitted to intensive care [3]. AKI is an independent risk factor for death, especially when renal replacement therapy is needed, and is associated with a mortality of 40–70% in critically ill patients [4,5]. Currently, there are no effective treatment strategies for AKI, and measures are supportive while recovery is awaited. Indeed, the kidney's capacity to recover after ischemic injury is remarkable but not perfect [6,7]. In mild injury, this repair process restores renal structure and function; however, when the injury is severe, the repair process can trigger fibrosis, increasing the risk of developing chronic kidney disease [8]. Understanding the link between the severity of injury and the regeneration process could lead to the development of treatments that enhance recovery. A possible link is autophagy, an evolutionary conserved intracellular degradation pathway with homeostatic and damage-mitigating functions.

Macroautophagy, the best studied type of autophagy (and hereafter simply referred to as "autophagy"), manifests as intracellular vesicles (autophagosomes) that envelop cytoplasmic material and subsequently transport and deliver their cargo to the lysosomes for degradation. It involves more than 30 autophagy (Atg) proteins for the initiation, formation, transportation, and fusion of autophagosomes towards lysosomes [9]. Its levels depend on input from various signaling pathways, including nutrient signaling through the mammalian target of rapamycin (mTOR) and energy status monitoring through adenosine monophosphate -activated kinase AMPK. Typically, autophagy is stimulated upon stress as a survival pathway. This way, autophagy recycles damaged and toxic cytoplasmic material into cellular building blocks, which are then used to support anti-stress responses and energy maintenance. Moreover, autophagy is able to degrade damaged mitochondria, preventing the initiation of apoptosis, and therefore might reduce IR injury [10,11]. However, in addition to necrosis and apoptosis [12–14], autophagy has also been positively associated with injury during renal IR [15–19]. Indeed, autophagy can both prevent and assist cell death, depending on the type and duration of the stress, due to the molecular crosstalks between autophagy and cell death mechanisms such as apoptosis and necrosis (reviewed in [20,21]). This autophagy paradox—damaging on the one hand, protecting on the other—implies that the role and dynamics of autophagy during renal IR injury are not well understood [22]. We hypothesized earlier that the role of autophagy in renal IR injury depends on the duration of ischemia, where autophagy can switch from a protective to an injuring mechanism with an increasing ischemia time [23,24].

We now examined this hypothesis by evaluating the dynamics of autophagy, apoptosis, and injury in a rat renal IR model. Subsequently, we assessed the effects of autophagy stimulation on renal IR injury by the administration of trehalose, a naturally occurring disaccharide known to stimulate autophagy [25].

## 2. Results

### 2.1. Transient Renal Injury Following Mild Ischemia

All Sham and I45 rats (subjected to 45 min of mild ischemia) survived 90 days of reperfusion (R90d). The plasma creatinine was higher after I45 compared to the Sham rats up to R7d (Figure 1A), as were plasmatic aspartate aminotransferase (AST) and heart-fatty acid binding protein (h-FABP), especially early post reperfusion (Figure 1B,C). Terminal deoxynucleotidyl transferase end labeling (TUNEL) staining gradually increased with increasing reperfusion time, with the strongest signal at R6h (Figure S1a). The positive area originated around the blood vessels (R1h) and migrated towards the tubuli at R6h and R24h. Cortical areas were most prominently stained, although some disperse staining was observed in the medulla. It should be noted that besides the expected TUNEL staining of the nuclei, we observed most prominently the staining of the tubular lumen, as previously described [26,27]. TEM revealed swollen and damaged mitochondria at R3h (Figure S1b) in the kidney, confirming the occurrence of intracellular damage. TEM also revealed possible early and late autophagosomes, but clear differences between the Sham and I45 group were not observed. In addition, the mRNA transcription of inflammatory factors intracellular adhesion molecule-1 (ICAM-1) (Figure 1D), interleukins IL-6 and IL-10 (Figure S1c,d) and stress marker heat shock protein 70 (Hsp70) (Figure 1E) significantly increased, with a peak around R3h. These results thus indicate that the kidneys are transiently injured in the I45 model, concomitant with decreased function, enhanced inflammation, and with sustained survival.

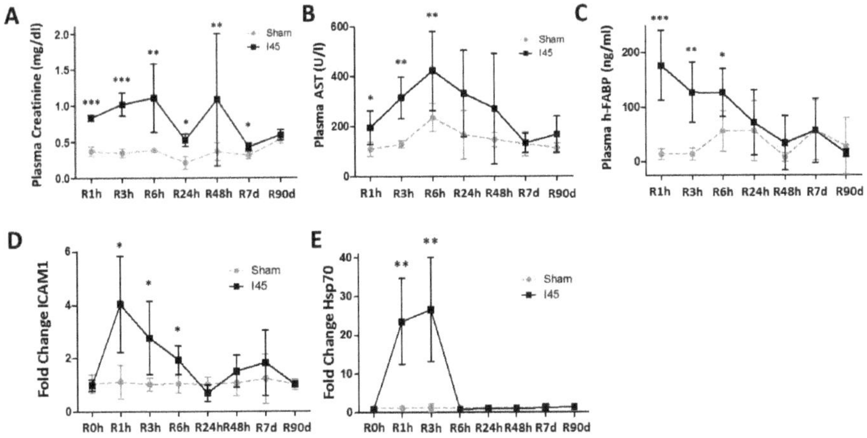


**Figure 1.** Kidney function is reduced, injury is increased, and tissue inflammatory processes are activated after mild ischemia and reperfusion. Rats, either Sham-operated (Sham) or subjected to 45 min of renal ischemia (I45), were sacrificed at various time points post reperfusion (R0h, R1h, R3h, R6h, R24h, R48h, R7d, and R90d). Plasma was collected to measure the creatinine (**A**), aspartate aminotransferase (AST) (**B**), and heart-fatty acid binding protein (h-FABP) (**C**). Kidneys were collected and analyzed for the mRNA expression of intracellular adhesion molecule-1 (ICAM-1) (**D**) and heat shock protein 70 (Hsp70) (**E**). * $p < 0.05$, ** $p < 0.01$, *** $p < 0.001$. $N = 6$.

### *2.2. Autophagy Is Suppressed during Ischemia and Reperfusion Following Mild Ischemia*

This rat IR model was now exploited to investigate the autophagic response to mild ischemia. Autophagy markers were assessed by Western blotting on Sham and I45 rat kidney lysates at several time points during reperfusion (R0h, R1h, R3h, R6h, R24h, R48h, R7d, and R90d) (Figure S2). During autophagy, LC3-I is converted into LC3-II, which then recruits to the autophagosomal membrane. As such, the LC3-II levels represent the amount of autophagosomes present at the time of kidney collection. As recommended in the literature, we quantified the ratio of LC3-II over the housekeeping protein Glyceraldehyde 3-phosphate dehydrogenase (GAPDH) [28]. Interestingly, ischemia alone (R0h) led to a reduction in LC3-II (Figure 2A). Since LC3-II eventually is degraded in the lysosomes, a decrease in LC3-II can signify reduced autophagosome formation or enhanced autophagosome clearance [28]. To establish the overall results of IR for the autophagic degradation rate, we also assessed the levels of Sequestosome 1 (Sqstm1/p62), a substrate for autophagic degradation. Ischemia alone (R0h) resulted in an elevation of p62, concomitant with the decrease in LC3-II (Figure 2B), suggesting suppressed autophagy. Since mTOR is the canonical signaling kinase negatively regulating autophagy, we evaluated the phosphorylation of ribosomal protein S6, which is indirectly phosphorylated by mTOR via the activation of p70S6 kinase. Reduced S6 phosphorylation was observed at R0h (Figure 2C), suggesting that the suppression of autophagy during ischemia could be mTOR-independent.

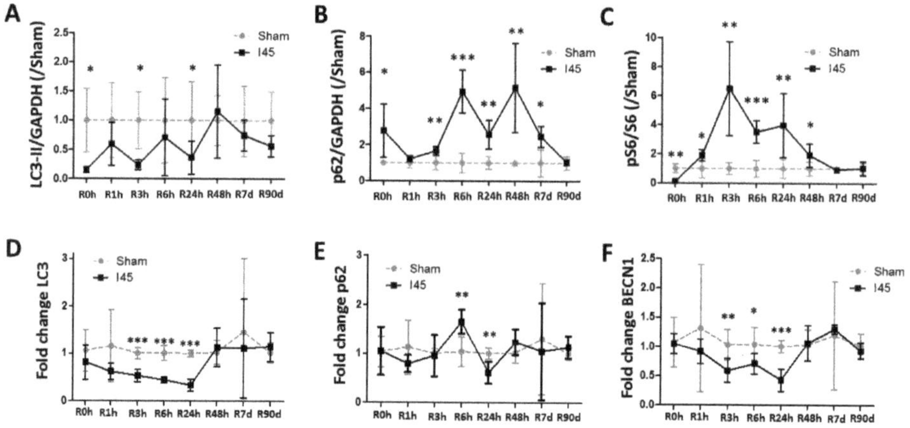


**Figure 2.** Autophagy is suppressed post reperfusion following mild ischemia. Rats, either Sham-operated (Sham) or subjected to 45 min of renal ischemia (I45), were sacrificed at various time points post reperfusion (R0h, R1h, R3h, R6h, R24h, R48h, R7d, and R90d). Kidney tissue was collected and analyzed by Western blotting for LC3 (**A**), p62 (**B**), S6, and phosphorylated S6 (pS6) (**C**), and by qPCR for the mRNA expression of LC3 (**D**), p62 (**E**), and BECN1 (**F**). * $p$ <0.05, ** $p < 0.01$, *** $p < 0.001$. $N = 6$.

Following mild ischemia, a decrease in LC3-II was generally detected compared to the Sham group, with significant reductions at R0h, R3h, and R24h (Figure 2A). Corresponding with a decrease in LC3-II, the p62 levels were significantly upregulated post reperfusion (Figure 2B), indicating that autophagy is suppressed during reperfusion in this model. Although phosphorylated S6 was decreased during ischemia (R0h), it was strongly increased post reperfusion (Figure 2C), suggesting that the decrease in autophagy could be partially explained by the negative regulation of autophagy by mTOR. It should be noted, however, that S6 can be phosphorylated by other kinases as well [29].

Next, we analyzed whether the results observed on the protein level were also reflected in the mRNA expression of LC3, p62, and BECN1. Interestingly, the LC3 and BECN1 expression were significantly reduced between R3h and R24h (Figure 2D,F). The sqstm1/p62 mRNA levels remained relatively stable, despite an increase at R6h, followed by a decrease at R24h (Figure 2E). As such, it is unlikely that the increase in the p62 levels on a protein level have a transcriptional cause, and most likely reflect the reduction in the autophagic degradation of the p62 protein. In conclusion, these data suggest that autophagy is most prominently suppressed during reperfusion in rats subjected to 45 min of ischemia.

### 2.3. *Apoptosis Is Enhanced during Reperfusion Following Mild Ischemia*

We further investigated the apoptotic pathway post reperfusion. Therefore, Western blotting was performed for pro- (Bax, cleaved caspase 3) and anti-apoptotic (Bcl-2) markers on kidney protein lysates from Sham and I45 rats (Figure S3). Despite the reduction in autophagy, apoptosis was not affected following ischemia alone (R0h) (Figure 3A–C). While the Bax protein levels were significantly elevated between R1h and R7d (Figure 3A), the Bcl-2 levels remained stable (Figure 3B). Despite the fast increase in Bax, the levels of cleaved Caspase 3 did not increase before R48h (Figure 3C). Interestingly, a similar trend was observed for the mRNA expression of Bim, a pro-apoptotic BH3-only protein (Figure 3F). Unlike the protein levels, the Bax mRNA expression decreased in I45 rats at R24h and increased at R48h and R90d (Figure 3D). The expression of anti-apoptotic Bcl-2 mRNA was reduced at most time points post reperfusion in I45 rats (Figure 3E). Taken together, these results indicate that the apoptotic machinery is activated late post reperfusion (after 24 h) following mild ischemia in rat kidneys.

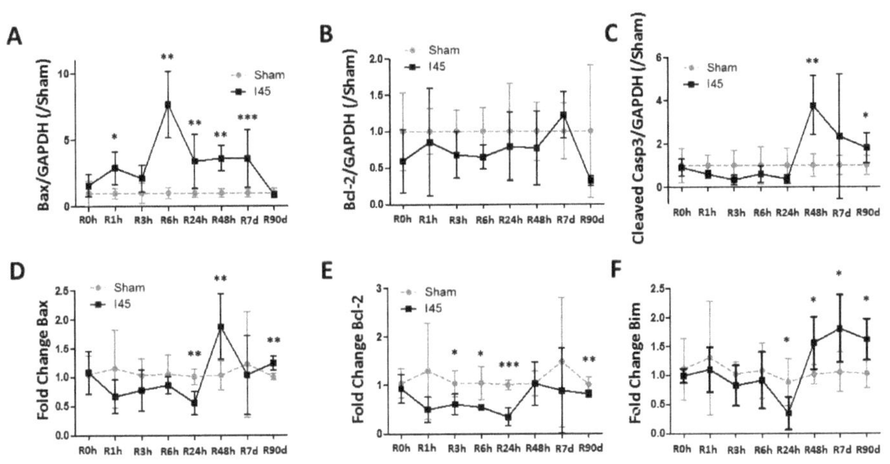


**Figure 3.** Apoptosis increases post reperfusion following mild ischemia. Rats, either Sham-operated (Sham) or subjected to 45 min of renal ischemia (I45), were sacrificed at various time points post reperfusion (R0h, R1h, R3h, R6h, R24h, R48h, R7d, and R90d). Kidney tissue was collected and analyzed by Western blotting for Bax (**A**), Bcl-2 (**B**), and Cleaved Caspase 3 (**C**), and by qPCR for the mRNA expression of Bax (**D**), Bcl-2 (**E**), and Bim (**F**). * $p < 0.05$, ** $p < 0.01$, *** $p < 0.001$. $N = 6$.

### 2.4. More Severe Ischemia Increases Kidney Damage

To understand whether autophagy is protective or detrimental for renal IR injury, we first compared the autophagic response in rats subjected to mild (I45) and severe (I60) ischemia. First, in the I60 group, 4/6 rats died within seven days following IR, while in both the I45 and Sham group, all the rats survived. Moreover, the plasma creatinine and AST were also higher in I60 compared to I45 at R3h and R24h (Figure 4A,B), while the plasma h-FABP was only significantly different at R3h (Figure 4C). In addition, the mRNA expression of inflammatory and stress markers ICAM-1 and Hsp70 were higher in I60 versus I45 at R3h (Figure 4D,E). The expressions of IL-6 and -10, however, were lower in I60 compared to I45 (Figure S4a,b). Altogether, the I60 rat model inflicted more kidney damage and inflammation compared to the I45 model.

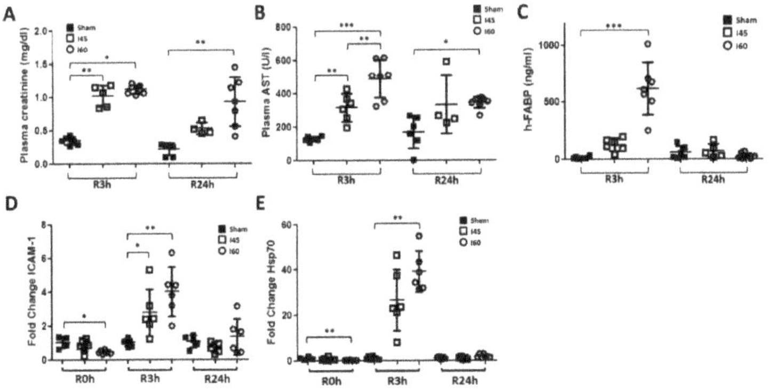


**Figure 4.** Kidney function is reduced and injury is increased following severe compared to mild or no ischemia. Rats, either Sham-operated (Sham) or subjected to 45 min (I45) or 60 min (I60) of renal ischemia, were sacrificed at various time points post reperfusion (R0h, R3h, and R24h). Plasma was collected to measure the creatinine (**A**), AST (**B**), and h-FABP (**C**). Kidneys were collected and analyzed for the mRNA expression of ICAM-1 (**D**) and Hsp70 (**E**). * $p < 0.05$, ** $p < 0.01$, *** $p < 0.001$. $N = 6$.

### 2.5. More Autophagy upon Severe Compared to Mild Ischemia

In the I60 model of severe ischemia, we then explored autophagy and apoptosis markers in the kidney. The results observed in the I60 model at the post-reperfusion times R0h, R3h, and R24h (Figure S5a–c) were compared with these time points in the mild ischemia (I45) model. LC3-II decreased in both I45 and I60 in a similar trend, but its levels at R24h were significantly higher in I60 versus I45 (Figure 5A). Interestingly, this was associated with lower p62 levels in the I60 model (Figure 5B and Figure S5b), suggesting a higher autophagic activity in I60 compared to I45. The phosphorylated S6 levels did not significantly differ between I45 and I60 (Figure 5C). On the mRNA level, the LC3 expression was, similarly to the protein levels, increased in I60 versus I45 (Figure 5D), while the p62 levels remained unaltered between the two groups (Figure 5E). The BECN1 expression was significantly lower in I60 versus I45 at R0h, but remained similarly downregulated in both groups afterwards (Figure 5F). Despite these changes in autophagy, no clear trend was observed in the apoptosis markers comparing I60 and I45 (Figure S5d–i). These data thus indicate elevated autophagy upon severe ischemia compared to mild ischemia.

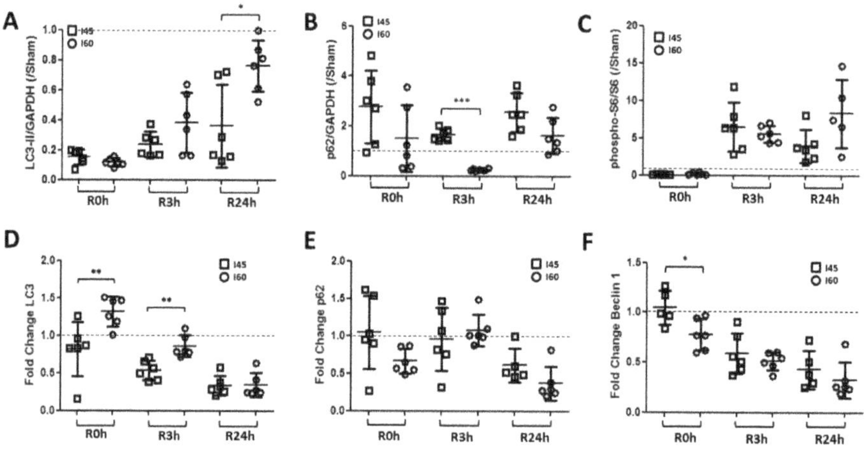


**Figure 5.** Autophagy is increased during ischemia and after reperfusion following severe ischemia compared to mild ischemia. Rats, either Sham-operated (Sham) or subjected to 45 min (I45) or 60 min (I60) of renal ischemia, were sacrificed at various time points post reperfusion (R0h, R3h, and R24h). Kidneys were collected and analyzed by Western blotting and qPCR for LC3 (**A**), p62 (**B**), S6, and phosphorylated S6 (pS6) (**C**), and by qPCR for the mRNA expression of LC3 (**D**), p62 (**E**), and BECN1 (**F**).The relative change in I45 and I60 compared to the corresponding Sham group (represented by the dashed line at y = 1) was plotted. * $p < 0.05$, ** $p < 0.01$, *** $p < 0.001$. $N = 6$.

### 2.6. Trehalose Stimulates Autophagy and Reduces IR Injury in the Kidney

To evaluate whether autophagy modulation would alter IR injury, rats were given 2 g/kg body weight trehalose by intraperitoneal injection 48 and 24 h prior to 60 min of ischemia, followed by 24 h or 7 days of reperfusion. Trehalose is a naturally occurring sugar synthesized by bacteria, fungi, and invertebrates, consisting of two glucose molecules connected by a 1-1 $\alpha$ bond. It is an mTOR-independent autophagy inducer that acts partially by inhibiting glucose transport [30]. The kidneys of trehalose-treated rats displayed higher LC3-I and LC3-II levels compared to vehicle-treated rats following 60 min of ischemia and 24 h of reperfusion, without affecting phosphorylated S6, suggesting no change in the mTOR activity and apoptosis (Figure 6A,B). Despite an improvement in survival after R7d (vehicle 50%; trehalose 83%), trehalose did not reduce renal injury at R24h, as evidenced by the similar TUNEL staining (Figure 6C) and plasma AST levels (Figure 6D). The mRNA expression of ICAM-1, Hsp70, and IL-10 even displayed an increasing trend upon trehalose treatment (Figure S6a–d). In addition, the plasma creatinine was increased in the trehalose-treated rats (Figure 6E), suggesting reduced kidney function. However, at R7d, the trehalose-treated rat kidneys showed reduced TUNEL staining (Figure 6F) and an overall improved kidney structure with less dilated tubules (Figure 6G). Together, this suggests that trehalose-induced autophagy does not reduce AKI but improves the repair of the affected tissue.

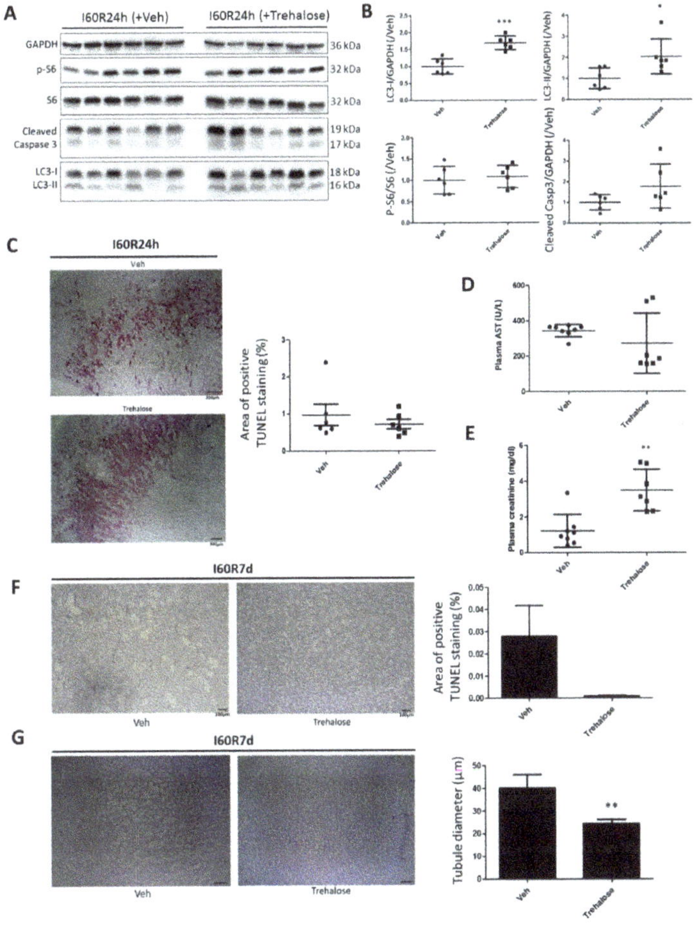


**Figure 6.** Trehalose induces autophagy and improves the renal structure post reperfusion following severe ischemia. Rats were injected with vehicle (Veh) or trehalose 48 h and 24 h prior to 60 min of renal ischemia (I60), and sacrificed 24 h (I60R24h) or 7 days (I60R7d) post reperfusion. Kidneys of I60R24h were analyzed by Western blotting for the annotated markers (**A**) and compared between Veh- and trehalose-treated for LC3-I, LC3-II, phosphorylated S6 (pS6), and cleaved caspase 3 (**B**). Kidney sections of I60R24h were also stained with TUNEL (**C**) and the plasma levels of AST (**D**) and creatinine (**E**) were determined. In the kidney sections of I60R7d, TUNEL staining was performed (**F**) and the average tubule diameter was assessed (**G**). * $p < 0.05$, ** $p < 0.01$, *** $p < 0.001$. $N = 6$.

## 3. Discussion

Renal IR injury is a common clinical complication and is the leading cause of AKI. With no effective treatment available to alleviate renal IR injury, it may progress into acute renal failure and increase mortality rates. Therefore, understanding the underlying mechanisms of this injury is crucial to reveal new therapeutic approaches. A central pathway in the progress of renal IR injury is autophagy, an evolutionary conserved intracellular catabolic pathway regulating cellular homeostasis and survival during stress. However, the exact role of autophagy in renal IR injury is still undetermined, as both protective and detrimental effects have been described [23,24]. Indeed, in certain conditions autophagy-dependent cell death can occur. This is suggested to be dependent on the dynamics of autophagy, where excessive or uncontrolled autophagy could trigger the initiation of cell death [19]. The role of autophagy in renal IR injury could therefore be dependent on the ischemic duration of the model, with mild ischemia triggering moderate, protective autophagy and severe ischemia triggering excessive, detrimental autophagy [23,24]. Here, we observed that autophagy dynamics are indeed strongly influenced by these parameters.

First, autophagy was attenuated very rapidly following ischemia (Figure 2). This was not expected, as the lack of oxygen and subsequently energy reduction during ischemia should activate autophagy through AMPK [31]. However, AMPK-dependent autophagy activation occurs upon subtle changes in ATP production, while warm ischemia in rat kidneys leads to a fast and sudden fall in the ATP levels [32]. In view of the ATP dependency of the conjugation reactions leading to the autophagy-specific lipidation of LC3-I into LC3-II [33], this sudden lack of ATP is possibly the cause of the observed decrease in autophagy during ischemia. Similar observations of reduced LC3-II levels have also been observed following renal ischemia in mice [34].

Second, autophagy fluctuated during reperfusion (Figure 2), but overall the attenuation of autophagy during ischemia continues during reperfusion. This effect post reperfusion is most likely due to increased mTOR activity, in which the re-introduction of nutrients during reperfusion likely stimulates mTOR after a suppression caused by nutrient absence during ischemia [35]. This is reflected in the levels of phosphorylated S6, an indirect target of mTOR (Figure 2C). However, it should be noted that the phosphorylation status of S6 is the sum of multiple kinase activities (including mTOR and protein kinase A) and the activity of protein phosphatase-1 [29]. Ideally, the phosphorylation of ULK-1 at Ser757 should be assessed to determine the link between mTOR activity and autophagy [36].

Despite the dynamics of injury and autophagy, apoptosis occurred rather late post reperfusion (R48h). Although TUNEL staining was mostly observed early post reperfusion (R3–6h), this did not correspond with the levels of cleaved caspase 3. In addition, this staining was not typically nucleus-specific, as has been observed previously [26,27]. This suggests that TUNEL staining is indicative of apoptosis-independent DNA damage during renal IR. Indeed, massive reactive oxygen species production has been suggested to induce DNA damage independent of necrosis and apoptosis [37]. These data, therefore, suggest that that the initial (acute) injury post reperfusion is likely more associated with other (inflammatory) types of cell death (e.g., necrosis, caspase3-independent pyrroptosis, ferroptosis, or necroptosis) rather than apoptosis [38,39]. Indeed, in previous work we have shown that necroptosis inhibitor Nec-1 reduces the positive TUNEL staining 3 h post reperfusion in our model [26], suggesting that necroptosis is activated shortly following reperfusion. However, since Nec-1 did not affect the injury markers AST and h-FABP and the plasma creatinine levels, other types of cell death are likely to be activated as well. As such, the observed late apoptosis enhancement 48 h post reperfusion could therefore rather represent a mechanism to remove damaged cells associated with tissue repair.

Third, the autophagy levels are higher when the ischemic duration increases (Figure 5). In general, these data suggest that more severe ischemia is associated with higher autophagy levels and that autophagy dynamics are dependent on the ischemia and reperfusion duration. This could explain the differences in autophagy regulation observed in the literature, as reports often focus on one or few time points post-reperfusion [23]. These differences in the literature are further complicated by the dependency of the IR-induced autophagic response on the gender and age of the model [40], as well as the differences between species. In this context, it is important to note that cell death responses to anoxia-reoxygenation differ between rodent and human cells [41], and that this will likely be reflected in the autophagy dynamics as well. Moreover, in the clinical AKI setting the ischemic time is longer than that in the model presented here. The fact that autophagy dynamics are very dependent on the species and ischemia/reperfusion time, as this study suggests, warrants the need for further evaluation in AKI patients.

As severe ischemia is associated with decreased survival and elevated autophagy, these results bring into question whether autophagy plays an active role in renal damage or is stimulated to prevent renal IR injury. In this respect, trehalose, an autophagy inducer, seemed to have a dual effect following severe ischemia: a (slight) exacerbation of renal injury 24 h post reperfusion on the one hand and an improvement in the kidney tubular structure and reduced apoptosis 7 days following the ischemia on the other (Figure 6 and Figure S6). A similar autophagy-dependent stimulation of tissue remodeling was observed following cardiac injury, in which the beneficial effects of trehalose were blunted by the suppression of autophagy [42]. These observations, together with the lower autophagy levels associated with mild ischemia (Figure 2), suggest that autophagy may be detrimental in the acute phase of IR injury, but protective by promoting tissue repair in the recovery phase. This opens prospects for possible clinical applications of autophagy modulators such as trehalose; for example, as it functions in the repair process following injury, it could be administered peri- or post-operatively during kidney transplantation. In this respect, it is important to note that trehalose is an essential component of the "extracellular type" ET-Kyoto organ preservation solution, which is used in clinical lung transplantation [43], and which was found to be superior in the preservation of rat livers compared to the University of Wisconsin solution [44]. The molecular mechanisms of the beneficial effects of trehalose in renal IR injury, whether this is autophagy-dependent and whether this could be used in the clinical setting, require more investigation.

Due to the limitations of the rat model in this study, autophagy was only analyzed with the Western blotting and qPCR techniques. Nevertheless, it is recommended to analyze autophagy through a series of techniques [28]. Although TEM analysis revealed autophagic vesicles in the kidney tissue (Figure S1b), no clear differences were observed between the Sham and I45 rats. However, TEM is performed on a very small section of the kidney, while the altered autophagy responses are likely restricted to certain renal zones (cf. positive TUNEL staining in the corticomedullary area). Similar experiments in GFP- or RFP-GFP-LC3 mice subjected to various durations of ischemia and reperfusion should gain more insight in the exact dynamics of autophagy. Nonetheless, the combination of the autophagosome marker LC3-II and autophagy degradation marker p62 analyzed in our experiments revealed the expected inverse correlation of LC3-II and p62 dynamics, indicating that these levels indeed reflected autophagy alterations in response to renal ischemia and reperfusion.

In conclusion, the differential dynamics observed in these different IR models thus partially explain the conflicting findings in the literature regarding the role of autophagy in renal IR injury, which is dependent on ischemic duration and the time of reperfusion. As such, it is important to investigate multiple time points post reperfusion and various ischemic lengths. Additionally, modulation with trehalose revealed that autophagy stimulation likely has different outcomes in tissue repair (protective) and in acute IR injury (detrimental). This information is crucial in light of the possible clinical application of (trehalose-dependent) autophagy stimulation in acute kidney injury or kidney transplantation.

## 4. Materials and Methods

### 4.1. Ischemia-Reperfusion Injury Model

Female Sprague-Dawley rats (200–250 g; 8–10 weeks old) were housed at the KU Leuven animal facility. After at least 1 week of acclimatization, they were anesthetized by an intraperitoneal injection of 7.5 mg/kg of ketamin (Anesketin®, Eurovet Animal Health BV, Bladel, The Netherlands) and 2.5 mg/kg of xylazin (Xyl-M 2%®, Van Miert & Dams Chemie (VMD), Arendonk, Belgium). Both renal pedicles were dissected free through a midline abdominal incision and clamped "en bloc" with microaneurysm clamps to induce ischemia. Reperfusion was initiated by the removal of the clamps. Sham-operated rats underwent the same surgery without the clamping of the pedicles. Analgesics were administered daily (Vetergesic 0.1 mg/kg, CEVA, Libourne, France) following surgery. At the end of the experiment, pentobarbital (Nembutal 60 mg/kg, CEVA) was injected intraperitoneally and the rats were sacrificed by exsanguination, which allowed plasma sampling directly from the aorta. Plasma was spun down (1000× *g*; 10 min) and snap-frozen. Kidneys were collected and processed immediately, as described below. For the trehalose experiments, sterile PBS (Vehicle) or 2 g/kg bodyweight of trehalose in PBS (in a total volume of ca. 500 µL) was injected intraperitoneally 48 h and 24 h prior to surgery. The rat survival, behavior, and humane endpoints were monitored thrice daily. The animal care and experimental protocols were in accordance with the European guidelines and approved by the Ethical Committee for Animal Experimentation of KU Leuven (P053/2016).

### 4.2. Experimental Groups

First, to analyze the dynamics of autophagy during reperfusion, Sham-operated rats (Sham) and rats subjected to 45 min of ischemia (I45-mild ischemia) were divided into subgroups with various reperfusion (R) times: R0h, R1h, R3h, R6h, R24h, R48h, R7d, or R90d. Next, to assess the effects of the ischemic time, we compared the I45 mild ischemia group with rats subjected to 60 min of ischemia (severe ischemia-I60), followed by 0 h, 3 h, 24 h, and 7 days of reperfusion. Six rats were included per subgroup.

### 4.3. Kidney Function and Injury

Kidney function was assessed by plasma creatinine, measured by the kinetic Jaffé method (Hitachi/Roche Modular P, Roche Diagnostics, Diegem, Belgium) by the central laboratory of our University Hospitals. The cellular injury markers aspartate aminotransferase [26,45] (AST, colorimetric method on Hitachi/Roche Modular P) and heart-fatty acid binding protein [26,45,46] (h-FABP, enzyme-linked immunosorbant assay (ELISA)) were assessed according to the manufacturer's instructions (HK414-Hycult Biotech, Uden, The Netherlands).

### 4.4. Transmission Electron Microscopy

Small samples of the cortex (ca. 1 $mm^3$) were fixed in 2.5% glutaraldehyde, 0.1 M of sodium cacodylate, and 0.05% $CaCl_2$ (pH 7.4) and further processed for transmission electron microscopy, as described previously [47], with minor modifications (extra staining with 1% tannic acid in veronal acetate for 1h after OsO4 postfixation). A FEI Tecnai microscope was used to examine ultrathin sections at 80–120 kV.

### 4.5. Western Blotting

Snap-frozen kidney samples were homogenized in a radioimmunoprecipitation assay buffer (RIPA) lysis buffer containing 50 mM of Tris-HCl (pH 7.4); 150 mM of NaCl; 1 mM of EDTA; 1% Ipegal; protease, and phosphatase inhibitors (Roche, Basel, Switzerland). The protein concentration was determined through use of a Bradford protein assay (Sigma-Aldrich, Saint-Louis, MO, USA). Samples were prepared with Laemmli buffer containing β-mercaptoethanol, heated at 95 °C for 3 min and loaded on Any kD Mini-Protean TGX Precast Gel (Bio-Rad Laboratories, Hercules, CA, USA). SDS-PAGE was performed with a constant voltage of 150 V. Next, the proteins were blotted on polyvinylidene difluoride (PVDF) membranes using the semi-dry Trans-Blot Turbo Transfer system (Bio-Rad Laboratories). Membranes were blocked for 1h at room temperature with PBS-Tween (0.1%) containing 5% milk powder (MP), followed by incubation with the primary antibody diluted in PBS-T and 2% MP overnight at 4 °C. Next day, the membranes were washed 3 times with PBS-T and then incubated with the secondary horseradish peroxidase (HRP)-coupled antibody for 45 min with PBS-T + 2% MP. After washing three times with PBS-T, immunoreactive bands were visualized through enhanced chemoluminescence (Pierce ECL Western Blotting Substrate, Thermo Fisher Scientific, Waltham, MA, USA), followed by detection and band intensity quantification using the Chemidoc MP technology and associated Imagelab software (Bio-Rad Laboratories).

### 4.6. Antibodies

The following antibodies and reagents were used for the Western blotting experiments. Anti-LC3 (5F10, Nanotools), anti-S6 (2217, Cell Signaling Technology, Danvers, MA, USA), anti-phospho-S6 (4858, Cell Signaling Technology), anti-cleaved caspase 3 (9664, Cell Signaling Technology), anti-SQSTM1/p62 (P0067, Sigma-Aldrich, Saint-Louis, MO, USA), anti-Bcl-2 (sc-492, Santa Cruz Biotechnology, Dallas, TX, USA), and anti-Bax (sc-493, Santa Cruz Biotechnology). Anti-GAPDH (G8715, Sigma-Aldrich) served as an internal control. Secondary antibodies are HRP-linked anti-mouse IgG (7076, Cell Signaling Technology) and HRP-linked anti-rabbit IgG (1706515, Bio-Rad Laboratories, Hercules, CA, USA).

### 4.7. Quantitative Real-Time Polymerase Chain Reaction

RNA was extracted from kidney tissues using Trizol reagent and chloroform, followed by an additional purification step with the RNeasy mini kit (Qiagen, Hilden, Germany), according to the manufacturer's protocol. The mRNA expression levels in kidney tissues were analyzed using quantitative real-time polymerase chain reaction (Q-RT-PCR). Reverse transcription was performed at 37 °C for 1 h with the M-MLV Reverse Transcriptase along with FSBuffer and Rnase out (Life Technologies, Carlsbad, CA, USA). Q-RT-PCR was performed with the PCR mastermix of Applied Biosystems (1.503.193, Foster City, CA, USA). Thermal cycling conditions were composed of cDNA initially denatured at 95 °C for 60 s, and then amplified by PCR for 45 cycles (95 °C for 5 s, 60 °C for 30 s). Experiments were carried out in duplicates. Using the 2-ΔΔCt method [48], the relative quantification in gene expression was determined. Data are expressed as the relative differences (fold change) between the sham and IR samples after correction for GAPDH expression.

### 4.8. qPCR Taqman Probes

The following reagents from TaqMan Gene Expression Assays (Applied biosystems, Foster Cyti, CA, USA) were used for RT-PCR experiments: GAPDH (Rn01775763_g1), BECN1 (Rn00586976_m1), LC3 (Rn02132764_S1), p62 (Rn00709977_m1), Bcl-2 (Rn99999125_m1), Bax (Rn01480160_g1), Bim (Rn00674175_m1), Hsp70 (Rn00583013_S1), ICAM-1 (Rn00564227_m1), IL-10 (Rn00563409_m1), and IL-6 (Rn01410330_m1).

### 4.9. Terminal Deoxynucleotidyl Transferase End Labeling

For the detection of oligonucleosomal DNA cleavage via terminal deoxynucleotidyl transferase end labeling (TUNEL), tissue sections were deparaffinized in toluene (2 × 5 min), rehydrated in distilled water (5 min), and pretreated with 3% citric acid (60 min) to remove tissue calcification. Endogenous peroxidase was quenched by incubating sections for 15 min in 0.9% hydrogen peroxide. Thereafter, TUNEL was performed using an ApopTag Plus Peroxidase In Situ Apoptosis Detection Kit (Merck-Millipore, Burlington, MA, USA) according to the instructions of the manufacturer. Slides were observed with an Olympus BX61 microscope at 20× magnification, and pictures were taken with the Olympus Stream Essentials 1.9 software. Quantification of the TUNEL staining was performed with the "color threshold" function of ImageJ, using the color space RGB and the same parameters for each analyzed picture.

### 4.10. Statistical Analysis

If data were normally distributed, unpaired t-tests were used for the comparison of 2 groups (Sham versus IR group) or a one-way ANOVA for 3 groups (Sham, I45, and I60) with Tukey Multiple Comparison test post-hoc. F-test was performed to compare variances. If the variances were significantly different, Welch's correction was applied. If a group was not normally distributed, non-parametric tests (Mann–Whitney or Kruskal–Wallis test with Dunns post-hoc) were performed. For relative Western blotting and qPCR data, values were normalized to the mean of the control Sham group. Outliers were removed based on the Grubb's test. Normal distribution was analyzed with the Kolmogorov–Smirnov test (for small sample sizes).

**Supplementary Materials:** Supplementary materials can be found at http://www.mdpi.com/1422-0067/21/19/7185/s1.

**Author Contributions:** Conceptualization J.-P.D. and I.J.; methodology, J.-P.D. and W.M.; validation, J.-P.D., D.M., J.P., and I.J.; formal analysis, J.-P.D. and S.H.; investigation, J.-P.D., S.H., and I.J.; resources, J.-P.D., D.M., J.P., and I.J.; data curation, J.-P.D.; writing—original draft preparation, J.-P.D.; writing—review and editing, S.H., D.M., W.M., J.P., and I.J.; visualization, J.-P.D.; supervision, J.P. and I.J.; funding acquisition, J.-P.D., D.M., J.P., and I.J. All authors have read and agreed to the published version of the manuscript.

**Funding:** This work was supported by a Research Grant of the Research Foundation Flanders (FWO-KaN 1518914N). At the time of the research, J.-P.D. was a fellow with ERA-EDTA.

**Acknowledgments:** We would like to thank Veerle Heedfeld and Tine Wylin (Abdominal Transplantation) for their practical help with the rat and laboratory experiments.

**Conflicts of Interest:** The authors declare no conflict of interest.

## Abbreviations

| | |
|---|---|
| AKI | Acute kidney injury |
| AMPK | 5′ adenosine monophosphate-activated protein kinase |
| AST | Aspartate transaminase |
| Bcl-2 | B-Cell lymphoma 2 |
| hFABP | heart-type fatty acid binding protein |
| Hsp70 | Heat shock protein 70 |
| ICAM | Intracellular adhesion molecule |
| IL | Interleukin |
| IR | Ischemia-reperfusion |
| LC3 | (microtubule-associated protein 1) Light chain 3 |
| mTOR | mammalian target of rapamycin |
| Sqstm1 | Sequestosome 1 |
| TEM | transmission electron microscopy |
| TUNEL | Terminal deoxynucleotidyl transferase dUTP nick end labeling |
| ULK-1 | Unc51-like kinase-1 |

## References

1. Bellomo, R.; Kellum, J.A.; Ronco, C. Acute kidney injury. *Lancet* **2012**, *380*, 756–766. [CrossRef]
2. Lameire, N.; Bagga, A.; Cruz, D.; De Maeseneer, J.; Endre, Z.H.; Kellum, J.A.; Liu, K.D.; Mehta, R.L.; Pannu, N.; Van Biesen, W.; et al. Acute kidney injury: An increasing global concern. *Lancet* **2013**, *382*, 170–179. [CrossRef]
3. Hoste, E.; Kellum, J.A.; Selby, N.M.; Zarbock, A.; Palevsky, P.M.; Bagshaw, S.M.; Goldstein, S.L.; Cerdá, J.; Chawla, L.S. Global epidemiology and outcomes of acute kidney injury. *Nat. Rev. Nephrol.* **2018**, *14*, 607–625. [CrossRef] [PubMed]
4. RENAL Replacement Therapy Study Investigators; Bellomo, R.; Cass, A.; Cole, L.; Finfer, S.; Gallagher, M.; Billot, L.; McArthur, C.; McGuinness, S.; Myburgh, J.A.; et al. Intensity of continuous renal-replacement therapy in critically ill patients. *N. Engl. J. Med.* **2009**, *361*, 1627–1638. [PubMed]
5. Palevsky, P.M.; Zhang, J.H.; O'Connor, T.Z.; Chertow, G.M.; Crowley, S.T.; Choudhury, D.; Finkel, K.; Kellum, J.A.; Paganini, E.; Schein, R.M.H.; et al. Intensity of renal support in critically ill patients with acute kidney injury. *N. Engl. J. Med.* **2008**, *359*, 7–20. [PubMed]
6. Bonventre, J.V.; Yang, L. Cellular pathophysiology of ischemic acute kidney injury. *J. Clin. Investig.* **2011**, *121*, 4210–4221. [CrossRef]
7. Sharfuddin, A.A.; Molitoris, B.A. Pathophysiology of ischemic acute kidney injury. *Nat. Rev. Nephrol.* **2011**, *7*, 189–200. [CrossRef]

8. Chawla, L.S.; Kimmel, P.L. Acute kidney injury and chronic kidney disease: An integrated clinical syndrome. *Kidney Int.* **2012**, *82*, 516–524. [CrossRef]
9. Parzych, K.R.; Klionsky, D.J. An Overview of Autophagy: Morphology, Mechanism, and Regulation. *Antioxid Redox Signal.* **2014**, *20*, 460–473. [CrossRef]
10. Pallet, N.; Livingston, M.; Dong, Z. Emerging Functions of Autophagy in Kidney Transplantation. *Am. J. Transplant.* **2013**, *14*, 13–20. [CrossRef]
11. Eltzschig, H.K.; Carmeliet, P. Hypoxia and inflammation. *N. Engl. J. Med.* **2011**, *364*, 656–665. [CrossRef] [PubMed]
12. Daemen, M.A.; Veer, C.v.; Denecker, G.; Heemskerk, V.H.; Wolfs, T.G.A.M.; Clauss, M.; Vandenabeele, P.; Buurman, W.A. Inhibition of apoptosis induced by ischemia-reperfusion prevents inflammation. *J. Clin. Investig.* **1999**, *104*, 541–549. [CrossRef] [PubMed]
13. Daemen, M.A.; de Vries, B.; Buurman, W.A. Apoptosis and inflammation in renal reperfusion injury. *Transplantation* **2002**, *73*, 1693–1700. [CrossRef] [PubMed]
14. Yang, B.; Hosgood, S.A.; Nicholson, M.L. Naked small interfering RNA of caspase-3 in preservation solution and autologous blood perfusate protects isolated ischemic porcine kidneys. *Transplantation* **2011**, *91*, 501–507. [CrossRef] [PubMed]
15. Nakagawa, S.; Nishihara, K.; Inui, K.; Masuda, S. Involvement of autophagy in the pharmacological effects of the mTOR inhibitor everolimus in acute kidney injury. *Eur. J. Pharmacol.* **2012**, *696*, 143–154. [CrossRef] [PubMed]
16. Chien, C.T.; Shyue, S.K.; Lai, M.K. Bcl-xL augmentation potentially reduces ischemia/reperfusion induced proximal and distal tubular apoptosis and autophagy. *Transplantation* **2007**, *84*, 1183–1190. [CrossRef]
17. Isaka, Y.; Suzuki, C.; Abe, T.; Okumi, M.; Ichimaru, N.; Imamura, R.; Kakuta, Y.; Matsui, I.; Takabatake, Y.; Rakugi, H.; et al. Bcl-2 protects tubular epithelial cells from ischemia/reperfusion injury by dual mechanisms. *Transplant. Proc.* **2009**, *41*, 52–54. [CrossRef]
18. Yeh, C.H.; Hsu, S.P.; Yang, C.C.; Chien, C.T.; Wang, N.P. Hypoxic preconditioning reinforces HIF-alpha-dependent HSP70 signaling to reduce ischemic renal failure-induced renal tubular apoptosis and autophagy. *Life Sci.* **2010**, *86*, 115–123. [CrossRef]
19. Wu, H.H.; Hsiao, T.Y.; Chien, C.T.; Lai, M.K. Ischemic conditioning by short periods of reperfusion attenuates renal ischemia/reperfusion induced apoptosis and autophagy in the rat. *J. Biomed. Sci.* **2009**, *16*, 19. [CrossRef]
20. Mariño, G.; Niso-Santano, M.; Baehrecke, E.H.; Kroemer, G. Self-consumption: The interplay of autophagy and apoptosis. *Nat. Rev. Mol. Cell Biol.* **2014**, *15*, 81–94. [CrossRef]
21. Chen, Q.; Kang, J.; Fu, C. The independence of and associations among apoptosis, autophagy, and necrosis. *Signal Transduct. Target. Ther.* **2018**, *3*, 18. [CrossRef]
22. Liu, Y.; Levine, B. Autosis and autophagic cell death: The dark side of autophagy. *Cell Death Differ.* **2015**, *22*, 367–376. [CrossRef] [PubMed]
23. Decuypere, J.P.; Pirenne, J.; Jochmans, I. Autophagy in Renal Ischemia-Reperfusion Injury: Friend or Foe? *Am. J. Transplant.* **2014**, *14*, 1464–1465. [CrossRef] [PubMed]
24. Decuypere, J.P.; Ceulemans, L.J.; Agostinis, P.; Monbaliu, D.; Naesens, M.; Pirenne, J.; Jochmans, I. Autophagy and the kidney: Implications for ischemia-reperfusion injury and therapy. *Am. J. Kidney Dis.* **2015**, *66*, 699–709. [CrossRef] [PubMed]
25. Sarkar, S.; Davies, J.E.; Huang, Z.; Tunnacliffe, A.; Rubinsztein, D.C. Trehalose, a novel mTOR-independent autophagy enhancer, accelerates the clearance of mutant huntingtin and alpha-synuclein. *J. Biol. Chem.* **2007**, *82*, 5641–5652. [CrossRef]
26. Decuypere, J.P.; Ceulemans, L.J.; Wylin, T.; Martinet, W.; Monbaliu, D.; Pirenne, J.; Jochmans, I. Plasmatic Villin 1 Is a Novel In Vivo Marker of Proximal Tubular Cell Injury During Renal Ischemia-Reperfusion. *Transplantation* **2017**, *101*, e330–e336. [CrossRef] [PubMed]
27. Ikegami, Y.; Goodenough, S.; Inoue, Y.; Dodd, P.R.; Wilce, P.A.; Matsumoto, I. Increased TUNEL positive cells in human alcoholic brains. *Neurosci. Lett.* **2003**, *349*, 201–205. [CrossRef]
28. Klionsky, D.J.; Abdelmohsen, K.; Abe, A.; Abedin, J.; Abeliovich, H.; Arozena, A.A.; Adachi, H.; Adams, C.M.; Adams, P.D.; Adeli, K.; et al. Guidelines for the use and interpretation of assays for monitoring autophagy (3rd edition). *Autophagy* **2016**, *12*, 1–222. [CrossRef]
29. Biever, A.; Valjent, E.; Puighermanal, E. Ribosomal Protein S6 Phosphorylation in the Nervous System: From Regulation to Function. *Front. Mol. Neurosci.* **2015**, *8*, 75. [CrossRef]
30. Mardones, P.; Rubinsztein, D.C.; Hetz, C. Mystery solved: Trehalose kickstarts autophagy by blocking glucose transport. *Sci. Signal.* **2016**, *9*, fs2. [CrossRef]

31. Zhao, M.; Klionsky, D.J. AMPK-dependent phosphorylation of ULK1 induces autophagy. *Cell Metab.* **2011**, *13*, 119–120. [CrossRef] [PubMed]
32. Bore, P.J.; Papatheofanis, I.; Sells, R.A. Adenosine triphosphate regeneration and function in the rat kidney following warm ischaemia. *Transplantation* **1979**, *27*, 235–237. [CrossRef] [PubMed]
33. Glick, D.; Barth, S.; Macleod, K.F. Autophagy: Cellular and molecular mechanisms. *J. Pathol.* **2010**, *221*, 3–12. [CrossRef] [PubMed]
34. Jiang, M.; Liu, K.; Luo, J.; Dong, Z. Autophagy is a renoprotective mechanism during in vitro hypoxia and in vivo ischemia-reperfusion injury. *Am. J. Pathol.* **2010**, *176*, 1181–1192. [CrossRef] [PubMed]
35. Aoyagi, T.; Kusakari, Y.; Xiao, C.-Y.; Inouye, B.T.; Takahashi, M.; Scherrer-Crosbie, M.; Rosenzweig, A.; Hara, K.; Matsui, T. Cardiac mTOR protects the heart against ischemia-reperfusion injury. *Am. J. Heart Physiol. Circ. Physiol.* **2012**, *303*, H75–H85. [CrossRef] [PubMed]
36. Kim, J.; Kundu, M.; Viollet, B.; Guan, K.L. AMPK and mTOR regulate autophagy through direct phosphorylation of Ulk1. *Nat. Cell Biol.* **2011**, *13*, 132–141. [CrossRef]
37. Mulay, S.R.; Thomasova, D.; Ryu, M.; Anders, H.J. MDM2 (murine double minute 2) links inflammation and tubular cell healing during acute kidney injury in mice. *Kidney Int.* **2012**, *81*, 1199–1211. [CrossRef]
38. Linkermann, A.; Chen, G.; Dong, G.; Kunzendorf, U.; Krautwald, S.; Dong, Z. Regulated Cell Death in AKI. *J. Am. Soc. Nephrol.* **2014**, *25*, 2689–2701. [CrossRef]
39. Belavgeni, A.; Meyer, C.; Stumpf, J.; Hugo, C.; Linkermann, A. Ferroptosis and Necroptosis in the Kidney. *Cell Chem. Biol.* **2020**, *27*, 446–462. [CrossRef]
40. Van Erp, A.C.; Hoeksma, D.; Rebolledo, R.A.; Ottens, P.J.; Jochmans, I.; Monbaliu, D.; Pirenne, J.; Leuvenink, H.; Decuypere, J.-P. The Crosstalk between ROS and Autophagy in the Field of Transplantation Medicine. *Oxidative Med. Cell. Longev.* **2017**, *2017*, 7120962. [CrossRef]
41. Eleftheriadis, T.; Pissas, G.; Antoniadi, G.; Liakopoulos, V.; Stefanidis, I. Cell Death Patterns Due to Warm Ischemia or Reperfusion in Renal Tubular Epithelial Cells Originating from Human, Mouse, or the Native Hibernator Hamster. *Biology* **2018**, *7*, 48. [CrossRef] [PubMed]
42. Sciarretta, S.; Yee, D.; Nagarajan, N.; Bianchi, F.; Saito, T.; Valenti, V.; Tong, M.; Del Re, M.P.; Vecchione, C.; Schirone, L.; et al. Trehalose-Induced Activation of Autophagy Improves Cardiac Remodeling After Myocardial Infarction. *J. Am. Coll. Cardiol.* **2018**, *71*, 1999–2010. [CrossRef] [PubMed]
43. Ikeda, M.; Bando, T.; Yamada, T.; Sato, M.; Menjyu, T.; Aoyama, A.; Sato, T.; Chen, F.; Sonobe, M.; Omasa, M.; et al. Clinical application of ET-Kyoto solution for lung transplantation. *Surg. Today* **2015**, *45*, 439–443. [CrossRef]
44. Zhao, X.; Koshiba, T.; Nakamura, T.; Tsuruyama, T.; Li, Y.; Bando, T.; Wada, H.; Tanaka, K. ET-Kyoto solution plus dibutyryl cyclic adenosine monophosphate is superior to University of Wisconsin solution in rat liver preservation. *Cell Transplant.* **2008**, *17*, 99–109. [CrossRef]
45. Jochmans, I.; Lerut, E.; Van Pelt, J.; Monbaliu, D.; Pirenne, J. Circulating AST, H-FABP, and NGAL are early and accurate biomarkers of graft injury and dysfunction in a preclinical model of kidney transplantation. *Ann. Surg.* **2011**, *254*, 784–791. [CrossRef]
46. Shirakabe, A.; Kobayashi, N.; Hata, N.; Shinada, T.; Tomita, K.; Tsurumi, M.; Okazaki, H.; Matsushita, M.; Yamamoto, Y.; Yokoyama, S.; et al. The serum heart-type fatty acid-binding protein (HFABP) levels can be used to detect the presence of acute kidney injury on admission in patients admitted to the non-surgical intensive care unit. *BMC Cardiovasc. Disord.* **2016**, *16*, 174. [CrossRef] [PubMed]
47. Martinet, W.; Timmermans, J.P.; De Meyer, G.R.Y. Methods to assess autophagy in situ—Transmission electron microscopy versus immunohistochemistry. *Methods Enzymol.* **2014**, *543*, 89–114.
48. Livak, K.J.; Schmittgen, T.D. Analysis of relative gene expression data using real-time quantitative PCR and the 2(-Delta Delta C(T)) Method. *Methods* **2001**, *25*, 402–408. [CrossRef]

International Journal of
*Molecular Sciences*

MDPI

*Article*

# ND-13, a DJ-1-Derived Peptide, Attenuates the Renal Expression of Fibrotic and Inflammatory Markers Associated with Unilateral Ureter Obstruction

**Carmen De Miguel [1,*], Abigayle C. Kraus [1], Mitchell A. Saludes [2], Prasad Konkalmatt [2], Almudena Ruiz Domínguez [3], Laureano D. Asico [2], Patricia S. Latham [4], Daniel Offen [5], Pedro A. Jose [2] and Santiago Cuevas [3,*]**

1 Section of Cardio-Renal Physiology and Medicine, Division of Nephrology, Department of Medicine, University of Alabama at Birmingham, AL 35233, USA; abkraus@uab.edu
2 Department of Medicine, Division of Renal Diseases & Hypertension and Pharmacology/Physiology, The George Washington University School of Medicine and Health Sciences, Washington, DC 20052, USA; mtsaludes@live.com (M.A.S.); prk@email.gwu.edu (P.K.); lasico@email.gwu.edu (L.D.A.); pjose@mfa.gwu.edu (P.A.J.)
3 Molecular Inflammation Group, Biomedical Research Institute of Murcia (IMIB), University Clinical Hospital Virgen Arrixaca, 30120 Murcia, Spain; almuruiz_8@hotmail.com
4 Pathology and Internal Medicine The George Washington University School of Medicine and Health Sciences, Washington, DC 20052, USA; pslath@gwu.edu
5 Neuroscience Laboratory, The Felsenstein Medical Research Center, Sackler School of Medicine, Tel-Aviv University, Tel-Aviv 6997801, Israel; danioffen@gmail.com
* Correspondence: cdemigue@uab.edu (C.D.M.); santiago.cuevas@imib.es (S.C.); Tel.: +1-(205)-934-2430 (C.D.M.); +34-(868)-885-038 (S.C.)

Received: 1 September 2020; Accepted: 22 September 2020; Published: 24 September 2020

check for updates

**Abstract:** DJ-1 is a redox-sensitive chaperone with reported antioxidant and anti-inflammatory properties in the kidney. The 20 amino acid (aa) peptide ND-13 consists of 13 highly conserved aas from the DJ-1 sequence and a TAT-derived 7 aa sequence that helps in cell penetration. This study aimed to determine if ND-13 treatment prevents the renal damage and inflammation associated with unilateral ureter obstruction (UUO). Male C57Bl/6 and *DJ-1*$^{-/-}$ mice underwent UUO and were treated with ND-13 or vehicle for 14 days. ND-13 attenuated the renal expression of fibrotic markers *TGF-β* and *collagen1a1* (*Col1a1*) and inflammatory markers *TNF-α* and *IL-6* in C57Bl/6 mice. *DJ-1*$^{-/-}$ mice treated with ND-13 presented similar decreased expression of *TNF-α*, *IL-6* and *TGF-β*. However, in contrast to C57Bl/6 mice, ND-13 failed to prevent renal fibrosis or to ameliorate the expression of *Col1a1* in this genotype. Further, UUO led to elevated urinary levels of the proximal tubular injury marker neutrophil gelatinase-associated lipocalin (NGAL) in *DJ-1*$^{-/-}$ mice, which were blunted by ND-13. Our results suggest that ND-13 protects against UUO-induced renal injury, inflammation and fibrosis. These are all crucial mechanisms in the pathogenesis of kidney injury. Thus, ND-13 may be a new therapeutic approach to prevent renal diseases.

**Keywords:** renal disease; DJ-1; ND-13; renal inflammation; oxidative stress; UUO; fibrosis

## 1. Introduction

Renal oxidative stress and inflammation are two of the most important factors involved in the pathogenesis of renal diseases and other cardiovascular disease complications [1]. Inflammation, the consequent oxidative stress, and vice versa, are considered major factors triggering fibrosis, and are key components in the development and progression of renal failure [2]. Renal fibrosis is caused, in part, by excess deposition of extracellular matrix, and inflammation is one of the main pathways that trigger this mechanism [3]. The inflammatory response during the initial stages of renal disease is characterized by glomerular and tubulo-interstitial infiltration of immune cells, including neutrophils and macrophages [4]. Furthermore, the activation of neutrophils during these early stages results in the release of proinflammatory and profibrogenic cytokines [4], followed by the infiltration of macrophages and T and B lymphocytes into the tissues. Macrophages are a major source of TGF-β in fibrotic organs [5,6], and recruitment of T and B lymphocytes to the site of injury further facilitates the secretion of fibrogenic cytokines [7,8]. TGF-β is also a potent chemoattractant involved in the recruitment of inflammatory cells [9] and, thereby, facilitates the expansion of the inflammatory process. Renal inflammation plays a central role in the initiation and progression of fibrosis in chronic kidney disease. Therefore, attenuation of the inflammatory response may be a critical step for the restoration of the proper balance between pro and antifibrotic signaling pathways [10,11] in the kidney and other organs.

DJ-1, also known as Park 7, is a multifunctional oxidative stress response protein. *DJ-1* was initially identified as an autosomal recessive gene associated with Parkinson's disease, and it has been shown to be expressed in the brain, heart, kidney, liver, pancreas, and skeletal muscle in rodents as well as in humans [12]. DJ-1 functions as a redox-sensitive chaperone with intrinsic antioxidant properties, especially in the mitochondria, and it regulates the expression of several antioxidant genes such as glutathione and heat shock protein 70 in dopaminergic neurons [13,14]. DJ-1 is mainly present in the cytoplasm and, to a lesser extent, in the mitochondria. However, upon an oxidant challenge, DJ-1 translocates from the cytoplasm to the mitochondria where it protects mitochondrial function [15]. In a previous report, our group demonstrated that renal DJ-1 plays a critical role in the regulation of oxidative stress-dependent hypertension in mice [16].

Nrf2 (nuclear factor erythroid 2-related factor 2) is a transcription factor that regulates the expression of several antioxidant genes and also inhibits the development and progression of acute kidney injury caused by heavy metals, ischemia and xenobiotics such as cyclosporin A and cisplatin [17]. Nrf2 attenuates the NFκB-inflammatory pathway and suppresses proinflammatory cell signaling [18,19]. We previously reported that the kidney-selective silencing of *DJ-1* in mice leads to impairment of the antioxidant response mediated by the dopamine receptor 2 and increases in blood pressure associated with decreased Nrf2 expression and activity in the kidney [16,20]. In addition, mice with *DJ-1* selectively silenced in the kidney, and mice with germline deletion of *DJ-1* ($DJ\text{-}1^{-/-}$ mice), develop high blood pressure, renal damage and decreased kidney expression and activity of Nrf2 [20], suggesting that DJ-1 inhibits the production of renal reactive oxygen species (ROS), at least in part, via the activation of Nrf2-controlled antioxidant genes. We also recently demonstrated the important role of the antioxidant protein UCP2 in hypertension associated with the depletion of DJ-1 [21]. Moreover, other reports also implicated the DJ-1/Nrf2 pathway in the pathogenesis of several renal diseases, such as diabetic nephropathy in rats [22].

Dr. Daniel Offen's laboratory, at the University of Tel Aviv, developed a 13 aa-long peptide derived from the most conserved sequence of DJ-1 [23]. To achieve cell permeability, this 13 aa chain was fused to a 7 aa TAT sequence (YGRKKRR). The resulting 20 amino acid compound was named ND-13 and was demonstrated to be effective in protecting neuronal cultures from the effects of relevant neurotoxins in the setting of Parkinson's disease, amyotrophic lateral sclerosis or multiple system atrophy [23–25]. ND-13 exerts these protective effects by reducing apoptosis and by inactivating the proapoptotic protein caspase-3 in neuronal cell lines exposed to these neurotoxic insults. In those studies, ND-13 treatment led to the activation of the Nrf2 pathway and the consequent increased expression of Nrf2-induced antioxidant genes [23], similar observations to our previous findings in the kidney of $DJ\text{-}1^{-/-}$ mice [20]. However, the potential protective effects of ND-13 against the development of renal disease remain unknown. Therefore, the goal of these studies was to determine if ND-13 prevents the renal damage and inflammation associated with an animal model of progressive kidney fibrosis, the unilateral ureter obstruction (UUO) model, and if this protection is mediated by the activation of the DJ-1/Nrf2 pathway.

## 2. Results

### 2.1. ND-13 Treatment Reduces UUO-Induced Renal Fibrosis in WT Mice, but Not in $DJ\text{-}1^{-/-}$ Mice

Because UUO is a classical model of progressive renal fibrosis, we evaluated by RT-PCR the expression levels of markers of fibrosis in the cortex of wild type (WT) mice that underwent sham or UUO surgery and were treated with ND-13 or vehicle for 14 days. We found that after UUO surgery, WT mice treated with vehicle presented a significant upregulation of the markers of fibrosis *Col1a1* and *TGF-β* (~70-fold increase for *Col1α1* and ~7-fold increase for *TGF-β* $p < 0.05$; Figure 1) in the renal cortex. Importantly, daily treatment with ND-13 significantly decreased the cortical expression of both markers of fibrosis, suggesting a protective effect of this peptide against the development of the cortical fibrosis typically induced by UUO.

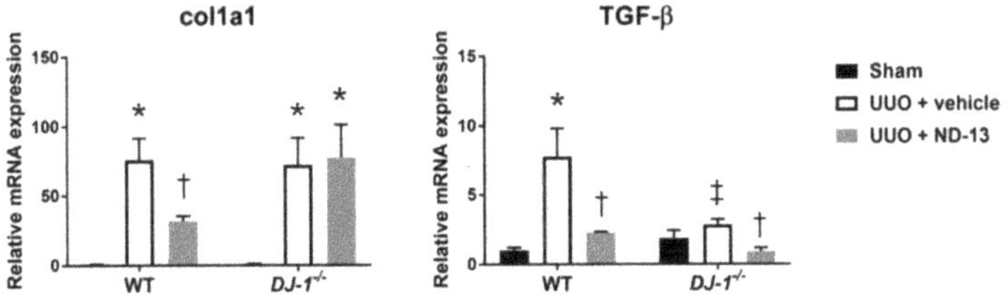


**Figure 1.** Treatment with ND-13 reduces the unilateral ureter obstruction (UUO)-induced renal expression of fibrotic markers in wild type (WT) mice, but not in $DJ\text{-}1^{-/-}$ mice. Relative mRNA expression of markers of fibrosis *col1a1* and *TGF-β* in renal cortex of WT and $DJ\text{-}1^{-/-}$ mice that underwent sham surgery, UUO and vehicle treatment or UUO and ND-13 treatment. $N$ = 4–5/group; * $p < 0.05$ vs. same genotype sham, † $p < 0.05$ vs. same genotype UUO + vehicle, ‡ $p < 0.05$ vs. WT UUO + vehicle; two-way ANOVA with Tukey's post-hoc test.

In order to characterize the role of DJ-1 in the development of the renal fibrosis associated with UUO, we performed similar studies using the *DJ-1* global knockout ($DJ\text{-}1^{-/-}$) mouse. In response to UUO, and similar to our findings in the WT mice, $DJ\text{-}1^{-/-}$ mice significantly upregulated the mRNA expression of the marker of fibrosis *Col1a1* compared to the levels that the sham group presented (Figure 1). However, and contrary to the results found in WT mice, treatment of $DJ\text{-}1^{-/-}$ mice with ND-13 failed to prevent the elevation of *Col1a1* in the cortex after UUO. In contrast, the cortical levels of *TGF-β* after UUO did not significantly increase in the $DJ\text{-}1^{-/-}$ mice compared to sham controls, but interestingly, treatment with ND-13 was efficient in decreasing the mRNA expression of *TGF-β* in the renal cortex (Figure 1).

Similar to the results obtained by RT-PCR, Masson's blue trichrome histological staining demonstrated extensive interstitial fibrosis in the cortex, outer and inner medulla in WT mice treated with vehicle, as indicated by the homogeneous presence of blue staining in Figure 2A. Although deposition of fibrotic material was also apparent in the WT mice treated with ND-13, examination of the tissue at higher magnification revealed that the cortical fibrosis was not as homogenously distributed, and tended to be localized to certain areas of the cortex while other areas appeared fibrosis-free (Figures 2A and 3A), suggesting that treatment with ND-13 may be blunting the accumulation of fibrotic material in the renal cortex. Despite these observations of the extension of fibrosis and the clear trend of the results, no significant difference in the cortical fibrosis quantification was found among the WT groups (relative fibrosis: sham: 1 ± 0.4, UUO + vehicle: 2.1 ± 0.3 and UUO + ND-13: 1.0 ± 0.4, $p > 0.05$, $n$ = 4–5/group, Figure 2B).

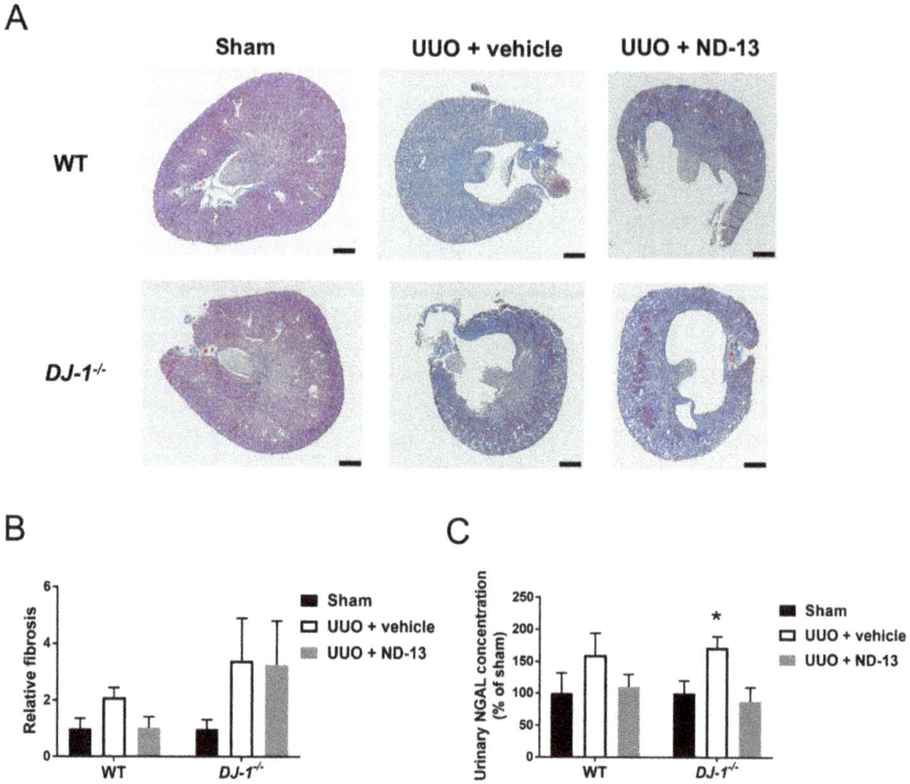


**Figure 2.** Treatment with ND-13 reduces UUO-induced renal fibrosis in WT mice. (**A**) Representative full scan images of Masson's blue trichrome-stained kidneys obtained from WT and *DJ-1*$^{-/-}$ mice that underwent sham surgery, UUO and vehicle treatment or UUO and ND-13 treatment (scale bar = 500 μm). (**B**) Quantification of collagen deposition in renal cortex of WT and *DJ-1*$^{-/-}$ mice that underwent sham surgery, UUO and vehicle treatment or UUO and ND-13 treatment. (**C**) Urinary concentration of the proximal tubule marker NGAL in WT and *DJ-1*$^{-/-}$ mice that underwent sham surgery, UUO and vehicle treatment or UUO and ND-13 treatment. $n$ = 4–5/group; * $p < 0.05$ vs. same genotype sham, two-way ANOVA with Tukey's post hoc test.

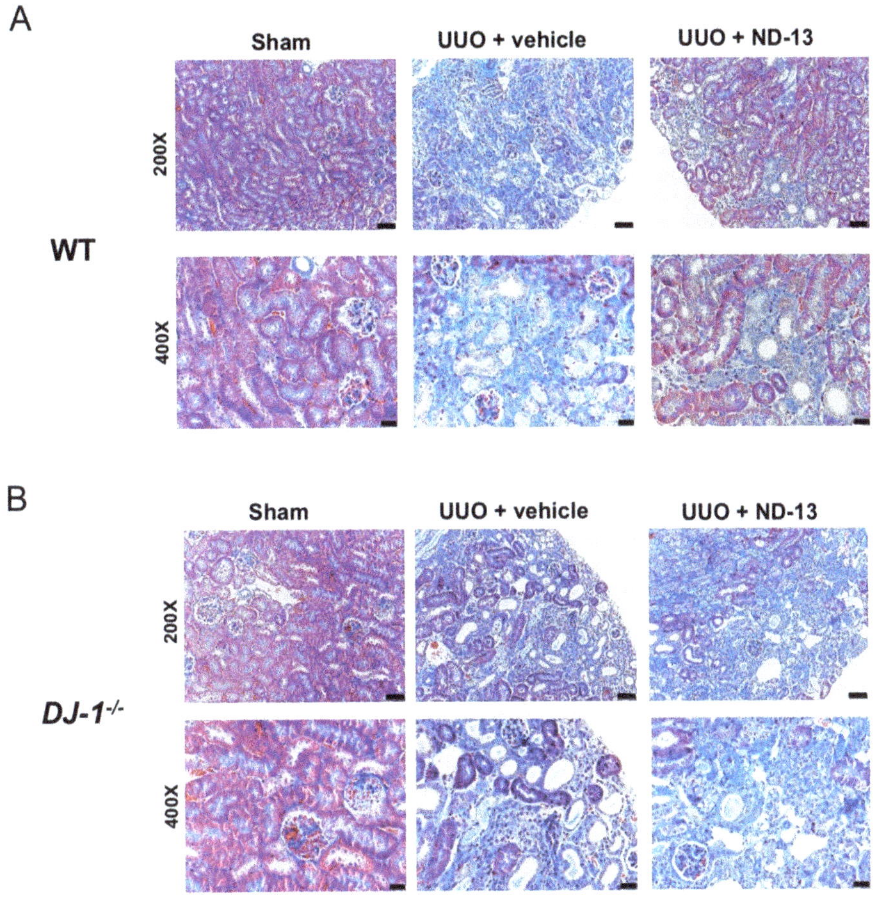


**Figure 3.** Treatment with ND-13 seems to blunt the spread of UUO-induced fibrosis accumulation in the cortex of WT mice but fails to do so in *DJ-1*$^{-/-}$ mice. (**A**) Representative Masson's blue trichrome images of renal cortex of WT mice that underwent sham surgery, UUO and vehicle treatment or UUO and ND-13 treatment: 200× (upper panels; scale bar = 50 μm) and 400× magnification (bottom panels; scale bar = 20 μm). (**B**) Representative Masson's blue trichrome images of renal cortex of *DJ-1*$^{-/-}$ mice that underwent sham surgery, UUO and vehicle treatment or UUO and ND-13 treatment: 200× (upper panels; scale bar = 50 μm) and 400× magnification (bottom panels; scale bar = 20 μm).

Likewise, histological evaluation of cortical tissue obtained from *DJ-1*$^{-/-}$ mice after the UUO protocol supported the molecular findings in this genotype, as ND-13 treatment had no effect on the amount of collagen deposition detected by trichrome blue staining in this region of the kidney (relative fibrosis, UUO + vehicle vs. UUO + ND-13: 3.4 ± 1.5 vs. 3.3 ± 1.5; Figure 2A,B and Figure 3B). The renal fibrosis in *DJ-1*$^{-/-}$ mice was found to be evenly distributed across the cortical region (Figure 3B).

To determine the extent of renal damage, the concentration of neutrophil gelatinase-associated lipocalin (NGAL), a marker of proximal tubule damage, was measured in urine. We found that the urinary concentrations of NGAL were similar among the three experimental groups of WT mice, suggesting that these groups presented similar levels of renal damage (Figure 2C). On the other hand, fourteen days after UUO, *DJ-1*$^{-/-}$ mice presented significantly greater amounts of urinary NGAL compared to *DJ-1*$^{-/-}$ mice that underwent sham surgery, and daily treatment of these mice with ND-13 resulted in a normalization of these urinary values to sham levels (Figure 2C). These results suggest that *DJ-1*$^{-/-}$ mice are more sensitive to UUO-induced kidney damage, and that ND-13 ameliorates the damage inflicted to the proximal tubules by UUO.

### 2.2. Treatment with ND-13 Does Not Prevent UUO-Induced Cell Death in the Kidney

To determine if treatment with ND-13 effectively protected against kidney cell death in response to the UUO protocol, the presence of Terminal Deoxynucleotidyl Transferase-Mediated dUTP Nick-End Labeling (TUNEL)-positive areas in kidney cortex and medulla was quantified in both genotypes. As shown in Figure 4A, and as expected, WT and *DJ-1*$^{-/-}$ sham animals hardly presented any TUNEL-positive cells in the kidney cortex. UUO induced cell death in mice of both genotypes treated with vehicle, although the elevation in the percentage area of the kidney that stained positive for TUNEL only reached significance in the *DJ-1*$^{-/-}$ mice, and appeared to be greater than in WT mice ($p > 0.05$, Figure 4B). Upon closer examination, the cortical TUNEL-positive stain was observed in glomeruli, tubular cells and interstitial cells in both genotypes. Treatment with ND-13 was unable to prevent cortical cell death in either genotype, as the percentage area of the kidney stained for TUNEL remained elevated in both. No differences between the treatments and genotypes were observed in the renal medulla (Figure 4B).

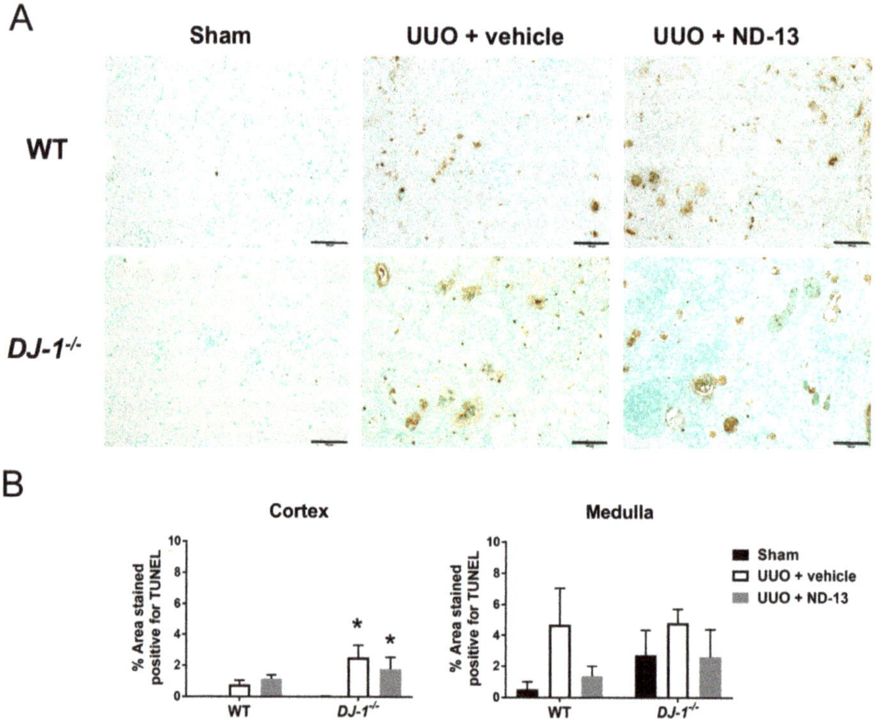


**Figure 4.** ND-13 does not protect against UUO-induced cell death. (**A**) Representative images of TUNEL stained (brown color) kidney cortex from WT (upper panels) and *DJ-1*$^{-/-}$ mice that underwent sham surgery, UUO and vehicle treatment or UUO and ND-13 treatment (scale bar = 100 μm). (**B**) Quantification of cell death (% TUNEL-positive area) in kidney cortex and medulla of WT and *DJ-1*$^{-/-}$ mice that underwent sham surgery, UUO and vehicle treatment or UUO and ND-13 treatment. $n$ = 4–5/group; * $p < 0.05$ vs. same genotype sham, two-way ANOVA with Tukey's post-hoc test.

### *2.3. Renal Expression of Cytokine and Chemokine Genes Associated with UUO Is Ameliorated in Mice Treated with ND-13*

Renal inflammation has been proven to be intimately associated with the development of kidney damage [2]. Therefore, we evaluated the level of kidney inflammation in our experimental animals and found that WT mice that underwent UUO, and were treated with vehicle, had significantly upregulated expression of cytokines *TNF-α* and *IL-6* and chemokine *CCL25* in the renal cortex (Figure 5). Interestingly, daily treatment with ND-13 led to a significant attenuation in the expression of these markers of inflammation, bringing their expression levels to values similar to those found in the sham WT group.

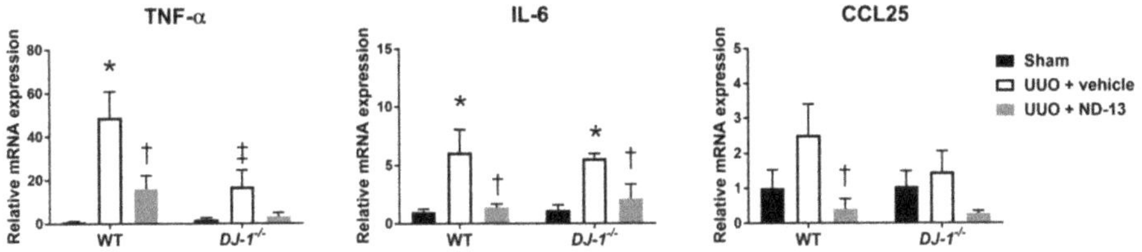


**Figure 5.** Expression of cytokine and chemokine genes associated with UUO is attenuated in kidneys obtained from WT mice treated with ND-13. Relative mRNA expression of cytokines *TNF-α* and *IL-6* and chemokine *CCL25* in renal cortex of WT mice and $DJ\text{-}1^{-/-}$ mice that underwent sham surgery, UUO and vehicle treatment or UUO and ND-13 treatment. $n$ = 4–5/group; * $p < 0.05$ vs. same genotype sham, † $p < 0.05$ vs. same genotype UUO + vehicle, ‡ $p < 0.05$ vs. WT UUO + vehicle; two-way ANOVA with Tukey's post-hoc test.

Similar to the trends found in WT mice, ND-13 had anti-inflammatory effects on $DJ\text{-}1^{-/-}$ mice that underwent UUO surgery, as indicated by the blunted expression of *TNF-α*, *CCL25* and *IL-6* in the renal cortex compared to the values observed in the vehicle-treated group (Figure 5). Of note, the *TNF-α* response to UUO was significantly smaller in $DJ\text{-}1^{-/-}$ mice treated with vehicle than the response observed in WT mice treated with vehicle (Figure 5).

### *2.4. ND-13 Treatment Attenuates the UUO-Induced Cortical Macrophage Inflammation in WT Mice, but Not in $DJ\text{-}1^{-/-}$ Mice, While Not Preventing the Infiltration of T-Lymphocytes in Either Genotype*

As expected, the population of T-lymphocytes ($CD3^+$ cells) in the cortex was elevated in WT mice after UUO, although it did not reach statistical significance from the levels shown in mice that underwent sham surgery (sham vs. UUO + vehicle: 4.6 ± 0.7 vs. 14.9 ± 4.6 cells/field, $p > 0.05$, $n$ = 4–5/group). Daily treatment with ND-13 failed to normalize the kidney T-cell inflammation in WT mice (16.1 ± 2.8 cells/field; Figure 6). Similarly, $DJ\text{-}1^{-/-}$ mice showed an increased infiltration of T-lymphocytes in the renal cortex (Figure 6) in response to UUO (sham vs. UUO + vehicle: 3.7 ± 0.3 vs. 24.9 ± 2.2 cells/field, $p < 0.05$, $n$ = 4–5/group). However, the magnitude of T cell accumulation in the cortex of $DJ\text{-}1^{-/-}$ mice was greater than in WT mice (WT mice vs. $DJ\text{-}1^{-/-}$ mice: 14.9 ± 4.6 vs. 24.9 ± 2.2 cells/field), and it remained elevated despite the ND-13 treatment (26.0 ± 8.3 cells/field). Raw data for the T cell numbers in each of the 10 fields evaluated per animal, as well as the mean and SEM per animal, are provided in Supplementary Table S1.

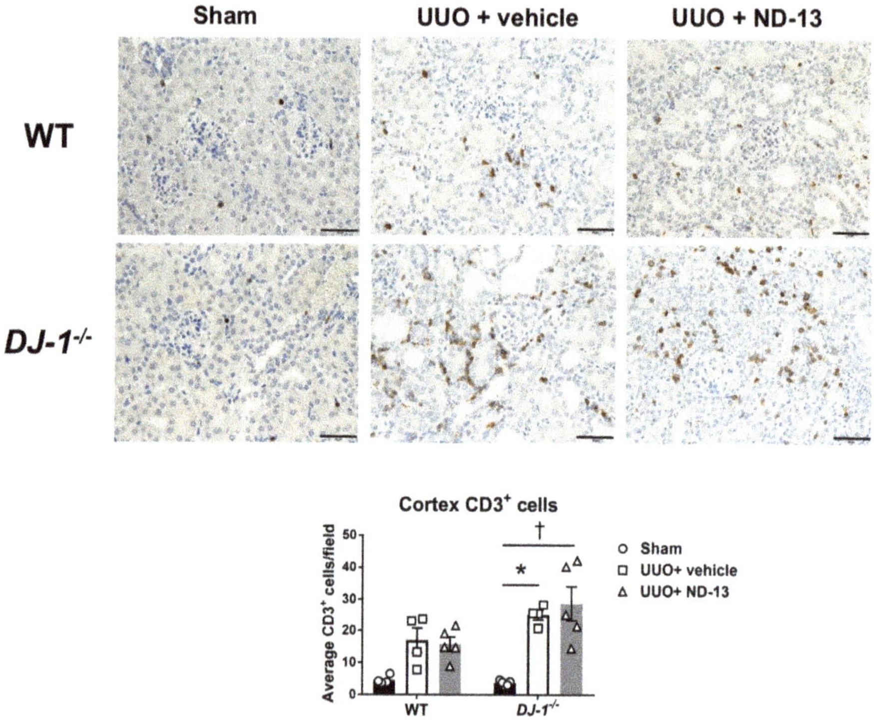


**Figure 6.** Treatment with ND-13 does not prevent the UUO-induced infiltration of T cells into the kidney cortex of mice that underwent UUO. Representative images and quantification of T cell ($CD3^+$ cells) infiltration in renal cortex of WT (upper panels) and *DJ-1*$^{-/-}$ (bottom panels) mice that underwent sham surgery, UUO and vehicle treatment or UUO and ND-13 treatment (scale bar = 20 μm). * $p < 0.05$ vs. same genotype sham, † $p < 0.05$ vs. same genotype UUO + vehicle; two-way ANOVA with Tukey's post hoc test.

Similar to what was found with T cells, the number of macrophages infiltrating the cortex was elevated fourteen days after UUO surgery (sham vs. UUO + vehicle: 0.1 ± 0.0 vs. 2.4 ± 1.1 % area stained positive for F4/80, $p > 0.05$, $n$ = 4–5/group). However, treatment with ND-13 only tended to attenuate those numbers (0.7 ± 0.3 % area stained positive; Figure 7). Evaluation of the macrophage population in the renal cortex of *DJ-1*$^{-/-}$ mice also revealed elevated numbers of these immune cells after UUO (sham vs. UUO + vehicle: 0.2 ± 0.1 vs. 6.5 ± 1.2 % area stained positive for F4/80, $p < 0.05$, $n$ = 4–5/group); however, in contrast to WT mice, treatment with ND-13 failed to prevent macrophage infiltration in these mice, and the numbers of macrophages were similar to those found in mice treated with vehicle (7.0 ± 2.0 % area stained positive) (Figure 7). Of note, the magnitude of the cortical infiltration of macrophages after UUO was significantly worse in the case of the *DJ-1*$^{-/-}$ mice compared to WT mice (UUO + vehicle, WT mice vs. *DJ-1*$^{-/-}$ mice: 2.4 ± 1.1 vs. 6.5 ± 1.2 % area stained positive, $p < 0.05$, $n$ = 4–5/group). Raw data for the percentage area stained positive for F4/80 quantified in each of the 10 fields/animal, as well as the mean and SEM per animal, are provided in Supplementary Table S2.

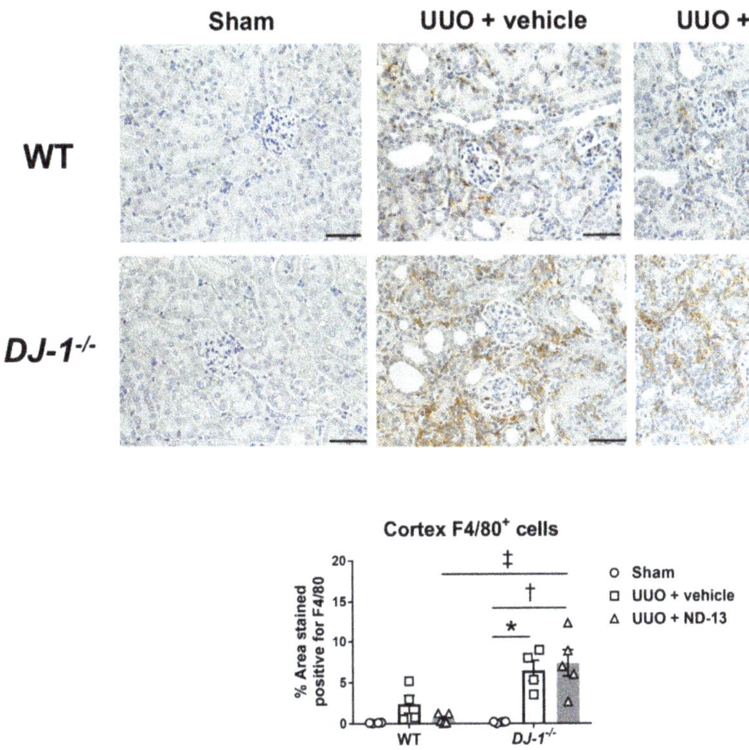


**Figure 7.** Treatment with ND-13 tends to decrease the UUO-induced macrophage infiltration into the renal cortex of WT mice that underwent UUO but fails to prevent this inflammation in *DJ-1*$^{-/-}$ mice that underwent UUO. Representative images and quantification of macrophage infiltration (% area stained for F4/80) in renal cortex of WT mice that underwent sham surgery, UUO and vehicle treatment or UUO and ND-13 treatment (scale bar = 20 μm). * $p < 0.05$ vs. same genotype sham, † $p < 0.05$ vs. same genotype UUO + vehicle, ‡ $p < 0.05$ vs. WT UUO + vehicle; two-way ANOVA with Tukey's post hoc test.

### *2.5. ND-13 Does Not Improve the Renal Damage Score in UUO Mice*

The tubular damage and neutrophilic infiltrates present in the kidneys obtained from the experimental mice were evaluated using hematoxylin and eosin (H&E) stained sections and given a combined renal damage score. Kidneys obtained from UUO mice showed epithelial flattening and focally dilated tubules, with moderate proteinaceous contents and casts, and showed no difference between genetic backgrounds or treatment conditions. The glomerular morphology presented unremarkable changes in all groups. The renal damage score based on H&E staining showed a very small, insignificant protective effect of ND-13 on the extent of the neutrophilic infiltrate in the cortex. The means and standard errors of these inflammation scores, adjusted by density, are the following: C57BL/6 mice with UU0 + vehicle: 1.45 ± 0.83 vs. UU0 + N-13: 1.15 ± 0.81; *DJ-1*$^{-/-}$ mice with UU0 + vehicle: 3.13 ± 1.04 vs UU0 + N-13: 2.31 ± 1.14. Significant differences were not found between the groups. No inflammation was found in the control mice and no apparent morphological changes were found in the contralateral kidneys.

## 3. Discussion

The major finding of this study is that treatment with ND-13 is effective in preventing the exaggerated expression of kidney fibrotic and inflammatory markers that normally develop as consequences of UUO. We demonstrated that ND-13 significantly reduced the expression of fibrotic markers col1a1 and TGF-β and prevented the accumulation of macrophages in the kidney of C57Bl/6J mice after UUO. The fact that ND-13 did not protect *DJ-1*$^{-/-}$ mice against the UUO-induced renal damage highlights the critical role of DJ-1 as an important mediator of this protective mechanism. To our knowledge, this is the first report to evaluate the protective effects of ND-13 in renal diseases.

According to the Center for Disease Control, 37 million Americans suffered from chronic kidney disease in 2019, with associated health costs of about $114 billion to care for these patients [26]. Current therapies are not effective in preventing the development of renal disease [27]. Thus, new therapeutic alternatives are urgently needed. There is abundant evidence in the literature that demonstrates that renal inflammation and renal fibrosis precede the development of chronic kidney disease [28], highlighting the critical involvement of these two factors in the pathogenesis of renal damage. Among other kidney diseases, inflammation and fibrosis are involved in the progression of glomerulonephritis [29], acute kidney injury [7], polycystic kidney disease [30], renal artery stenosis [31], lupus nephritis [32] and diabetic nephropathy [33]. Accordingly, pharmacological therapies aimed at the attenuation of inflammatory and fibrotic processes may be an appropriate approach in the prevention of these renal pathologies.

UUO is a model of progressive kidney fibrosis and inflammation that is characterized by tubular dilation, loss of proximal tubular mass, interstitial expansion, hypertrophy, hydronephrosis and tubular epithelial cell death [34]. The mechanical stretching induced by the tying of the ureter stimulates a massive production of reactive oxygen species (ROS) and cellular apoptosis in the affected kidney that, in turn, result in alterations of the hemodynamic status and significant inflammation and fibrosis [34]. Therefore, UUO is an ideal experimental model to evaluate the putative preventive effects of ND-13 against renal damage and, particularly, on kidney fibrosis.

To examine DJ-1 as a possible novel therapeutic target for renal diseases, we used the 20 aa peptide known as ND-13 [23]. Treatment of WT mice with ND-13 blunted the UUO-induced upregulation in the kidney expression of *TGF-β* and *Col1a1*, and also decreased the kidney expression of inflammatory markers *TNF-α*, *IL-6* and *CCL25*. Interestingly, the ND-13-mediated decrease in fibrotic marker expression was not accompanied by a significant improvement in the deposition of collagen in the kidney. These seemingly contradictory findings could be due to the long timeline in our studies, where the animals were examined a full two weeks after the UUO protocol. This timeline, compared to shorter postsurgical times, is known to induce severe injury to the kidney and stimulate extreme deposition of collagen in this organ [34–36]. The protective effects of ND-13 against collagen deposition may have been hindered by starting the treatment at the same time as the UUO pathology. Interestingly, and although it did not reach statistical significance, we observed that the cortical fibrosis in the WT mice treated with ND-13 was not as generalized as it was in mice treated with vehicle, possibly suggesting that treatment with ND-13 may have slightly slowed down the fibrotic deposition. Considering the profound reduction in kidney fibrotic marker expression induced by ND-13, it is likely that its effects on kidney fibrosis would have been different if the animals were treated with this peptide for a period of time prior to the UUO protocol. This is a research avenue that our group will investigate in the future. Similarly, the protective effects of ND-13 did not extend to the renal T cell infiltration, which remained elevated. However, it seemed to prevent the macrophage influx into this organ. It is possible that ND-13 shifted the phenotype of the T cell and macrophage populations present in the kidney from a proinflammatory type to an anti-inflammatory type (i.e., Tregs vs. Th17 cells, or M1 vs. M2 macrophages) attenuating the inflammatory response and renal damage. Future follow-up studies will focus on the further evaluation of immune cell subtypes present in the kidneys of these animals in order to completely understand the effects of ND-13 in proinflammatory versus anti-inflammatory immune populations in the kidney after UUO. Moreover, these results suggest promising protective effects of ND-13 that could be more evident in less aggressive animal models of kidney disease with pathogenic mechanisms more similar to human renal disease.

On the other hand, and despite the attenuation in the expression of inflammatory cytokines that we observed in *DJ-1*$^{-/-}$ mice that underwent UUO and were treated with ND-13, we did not find differences in kidney fibrosis nor collagen deposition in these mice when compared with the shams. The fact that treatment with ND-13 did not decrease kidney fibrosis in *DJ-1*$^{-/-}$ mice, but it did in WT mice, strongly underlines the essential role of renal DJ-1 in the prevention of renal damage.

Our group previously reported the effects that deletion of *DJ-1* has on renal oxidative stress and injury as well as on blood pressure [16,20,21] and a protective role of DJ-1 in endotoxin-induced acute kidney injury was recently described [36]. We demonstrated that silencing *DJ-1* expression in mouse kidneys, and in mouse proximal tubule cells specifically, attenuates the expression and activity of Nrf2 and results in increased ROS production [20]. Nrf2 is a master regulator of antioxidant and anti-inflammatory factors [19], and its activity and expression is regulated by ROS production [37]. Moreover, genetic deletion of *DJ-1* leads to increased ubiquitination of Nrf2, suggesting that the renal protection exerted by DJ-1 is mediated by preventing the degradation of Nrf2 [20]. Interestingly, both DJ-1 and Nrf2 are activated in acute kidney injury [38], and Nrf2 has been proven to inhibit the development and progression of several diseases affecting the kidney [17,39]. In previous studies, we also demonstrated that DJ-1 increases Nrf2 expression and activity only under pathological conditions and has no effects on Nrf2 in the physiological setting.

Consistent with our results, previous studies demonstrated that DJ-1 stabilized Nrf2 by preventing binding to Keap1 and Nrf2's subsequent ubiquitination [40]. DJ-1 may amplify Nrf2 activity by avoiding its degradation. However, the ability of DJ-1 to stimulate directly the Nrf2 pathway has not been demonstrated [41]. We speculate that ND-13 prevents the undesirable consequences of chronic Nrf2 activation. Thereby, ND-13 may be an appropriate therapeutic approach to enhance the actions of Nrf2, and it could be used to minimize the side effects associated with treatment of chronic Nrf2 activation by other Nrf2 inducers i.e., bardoxolone [42,43] in humans. Our working hypothesis is that the ROS and inflammation that are induced by UUO lead to increased levels of interleukins and chemokines and, in turn, to the activation of the immune response in the kidney. This inflammatory and oxidative milieu creates a vicious cycle that leads to fibrosis and promotes kidney damage and kidney dysfunction. In this setting, DJ-1 prevents the ubiquitination of Nrf2, amplifying this molecule's antioxidant response. We speculate that Nrf2 would attenuate oxidative stress and inflammation in the kidney, leading to reduced cytokine expression and thereby preventing inflammation and preserving renal function (Figure 8).

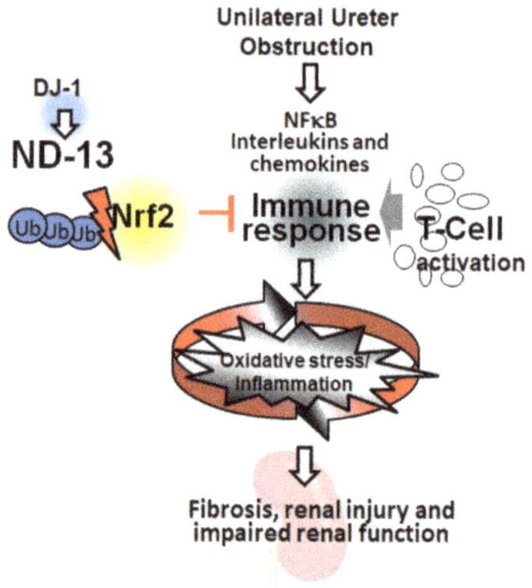


**Figure 8.** Working hypothesis. ROS and inflammation induced by unilateral ureter obstruction increase interleukin and chemokine expression activating the immune response. This inflammatory/oxidative environment leads to a vicious cycle, which may produce fibrosis and induce renal damage and kidney dysfunction. DJ-1 prevents the ubiquitination of Nrf2 and amplifies its response. Nrf2 may be acting by attenuating the oxidative stress and inflammation, leading to a reduced cytokine expression and preventing inflammation, resulting in protection of the renal function.

In summary, these data suggest that ND-13 prevents the renal inflammation and fibrosis associated with the acute renal damage induced by UUO. Further studies are needed to confirm if ND-13 treatment may be a new therapeutic approach for the prevention of renal injury, fibrosis and inflammation in human renal disease.

## 4. Materials and Methods

### 4.1. Animal Studies

All protocols were conducted in accordance with the Guide for the Care and Use of Laboratory Animals, and were approved by the Institutional Animal Care and Use Committee of the George Washington University (project identification numbers A353 and A412, approved on 26 February 2019 and 21 February 2019, respectively). Eight to nine-week old male C57Bl/6J (Jax Labs, Bar Harbor, ME) or *DJ-1*$^{-/-}$ mice (from our in-house colony) were used in these studies. Mice of each genotype underwent sham or unilateral ureter obstruction (UUO) surgery. In short, mice were anesthetized, the lower abdomen was opened and the left ureter was completely tied off using suture [44]. In those mice in the sham group, the abdomen was opened, the left ureter touched with a cotton tipped applicator and the abdomen was then sutured. The mice that underwent UUO surgery received either ND-13 (3 mg/kg/day, s.c.) or vehicle (scrambled peptide; 3 mg/kg/day, s.c.) starting from the day after surgery until the end of the study. Twelve days into the study, mice were placed in metabolic cages, acclimated to the cages for one day, and 24 h-urine was collected on the second day on the metabolic cages. On day 14 of the study, the mice were sacrificed, and kidneys harvested. One of the kidneys was snap-frozen in liquid nitrogen, while the other was placed in formalin for histological studies. No significant differences were found among the experimental groups regarding body weight, food intake, water intake or urine production (Table 1).

**Table 1.** Physical characteristics of the experimental groups.

| | Body Weight (g) | | | | | |
|---|---|---|---|---|---|---|
| | Pre | | Post | | Gain/Loss | |
| | Mean | SEM | Mean | SEM | Mean | SEM |
| WT sham | 28.75 | 3.22 | 28.85 | 2.90 | 0.10 | 0.38 |
| DJ-1$^{-/-}$ sham | 25.38 | 1.58 | 25.74 | 1.62 | 0.36 | 0.09 |
| WT vehicle | 23.30 | 2.05 | 23.94 | 2.00 | 0.64 | 0.31 |
| DJ-1$^{-/-}$ vehicle | 26.20 | 3.12 | 26.40 | 3.18 | 0.20 | 0.16 |
| WT ND-13 | 28.72 | 2.89 | 29.26 | 2.76 | 0.54 | 0.76 |
| DJ-1$^{-/-}$ ND-13 | 24.80 | 3.40 | 25.02 | 4.01 | 0.22 | 0.34 |
| | Food Intake (g) | | | | | |
| | Pre | | Post | | Net | |
| | Mean | SEM | Mean | SEM | Mean | SEM |
| WT sham | 75.85 | 0.57 | 72.40 | 2.95 | 3.45 | 2.57 |
| DJ-1$^{-/-}$ sham | 74.00 | 3.74 | 70.84 | 2.99 | 3.16 | 1.14 |
| WT vehicle | 70.66 | 3.89 | 64.80 | 3.87 | 5.86 | 1.88 |
| DJ-1$^{-/-}$ vehicle | 74.50 | 4.08 | 71.70 | 4.16 | 2.80 | 0.42 |
| WT ND-13 | 71.06 | 3.14 | 65.56 | 3.76 | 5.50 | 1.29 |
| DJ-1$^{-/-}$ ND-13 | 71.78 | 3.02 | 68.53 | 3.21 | 3.25 | 1.41 |
| | Water Intake (mL) | | | | | |
| | Pre | | Post | | Net | |
| | Mean | SEM | Mean | SEM | Mean | SEM |
| WT sham | 53.43 | 6.34 | 50.73 | 7.44 | 2.70 | 1.31 |
| DJ-1$^{-/-}$ sham | 55.44 | 4.97 | 51.48 | 3.90 | 3.96 | 1.60 |
| WT vehicle | 55.08 | 2.22 | 49.98 | 3.89 | 5.10 | 1.82 |
| DJ-1$^{-/-}$ vehicle | 57.90 | 6.12 | 54.25 | 6.02 | 3.65 | 0.53 |
| WT ND-13 | 56.08 | 1.93 | 50.34 | 2.28 | 5.74 | 0.57 |
| DJ-1$^{-/-}$ ND-13 | 59.58 | 2.75 | 55.45 | 2.22 | 4.13 | 1.97 |
| | | | Urine (mL) | | | |
| | | | Mean | SEM | | |
| WT sham | | | 0.63 | 0.28 | | |
| DJ-1$^{-/-}$ sham | | | 0.69 | 0.32 | | |
| WT vehicle | | | 1.10 | 0.36 | | |
| DJ-1$^{-/-}$ vehicle | | | 1 18 | 0.28 | | |
| WT ND-13 | | | 1.86 | 0.65 | | |
| DJ-1$^{-/-}$ ND-13 | | | 1.38 | 0.51 | | |

M: mean; SEM: standard error of the mean.

### 4.2. Quantitative RT-PCR

RNeasy mini kit (Qiagen, Valencia, CA, USA) was used to extract RNA from the kidney cortex. The amount of extracted RNA was quantified by spectrophotometry (NanoDrop ND-1000, Thermo Scientific, Waltham, MA, USA). RNA reverse transcription was performed using Quantitect Reverse Transcription kit (Qiagen) and following manufacturer's instructions. Primers were purchased from QuantiTect (Qiagen): *Col1a1* (QT00371308), *TGF-β* QT00371308), *TNF-α*QT00371308), *CCL25* (QT00371308) and *IL-6* (QT00371308). GAPDH was used as housekeeping gene (QT01658692). RNA expression was detected by the Quantitect SYBR green kit (Qiagen) and using a CFX96 Touch RT-PCR detection system (Bio-Rad, Hercules, CA, USA).

### *4.3. Histology and Fibrosis Quantification*

Kidneys were fixed overnight in 4% buffered formalin solution at room temperature, transferred to 70% ethanol for 24 h, and paraffin-embedded. Tissues were cut longitudinally into 4 µm-thick sections and mounted on Superfrost slides. Masson's trichrome blue staining was used to visualize renal fibrosis using bright-field microscopy (Olympus BX40 with 10× eyepiece lens; Olympus America, Melville, NY, USA). Full scans of the kidneys were obtained using a microscope fitted with a motorized XY stage and a digital camera (Olympus DP71), with sequential 20× images of each kidney taken and digitally stitched together with CellSense imaging software (Olympus). The cortical area of each full kidney scan was outlined and the percentage of blue fibrotic deposition within the outlined area was quantified using MetaMorph software (Molecular Devices LLC., San Jose, CA, USA). The average percentage fibrotic area for each experimental group was calculated and then normalized to the sham group. Data are presented as relative fibrosis compared to sham group.

### *4.4. Immunohistochemistry and Quantification of Immune Cell Infiltration in the Kidney*

Tissue sections were stained with primary antibodies specific for CD3 (1:600; Abcam, Cambridge, MA, USA) and F4/80 (1:200; Bio-Rad, Hercules, CA, USA) and detected with polymer conjugated secondary antibody (Biocare Medical, Concord, CA, USA). Quantification of renal T-lymphocyte ($CD3^+$ cells) infiltration was performed by blindly counting 10 microscopic fields (200 × 200 µm, 400× magnification) in each renal cortex. Infiltrating T cell numbers are reported as the average of the counts in the 10 fields per renal cortex. Quantification of renal macrophages ($F4/80^+$ cells) was performed by taking 10 cortical images from each animal at 400× magnification. The percentage of cortical area stained positive for F4/80 was quantified in each image using MetaMorph software and the average expression per animal was calculated. The data are reported as the average percentage area that stained positively for F4/80 per experimental group.

### *4.5. Terminal Deoxynucleotidyl Transferase-Mediated dUTP Nick-End Labeling (TUNEL) Assay and Quantification*

Tissue sections were stained using the Apoptag® Plus Peroxidase In Situ Apoptosis Kit (S7101, MP Biomedicals, Santa Ana, CA, USA) in order to detect dead cells. Ten microscopy images were taken of each kidney cortex and medulla (400 × 400 µm fields at 200× magnification) and the area stained positively with TUNEL in each image was quantified using Metamorph software and averaged per kidney region and animal. The data are reported as the average percentage area that stained positive for TUNEL in cortex and medulla per experimental group.

### *4.6. Urinary NGAL Measurements*

Urine collected on day two of the metabolic cage study was analyzed for concentration levels of the proximal tubular injury marker neutrophil gelatinase-associated lipocalin (NGAL) using an ELISA kit (Abcam). Average concentration per experiment group was calculated and the data are presented as percentage of sham group.

### *4.7. Renal Damage Evaluation*

Five images per mouse kidney section stained with H&E were evaluated by a blinded pathologist and each mouse was assigned a renal damage score based on the following criteria: inflammatory involvement (1 = <25%, 2 = 25–50%, 3 = 50–75%, 4 = >75%), inflammatory density (1 = mild, 2 = mild-moderate, 3 = moderate-severe, 4 = severe), dilation of tubules and tubular injury with neutrophilic infiltrates (PMNs) (1 = <2, 2 = 2–4, 3 = several, 4 = many) and casts (1 = <3, 2 = easily found; 3 = many).

### 4.8. Statistical Analysis

All data are expressed as mean ± SEM. Differences between groups were analyzed by two-way analysis of variance with a Tukey's post hoc test. A $p < 0.05$ was considered statistically significant. All statistical analyses were conducted using SigmaPlot 11 (Systat Software, Inc., San Jose, CA, USA).

**Supplementary Materials:** The following are available online at http://www.mdpi.com/1422-0067/21/19/7048/s1.

**Author Contributions:** Conceptualization, C.D.M. and S.C.; methodology, C.D.M., S.C. and D.O.; formal analysis, C.D.M. and S.C.; investigation, C.D.M., A.C.K., M.A.S., P.K., A.R.D., L.D.A., P.S.L. and S.C.; resources, C.D.M. and P.A.J.; writing—original draft preparation, C.D.M. and S.C.; writing—review and editing, C.D.M., S.C., P.A.J., P.S.L. and D.O.; visualization, C.D.M. and S.C.; supervision, C.D.M. and S.C.; funding acquisition, C.D.M., S.C. and P.A.J. All authors have read and agreed to the published version of the manuscript.

**Funding:** This work was funded in part by K01HL145324 and T32DK007545 to C.D.M., Seneca Foundation 21090/SF/19 to S.C. and 5P01 HL074940-10 and 7R01 DK039308-31 to P.A.J.

**Acknowledgments:** The authors thank the Histology Services at the George Washington University Research Pathology Core Lab for their expertise.

**Conflicts of Interest:** The authors declare that co-authors Santiago Cuevas, Pedro A. Jose and Daniel Offen hold a provisional patent in the United States on the effect of ND-13 in renal disorders.

## Abbreviations

| | |
|---|---|
| UUO | Unilateral ureter obstruction |
| Col1a1 | Collagen 1a1 |
| Nrf2 | Nuclear factor erythroid 2-related factor 2 |

## References

1. Giacco, F.; Brownlee, M. Oxidative stress and diabetic complications. *Circ. Res.* **2010**, *107*, 1058–1070. [CrossRef] [PubMed]
2. Navarro-Gonzalez, J.F.; Mora-Fernandez, C. The role of inflammatory cytokines in diabetic nephropathy. *J. Am. Soc. Nephrol.* **2008**, *19*, 433–442. [CrossRef] [PubMed]
3. Lee, S.B.; Kalluri, R. Mechanistic connection between inflammation and fibrosis. *Kidney Int.* **2010**, *78*, S22–S26. [CrossRef] [PubMed]
4. Imig, J.D.; Ryan, M.J. Immune and inflammatory role in renal disease. *Compr. Physiol.* **2013**, *3*, 957–976. [CrossRef]
5. Anders, H.J.; Ryu, M. Renal microenvironments and macrophage phenotypes determine progression or resolution of renal inflammation and fibrosis. *Kidney Int.* **2011**, *80*, 915–925. [CrossRef] [PubMed]
6. Duffield, J.S. Macrophages and immunologic inflammation of the kidney. *Semin. Nephrol.* **2010**, *30*, 234–254. [CrossRef]
7. Cao, Q.; Harris, D.C.; Wang, Y. Macrophages in kidney injury, inflammation, and fibrosis. *Physiology* **2015**, *30*, 183–194. [CrossRef] [PubMed]
8. Kisseleva, T.; Brenner, D.A. Fibrogenesis of parenchymal organs. *Proc. Am. Thorac. Soc.* **2008**, *5*, 338–342. [CrossRef]
9. Brenmoehl, J.; Miller, S.N.; Hofmann, C.; Vogl, D.; Falk, W.; Scholmerich, J.; Rogler, G. Transforming growth factor-beta 1 induces intestinal myofibroblast differentiation and modulates their migration. *World J. Gastroenterol.* **2009**, *15*, 1431–1442. [CrossRef]
10. Meng, X.M.; Nikolic-Paterson, D.J.; Lan, H.Y. Inflammatory processes in renal fibrosis. *Nat. Rev. Nephrol.* **2014**, *10*, 493–503. [CrossRef]
11. Lv, W.; Booz, G.W.; Wang, Y.; Fan, F.; Roman, R.J. Inflammation and renal fibrosis: Recent developments on key signaling molecules as potential therapeutic targets. *Eur. J. Pharmacol.* **2018**, *820*, 65–76. [CrossRef] [PubMed]
12. Nagakubo, D.; Taira, T.; Kitaura, H.; Ikeda, M.; Tamai, K.; Iguchi-Ariga, S.M.; Ariga, H. DJ-1, a novel oncogene which transforms mouse NIH3T3 cells in cooperation with ras. *Biochem. Biophys. Res. Commun.* **1997**, *231*, 509–513. [CrossRef] [PubMed]

13. Liu, F.; Nguyen, J.L.; Hulleman, J.D.; Li, L.; Rochet, J.C. Mechanisms of DJ-1 neuroprotection in a cellular model of Parkinson's disease. *J. Neurochem.* **2008**, *105*, 2435–2453. [CrossRef] [PubMed]
14. Zhou, W.; Freed, C.R. DJ-1 up-regulates glutathione synthesis during oxidative stress and inhibits A53T alpha-synuclein toxicity. *J. Biol. Chem.* **2005**, *280*, 43150–43158. [CrossRef] [PubMed]
15. Junn, E.; Jang, W.H.; Zhao, X.; Jeong, B.S.; Mouradian, M.M. Mitochondrial localization of DJ-1 leads to enhanced neuroprotection. *J. Neurosci. Res.* **2009**, *87*, 123–129. [CrossRef]
16. Cuevas, S.; Zhang, Y.; Yang, Y.; Escano, C.; Asico, L.; Jones, J.E.; Armando, I.; Jose, P.A. Role of renal DJ-1 in the pathogenesis of hypertension associated with increased reactive oxygen species production. *Hypertension* **2012**, *59*, 446–452. [CrossRef]
17. Shelton, L.M.; Park, B.K.; Copple, I.M. Role of Nrf2 in protection against acute kidney injury. *Kidney Int.* **2013**, *84*, 1090–1095. [CrossRef]
18. Li, W.; Khor, T.O.; Xu, C.; Shen, G.; Jeong, W.S.; Yu, S.; Kong, A.N. Activation of Nrf2-antioxidant signaling attenuates NFkappaB-inflammatory response and elicits apoptosis. *Biochem. Pharmacol.* **2008**, *76*, 1485–1489. [CrossRef]
19. Kobayashi, E.H.; Suzuki, T.; Funayama, R.; Nagashima, T.; Hayashi, M.; Sekine, H.; Tanaka, N.; Moriguchi, T.; Motohashi, H.; Nakayama, K.; et al. Nrf2 suppresses macrophage inflammatory response by blocking proinflammatory cytokine transcription. *Nat. Commun.* **2016**, *7*, 11624. [CrossRef]
20. Cuevas, S.; Yang, Y.; Konkalmatt, P.; Asico, L.D.; Feranil, J.; Jones, J.; Villar, V.A.; Armando, I.; Jose, P.A. Role of nuclear factor erythroid 2-related factor 2 in the oxidative stress-dependent hypertension associated with the depletion of DJ-1. *Hypertension* **2015**, *65*, 1251–1257. [CrossRef]
21. De Miguel, C.; Hamrick, W.C.; Sedaka, R.; Jagarlamudi, S.; Asico, L.D.; Jose, P.A.; Cuevas, S. Uncoupling Protein 2 Increases Blood Pressure in DJ -1 Knockout Mice. *J. Am. Heart Assoc.* **2019**, *8*, e011856. [CrossRef] [PubMed]
22. Sun, Q.; Shen, Z.Y.; Meng, Q.T.; Liu, H.Z.; Duan, W.N.; Xia, Z.Y. The role of DJ-1/Nrf2 pathway in the pathogenesis of diabetic nephropathy in rats. *Renal Fail.* **2016**, *38*, 294–304. [CrossRef] [PubMed]
23. Lev, N.; Barhum, Y.; Ben-Zur, T.; Aharony, I.; Trifonov, L.; Regev, N.; Melamed, E.; Gruzman, A.; Offen, D. A DJ-1 Based Peptide Attenuates Dopaminergic Degeneration in Mice Models of Parkinson's Disease via Enhancing Nrf2. *PLoS ONE* **2015**, *10*, e0127549. [CrossRef] [PubMed]
24. Glat, M.J.; Ben-Zur, T.; Barhum, Y.; Offen, D. Neuroprotective Effect of a DJ-1 Based Peptide in a Toxin Induced Mouse Model of Multiple System Atrophy. *PLoS ONE* **2016**, *11*, e0148170. [CrossRef] [PubMed]
25. Lev, N.; Barhum, Y.; Lotan, I.; Steiner, I.; Offen, D. DJ-1 knockout augments disease severity and shortens survival in a mouse model of ALS. *PLoS ONE* **2015**, *10*, e0117190. [CrossRef]
26. Centers for Disease Control and Prevention. *Chronic Kidney Disease in the United States, 2019*; US Department of Health and Human Services, Centers for Disease Control and Prevention: Atlanta, GA, USA, 2019.
27. Higgins, G.C.; Coughlan, M.T. Mitochondrial dysfunction and mitophagy: The beginning and end to diabetic nephropathy? *Br. J. Pharmacol.* **2014**, *171*, 1917–1942. [CrossRef]
28. Mihai, S.; Codrici, E.; Popescu, I.D.; Enciu, A.M.; Albulescu, L.; Necula, L.G.; Mambet, C.; Anton, G.; Tanase, C. Inflammation-Related Mechanisms in Chronic Kidney Disease Prediction, Progression, and Outcome. *J. Immunol. Res.* **2018**, *2018*, 2180373. [CrossRef]
29. Han, Y.; Ma, F.Y.; Tesch, G.H.; Manthey, C.L.; Nikolic-Paterson, D.J. Role of macrophages in the fibrotic phase of rat crescentic glomerulonephritis. *Am. J. Physiol. Renal Physiol.* **2013**, *304*, F1043–F1053. [CrossRef]
30. Song, C.J.; Zimmerman, K.A.; Henke, S.J.; Yoder, B.K. Inflammation and Fibrosis in Polycystic Kidney Disease. *Results Probl. Cell Differ.* **2017**, *60*, 323–344. [CrossRef]
31. Ma, Z.; Jin, X.; He, L.; Wang, Y. CXCL16 regulates renal injury and fibrosis in experimental renal artery stenosis. *Am. J. Physiol. Heart Circ. Physiol.* **2016**, *311*, H815–H821. [CrossRef]
32. Hill, G.S.; Delahousse, M.; Nochy, D.; Thervet, E.; Vrtovsnik, F.; Remy, P.; Glotz, D.; Bariety, J. Outcome of relapse in lupus nephritis: Roles of reversal of renal fibrosis and response of inflammation to therapy. *Kidney Int.* **2002**, *61*, 2176–2186. [CrossRef] [PubMed]
33. Brennan, E.P.; Cacace, A.; Godson, C. Specialized pro-resolving mediators in renal fibrosis. *Mol. Asp. Med.* **2017**, *58*, 102–113. [CrossRef] [PubMed]
34. Martinez-Klimova, E.; Aparicio-Trejo, O.E.; Tapia, E.; Pedraza-Chaverri, J. Unilateral Ureteral Obstruction as a Model to Investigate Fibrosis-Attenuating Treatments. *Biomolecules* **2019**, *9*. [CrossRef] [PubMed]

35. Chevalier, R.L.; Forbes, M.S.; Thornhill, B.A. Ureteral obstruction as a model of renal interstitial fibrosis and obstructive nephropathy. *Kidney Int.* **2009**, *75*, 1145–1152. [CrossRef]
36. Leeds, J.; Scindia, Y.; Loi, V.; Wlazlo, E.; Ghias, E.; Cechova, S.; Portilla, D.; Ledesma, J.; Swaminathan, S. Protective Role of DJ-1 in Endotoxin-induced Acute Kidney Injury. *Am. J. Physiol. Renal Physiol.* **2020**. [CrossRef]
37. Niture, S.K.; Khatri, R.; Jaiswal, A.K. Regulation of Nrf2-an update. *Free Rad. Biol. Med.* **2014**, *66*, 36–44. [CrossRef]
38. Sun, Q.; Shen, Z.Y.; Duan, W.N.; Meng, Q.T.; Xia, Z.Y. Mechanism of myocardial ischemia/reperfusion-induced acute kidney injury through DJ-1/Nrf2 pathway in diabetic rats. *Exp. Ther. Med.* **2017**, *14*, 4201–4207. [CrossRef]
39. Schmidlin, C.J.; Dodson, M.B.; Zhang, D.D. Filtering through the role of NRF2 in kidney disease. *Arch. Pharm. Res.* **2019**. [CrossRef]
40. Clements, C.M.; McNally, R.S.; Conti, B.J.; Mak, T.W.; Ting, J.P. DJ-1, a cancer- and Parkinson's disease-associated protein, stabilizes the antioxidant transcriptional master regulator Nrf2. *Proc. Natl. Acad. Sci. USA* **2006**, *103*, 15091–15096. [CrossRef]
41. Gan, L.; Johnson, D.A.; Johnson, J.A. Keap1-Nrf2 activation in the presence and absence of DJ-1. *Eur. J. Neurosci.* **2010**, *31*, 967–977. [CrossRef]
42. Himmelfarb, J.; Tuttle, K.R. New therapies for diabetic kidney disease. *N. Engl. J. Med.* **2013**, *369*, 2549–2550. [CrossRef] [PubMed]
43. Rossing, P. Diabetic nephropathy: Could problems with bardoxolone methyl have been predicted? *Nat. Rev. Nephrol.* **2013**, *9*, 128–130. [CrossRef] [PubMed]
44. Li, Z.; Xie, W.B.; Escano, C.S.; Asico, L.D.; Xie, Q.; Jose, P.A.; Chen, S.Y. Response gene to complement 32 is essential for fibroblast activation in renal fibrosis. *J. Biol. Chem.* **2011**, *286*, 41323–41330. [CrossRef] [PubMed]

International Journal of
*Molecular Sciences*

MDPI

*Article*

# Growth Differentiation Factor 15 Ameliorates Anti-Glomerular Basement Membrane Glomerulonephritis in Mice

**Foteini Moschovaki-Filippidou [1], Stefanie Steiger [1], Georg Lorenz [2], Christoph Schmaderer [2], Andrea Ribeiro [1], Ekaterina von Rauchhaupt [1], Clemens D. Cohen [1], Hans-Joachim Anders [1], Maja Lindenmeyer [3] and Maciej Lech [1,*]**

[1] LMU Klinikum, Medizinische Klinik und Poliklinik IV, Ludwig-Maximilians-Universität Munich, 80336 München, Germany; foteini.moschovaki@gmail.com (F.M.-F.); stefanie.steiger@med.uni-muenchen.de (S.S.); andrea.sof@gmail.com (A.R.); katjats95@gmail.com (E.v.R.); C.Cohen@med.uni-muenchen.de (C.D.C.); hjanders@med.uni-muenchen.de (H.-J.A.)

[2] Klinikum rechts der Isar, Department of Nephrology, Technical University Munich, 81675 München, Germany; georg.lorenz.gl@googlemail.com (G.L.); christoph.schmaderer@mri.tum.de (C.S.)

[3] III. Department of Medicine, University Medical Center Hamburg-Eppendorf, 20246 Hamburg, Germany; m.lindenmeyer@uke.de

* Correspondence: maciej.lech@med.uni-muenchen.de

check for updates

Received: 28 August 2020; Accepted: 21 September 2020; Published: 23 September 2020

**Abstract:** Growth differentiation factor 15 (GDF15) is a member of the transforming growth factor-β (TGF-β) cytokine family and an inflammation-associated protein. Here, we investigated the role of GDF15 in murine anti-glomerular basement membrane (GBM) glomerulonephritis. Glomerulonephritis induction in mice induced systemic expression of GDF15. Moreover, we demonstrate the protective effects for GDF15, as GDF15-deficient mice exhibited increased proteinuria with an aggravated crescent formation and mesangial expansion in anti-GBM nephritis. Herein, GDF15 was required for the regulation of T-cell chemotactic chemokines in the kidney. In addition, we found the upregulation of the CXCR3 receptor in activated T-cells in GDF15-deficient mice. These data indicate that CXCL10/CXCR3-dependent-signaling promotes the infiltration of T cells into the organ during acute inflammation controlled by GDF15. Together, these results reveal a novel mechanism limiting the migration of lymphocytes to the site of inflammation during glomerulonephritis.

**Keywords:** inflammation; T cells; glomerulonephritis; innate immunity; chemokines

## 1. Introduction

Anti-glomerular basement membrane glomerulonephritis (anti-GBM nephritis) is a severe acute kidney disease characterized by a variety of lesion patterns, including crescents, vascular loop necrosis, and mesangial expansion, suggesting multiple pathogenic mechanisms [1–4]. The upstream role of the adaptive immune system in failing to maintain immune tolerance and its downstream role in causing antigen-specific immunopathology in the glomerular compartment of the kidney has been widely recognized [3,5–7]. Experimental and clinical studies confirmed that various pro-inflammatory mediators are involved in this process [8–10]. For example, chemokines and transforming growth factor-β (TGF-β) family members regulate the inflammatory process and determine the progression and outcome of anti-GBM nephritis [11–14].

Growth differentiation factor 15 (GDF15, also known as macrophage inhibitory cytokine-1, MIC-1) is produced as a 35 kDa full-length form, cleaved in the N-terminus and secreted as a 25 kDa mature form [15]. GDF15 is a divergent member of the TGF- β superfamily and shows several structural differences compared to the rest of the superfamily. GDF15 is a regulator of inflammatory response dendritic cells maturation [16] and peripheral blood mononuclear proliferation [17]. Moreover, its role was suggested in cervical cancer, glioblastoma, cardiovascular ischemic stress, obesity, and metabolic disease, such as mitochondrial myopathies [18–24]. However, the knowledge of its role in progression of glomerulonephritis (GN) and mechanisms of function is still limited and requires further investigation. T cell-driven effector mechanisms play an important role, particularly in crescentic GN [25], and understanding the function of T-cells in the disease can be beneficial in future therapies for glomerular injury. Some studies showed a functional role for CD4+ T cells as effector cells participating in the development of crescentic GN by executing delayed-type hypersensitivity [26]. Others identified CD4+ cells but not CD8+ cells as crucial for the development of crescentic GN in mice [27]. By contrast, some findings suggest that glomerular injury in anti-GBM GN is driven by macrophage recruitment, which depends on both CD4+ and CD8+ T cells, and that T cell cytotoxicity does not play a role in the progression of the disease [28]. However, an anti-CD8 monoclonal antibody therapy was effective in both the prevention and treatment of experimental autoimmune glomerulonephritis [29], which could be associated with the effects of CD8+ cells on ICAM-1 and cytokine expression in crescentic glomerulonephritis [30]. Until now, systemic GDF15 levels have been shown to correlate with the progression of chronic kidney disease (CKD). Recombinant GDF15 protein reduced fibroblast activation and interstitial fibrosis in a model of unilateral ureter obstruction (UUO), possibly by blocking the TGF-β receptor and N-Myc signaling pathways [31]. Moreover, GDF15 reduces the expression of MHC class II and co-stimulatory molecules, as well as NF-kB family members Rel A and Rel B, IL-2, IFN-γ, and IL-12p40, and increases expression of TGF-β, and IL-10 [32]. In general, GDF15 is believed to be associated with stress responses, but its precise biological functions remain to be elucidated. Although GDF15 has been shown to affect aspects of chronic diseases (both inflammation and fibrosis), whether it controls glomerular disease progression is unclear [31,33,34].

In the present study, we used GDF15-deficient mice to investigate the role of GDF15 in anti-GBM nephritis. We hypothesized that GDF15 ameliorates the anti-Glomerular Basement Membrane (GBM) glomerulonephritis by limiting the inflammation and infiltration of the immune cells into the kidney.

## 2. Results

### 2.1. Experimental Anti-GBM Nephritis Is Associated with Higher Systemic and Intrarenal Expression of GDF15

We first asked if we could detect increased levels of GDF15 in mice following anti-GBM nephritis. To develop a reliable model, we tested several protocols and chose one with significant proteinuria and histopathological changes (Figure 1A). The nephrotoxic potential of the GBM antiserum in C57BL/6 mice (without pre-immunization) was previously assessed [35]. To implement the autologous adaptive immune response, we immunized mice with sheep-IgG 7 days prior to anti-GBM serum injection. We compared the development of albuminuria from day 0 to 21 in order to define the time-point with stable glomerular injury (Figure 1A). Moreover, we compared the amount of albuminuria of pre-immunized mice with mice without pre-immunization (heterologous model). Pre-immunization and the administration of anti-GBM serum resulted in a significant increase in albuminuria at 7 and 14 days. RT-PCR analysis of *Gdf15* and serum analysis of the protein revealed a low basal expression level, which was significantly upregulated 14 days upon anti-GBM serum injection (Figure 1B,C). We conclude that GDF15 is induced anti-GBM nephritis and that our protocol (7 + 14 days) of autologous anti-GBM nephritis is suitable to study the role of GDF15 in glomerular inflammation.

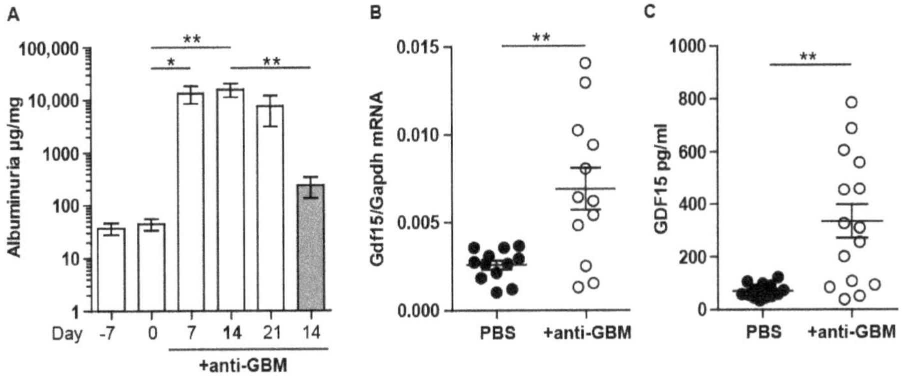


**Figure 1.** Evaluation of the anti-GBM model and expression of GDF15. (**A**) We used the commercially available GBM antiserum that was raised in sheep against rat GBM. We first examined its nephritogenic potential in C57BL/6 mice by assessing albuminuria 7, 14, and 21 days after a single intravenous injection of antiserum in pre-immunized mice, as well as in mice without pre-immunization (gray bar, 14 days). ($n = 5$, one-way ANOVA). (**B**) Total RNA isolated from kidneys of saline- or antiserum-injected C57BL/6 mice underwent quantitative real-time RT-PCR analysis and revealed significantly higher expression of Gdf15 in treated mice. (**C**) Serum GDF15 level was significantly increased in antiserum-injected C57BL/6 mice ($n = 12$, Student's $t$-Test). Data are mean ± SEM. * $p < 0.05$; ** $p < 0.01$.

### *2.2. GDF15 Deficiency Aggravates Albuminuria, Kidney Function Loss, and More Severe Tubular and Glomerular Injury in Anti-GBM Nephritis*

In order to address the role of GDF15 in glomerular inflammation, we applied the same protocol to C57BL/6 mice and *Gdf15-/-* mice. Plasma levels of multiple cytokines revealed an increased pro-inflammatory systemic signature. We detected significantly increased levels of IL-6, IL-12, TNF-α, and IFN-γ in the serum of GDF15-deficient mice (Figure 2A). Significantly increased glomerular filtration markers such as serum creatinine and blood urea nitrogen, glomerular injury markers-i.e., albuminuria (albumin/urine creatinine ratio), and tubular injury markers-i.e., urinary lipocalin-2 (NGAL) were noted in *Gdf15-/-* mice compared with wild type controls, which indicates more severe kidney disease in knockout mice (Figure 2B).

Based on these data, we assumed that GDF15 might play a protective role in anti-GBM nephritis. Both ongoing inflammation and severe glomerular injury can cause tubular injury. As expected, kidney sections stained with Periodic acid Schiff (PAS) reagent revealed increased tubular cast formation and tubular atrophy (scored as tubular injury TI) in nephritic GDF15-deficient animals compared to nephritic wild type animals (Figure 2D). These results demonstrate that the systemic deletion of *Gdf15* ameliorates proteinuria and renal tubular injury in anti-GBM nephritis. We did not observe any significant differences in total IgG levels in the blood of wild type and knockout mice. Consequently, the whole IgG staining of renal tissue did not reveal significant differences between the two treated groups (Figure 2C).

Because the majority of patients with an anti-GBM disease develop widespread glomerular crescent formation followed by features of rapidly progressive glomerulonephritis, we quantified the number of glomerular crescents of $n = 8$ mice per group. We showed that GDF15-deficient mice displayed enhanced crescent formation (Figure 3A). As endothelial cells (ECs) are involved in the inflammatory process in glomeruli and the progression of glomerulonephritis, we investigated by immunohistochemistry the expression of CD31. Glomerular endothelial injury leads to podocyte loss and proteinuria. A cross-sectional evaluation revealed that the glomeruli of *Gdf15-/-* mice strongly expressed the CD31 marker (Figure 3B). Importantly, we observed the differences in glomerular architecture between wild type and knockout mice, indicating distinct stages of glomerulonephritis. To assess the cellular (including endothelial cell) proliferative responses, we stained renal sections with the antibody against Ki67. We observed increased proliferation of the cells in glomeruli as in the other renal compartments. This indicates the higher rearrangement (triggered by higher injury) of the tissue of knockout mice compared to wild types (Figure 3C). Furthermore, *Gdf15-/-* mice with anti-GBM nephritis exhibited a decreased number of WT1 positive podocytes in the glomeruli (Figure 3D). These pathological features explained massive albuminuria, increased BUN, and serum creatinine observed (Figure 2B). Together, lack of GDF15 induces severe renal disease upon anti-GBM serum treatment, whereas control mice (WT anti-GBM) displayed a less severe phenotype. These data emphasize an indispensable role for GDF15 in kidney disease.

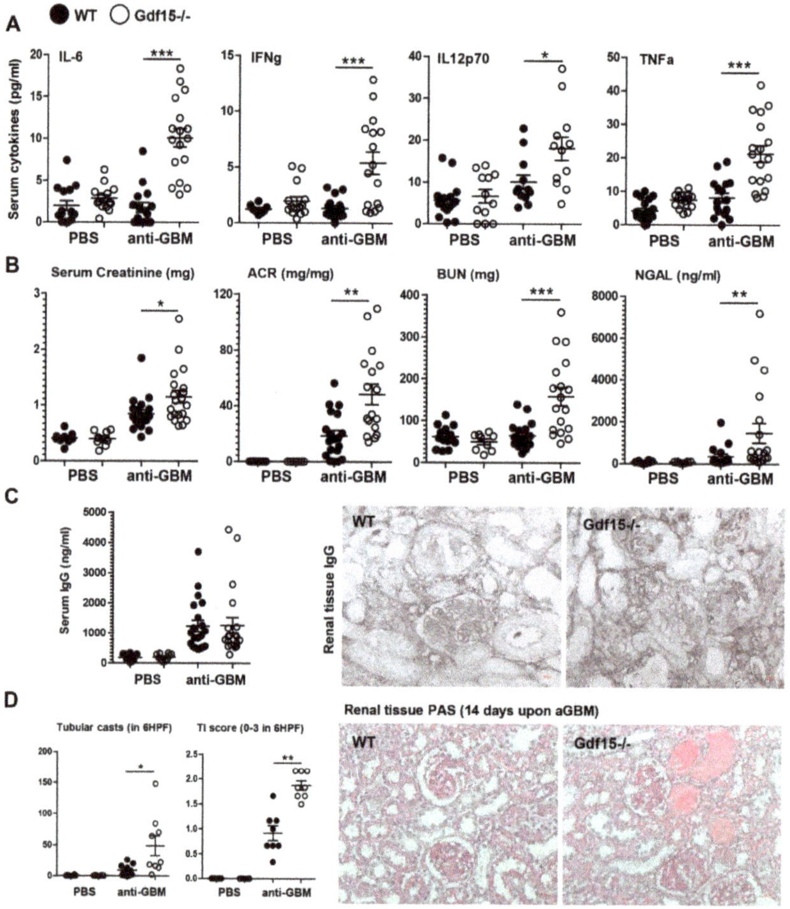


**Figure 2.** Systemic inflammation, kidney function, and histopathology of anti-GBM nephritis. (**A**) Sera were obtained from wild type or GDF15-deficient C57BL/6 mice on day 14 after saline or antiserum (anti-GBM) injection. Cytokine levels were quantified by flow cytometry ($n = 15$–17, one-way ANOVA). (**B**) Renal function parameter ($n = 15$–17, one-way ANOVA). (**C**) Serum IgG levels ($n = 15$–17, one-way ANOVA) and immunohistochemistry staining for IgG on kidney sections were quantified. (**D**) Kidneys from WT or KO mice were paraffin-embedded, stained with Periodic acid-Schiff (PAS) reagent, and quantified to assess tubular casts formation and tubular injury score ($n = 8$ mice per group, one-way ANOVA). Representative images of renal sections (original magnification 400×). Data are mean ± SEM. * $p < 0.05$; ** $p < 0.01$; *** $p < 0.001$.

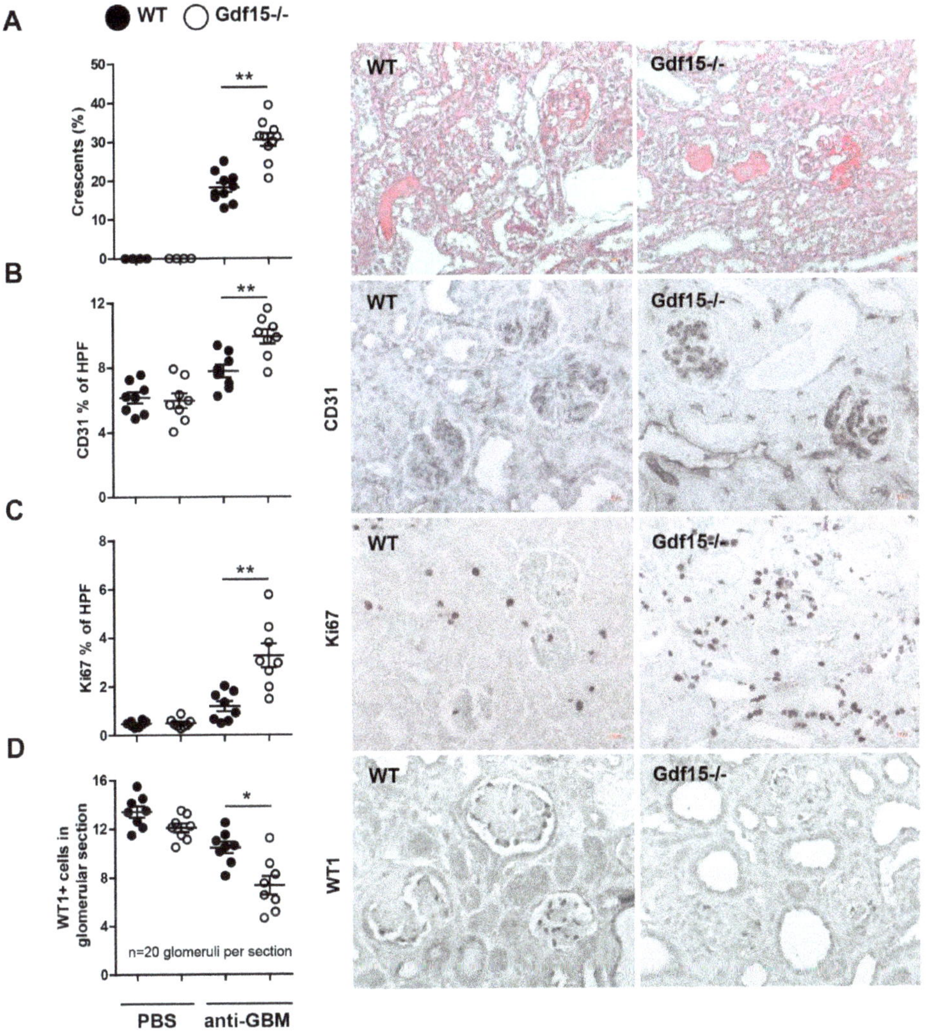


**Figure 3.** Kidney histopathology of anti-GBM nephritis. Sections were obtained from wild type or GDF15-deficient C57BL/6 mice on day 14 after saline or antiserum (anti-GBM) injection. Kidneys from WT or KO mice were paraffin-embedded and stained either with (**A**) PAS, (**B**) anti-CD31 antibody, (**C**) anti-ki67 antibody and (**D**) anti-WT1 antibody, and quantified ($n$ = 8 mice per group, one-way ANOVA). Representative images of renal sections (original magnification 400×). Data are mean ± SEM. * $p < 0.05$; ** $p < 0.01$.

### 2.3. *Gdf15-Deficient Mice Exhibit Increased Renal Inflammation in Anti-GBM Nephritis Model*

Further, we investigated the impact of GDF15 on renal inflammation as one of the key determinants of glomerular damage and albuminuria in the early phase of anti-GBM nephritis. We hypothesized that the mechanism underlying severe glomerulonephritis in *Gdf15-/-* mice could be associated with T cells. T-cells play a crucial role in proliferative and crescentic glomerulonephritis and can be a trigger of severe and rapid damage even in the absence of glomerular antibody deposition [3,8,36]. Indeed, we observed a significant increase in the number of CD3+ T cells, neutrophils, and macrophages on kidney sections from anti-GBM-treated *Gdf15-/-* mice compared with WT mice (Figure 4A). At the preselected mRNA level, the expression of the glomerular extracellular matrix proteins, matrix remodeling enzymes matrix metalloproteinase-7 and matrix metalloproteinase-9, as well as inflammation markers, was higher in anti-GBM-treated *Gdf15-/-* mice compared with WT mice on day 14 (Figure 4B). However, the further quantification of samples revealed that the expression of chemokines/cytokines *Ccl2, Ccl5, Cxcl1, Cxcl10, Ctgf, and Il2,* as well as adhesion molecules *Icam1* and *Vcam1*, were significantly more expressed in GDF15-deficient mice compared to wild type mice upon anti-GBM serum treatment. Together, the systemic lack of GDF15 leads to an increased progression of renal disease by orchestrating inflammation and immune cell influx.

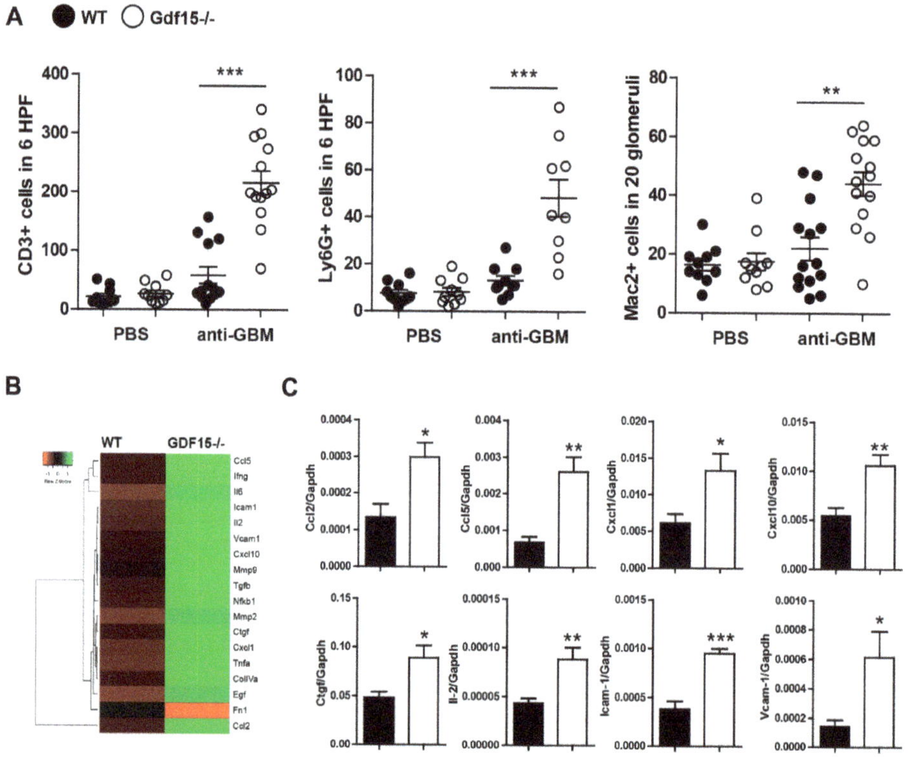


**Figure 4.** Kidney inflammation in wild type and *Gdf15* KO mice with anti-GBM nephritis. (**A**) Kidney sections were stained with anti- CD3, Ly6G, or Mac2 antibodies and quantified by counting, as indicated on graphs and in material and methods ($n$ = 9–15 mice per group, one-way ANOVA). (**B**) Heat map depicting kidney expression of pre-selected genes of wild type and GDF15-deficient mice upon anti-GBM serum treatment. (**C**) Gene expression levels in kidneys were quantified by real-time PCR. Data are shown as means of the ratio of the specific mRNA vs. that of *Gapdh* mRNA ($n$ = 6–8 samples per group, Student's *t*-Test). Data are mean ± SEM. * $p < 0.05$; ** $p < 0.01$; *** $p < 0.001$ versus control mice.

## 2.4. T Cells from Wild Type and Knockout Mice Display No Differences in Expression of Adhesions Markers

Due to the observed kidney influx of CD3+ cells and the increased IL-2 expression (crucial T-cell cytokine), we hypothesized that T cells from *Gdf15-/-* mice could also have an adhesion associated phenotype. To evaluate the effect of GDF15-deficiency on the adhesive capacity of T cells, we established an in vitro system in order to analyze the expression of several adhesion markers on T cells isolated from spleens. After the activation of naïve T cells with LPS, we did not observe increased expression of

CD28, CD154, CD62L, and CD11a/CD18 in CD4+ T cells (Figure 5B) nor CD8+ T cells (Figure 5C) in comparison with unprimed vehicle-treated cells. We did not see any significant differences between WT and KO cells. After in vitro stimulation, T cells from wild type and *Gdf15-/-* mice showed no differences in TCR internalization, evidenced by the reduction in CD3 MFI (data not shown). Interestingly, we observed a shift towards CD8+ cytotoxic T cells in primed GDF15-deficient cells (Figure 5A). The accumulation of effector CD8+ T lymphocytes may suggest increased damage to the surrounding tissue.

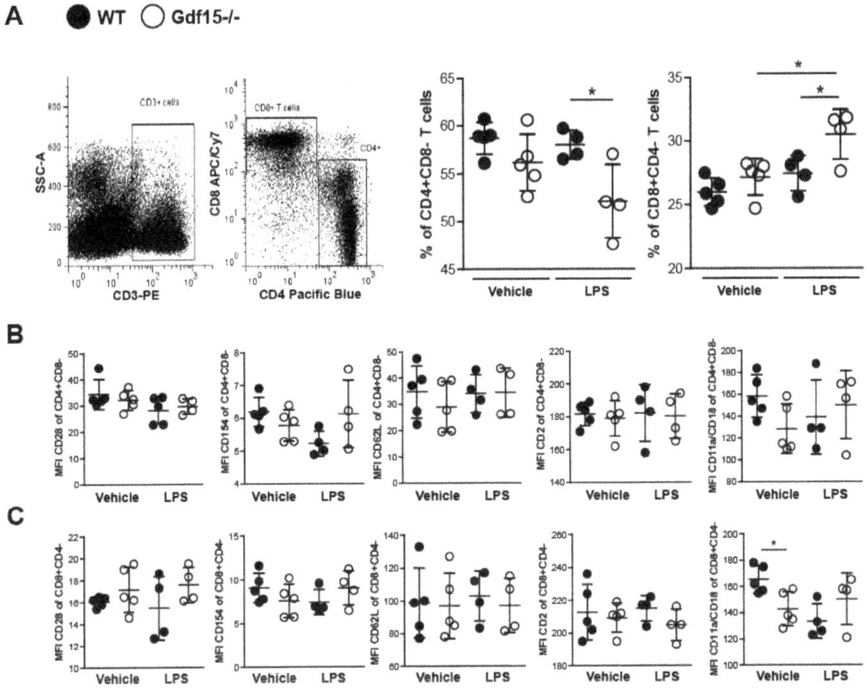


**Figure 5.** Stimulation of splenic T cells from WT and *Gdf15* KO mice with or without LPS ex vivo. (**A**) T cells were isolated from WT and *Gdf15* KO mice and stimulated with or without LPS for 24 h. The percentage of CD4+CD8- and CD8+CD4- T cells was quantified by flow cytometry (gating strategy, $n$ = 4–5 per group, one-way ANOVA). (**B**,**C**) Mean fluorescence intensity (MFI) of the surface markers CD28, CD154, CD62L, CD2, and CD11a/CD18 on LPS-stimulated or untreated CD4+CD8- T cells (**B**) and CD8+CD4- T cells (**C**) ($n$ = 4–5 per group, one-way ANOVA). Data are mean ± SD. * $p < 0.05$.

As the trafficking of T cells to tissues mainly depends on the tissue microenvironment, we decided to investigate the effect of chemokines that were highly expressed during anti-GBM nephritis on the migratory potential of T cells. We used both naïve and activated T cells (interaction with APC upon LPS treatment), and analyzed their migration towards the chemokines CXCL1, CXCL10, and CCL5 using migration chambers with micro-channels for 24 h. We observed a significant increase in the percentage of T cells from GDF15-deficient mice that migrated towards CXCL10 but not CXCL1 and CCL5 (Figure 6A). CXCL10 is known to be highly expressed during kidney disease [37–39]. Its receptor CXCR3 is expressed on effector T cells and crucial in T cell trafficking and function [40,41]. Moreover, IFNγ activates the Stat-dependent pathway in tissue-resident cells to enhance the production of CXCL10 during tissue injury. We previously observed high Cxcl10 expression in kidney tissue and high systemic levels of IFN-γ in treated *Gdf15* KO mice. We hypothesized that the elevated number of effector T cells might not only be associated with the CXCR3 receptor. Therefore, we looked at the level of Cxcr3 in naïve and activated T cells. Indeed, we found a significantly higher mRNA and protein levels of CXCR3 in T cells from GDF15-deficient mice upon activation (Figure 6B,C). Taken together, these data indicate that GDF15 plays a role in the migration of T cells to the side of inflammation via a CXCL10-CXCR3 dependent mechanism.

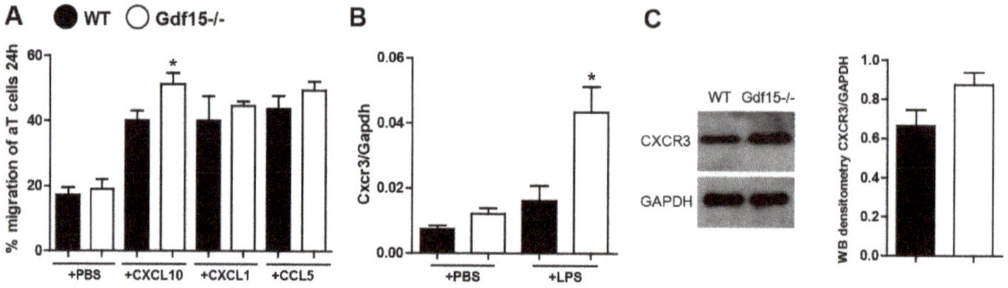


**Figure 6.** Quantification of T cell migration and CXCR3 expression. (**A**) T cells from the spleens of WT and GDF15-deficient mice were isolated and migration assays were performed. The percentage of migrated T cells towards the chemokines CXCL10, CXCL1, and CCL5 was quantified after 24 h ($n = 4$ per group, one-way ANOVA, * $p < 0.05$). (**B**) Cxcr3 expression levels in LPS-stimulated or untreated T cells were quantified by real-time PCR. Data are shown as means of the ratio of the Cxcr3 mRNA vs. Gapdh mRNA ($n = 4$ per group, one-way ANOVA, * $p < 0.05$). (**C**) CXCR3 protein expression levels in LPS-activated T cells were quantified by Western blot. The histogram shows the densitometry of two independent experiments; no statistical analysis was performed. Data are mean ± SEM.

### *2.5. Gene Expression Analysis of GDF15, CXCL10 and CXCR3 in Patients with RPGN*

In order to estimate the transferability of our results to human disease, we assessed transcriptional levels of *GDF15*, *CXCL10*, and *CXCR3* in the glomerular and tubular compartment from human renal biopsy specimens using Affymetrix microarray expression data. For this project, we used biopsies of individuals with rapidly progressive glomerulonephritis (RPGN) versus living donor (LD) biopsy specimens (Figure 7). In both, the glomerular and the tubular compartment of the patient cohort, *GDF15* was significantly downregulated in patients with RPGN compared with controls. At the same time, the *CXCL10* and its receptor *CXCR3* were significantly upregulated it both the glomerular and tubular compartment. Together, genes that seem to be regulated by GDF15 in the experimental mouse model of anti-GBM were induced during rapidly progressive glomerulonephritis in the glomerular and tubular compartment of the kidney.

**A**

| | | Glom_LD7_RPGN7 | | |
|---|---|---|---|---|
| Entrez Gene | Gene Symbol | Fold change | Log Fold Change | q-value (%) |
| 2833 | CXCR3 | 1.133 | 0.180 | 4.322 |
| 3627 | CXCL10 | 4.377 | 2.130 | 0.013 |
| 9518 | GDF15 | 0.392 | -1.351 | 1.343 |

**B**

| | | Tub_LD7_RPGN7 | | |
|---|---|---|---|---|
| Entrez Gene | Gene Symbol | Fold change | Log Fold Change | q-value (%) |
| 2833 | CXCR3 | 1.082 | 0.114 | 4.917 |
| 3627 | CXCL10 | 5.509 | 2.462 | 0.000 |
| 9518 | GDF15 | 0.652 | -0.618 | 0.446 |

**Figure 7.** Gene expression analysis of *GDF15*, *CXCL10*, and *CXCR3* genes in (**A**) glomerular and (**B**) tubular

compartment of manually microdissected kidney biopsies from patients with RPGN. Values are expressed as a log2-fold change compared to controls (living donors, LD). All represented genes are significantly changed ($q < 0.05$). (**A**) Glomerular expression single hybridization (LD: $n = 18$, RPGN: $n = 23$), (**B**) Tubular compartment expression (LD: $n = 18$, RPGN: $n = 21$). Red represents upregulation and blue represents downregulation of the transcript.

## 3. Discussion

We hypothesized that a GDF-15-associated mechanism is responsible for the development of GBM. Our results now show that the cytokine GDF15 protects from kidney injury and inflammation in a mouse model of anti-GBM nephritis. Furthermore, we demonstrate that Gdf15 is induced locally as well as systemically in the injured kidney and that GDF15 acts as an anti-inflammatory cytokine by regulating systemic cytokine production. GDF15 is involved in the recruitment of T cells into the injured tissue, a phenomenon associated with CXCL10-CXCR3 signaling. This finding is in line with previous reports on the functional role of GDF15 demonstrating that this cytokine can regulate chemokine-triggered β2 integrin activation on myeloid cells [42]. We further expand this knowledge by reporting on the enhanced migratory capability of peripheral blood mononuclear cells towards CXCL10 ex vivo and provide evidence for increased numbers of infiltrating immune cells in kidneys of mice with anti-GBM nephritis. The accumulation of T lymphocytes within the kidney might display a key event contributing to kidney injury. Some of the studies evidenced that anti-GBM GN depends on both CD4 and CD8 T cells without direct T cell-mediated cytotoxicity [28]. Other investigations support the hypothesis that especially CD8+ T cells are important mediators of glomerulonephritis [43]. Nevertheless, chemokines and chemokine receptors play a role in the process of T cell recruitment to the site of inflammation. Here, we show that both CXCL10, as well as its receptor, might be regulated by GDF15. Previous studies highlighted the importance of CXCL10 during inflammation and showed that CXCL10 is critical for the recruitment of CXCR3-expressing effector T cells to the injured tissue [44]. In in vivo models, CXCR3-expressing CD4+ and CD8+ T cells did not migrate efficiently into inflamed tissues of CXCL10-deficient mice compared to wild type, suggesting that CXCR3 expression is crucial for the selection of cells that respond to CXCL10 [44]. Consistent with earlier studies, our data indicate that GDF15 limits the inflammatory response during injury by restricting immune cell infiltration. Kempf et al. showed that GDF15 protects against fatal cardiac rupture by counteracting chemokine-triggered β2 integrin activation on myeloid cells [42]. This, for the first time, implied that GDF15 might be involved in the regulation of cytoskeleton rearrangement. In our experiments, except for changes in inflammation and significant effects of GDF15 on chemokine production, we could observe significant upregulation of *Icam* and *Vcam* adhesion molecules in the injured kidneys of *Gdf15-/-* mice. This suggests pleiotropic effects of GDF15 in the process of progressive GN, whereby GDF15 orchestrates the migration of T cell populations into the kidney. Therefore, treatment with GDF15 seems to be more beneficial than blocking particular chemokines and chemokine receptors to inhibit the selective migration of defined cell populations to the site of inflammation.

Other mechanisms potentially contributing to exaggerated injury in GDF-15-deficient mice include the polarization of cytotoxic CD8 T cells. Although overall surface marker expression upon LPS stimulation was comparable to wild type, we observed a significant decrease in the number of CD4+ T cells but an increase in CD8+ T cells upon activation in knockout cells. This suggests a distinct immune response associated with specific T cell subsets and more severe clinical manifestations in GDF15-deficient mice. CD8+ cytotoxic T cells serve as a potent source of inflammation by producing perforin and granzymes and inducing apoptosis in target cells [45–47]. By contrast, CD4+ helper T cells support the immune responses by promoting the activation and/or proliferation of immune cells [48]. The polarization of T cells towards CD8+ T cells could be an additional explanation for the severe phenotype observed in knockout mice.

In addition, we observed a protective role of GDF15 in both the glomerular and tubular compartment as evidenced by increased macrophage infiltration and expression of inflammatory markers in *Gdf15-/-* mice, indicating that glomerular inflammation in autologous anti-GBM disease involves both innate and adaptive immunity [49,50] and that GDF15 could act as a regulator of both immune responses. Currently, it is unclear whether the injured glomeruli cause tubular damage or whether both processes occur independently of each other due to the accumulation of immunoglobulins and immune complexes in the kidney. In our model, the glomerular damage is accompanied by tubule interstitial damage and both seem to depend on GDF15, because the injury in knockout mice is significantly higher. Therefore, we investigated both the tubular and glomerular compartment of patients with RPGN. RPGN is associated with a high frequency of crescentic glomerulonephritis [51]. Since we observed significant changes in GDF15 in an experimental anti-GBM model, as well as enhanced CXCL10-CXCR3 signaling, we chose to compare the expression of these three transcripts. Our analysis revealed the significant downregulation of GDF15 and at the same time the upregulation of CXCL10 and CXCR3. In support of our experimental findings, the human data suggest that the level of GDF15 affects the infiltration of CXCR3-expressing T cells to the site of injury. For instance, Dai et al. showed that the anti-CXCR3 treatment of mice inhibits autoreactive CD8+ T cells in the skin and peripheral lymphoid tissues [52]. Moreover, in a mouse model of vitiligo, CXCL10-/- unlike CXCL9-/- mice did not develop depigmentation, indicating that the CXCL10-CXCR3 axis is responsible for this disease [53]. In humans, the blockade of CXCL10 showed positive effects on the progression of rheumatoid arthritis, indicating a therapeutic approach in blocking the CXCL10-CXCR3 axis not only in experimental mouse models but also in human disease [54].

Stable and accurate noninvasive markers, as well as a better understanding of the pathophysiology of rapidly progressive GN could enable fast, precise diagnosis and appropriate treatment of the disease. Until now, several studies showed that GDF15 is associated with a rapid decline in kidney function, suggesting that might be a useful predictor for the development of kidney disease. For instance, recent investigations of two independent cohorts showed that systemic GDF15 levels correlate with the intrarenal expression of *GDF15* and are significantly associated with the progression of kidney disease [55]. Enhanced GDF15 levels correlate not only with increased mortality in hemodialysis and diabetic nephropathy (DN) patients [56,57] but also with all-cause mortality [58,59]. Moreover, in DN patients, high levels of GDF15 are associated with a decline in estimated glomerular filtration rate and faster progression to kidney failure [57]. Surely, the enhanced levels of GDF15 can deliver information about the deterioration of kidney function [60–62]. However, the suitability of GDF15 as a precise marker for kidney disease needs further investigation. Moreover, its role as a urinary marker on the progression of kidney disease, as well as the correlation of plasma and urine GDF15 levels, needs to be elucidated [63]. Our experimental study with GDF15-deficient mice proves the strong impact of the protein on the outcome of kidney disease and shows increased systemic and kidney expression of GDF15 during experimental GN. This increase in GDF15 levels during kidney diseases is associated with the increased production of GDF15 in response to stress (unpublished data) rather than with decreased protein clearance from circulation. Collectively, our data suggest that GDF15 reduces the outcome of experimental GN and contributes to pathogenesis by modulating T cell phenotypes and reducing the accumulation of T cells in the kidney. GDF15 may serve as a useful therapeutic molecule that could reduce disease progression by its effect on CXCL10 and CXCR3. The wide range of reported effects is diverse and the inconsistency of the published functions can be referred to by the commercial source of recombinant GDF15, which was contaminated with bioactive concentrations of TGF-$\beta$1 [64]. To avoid this issue, we used mice deficient in the GDF15 protein, which consistently proves the immunomodulatory functions of GDF15 in glomerular disease.

## 4. Materials and Methods

Animal studies: GDF15-deficient mouse strain (MGI: 2386300, *Gdf15tm1Sjl*) were backcrossed to the C57BL/6 strain. Female and male mice were housed in sterile filter top cages with a 12 h dark/light cycle. The study was carried out following the principles of the Directive 2010/63/EU on the Protection of Animals Used for Scientific Purpose and with approval by the local government authorities (27.02.2015; ROB 55.2-1-54-2532-63-12). Induction of anti-GBM nephritis: For the induction of anti-GBM nephritis, mice were pre-immunized subcutaneously with 100 µL of 2 mg/mL sheep IgG (Jackson ImmunoResearch Laboratories Inc., West Grove, PA, USA), dissolved in complete Freund's adjuvant (Sigma-Aldrich, St. Louis, MI, USA). Five days later, sheep anti-rat glomeruli (GBM) serum (Probetex, San Antonio, TX, USA) was injected via the tail vein.

Kidney parameters: Urinary albumin excretion was evaluated by a double-sandwich ELISA. First, 96-well plates were coated with goat anti-mouse albumin antibody A90-13A-5 (Bethyl Laboratories, Montgomery, TX, USA) and plates were incubated overnight at 4 °C. After blocking for half an hour at room temperature in 0.5% BSA in PBS with 0.05% Tween20, urine samples, and mouse albumin standard (Sigma-Aldrich, St. Louis, MI, USA) were added on the plate in triplicates for 2 h. Mouse urine samples were diluted in serial dilutions ranging from $1{:}10^2$ to $1{:}10^7$. As a secondary antibody, HRP-conjugated anti-mouse albumin antibody A90-134P-7 (Bethyl Laboratories) was used. Urinary Lipocalin-2/NGAL levels were determined using a commercially available mouse ELISA DuoSet kit (R&D Systems, Park Abingdon, UK), according to manufacturer's recommendations. The samples and standard curve dilutions were added on the plate in triplicates and incubated for two hours. Mouse urine samples were diluted in serial dilutions ranging from $1{:}10^3$ to $1{:}10^6$. TMB substrate solution (BD, Franklin Lakes, NJ, USA) was applied and the reaction was stopped after fifteen minutes with 2 M $H_2SO_4$. OD was measured at 450 nm and the calculation of the final concentrations was performed using a four-parameter logistic curve. Creatinine levels in urine and serum were determined using the creatinine assay DiaSys kit (Diagnostic Systems GmbH, Holzheim, Germany). Urine samples were prepared in dilutions of 1:10, while serum was used undiluted. According to the manufacturer's recommendations, 10 µL of sample or standard was pipetted on 96-well plates in triplicates. Then, 200 µL of prepared reagent provided by the kit was added and absorbance was measure at 492 nm 60 s later. Two more measurements were performed 120 s and 20 min later. Concentrations were calculated using a linear standard curve. Kidney function was determined by measuring serum blood urea nitrogen (DiaSys Diagnostic Systems) and serum creatinine levels determined by the Jaffe method (DiaSys Diagnostic Systems).

Evaluation of kidney histopathology: Organs were fixed in 4% buffered formalin and embedded in paraffin. For quantitative analysis, cells were counted in sections (from at least 8–16 mice per group) or analyzed using Adobe Photoshop CS4Extended (% of stained high power field). The PAS score evaluation was performed following a semi-quantitative scoring system with a scale from 0 to 3. Samples were blinded before evaluation. CD3 positive and Ly6G positive cell quantification was performed by counting the number of positive cells in six adjacent high-power fields (Hpf) of the renal cortex and medulla. For the evaluation of the Mac-2 staining, stained cells in 20 glomeruli per sample were counted.

Mouse IgG detection: The levels of mouse IgG in the serum were determined using the mouse IgG ELISA kit (Bethyl Laboratories), according to the manufacturer's recommendations. Briefly, 96-well plates were coated with coating antibody provided by the kit diluted (1:100) in 0.05 M Carbonate Bicarbonate with pH = 9.6 overnight at 4 °C. After 30 min blocking in 1% BSA in TrisNaCl samples and standard were added on the plate and incubated for one hour. Following five washing steps with TrisNaCl, the detection antibody was added on the plate in a dilution of 1:50,000. After the washing steps, TMB substrate solution (BD) was applied and the reaction was stopped with 2 M $H_2SO_4$. OD was measured at 450 nm and the calculation of the final concentrations was performed using a four-parameter logistic curve.

Flow cytometry: T cells were isolated from spleens of WT and *Gdf15-/-* mice and stimulated with or without LPS ex vivo for 24 h. After stimulation, T cells were collected, centrifuged, and resuspended in wash buffer (0.1% BSA, 0.01% sodium azide in D-PBS). After blocking the Fc receptor with anti-mouse CD16/32 (2.4G2) for 5 min, cells were stained with the surface antibodies FITC anti-mouse CD28, PacificBlue anti-mouse CD4, APC/Cy7 anti-mouse CD8a, PE anti-mouse CD3, PE/Cy7 anti-mouse CD154, PerCP/Cy5.5 anti-mouse CD2, APC anti-mouse CD11a/CD18, BV510 anti-mouse CD62L (all from BioLegend) for 30 min. After staining, cells were washed with wash buffer and flow cytometry was performed using the BD FACS Canto II (Becton Dickinson, New Jersey, USA). Data were analyzed with the software FlowJo 8.7 (Tree Star Inc., Ashland, OR, USA). For cytokine analysis of serum from mice or cell culture experiments, samples were prepared according to the instruction of the BD Cytometric Bead Array Mouse Inflammation Kit. The concentrations of the cytokines IL-6, IL-10, MCP-1, IFN-$\gamma$, TNF, and IL-12p70 in the samples were determined by the software FlowJo 8.7.

Real-time quantitative PCR: SYBR Green Dye detection system was used for quantitative real-time PCR on Light Cycler 480 (Roche, Mannheim, Germany). Gene-specific primers (225 nM, Metabion, Martinsried, Germany) were used. Standard controls for genomic DNA contamination, RNA quality, and general PCR performance were included. RNA was isolated from the samples using the Norgen Biotek Total RNA Purification kit (Thorold, ON, Canada) and MagNA Lyser Green beads (Roche, Basel, Switzerland) according to the manufacturer's instructions. The data were evaluated using the 2ΔΔCT method.

Patients and microarray analysis: Human kidney biopsy specimens and Affymetrix microarray expression data were procured within the framework of the European Renal cDNA Bank–Kröner–Fresenius Biopsy Bank. Biopsies were obtained from patients after informed consent and with the approval of the local ethics committees [65]. Following a renal biopsy, the tissue was transferred to RNase inhibitor and microdissected into glomeruli and tubulointerstitium. Total RNA was isolated from micro-dissected glomeruli, reverse transcribed, and linearly amplified according to a protocol previously reported [66]. CEL file normalization was performed with the Robust Multichip Average method using RMAExpress (Version 1.0.5) and the human Entrez-Gene custom CDF annotation from Brain Array version 18 (http://brainarray.mbni.med.umich.edu/Brainarray/default.asp). To identify differentially expressed genes, the SAM (Significance Analysis of Microarrays) method was applied using TiGR (MeV, Version 4.8.1) [67]. Published gene expression profiles from patients with RPGN as well as controls (living donors (LD)) were used in this study (GSE104954, GSE104948,).

Statistical analysis: Data were expressed as mean ± SEM. Data from wild type and knockout mice were compared with one-way ANOVA on ranks, followed by the Student–Newman–Keuls test using SigmaStat Software (Jandel Scientific, Erkrath, Germany). The student *t*-test was used for direct comparisons between single groups—i.e., wild type and knockout cells/mice in case of normally distributed data or samples size $n > 15$. Mann–Whitney U test was used to analyze data with small sample size and non-parametric distribution of data. We used GraphPad Prism software. A $p$-value $< 0.05$ indicated statistical significance. Statistical significance was indicated as follows: $p$-value of <0.05 (*); $p$-value of <0.01 (**); $p$-value of <0.001 (***).

**Author Contributions:** Conceptualization, F.M.-F. and M.L. (Maciej Lech); formal analysis, F.M.-F., S.S., G.L., A.R., E.v.R., M.L. (Maja Lindenmeyer) and M.L. (Maciej Lech); investigation, F.M.-F., S.S., G.L., A.R., E.v.R. and M.L. (Maciej Lech); resources, H.-J.A., C.D.C. and M.L. (Maciej Lech); writing—original draft preparation, M.L. (Maciej Lech); writing—review and editing, F.M.-F., S.S., G.L., A.R., E.v.R., H.-J.A., C.S., M.L. (Maja Lindenmeyer) and M.L. (Maciej Lech); visualization, F.M.-F., S.S., M.L. (Maja Lindenmeyer) and M.L. (Maciej Lech); supervision, M.L. (Maciej Lech); project administration, M.L. (Maciej Lech); funding acquisition, M.L. (Maciej Lech). All authors have read and agreed to the published version of the manuscript.

**Funding:** This research and APC were funded by DFG, Deutsche Forschungsgemeinschaft (LE2621/6-1, AN372/24-1).

**Acknowledgments:** We thank Karina Adamowicz and Jana Mandelbaum for expert technical support. This work is presented in part in the thesis project of E.vR to the Medical Faculty of the LMU Munich. The ERCB-KFB was supported by the Else Kröner–Fresenius Foundation. We also thank all participating centers of the European Renal cDNA Bank—Kröner–Fresenius biopsy bank (ERCB-KFB) and their patients for their cooperation. For active members at the time of the study see [68].

**Conflicts of Interest:** The authors declare no conflict of interest. The funders had no role in the design of the study; collection, analyses, or interpretation of data; writing of the manuscript, or decision to publish the results.

## Abbreviations

| | |
|---|---|
| MDPI | Multidisciplinary Digital Publishing Institute |
| DOAJ | Directory of open access journals |
| TLA | Three letter acronym |
| LD | Linear dichroism |

## References


1. McAdoo, S.P.; Pusey, C.D. Anti-Glomerular Basement Membrane Disease. *Clin. J. Am. Soc. Nephrol.* **2017**, *12*, 1162–1172. [CrossRef] [PubMed]
2. Canney, M.; O'Hara, P.V.; McEvoy, C.M.; Medani, S.; Connaughton, D.M.; Abdalla, A.A.; Doyle, R.; Stack, A.G.; O'Seaghdha, C.M.; Clarkson, M.R.; et al. Spatial and Temporal Clustering of Anti-Glomerular Basement Membrane Disease. *Clin. J. Am. Soc. Nephrol.* **2016**, *11*, 1392–1399. [CrossRef] [PubMed]
3. Kurts, C.; Panzer, U.; Anders, H.J.; Rees, A.J. The immune system and kidney disease: Basic concepts and clinical implications. *Nat. Rev. Immunol.* **2013**, *13*, 738–753. [CrossRef] [PubMed]
4. Kumar, S.V.; Kulkarni, O.P.; Mulay, S.R.; Darisipudi, M.N.; Romoli, S.; Thomasova, D.; Scherbaum, C.R.; Hohenstein, B.; Hugo, C.; Muller, S.; et al. Neutrophil Extracellular Trap-Related Extracellular Histones Cause Vascular Necrosis in Severe GN. *J. Am. Soc. Nephrol.* **2015**, *26*, 2399–2413. [CrossRef] [PubMed]
5. Artinger, K.; Kirsch, A.H.; Aringer, I.; Moschovaki-Filippidou, F.; Eller, P.; Rosenkranz, A.R.; Eller, K. Innate and adaptive immunity in experimental glomerulonephritis: A pathfinder tale. *Pediatr. Nephrol.* **2017**, *32*, 943–947. [CrossRef] [PubMed]
6. Suarez-Fueyo, A.; Bradley, S.J.; Klatzmann, D.; Tsokos, G.C. T cells and autoimmune kidney disease. *Nat. Rev. Nephrol.* **2017**, *13*, 329–343. [CrossRef]
7. Krebs, C.F.; Steinmetz, O.M. CD4(+) T Cell Fate in Glomerulonephritis: A Tale of Th1, Th17, and Novel Treg Subtypes. *Mediat. Inflamm.* **2016**, *2016*, 5393894. [CrossRef]
8. Summers, S.A.; Steinmetz, O.M.; Li, M.; Kausman, J.Y.; Semple, T.; Edgtton, K.L.; Borza, D.B.; Braley, H.; Holdsworth, S.R.; Kitching, A.R. Th1 and Th17 cells induce proliferative glomerulonephritis. *J. Am. Soc. Nephrol.* **2009**, *20*, 2518–2524. [CrossRef]
9. Hopfer, H.; Holzer, J.; Hunemorder, S.; Paust, H.J.; Sachs, M.; Meyer-Schwesinger, C.; Turner, J.E.; Panzer, U.; Mittrucker, H.W. Characterization of the renal CD4+ T-cell response in experimental autoimmune glomerulonephritis. *Kidney Int.* **2012**, *82*, 60–71. [CrossRef]
10. Odobasic, D.; Gan, P.Y.; Summers, S.A.; Semple, T.J.; Muljadi, R.C.; Iwakura, Y.; Kitching, A.R.; Holdsworth, S.R. Interleukin-17A promotes early but attenuates established disease in crescentic glomerulonephritis in mice. *Am. J. Pathol.* **2011**, *179*, 1188–1198. [CrossRef]
11. Paust, H.J.; Turner, J.E.; Riedel, J.H.; Disteldorf, E.; Peters, A.; Schmidt, T.; Krebs, C.; Velden, J.; Mittrucker, H.W.; Steinmetz, O.M.; et al. Chemokines play a critical role in the cross-regulation of Th1 and Th17 immune responses in murine crescentic glomerulonephritis. *Kidney Int.* **2012**, *82*, 72–83. [CrossRef] [PubMed]
12. Zhou, A.; Ueno, H.; Shimomura, M.; Tanaka, R.; Shirakawa, T.; Nakamura, H.; Matsuo, M.; Iijima, K. Blockade of TGF-beta action ameliorates renal dysfunction and histologic progression in anti-GBM nephritis. *Kidney Int.* **2003**, *64*, 92–101. [CrossRef] [PubMed]
13. Mesnard, L.; Keller, A.C.; Michel, M.L.; Vandermeersch, S.; Rafat, C.; Letavernier, E.; Tillet, Y.; Rondeau, E.; Leite-de-Moraes, M.C. Invariant natural killer T cells and TGF-beta attenuate anti-GBM glomerulonephritis. *J. Am. Soc. Nephrol.* **2009**, *20*, 1282–1292. [CrossRef] [PubMed]
14. Kanamaru, Y.; Nakao, A.; Mamura, M.; Suzuki, Y.; Shirato, I.; Okumura, K.; Tomino, Y.; Ra, C. Blockade of TGF-beta signaling in T cells prevents the development of experimental glomerulonephritis. *J. Immunol.* **2001**, *166*, 2818–2823. [CrossRef] [PubMed]
15. Bootcov, M.R.; Bauskin, A.R.; Valenzuela, S.M.; Moore, A.G.; Bansal, M.; He, X.Y.; Zhang, H.P.; Donnellan, M.; Mahler, S.; Pryor, K.; et al. MIC-1, a novel macrophage inhibitory cytokine, is a divergent member of the TGF-beta superfamily. *Proc. Natl. Acad. Sci. USA* **1997**, *94*, 11514–11519. [CrossRef]
16. Zhou, Z.; Li, W.; Song, Y.; Wang, L.; Zhang, K.; Yang, J.; Zhang, W.; Su, H.; Zhang, Y. Growth differentiation factor-15 suppresses maturation and function of dendritic cells and inhibits tumor-specific immune response. *PLoS ONE* **2013**, *8*, e78618. [CrossRef] [PubMed]

17. Soucek, K.; Slabakova, E.; Ovesna, P.; Malenovska, A.; Kozubik, A.; Hampl, A. Growth/differentiation factor-15 is an abundant cytokine in human seminal plasma. *Hum. Reprod* **2010**, *25*, 2962–2971. [CrossRef]
18. Rochette, L.; Meloux, A.; Zeller, M.; Cottin, Y.; Vergely, C. Functional roles of GDF15 in modulating microenvironment to promote carcinogenesis. *Biochim. Biophys. Acta Mol. Basis Dis.* **2020**, *1866*, 165798. [CrossRef]
19. Emmerson, P.J.; Wang, F.; Du, Y.; Liu, Q.; Pickard, R.T.; Gonciarz, M.D.; Coskun, T.; Hamang, M.J.; Sindelar, D.K.; Ballman, K.K.; et al. The metabolic effects of GDF15 are mediated by the orphan receptor GFRAL. *Nat. Med.* **2017**, *23*, 1215–1219. [CrossRef]
20. Baek, S.J.; Eling, T. Growth differentiation factor 15 (GDF15): A survival protein with therapeutic potential in metabolic diseases. *Pharmacol. Ther.* **2019**, *198*, 46–58. [CrossRef]
21. Tsai, V.W.W.; Husaini, Y.; Sainsbury, A.; Brown, D.A.; Breit, S.N. The MIC-1/GDF15-GFRAL Pathway in Energy Homeostasis: Implications for Obesity, Cachexia, and Other Associated Diseases. *Cell Metab.* **2018**, *28*, 353–368. [CrossRef] [PubMed]
22. Wang, W.; Yang, X.; Dai, J.; Lu, Y.; Zhang, J.; Keller, E.T. Prostate cancer promotes a vicious cycle of bone metastasis progression through inducing osteocytes to secrete GDF15 that stimulates prostate cancer growth and invasion. *Oncogene* **2019**, *38*, 4540–4559. [CrossRef] [PubMed]
23. Li, S.; Ma, Y.M.; Zheng, P.S.; Zhang, P. GDF15 promotes the proliferation of cervical cancer cells by phosphorylating AKT1 and Erk1/2 through the receptor ErbB2. *J. Exp. Clin. Cancer Res.* **2018**, *37*, 80. [CrossRef] [PubMed]
24. Emmerson, P.J.; Duffin, K.L.; Chintharlapalli, S.; Wu, X. GDF15 and Growth Control. *Front. Physiol.* **2018**, *9*, 1712. [CrossRef]
25. Kalluri, R.; Danoff, T.M.; Okada, H.; Neilson, E.G. Susceptibility to anti-glomerular basement membrane disease and Goodpasture syndrome is linked to MHC class II genes and the emergence of T cell-mediated immunity in mice. *J. Clin. Investig.* **1997**, *100*, 2263–2275. [CrossRef]
26. Huang, X.R.; Holdsworth, S.R.; Tipping, P.G. Evidence for delayed-type hypersensitivity mechanisms in glomerular crescent formation. *Kidney Int.* **1994**, *46*, 69–78. [CrossRef]
27. Tipping, P.G.; Huang, X.R.; Qi, M.; Van, G.Y.; Tang, W.W. Crescentic glomerulonephritis in CD4- and CD8-deficient mice. Requirement for CD4 but not CD8 cells. *Am. J. Pathol.* **1998**, *152*, 1541–1548.
28. Huang, X.R.; Tipping, P.G.; Apostolopoulos, J.; Oettinger, C.; D'Souza, M.; Milton, G.; Holdsworth, S.R. Mechanisms of T cell-induced glomerular injury in anti-glomerular basement membrane (GBM) glomerulonephritis in rats. *Clin. Exp. Immunol.* **1997**, *109*, 134–142. [CrossRef]
29. Reynolds, J.; Norgan, V.A.; Bhambra, U.; Smith, J.; Cook, H.T.; Pusey, C.D. Anti-CD8 monoclonal antibody therapy is effective in the prevention and treatment of experimental autoimmune glomerulonephritis. *J. Am. Soc. Nephrol.* **2002**, *13*, 359–369.
30. Fujinaka, H.; Yamamoto, T.; Feng, L.; Kawasaki, K.; Yaoita, E.; Hirose, S.; Goto, S.; Wilson, C.B.; Uchiyama, M.; Kihara, I. Crucial role of CD8-positive lymphocytes in glomerular expression of ICAM-1 and cytokines in crescentic glomerulonephritis of WKY rats. *J. Immunol.* **1997**, *158*, 4978–4983.
31. Kim, Y.I.; Shin, H.W.; Chun, Y.S.; Park, J.W. CST3 and GDF15 ameliorate renal fibrosis by inhibiting fibroblast growth and activation. *Biochem. Biophys. Res. Commun.* **2018**, *500*, 288–295. [CrossRef] [PubMed]
32. Zhang, Y.; Zhang, G.; Liu, Y.; Chen, R.; Zhao, D.; McAlister, V.; Mele, T.; Liu, K.; Zheng, X. GDF15 Regulates Malat-1 Circular RNA and Inactivates NFkappaB Signaling Leading to Immune Tolerogenic DCs for Preventing Alloimmune Rejection in Heart Transplantation. *Front. Immunol.* **2018**, *9*, 2407. [CrossRef] [PubMed]
33. Zhang, Y.; Jiang, M.; Nouraie, M.; Roth, M.G.; Tabib, T.; Winters, S.; Chen, X.; Sembrat, J.; Chu, Y.; Cardenes, N.; et al. GDF15 is an epithelial-derived biomarker of idiopathic pulmonary fibrosis. *Am. J. Physiol. -Lung Cell. Mol. Physiol.* **2019**, *317*, L510–L521. [CrossRef] [PubMed]
34. Luan, H.H.; Wang, A.; Hilliard, B.K.; Carvalho, F.; Rosen, C.E.; Ahasic, A.M.; Herzog, E.L.; Kang, I.; Pisani, M.A.; Yu, S.; et al. GDF15 Is an Inflammation-Induced Central Mediator of Tissue Tolerance. *Cell* **2019**, *178*, 1231–1244. [CrossRef]
35. Lichtnekert, J.; Kulkarni, O.P.; Mulay, S.R.; Rupanagudi, K.V.; Ryu, M.; Allam, R.; Vielhauer, V.; Muruve, D.; Lindenmeyer, M.T.; Cohen, C.D.; et al. Anti-GBM glomerulonephritis involves IL-1 but is independent of NLRP3/ASC inflammasome-mediated activation of caspase-1. *PLoS ONE* **2011**, *6*, e26778. [CrossRef]

36. Tipping, P.G.; Holdsworth, S.R. T cells in glomerulonephritis. *Springer Semin. Immunopathol.* **2003**, *24*, 377–393. [CrossRef]
37. Zhang, Y.; Thai, K.; Kepecs, D.M.; Winer, D.; Gilbert, R.E. Reversing CXCL10 Deficiency Ameliorates Kidney Disease in Diabetic Mice. *Am. J. Pathol.* **2018**, *188*, 2763–2773. [CrossRef]
38. Gniewkiewicz, M.S.; Czerwinska, M.; Gozdowska, J.; Czerwinska, K.; Sadowska, A.; Deborska-Materkowska, D.; Perkowska-Ptasinska, A.; Kosieradzki, M.; Durlik, M. Urinary levels of CCL2 and CXCL10 chemokines as potential biomarkers of ongoing pathological processes in kidney allograft: An association with BK virus nephropathy. *Pol. Arch. Intern. Med.* **2019**, *129*, 592–597. [CrossRef]
39. Nakaya, I.; Wada, T.; Furuichi, K.; Sakai, N.; Kitagawa, K.; Yokoyama, H.; Ishida, Y.; Kondo, T.; Sugaya, T.; Kawachi, H.; et al. Blockade of IP-10/CXCR3 promotes progressive renal fibrosis. *Nephron Exp. Nephrol.* **2007**, *107*, e12–e21. [CrossRef]
40. Groom, J.R.; Luster, A.D. CXCR3 in T cell function. *Exp. Cell Res.* **2011**, *317*, 620–631. [CrossRef]
41. Groom, J.R.; Luster, A.D. CXCR3 ligands: Redundant, collaborative and antagonistic functions. *Immunol. Cell Biol.* **2011**, *89*, 207–215. [CrossRef] [PubMed]
42. Kempf, T.; Zarbock, A.; Widera, C.; Butz, S.; Stadtmann, A.; Rossaint, J.; Bolomini-Vittori, M.; Korf-Klingebiel, M.; Napp, L.C.; Hansen, B.; et al. GDF-15 is an inhibitor of leukocyte integrin activation required for survival after myocardial infarction in mice. *Nat. Med.* **2011**, *17*, 581–588. [CrossRef] [PubMed]
43. Chang, J.; Eggenhuizen, P.; O'Sullivan, K.M.; Alikhan, M.A.; Holdsworth, S.R.; Ooi, J.D.; Kitching, A.R. CD8+ T Cells Effect Glomerular Injury in Experimental Anti-Myeloperoxidase GN. *J. Am. Soc. Nephrol.* **2017**, *28*, 47–55. [CrossRef]
44. Klein, R.S.; Lin, E.; Zhang, B.; Luster, A.D.; Tollett, J.; Samuel, M.A.; Engle, M.; Diamond, M.S. Neuronal CXCL10 directs CD8+ T-cell recruitment and control of West Nile virus encephalitis. *J. Virol.* **2005**, *79*, 11457–11466. [CrossRef] [PubMed]
45. Trapani, J.A.; Jans, D.A.; Jans, P.J.; Smyth, M.J.; Browne, K.A.; Sutton, V.R. Efficient nuclear targeting of granzyme B and the nuclear consequences of apoptosis induced by granzyme B and perforin are caspase-dependent, but cell death is caspase-independent. *J. Biol. Chem.* **1998**, *273*, 27934–27938. [CrossRef] [PubMed]
46. Trapani, J.A.; Smyth, M.J. Functional significance of the perforin/granzyme cell death pathway. *Nat. Rev. Immunol.* **2002**, *2*, 735–747. [CrossRef]
47. Nagata, S.; Golstein, P. The Fas death factor. *Science* **1995**, *267*, 1449–1456. [CrossRef]
48. Fung-Leung, W.P.; Schilham, M.W.; Rahemtulla, A.; Kundig, T.M.; Vollenweider, M.; Potter, J.; van Ewijk, W.; Mak, T.W. CD8 is needed for development of cytotoxic T cells but not helper T cells. *Cell* **1991**, *65*, 443–449. [CrossRef]
49. Brown, H.J.; Lock, H.R.; Wolfs, T.G.; Buurman, W.A.; Sacks, S.H.; Robson, M.G. Toll-like receptor 4 ligation on intrinsic renal cells contributes to the induction of antibody-mediated glomerulonephritis via CXCL1 and CXCL2. *J. Am. Soc. Nephrol.* **2007**, *18*, 1732–1739. [CrossRef]
50. Allam, R.; Anders, H.J. The role of innate immunity in autoimmune tissue injury. *Curr. Opin. Rheumatol.* **2008**, *20*, 538–544. [CrossRef]
51. Greenhall, G.H.; Salama, A.D. What is new in the management of rapidly progressive glomerulonephritis? *Clin. Kidney J.* **2015**, *8*, 143–150. [CrossRef] [PubMed]
52. Dai, Z.; Xing, L.; Cerise, J.; Wang, E.H.; Jabbari, A.; de Jong, A.; Petukhova, L.; Christiano, A.M.; Clynes, R. CXCR3 Blockade Inhibits T Cell Migration into the Skin and Prevents Development of Alopecia Areata. *J. Immunol.* **2016**, *197*, 1089–1099. [CrossRef] [PubMed]
53. Goebeler, M.; Toksoy, A.; Spandau, U.; Engelhardt, E.; Brocker, E.B.; Gillitzer, R. The C-X-C chemokine Mig is highly expressed in the papillae of psoriatic lesions. *J. Pathol.* **1998**, *184*, 89–95. [CrossRef]
54. Yellin, M.; Paliienko, I.; Balanescu, A.; Ter-Vartanian, S.; Tseluyko, V.; Xu, L.A.; Tao, X.; Cardarelli, P.M.; Leblanc, H.; Nichol, G.; et al. A phase II, randomized, double-blind, placebo-controlled study evaluating the efficacy and safety of MDX-1100, a fully human anti-CXCL10 monoclonal antibody, in combination with methotrexate in patients with rheumatoid arthritis. *Arthritis Rheum.* **2012**, *64*, 1730–1739. [CrossRef] [PubMed]
55. Nair, V.; Robinson-Cohen, C.; Smith, M.R.; Bellovich, K.A.; Bhat, Z.Y.; Bobadilla, M.; Brosius, F.; de Boer, I.H.; Essioux, L.; Formentini, I.; et al. Growth Differentiation Factor-15 and Risk of CKD Progression. *J. Am. Soc. Nephrol.* **2017**, *28*, 2233–2240. [CrossRef] [PubMed]

56. Breit, S.N.; Carrero, J.J.; Tsai, V.W.; Yagoutifam, N.; Luo, W.; Kuffner, T.; Bauskin, A.R.; Wu, L.; Jiang, L.; Barany, P.; et al. Macrophage inhibitory cytokine-1 (MIC-1/GDF15) and mortality in end-stage renal disease. *Nephrol. Dial. Transplant.* **2012**, *27*, 70–75. [CrossRef] [PubMed]
57. Lajer, M.; Jorsal, A.; Tarnow, L.; Parving, H.H.; Rossing, P. Plasma growth differentiation factor-15 independently predicts all-cause and cardiovascular mortality as well as deterioration of kidney function in type 1 diabetic patients with nephropathy. *Diabetes Care* **2010**, *33*, 1567–1572. [CrossRef]
58. Anand, I.S.; Kempf, T.; Rector, T.S.; Tapken, H.; Allhoff, T.; Jantzen, F.; Kuskowski, M.; Cohn, J.N.; Drexler, H.; Wollert, K.C. Serial measurement of growth-differentiation factor-15 in heart failure: Relation to disease severity and prognosis in the Valsartan Heart Failure Trial. *Circulation* **2010**, *122*, 1387–1395. [CrossRef]
59. Eggers, K.M.; Kempf, T.; Wallentin, L.; Wollert, K.C.; Lind, L. Change in growth differentiation factor 15 concentrations over time independently predicts mortality in community-dwelling elderly individuals. *Clin. Chem.* **2013**, *59*, 1091–1098. [CrossRef]
60. Na, K.R.; Kim, Y.H.; Chung, H.K.; Yeo, M.K.; Ham, Y.R.; Jeong, J.Y.; Kim, K.S.; Lee, K.W.; Choi, D.E. Growth differentiation factor 15 as a predictor of adverse renal outcomes in patients with immunoglobulin A nephropathy. *Intern. Med. J.* **2017**, *47*, 1393–1399. [CrossRef]
61. Ham, Y.R.; Song, C.H.; Bae, H.J.; Jeong, J.Y.; Yeo, M.K.; Choi, D.E.; Na, K.R.; Lee, K.W. Growth Differentiation Factor-15 as a Predictor of Idiopathic Membranous Nephropathy Progression: A Retrospective Study. *Dis. Markers* **2018**, *2018*, 1463940. [CrossRef] [PubMed]
62. Carlsson, A.C.; Nowak, C.; Lind, L.; Ostgren, C.J.; Nystrom, F.H.; Sundstrom, J.; Carrero, J.J.; Riserus, U.; Ingelsson, E.; Fall, T.; et al. Growth differentiation factor 15 (GDF-15) is a potential biomarker of both diabetic kidney disease and future cardiovascular events in cohorts of individuals with type 2 diabetes: A proteomics approach. *Upsala J. Med. Sci* **2020**, *125*, 37–43. [CrossRef] [PubMed]
63. Simonson, M.S.; Tiktin, M.; Debanne, S.M.; Rahman, M.; Berger, B.; Hricik, D.; Ismail-Beigi, F. The renal transcriptome of db/db mice identifies putative urinary biomarker proteins in patients with type 2 diabetes: A pilot study. *Am. J. Physiol. Renal Physiol.* **2012**, *302*, F820–F829. [CrossRef] [PubMed]
64. Olsen, O.E.; Skjaervik, A.; Stordal, B.F.; Sundan, A.; Holien, T. TGF-beta contamination of purified recombinant GDF15. *PLoS ONE* **2017**, *12*, e0187349. [CrossRef] [PubMed]
65. Cohen, C.D.; Frach, K.; Schlondorff, D.; Kretzler, M. Quantitative gene expression analysis in renal biopsies: A novel protocol for a high-throughput multicenter application. *Kidney Int.* **2002**, *61*, 133–140. [CrossRef] [PubMed]
66. Cohen, C.D.; Klingenhoff, A.; Boucherot, A.; Nitsche, A.; Henger, A.; Brunner, B.; Schmid, H.; Merkle, M.; Saleem, M.A.; Koller, K.P.; et al. Comparative promoter analysis allows de novo identification of specialized cell junction-associated proteins. *Proc. Natl. Acad. Sci. USA* **2006**, *103*, 5682–5687. [CrossRef]
67. Tusher, V.G.; Tibshirani, R.; Chu, G. Significance analysis of microarrays applied to the ionizing radiation response. *Proc. Natl. Acad. Sci. USA* **2001**, *98*, 5116–5121. [CrossRef]
68. Shved, N.; Warsow, G.; Eichinger, F.; Hoogewijs, D.; Brandt, S.; Wild, P.; Kretzler, M.; Cohen, C.D.; Lindenmeyer, M.T. Transcriptome-based network analysis reveals renal cell type-specific dysregulation of hypoxia-associated transcripts. *Sci. Rep.* **2017**, *7*, 8576. [CrossRef]

International Journal of
*Molecular Sciences*

MDPI

*Article*

# NOX1 Inhibition Attenuates Kidney Ischemia-Reperfusion Injury via Inhibition of ROS-Mediated ERK Signaling

**Hee-Yeon Jung †, Se-Hyun Oh †, Ji-Sun Ahn, Eun-Joo Oh, You-Jin Kim, Chan-Duck Kim, Sun-Hee Park, Yong-Lim Kim and Jang-Hee Cho ***

Division of Nephrology, Department of Internal Medicine, School of Medicine, Kyungpook National University, Kyungpook National University Hospital, Daegu 41944, Korea; hy-jung@knu.ac.kr (H.-Y.J.); ttily@nate.com (S.-H.O.); ggumsuni@hanmail.net (J.-S.A.); oej1124@naver.com (E.-J.O.); pinkqic1004@naver.com (Y.-J.K.); drcdkim@knu.ac.kr (C.-D.K.); sh-park@knu.ac.kr (S.-H.P.); ylkim@knu.ac.kr (Y.-L.K.)

* Correspondence: jh-cho@knu.ac.kr; Tel.: +82-10-6566-7551; Fax: +82-53-426-2046

† These authors contributed equally to this study.

Received: 25 August 2020; Accepted: 14 September 2020; Published: 21 September 2020

check for updates

**Abstract:** The protective effects of nicotinamide adenine dinucleotide phosphate (NADPH) oxidase (NOX) 1 inhibition against kidney ischemia-reperfusion injury (IRI) remain uncertain. The bilateral kidney pedicles of C57BL/6 mice were clamped for 30 min to induce IRI. Madin–Darby Canine Kidney (MDCK) cells were incubated with $H_2O_2$ (1.4 mM) for 1 h to induce oxidative stress. ML171, a selective NOX1 inhibitor, and siRNA against NOX1 were treated to inhibit NOX1. NOX expression, oxidative stress, apoptosis assay, and mitogen-activated protein kinase (MAPK) pathway were evaluated. The kidney function deteriorated and the production of reactive oxygen species (ROS), including intracellular $H_2O_2$ production, increased due to IRI, whereas IRI-mediated kidney dysfunction and ROS generation were significantly attenuated by ML171. $H_2O_2$ evoked the changes in oxidative stress enzymes such as SOD2 and GPX in MDCK cells, which was mitigated by ML171. Treatment with ML171 and transfection with siRNA against NOX1 decreased the upregulation of NOX1 and NOX4 induced by $H_2O_2$ in MDCK cells. ML171 decreased caspase-3 activity, the Bcl-2/Bax ratio, and TUNEL-positive tubule cells in IRI mice and $H_2O_2$-treated MDCK cells. Among the MAPK pathways, ML171 affected ERK signaling by ERK phosphorylation in kidney tissues and tubular cells. NOX1-selective inhibition attenuated kidney IRI via inhibition of ROS-mediated ERK signaling.

**Keywords:** NOX1; ML171; reactive oxygen species; ERK; ischemia-reperfusion injury; acute kidney injury

## 1. Introduction

Kidney ischemia/reperfusion injury (IRI), which is the interruption and restoration of blood flow, is a basic pathophysiology of acute kidney injury associated with high mortality and morbidity. IRI causes oxygen and nutrition deficiency, inflammatory cell infiltration, oxygen-derived reactive oxygen species (ROS) or nitrogen-derived reactive nitrogen species generation, microvascular damage, and ultimately tissue damage [1–3]. Excessive ROS is among the most important contributors of tissue damage by inducing oxidative damage of deoxyribonucleic acid, proteins, and lipids [4–8].

Nicotinamide adenine dinucleotide 3-phosphate (NADPH) oxidase (NOX) is a major enzyme that uses NADPH to catalyze oxygen conversion to superoxide and produce ROS. Seven NOX isoforms have been identified including NOX1–5, Duox1, and Duox2 [9]. In particular, NOX1-dependent ROS production contributes to cell signaling, cell growth, angiogenesis, motility, and blood pressure regulation [10–12]. Previous studies have reported that NOX1 upregulation was involved in cisplatin-induced kidney injury [13] and NOX1 inhibitor has a protective effect on lung IRI by suppressing inflammatory and autophagy activation [14]. Although several antioxidants and anti-inflammatory agents [15–19] have effects on ROS production and inflammatory reactions, and NOX4 inhibitor [20] has been used in experimental studies to prevent or decrease IRI-induced kidney damage, the protective effect of NOX1 inhibition against kidney IRI is not totally understood.

This study's aim is to identify the effect of NOX1 inhibition on the recovery from IRI through ROS suppression and related mechanisms. We used a pharmacological inhibitor specific for NOX1 (2-acetylphenothiazine, ML171) [21] and siRNA against NOX1.

## 2. Material and Methods

### 2.1. Animals

Eight-week-old male C57BL/6 mice that weighed 22–25 g (Samtako, Osan, Korea) were used. They were housed with a free access to standard chow and water and were kept in a 12 h light/dark cycle. They were divided randomly into six groups as follows: control vehicle (Con + Veh, $n$ = 5), control with 60 mg/kg ML171 (Con + ML171, $n$ = 5), sham operation with vehicle (Sham + Veh, $n$ = 6), sham operation with 60 mg/kg of ML171 (Sham + ML171, $n$ = 6), ischemia-reperfusion vehicle (IRI + Veh, $n$ = 8), and ischemia-reperfusion with 60 mg/kg of ML171 (IRI + ML171, $n$ = 8). ML171 (MedChemExpress, Monmouth Junction, NJ 08852, USA) was dissolved in 10% DMSO, 40% PEG300, 5% Tween-80, and 45% normal saline. Animals were injected intraperitoneally with a single daily dose of ML171 (60 mg/kg) or vehicle before 24 h for bilateral IRI and were sacrificed by cardiac puncture under anesthesia at 24 h after reperfusion. Blood and kidneys were harvested for the analyses. Animal experiments were performed according to the guidelines approved by the Animal Care and Use Committee at the Kyungpook National University (KNU-2017-0013).

### 2.2. Induction of Kidney IRI

For ischemia induction, the mice were anesthetized using isoflurane inhalation and kidney pedicles were completely occluded for 30 min using a microaneurysm clamp. After 30 min of ischemia, the artery clamp was removed to allow reperfusion, and the skin was closed. Identical surgical treatment was performed on sham-operated animals except for the clamping of the kidney pedicles. During the operation, animals were maintained at a temperature of 36.5–37 °C using a temperature-controlled heating device (Harvard Bioscience, Holliston, MA, USA).

### 2.3. Kidney Function and Histopathological Studies

In mouse serum, blood urea nitrogen (BUN) and creatinine (Cr) levels were evaluated by GCLabs (Yongin, Korea) using the Cobas 8000 modular analyzer system (Roche, Germany). Kidney tissues from each experimental group were immersion-fixed with 4% paraformaldehyde (pH 7.4) and then embedded in paraffin. Two-micrometer tissue sections were prepared and stained with periodic acid-Schiff (PAS) and Masson's trichrome using standard protocols for the determination of histological changes and collagen deposition, respectively. Immunohistochemical analysis of kidney tissues detected the Nox-1 (1:100, ab121009, Abcam) and Nox-4 proteins (1:100, MA5-32090, Invitrogen).

### 2.4. Cell Culture Treatment

Madin-Darby Canine Kidney (MDCK) cells were obtained from the American Type Culture Collection (CCL-34™, Manassas, VA, USA), which were maintained in Eagle's Minimum Essential Medium (EMEM, ATCC®30-2003™) and supplemented with 10% fetal bovine serum at 37 °C in a humidified atmosphere of 5% $CO_2$ and 95% air. Cultured MDCK cells were plated on 96-well plates ($1.0 \times 10^4$ cells/well) for intracellular ROS measurement and on 12-well plates ($1.0 \times 10^5$ cells/well) for real-time reverse transcriptase-polymerase chain reaction (RT-PCR) and on 6-well plates

($2.0 \times 10^5$ cells/well) for measurement of caspase-3 activity and immunoblot analysis. For each experiment, 80–85% confluent cells were incubated with serum-free media for 24 h and were placed into the 0.2% FBS-added medium, which were treated with (1) only medium, (2) ML171 (1 μM), (3) ML171 (2.5 μM), (4) $H_2O_2$ (1.4 mM), (5) $H_2O_2$ (1.4 mM) + ML171 (1 μM), or (6) $H_2O_2$ (1.4 mM) + ML171 (2.5 μM) for an additional 48 h and were pretreated with ML171 (1 μM or 2.5 μM) for 1 h and treated with $H_2O_2$ (1.4 mM). To further study the effect of Nox-1 inhibition, MDCK cells were transiently transfected with 100 nM siRNA against Nox-1 (AccuTarget™ SMART pool customized siRNA, Bioneer, Daejeon, Korea) or nontargeting siRNA (SignalSilence® Control siRNA, #6568, Cell signaling, Danvers, MA, USA) using Lipofectamine RNAiMax (Thermo Fisher Scientific, Waltham, MA, USA) for 6 h. Subsequently, cells were incubated with $H_2O_2$ (1.4 mM) for 48 h.

### *2.5. Hydrogen Peroxide Assay*

Extracellular $H_2O_2$ was measured using the Amplex Red Hydrogen Peroxide Assay Kit (Thermo Fisher Scientific) in accordance with the manufacturer's instructions. Briefly, to detect $H_2O_2$ released from mice kidney and treated MDCK cells, lysis buffer or culture media (50 mL) were reacted with the Amplex Red reagent, along with horseradish peroxidase, to produce resorufin, a red fluorescent oxidation product. Its fluorescence was determined at 530 nm excitation and 590 nm emission using a fluorescence microplate reader (Molecular Devices, Sunnyvale, CA, USA). The concentrations of $H_2O_2$ were calculated using standard curves.

### *2.6. Intracellular ROS Measurement*

Mice kidney and MDCK cells were stained using 10 μM 2′,7′-dichlorodihydrofluorescein diacetate ($H_2$DCFDA; Molecular Probes, Eugene, OR, USA) for 40 min and visualized using fluorescence microscopy (Nikon, Tokyo, Japan). To quantitatively measure fluorescence signal intensity, the stained kidney tissues and cells in 96-well plates were incubated with lysis buffer (0.1% Triton X-100 plus 0.5M EDTA in PBS), and the intensity was measured at 480 nm excitation and 520 nm emission using a fluorescence microplate reader (Molecular Devices Corp., Silicon Valley, CA, USA). The value of the fluorescence signal was normalized based on the total amount of cellular protein and then expressed as a percentage of the control.

### *2.7. Measurement of Caspase-3 Activity*

Caspase-3 activity in the mice kidney and MDCK cells was measured using a colorimetric assay kit (Sigma-Aldrich) in accordance with the manufacturer's protocol. In brief, kidney homogenates were incubated with the fluorometric caspase-3 substrate, Ac-DEVD-pNA, in the assay buffer. To account for nonspecific hydrolysis of the substrate, a control reaction mixture containing the caspase-3 inhibitor, acetyl-DEVD-CHO, in the assay buffer was used. Both mixtures were incubated for 90 min at 37 °C, with the absorbance being read at 405 nm.

### *2.8. TUNEL Assay*

Apoptosis was investigated by terminal deoxynucleotidyl transferase-mediated dUTP <nick end labeling (TUNEL) assay using the In Situ Cell Death Detection Kit (Roche, Mannheim, Germany), Fluorescein, for fluorescence and the Click-iT™ TUNEL colorimetric IHC Detection Kit (Life Technologies, Carlsbad, CA, USA) for immunohistochemistry. Briefly, treated cells were fixed with 4% paraformaldehyde for 1 h at room temperature and then permeabilized in the 0.1% Triton X-100/0.1% sodium citrate for 2 min at 4 °C. After washing with PBS, the cells were incubated with 50 uL TUNEL reagent mixture for 1 h at 37 °C and then counterstained with 4′,6-diamidino-2-phenylindole (DAPI; Sigma, St. Louis, MO, USA) to detect cell nucleus for 1 min. Finally, the cells were mounted with the Prolong Gold anti-fade reagent (Invitrogen, Eugene, OR, USA) and then observed under a confocal microscope (Carl Zeiss, Göttingen, Germany). The number of TUNEL-positive cells was randomly counted (three to five sections per experiment). The percentage of apoptotic cells was calculated

as a percentage of the TUNEL-positive cell-to-DAPI ratio. For immunohistochemistry of TUNEL assay, after treating with terminal deoxynucleotidyl transferase (TdT) reaction buffer for 10 min at 37 °C, the TdT reaction mixture was added for 60 min at 37 °C. The streptavidin-peroxidase conjugate solution was incubated for 30 min at room temperature. Then, the sections were washed and mixed with the 3,3′-diaminobenzidine (DAB) reaction to produce a brown color and then counterstained with Mayer's hematoxylin.

### 2.9. Quantitative RT-PCRs

Total RNA was extracted from treated MDCK cells and kidney tissues using Trizol (Invitrogen, Waltham, MA) in accordance to the manufacturer's instructions. One microgram of total RNA was reverse transcribed to cDNA using PrimeScript cDNA Synthesis kit (TaKaRa Shuzo Co., Ltd., Otsu, Japan). Quantitative PCR was performed in the synthesized cDNA using the StepOne Plus Real-time PCR system (Applied Biosystems, Foster City, CA, USA) with SYBER Green PCR master mix (Life Technologies, Carlsbad, CA, USA). The qRT-PCRs were performed in duplicate. The transcript level of target genes was calculated using the $2^{-\Delta\Delta CT}$ method. All primers used for qRT-PCR were designed using the Primer Express 3.0.1 software (Applied Biosystems, Foster City, CA, USA), which are listed in Table 1.

**Table 1.** Oligonucleotide primer sequences.

| Gene | Forward Primer (5′–3′) | Reverse Primer (5′–3′) |
|---|---|---|
| Mouse Nox-1 | CAG GCC ATG GAT GGA TCT CT | ATG TTT GGA GAC TGG ATG GGA TT |
| Mouse Nox-2 | GCT CTC TCT GAC ATC GGT GAC A | CGA GTC ACG GCC ACA TAC AG |
| Mouse Nox-4 | CAC CAA ACA CAG AAG CAC AAG AC | AAA GCA GGG TAT CAC TCC ATG AA |
| Mouse GAPDH | TAA AGG GCA TCC TGG GCT ACA CT | TTA CTC CTT GGA GGC CAT GTA GG |
| Dog Nox-1 | CCC CGC TGA GTC TTG GAA | TAA AAT CGG AGA ATC CTT TCA AGA A |
| Dog Nox-2 | GAC ACG CAC GCC TTT GAG T | CCT GCA TCT GGG TCT CTA GCA |
| Dog Nox-4 | CAC TCT TCG GAC TAT ACT GCA TGA TC | TCA TCC CCT GAG CCA AGA AT |
| Dog p40phox | GGG AAG ACA TCG CCC TGA AT | ACA GCA GCC GCA CCA GAT |
| Dog SOD2 | CGC CGC CTA CGT GAA CA | CTC CAG CGC CTC CAG ATA CT |
| Dog GPX | GAA TGT GGC GTC GCT CTG A | CGC TGC AGC TCG TTC ATC T |
| Dog GAPDH | GAT GCC CCC ATG TTT GTG A | TTT GGC TAG AGG AGC CAA GCA |

### 2.10. Immunoblot Analysis

Immunoblot analysis detected the marker proteins of apoptosis and mitogen-activated protein kinase (MAPK) pathway, and 20 µg of protein was separated using 10% SDS-polyacrylamide gel electrophoresis and transferred to a nitrocellulose membrane, which was blocked with 10% skimmed milk for 1 h at room temperature and incubated overnight at 4 °C with primary antibodies and then incubated with a horseradish peroxidase-conjugated secondary antibody (Dako, Glostrup, Denmark) for 1 h at room temperature and detected using advanced ECL reagents (Amersham Bioscience, Piscataway, NJ, USA). The intensity of the bands was quantified using the Scion Image software (Scion, Frederick, MD, USA). Primary antibodies that detect proteins are listed in Table 2.

**Table 2.** List of antibodies used in immunohistochemistry and immunoblotting.

| Antibodies | Cat. No. | Company |
|---|---|---|
| Dog Bcl-2 | ab117115 | Abcam |
| Dog Bax | 2772S | Cell signaling |
| Dog β-actin | A1978 | Sigma |
| Dog p-Erk1 (pT202/pY204) + p-Erk2(pT185/pY187) | ab4819 | Abcam |
| Dog Erk1+Erk2 | ab17942 | Abcam |
| Dog p-p38 (phospho T180+Y182) | ab4822 | Abcam |
| Dog p38 (M138) | ab31828 | Abcam |
| Dog p-JNK1 + p-JNK2 (phospho T183+Y185) | ab4821 | Abcam |
| Dog JNK1 + JNK2 + JNK3 | ab179461-1 | Abcam |
| Mouse Bcl-2 | 2876 | Cell signaling |
| Mouse Bax | 2772 | Cell signaling |
| Dog, mouse NOX-1 | Ab121009 | Abcam |
| Mouse NOX-4 | MA5-32090 | Invitroten |
| Mouse a-SMA | Ab5694 | Abcam |
| Mouse fibronectin | Ab2413 | Abcam |
| Mouse GAPDH | 2118S | Cell signaling |
| Mouse p-AKT (Ser473) | 9271 | Cell signaling |
| Mouse AKT | 9272 | Cell signaling |
| Mouse p-ERK (Thr202/Tyr204) | 4370S | Cell signaling |
| Mouse ERK | 9102 | Cell signaling |
| Mouse p-JNK (Thr183/Tyr185) | 9251S | Cell signaling |
| Mouse JNK | 9252S | Cell signaling |
| Mouse p-p38 (Thr180/Tyr182) | 9211S | Cell signaling |
| Mouse p38 | 9212S | Cell signaling |

### 2.11. Statistical Analysis

Data represent mean ± SEM. Statistical analyses were performed using GraphPad Prism 5.01 (GraphPad Software Inc., La Jolla, CA, USA). The difference among the groups was analyzed using a one-way nonparametric ANOVA followed by Tukey's multiple comparison test. Multiple comparison tests were only applied when a significant difference was determined using the ANOVA ($p < 0.05$).

## 3. Results

### 3.1. Effect of ML171 on Attenuation of Kidney Function and Histological Alteration in Kidney IRI

Figure 1A,B shows the results of kidney function after IRI with treatment of ML171. BUN and Cr levels were significantly increased by IRI compared to the control groups. The levels of serum BUN and Cr were decreased in IRI mouse pretreated with ML171. The PAS and trichrome staining evaluated the histological changes in IRI models (Figure 1C–F). The histological analyses revealed that ML171 attenuated tubular necrosis, loss of the brush border, and cast formation in IRI kidney. Treatment with ML171 decreased collagen deposition in the IRI model.

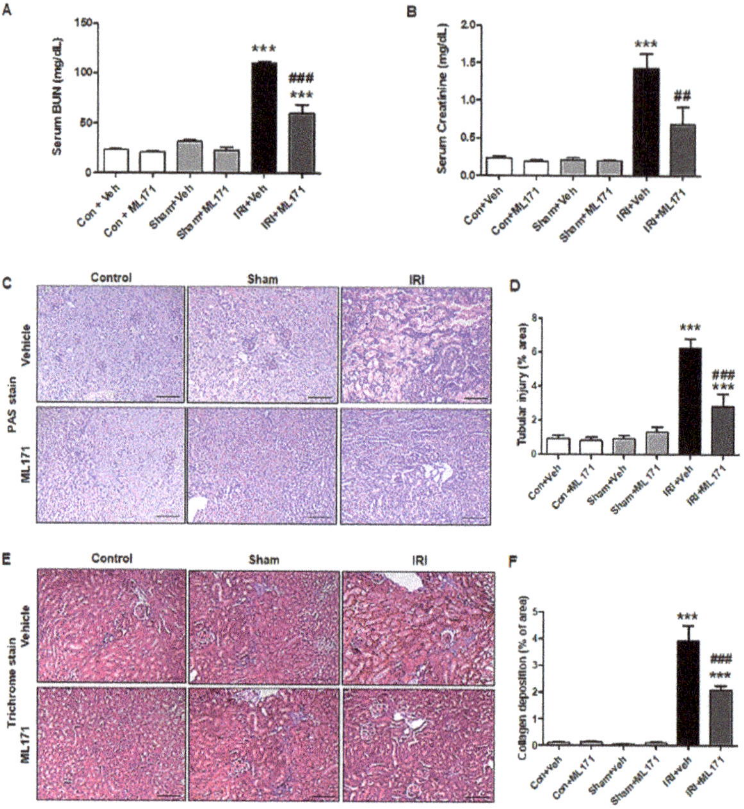


**Figure 1.** Effect of ML171 on attenuation of kidney function and histological alteration in renal ischemia-reperfusion injury (IRI). The levels of serum blood urea nitrogen (BUN) and creatinine were significantly reduced in ML171-pretreated IRI model (**A**,**B**). The periodic acid-Schiff (PAS)- and trichrome-stained kidney sections in IRI models showed that ML171 decreased tissue damage in renal tubular epithelial cells and collagen deposition (**C**–**F**). Data represent mean ± SEM. *** $p < 0.001$ vs. Con + Veh, ## $p < 0.01$, ### $p < 0.001$ vs. IRI + Veh. The difference among the groups was analyzed using a one-way nonparametric ANOVA followed by Tukey's multiple comparison test.

### 3.2. *Effect of ML171 on the Expression of NOX Family Subunits and Oxidative Stress Markers in IRI*

To investigate the changes in oxidative stress after IRI, the expression of NOX subunits and generation of ROS were evaluated. Among the NOX subunits, NOX1 and NOX4, but not NOX2 mRNA expression increased after IRI, which was significantly reduced by ML171 (Figure 2A–C). Immunohistochemical staining of NOX1 and NOX4 revealed an increased amount of NOX1 and NOX4 expression in the IRI model and a significant decrease by ML171 treatment (Figure 2D–G). ML171 attenuated the increase of intracellular $H_2O_2$ in the IRI kidney model (Figure 2H–I).

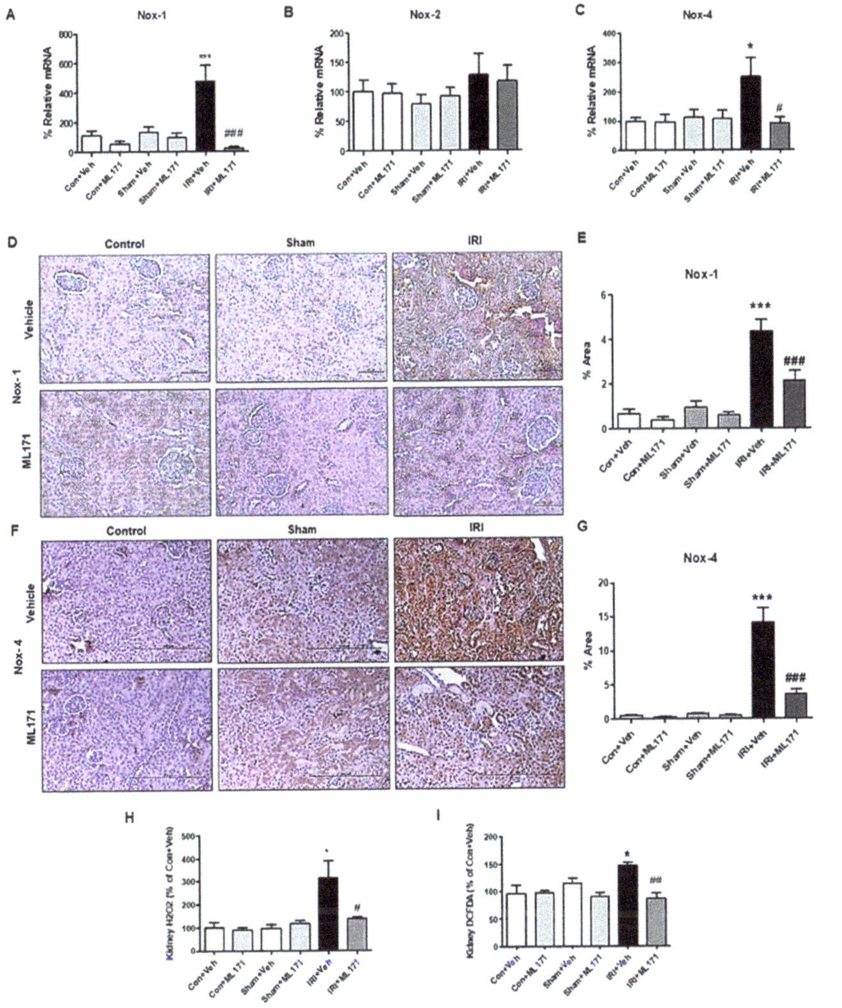


**Figure 2.** Effect of ML171 on nicotinamide adenine dinucleotide phosphate (NADPH) oxidase (NOX) family subunits and oxidative stress markers in IRI. The increased mRNA expression of NOX1 and NOX4 in IRI were significantly mitigated by ML171 (**A–C**). The immunohistochemical staining of NOX1 and NOX4 showed that the increased expression of NOX1 and NOX4 in IRI was decreased by ML171 (**D–G**). The increased reactive oxygen species (ROS) including $H_2O_2$ in the IRI model were significantly decreased by ML171 (**H**,**I**). Data represent mean ± SEM. * $p < 0.05$, *** $p < 0.001$ vs. Con + Veh, # $p < 0.05$, ## $p < 0.01$, ### $p < 0.001$ vs. IRI + Veh. The difference among the groups was analyzed using a one-way nonparametric ANOVA followed by Tukey's multiple comparison test.

## 3.3. Effect of ML171 on Apoptosis in Kidney Tubular Cells Following IRI

Caspase-3 activity decreased in the kidneys after ML171 treatment (Figure 3A), and TUNEL assay showed that apoptosis of kidney tubule cells decreased after MA171 treatment (Figure 3B). Figure 3C also showed that ML171 caused a significantly increased Bcl-2 level and Bcl-2/Bax ratio in the IRI model, suggesting the mitigating effect of ML171 on apoptosis.

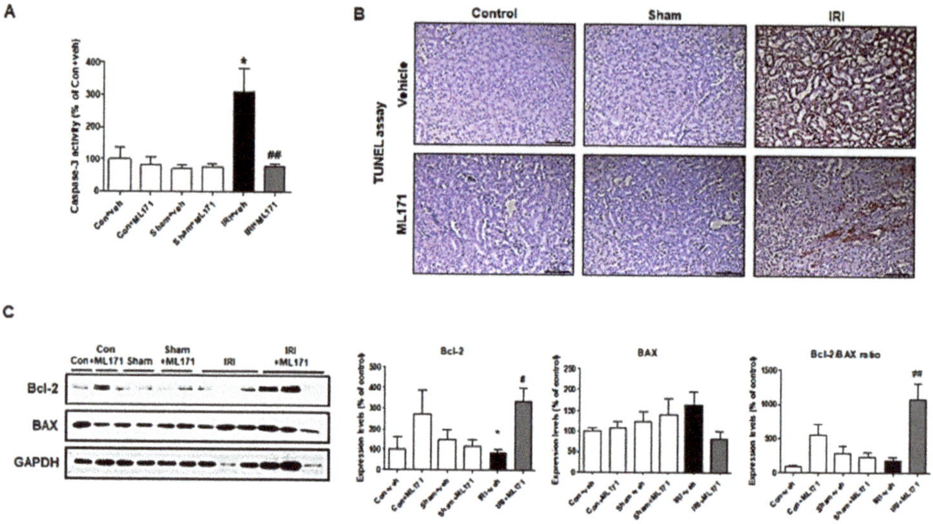


**Figure 3.** Effect of ML171 on apoptosis in kidney tubular cells following IRI. Caspase-3 activity was significantly decreased in IRI model after ML171 treatment (**A**). TUNEL assay showed that ML171 attenuated the apoptosis of kidney tubule cells (**B**). The Bcl-2 level and Bcl-2/Bax ratio were significantly increased in the IRI model after ML171 treatment (**C**). Data represent mean ± SEM. * $p < 0.05$ vs. Con + Veh, # $p < 0.05$, ## $p < 0.01$ vs. IRI + Veh. The difference among the groups was analyzed using a one-way nonparametric ANOVA followed by Tukey's multiple comparison test.

## 3.4. Changes in Phosphorylated Proteins of MAPK Signaling Pathways in Kidney Tissues

We identified MAPK pathway genes to determine the oxidative stress mechanism induced by IRI. The Western blot of MAPK genes revealed that the phosphorylated extracellular signal-regulated kinase (p-ERK) was significantly increased in the IRI model, which was effectively attenuated by ML171. However, no difference in the expression of phosphorylated p38 and JNK was noted (Figure 4).

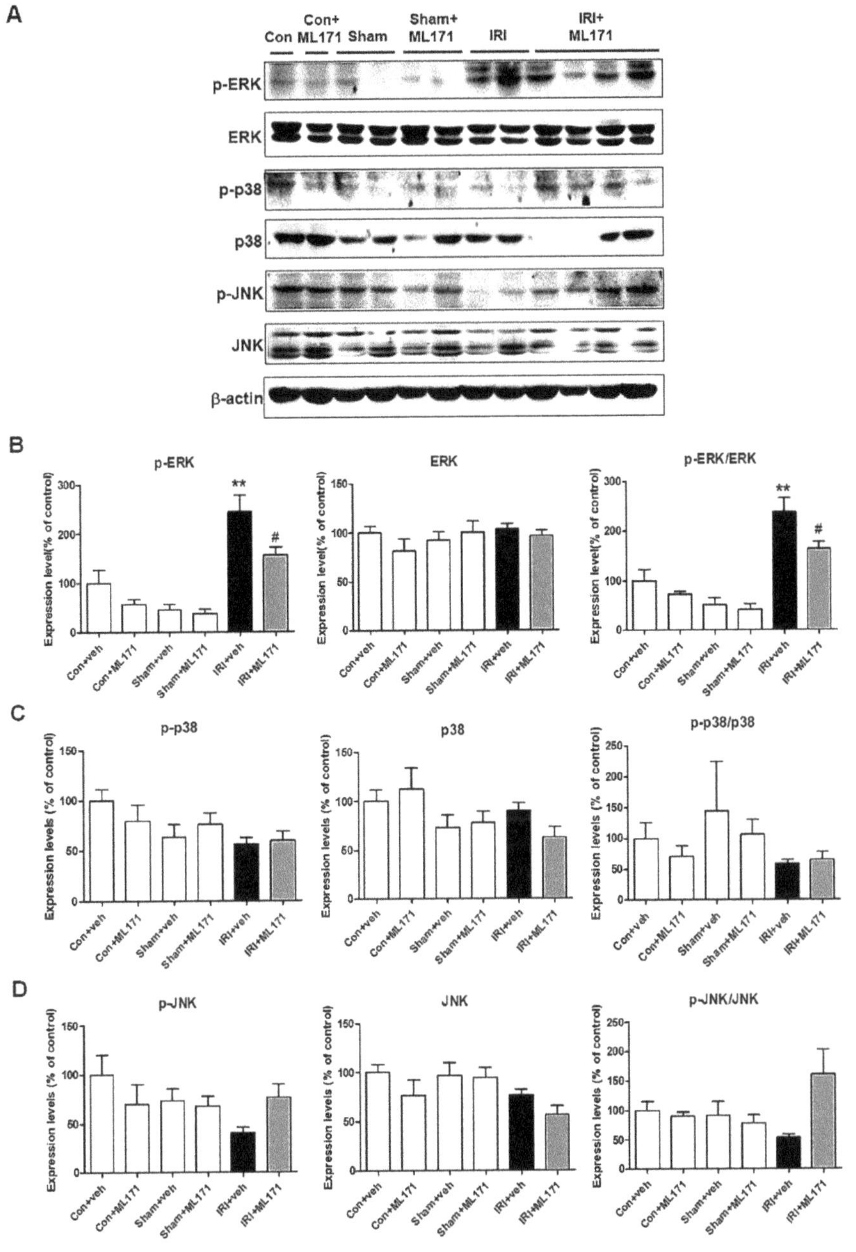


**Figure 4.** Changes in phosphorylated proteins of mitogen-activated protein kinase (MAPK) signaling pathways in kidney tissues. The genes of MAPK pathway determined the mechanism of oxidative stress-induced IRI. ML171 effectively attenuated increased p-ERK in the IRI model (**A**,**B**). The expression of phosphorylated p38 and JNK was not increased in the IRI model nor affected by ML171 (**C**,**D**). Data represent mean ± SEM. ** $p < 0.01$ vs. Con + Veh, # $p < 0.05$ vs. IRI + Veh. The difference among the groups was analyzed using a one-way nonparametric ANOVA followed by Tukey's multiple comparison test.

### 3.5. *Effect of ML171 on NOX Subunit Expression and ROS Generation in $H_2O_2$-Treated MDCK Cells*

MDCK cells were treated with $H_2O_2$ to induce NOX subunit expression and ROS generation. $H_2O_2$ increased expression of NOX1, NOX4, and p40$^{phox}$, but not NOX2. ML171 attenuated the increased expression of NOX subunits induced by $H_2O_2$ in MDCK cells. $H_2O_2$ evoked a change in oxidative stress-related enzymes of SOD2 and GPX production, which was mitigated by ML171 treatment (Figure 5).

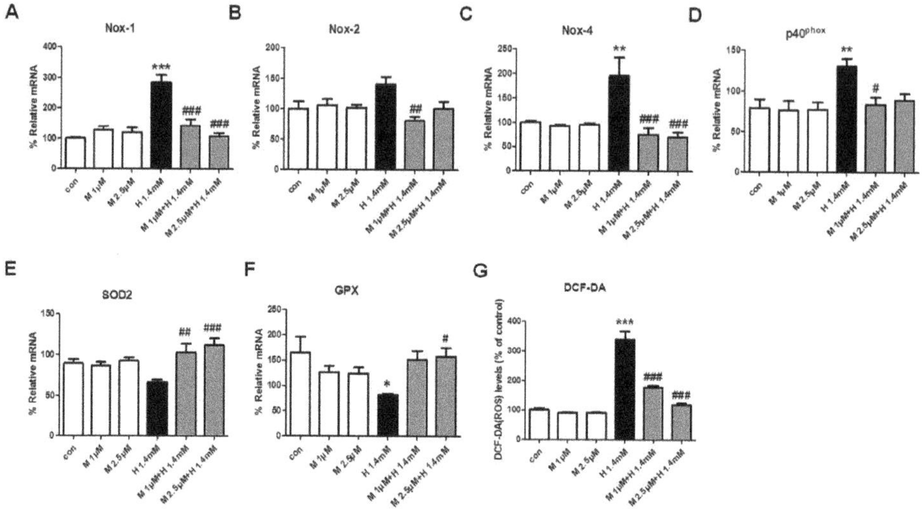


**Figure 5.** Effect of ML171 on $H_2O_2$-induced NOX subunit expression and ROS generation in MDCK cells. ML171 decreased NOX1, NOX4, and p40$^{phox}$ expression in $H_2O_2$-treated MDCK cells (**A–D**). Oxidative stress-related enzymes of SOD2 and GPX production were mitigated by ML171 treatment (**E–G**). Data represent mean ± SEM. * $p < 0.05$, ** $p < 0.01$, *** $p < 0.001$ vs. Con, # $p < 0.05$, ## $p < 0.01$, ### $p < 0.001$ vs. H 1.4 mM. The difference among the groups was analyzed using a one-way nonparametric ANOVA followed by Tukey's multiple comparison test.

### 3.6. *Effect of siRNA against NOX1 on $H_2O_2$-Treated MDCK Cells*

MDCK cells were transfected with siRNA against NOX1 to evaluate whether the protective effect of ML171 was mediated with NOX1 and the expression of NOX4 was related with that of NOX1 in MDCK cells. Compared to nontargeting siRNA, siRNA against NOX1 showed a decreased NOX1 expression after $H_2O_2$ induction. Transfection with siRNA against NOX1 also upregulated SOD2 and GPX mRNA, which is consistent with the effect of ML171 treatment. Surprisingly, $H_2O_2$-induced expression of NOX4 mRNA was inhibited in MDCK cells with siRNA against NOX1, whereas NOX2 and p40$^{phox}$ expression remained increased (Figure 6).

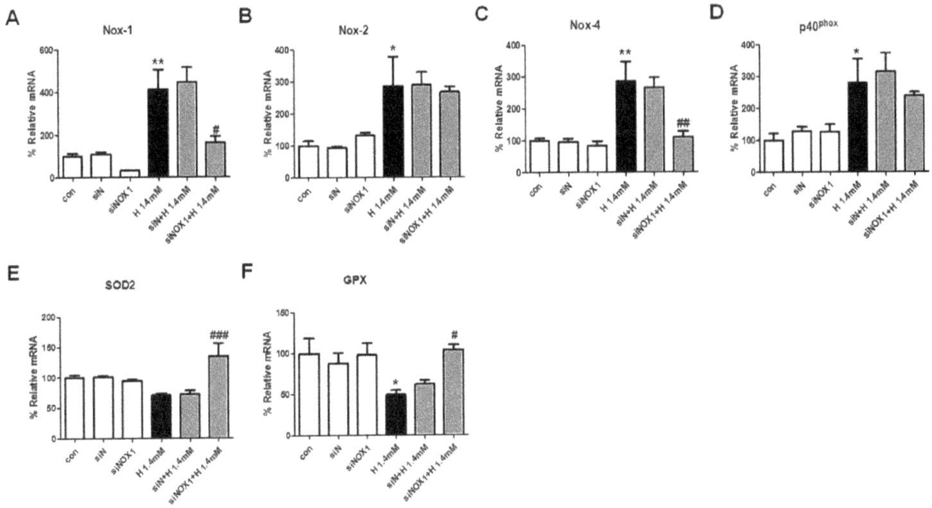


**Figure 6.** Effect of siRNA against NOX1 on $H_2O_2$-induced NOX subunit expression and ROS generation in MDCK cells. siRNA against NOX1 reduced NOX1 and NOX4 expression, however, did not affect NOX2 and $p40^{phox}$ expression (**A**–**D**). Oxidative stress-related enzymes of SOD2 and GPX production were upregulated by siRNA against NOX1 treatment (**E**,**F**). Data represent mean ± SEM. * $p < 0.05$, ** $p < 0.01$ vs. Con, # $p < 0.05$, ## $p < 0.01$, ### $p < 0.001$ vs. H 1.4 mM. The difference among the groups was analyzed using a one-way nonparametric ANOVA followed by Tukey's multiple comparison test.

### 3.7. Effect of ML171 on the Apoptosis Induced by $H_2O_2$ in MDCK Cells

The effect of ML171 on the apoptosis induced by oxidative stress was assessed in MDCK cells. Caspase-3 activity increased significantly after $H_2O_2$ treatment and decreased after ML171 treatment in MDCK cells (Figure 7A). ML171 also attenuated the changes in the expression of Bax and Bcl-2/Bax ratio in $H_2O_2$-treated MDCK cells (Figure 7B). The TUNEL assay showed that ML171 decreased the $H_2O_2$-induced apoptosis in tubule cells (Figure 7C,D).

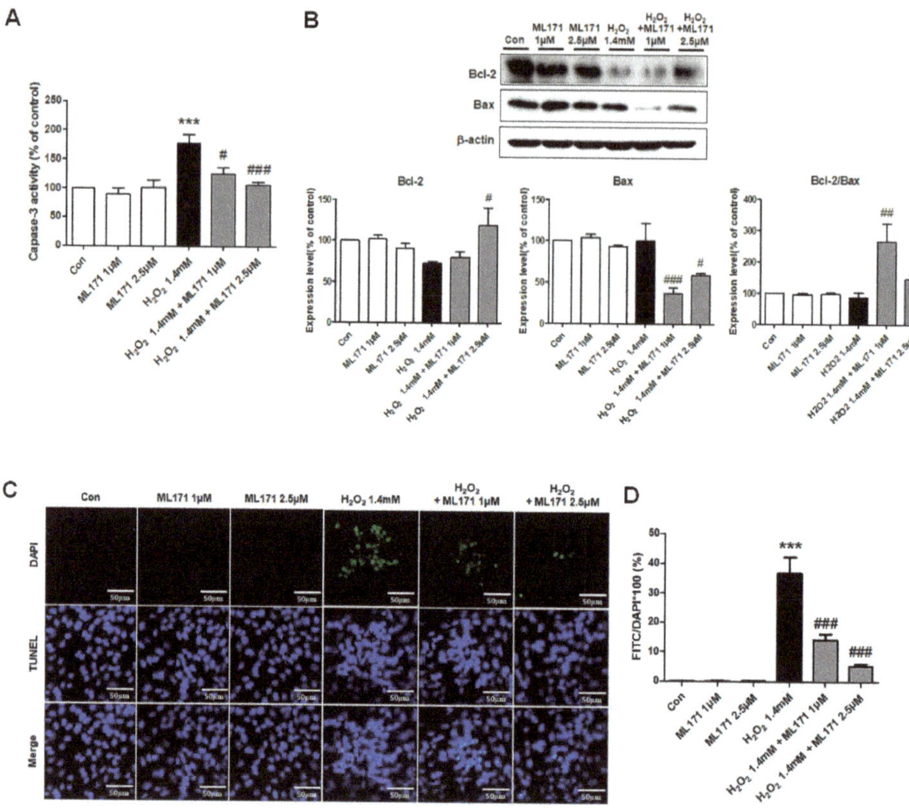


**Figure 7.** Effect of ML171 on the apoptosis induced by $H_2O_2$ in MDCK cells. Caspase-3 activity was significantly increased after $H_2O_2$ induced oxidative stress in MDCK cells and was significantly decreased by ML171 treatment (**A**). ML171 attenuated the changes in the expression of Bax and the Bcl-2/Bax ratio in $H_2O_2$-treated MDCK cells (**B**). TUNEL assay showed that $H_2O_2$-induced apoptosis was significantly reduced by ML171 treatment (**C**,**D**). Data represent mean ± SEM. *** $p < 0.001$ vs. Con, # $p < 0.05$, ## $p < 0.01$, ### $p < 0.001$ vs. H 1.4 mM. The difference among the groups was analyzed using a one-way nonparametric ANOVA followed by Tukey's multiple comparison test.

### 3.8. Changes in Phosphorylated Proteins of MAPK Signaling Pathways in MDCK Cells

We investigated the mechanism with which ML171 blocked oxidative stress and apoptosis in MDCK cells. The p-ERK and p-ERK/ERK ratio significantly increased after $H_2O_2$ treatment and was significantly reduced by ML171 in MDCK cells. p38 and JNK expressions were not affected by $H_2O_2$ and ML171, which was consistent with the in vivo experiment results (Figure 8).

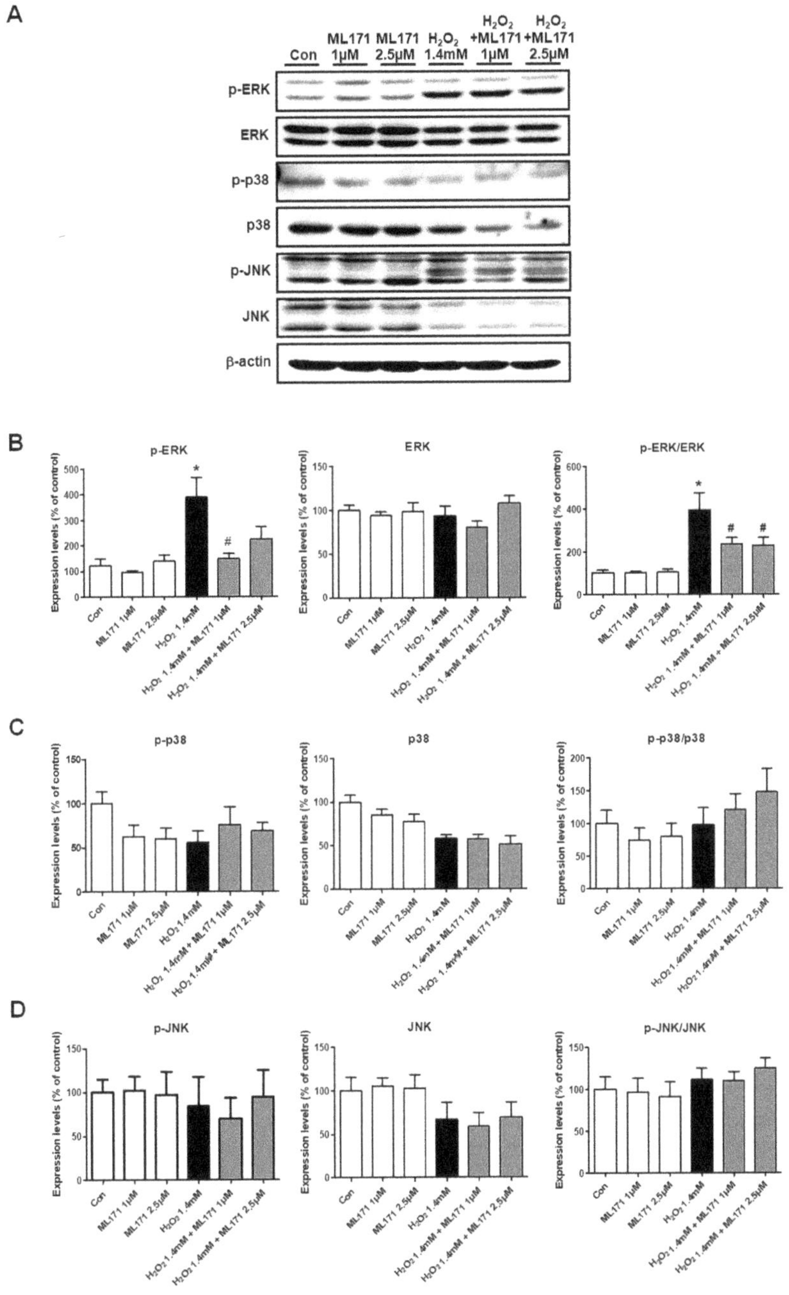


**Figure 8.** Changes in phosphorylated proteins of MAPK signaling pathways in MDCK cells. Consistent with the results from the in vivo experiment, the increased p-ERK and p-ERK/ERK ratio after $H_2O_2$ treatment was significantly decreased after ML171 treatment in MDCK cells (**A**,**B**). There were no significant differences in the expression of phosphorylated p38 and JNK after ML171 treatment (**C**,**D**). Data represent mean ± SEM. * $p < 0.05$ vs. Con, # $p < 0.05$ vs. H 1.4 mM. The difference among the groups was analyzed using a one-way nonparametric ANOVA followed by Tukey's multiple comparison test.

## 4. Discussion

The present study demonstrated that NOX1 inhibition by ML171 attenuated kidney IRI in the mouse model. The ischemic injury decreased significantly in the ML171-treated IRI group compared to that in the IRI group. The tissue injury was associated with the increased ROS production and NOX expression, which was reversed by ML171 treatment. $H_2O_2$ evoked changes in oxidative stress-related enzymes of SOD2 and GPX production in MDCK cells, which was mitigated by NOX1 inhibition with ML171 and siRNA against NOX1. Treatment with ML171 and transfection with siRNA against NOX1 decreased the expression of NOX1 induced by $H_2O_2$ exposure in MDCK cells. ML171 caused a significant increase in the Bcl-2 level and decrease in caspase-3 activity in IRI mice and $H_2O_2$-treated MDCK cells. ML171 affected ERK signaling by the phosphorylation of ERK in kidney tissues and tubular cells. The present study was the first to suggest that NOX1 inhibition could protect kidney IRI by inhibition of ROS-mediated ERK signaling.

Ischemic damage of the kidney causes acute kidney injury, which is responsible for the hypoxic damage induced by the production of ROS as well as the decrease in kidney blood flow [22,23]. ROS acts as signaling molecules including regulation of vascular tone, monitoring of oxygen tension, and signal transduction from membrane receptors in physiological situations, but in excess, it causes tissue damage [24–26]. NOX, one of the main sources of ROS, catalyzes the transfer of electrons from NADPH to molecular oxygen to produce ROS [27].

NOX4 is the most distributed NOX isoform in the kidney and has been studied in various kidney diseases. NOX4 expression in proximal tubular cells increased after exposure to high glucose, and NOX4 inhibition with GKT136901 decreased albuminuria in diabetic mice [28,29]. NOX4 deficiency was associated with the increased tubular injury after IRI [30], and hypoxia to kidney tubule cell upregulated NOX4 expression via a TGF-β1/Smad signaling pathway [31]. NOX2 also plays a role especially in the development of diabetic nephropathy, and its expression was upregulated in the kidneys of diabetic mice [32–34]. NOX2 is the classic phagocytic NOX and its main role is free radical generation [35,36]. It has been reported that NOX2 inhibition could prevent kidney damage and delayed graft function after IRI by the inhibition fibrosis and oxidative stress [37].

NOX1 is also expressed in the kidney cortex [38–40], and the associations with ischemic injury have been reported in other organs. NOX1 was a therapeutic target in ischemic retinopathy and IRI in the heart [41,42]. The role of NOX1 in kidney injury has been reported in cisplatin nephrotoxicity. Cardamonin, a flavone with anti-inflammatory activity, inhibited NOX1 expression in the cisplatin nephrotoxicity model, decreasing inflammation and apoptosis in the injured kidney [13]. The study on a NOX inhibitor has also revealed its protective effect in the kidney IRI. Apocynin, a nonspecific NOX inhibitor, ameliorated the histological damages after IRI by reducing oxidative stress markers, demonstrating that NOX1 was associated with kidney injury and downregulation of NOX could prevent kidney damage. However, it was difficult to attribute the action specifically to NOX1 inhibition, since two drugs did not selectively inhibit NOX1. In contrast, ML171 is a known potent NOX1 inhibitor with isoform selectivity only for NOX1 [21]. In the present study, NOX1 expression significantly increased in the kidney after IRI and MDCK cells treated with $H_2O_2$. ML171 effectively suppressed NOX1 upregulation induced by IRI, and the suppression of NOX1 by ML171 was also observed in $H_2O_2$-treated tubular cells, which are the main site of IRI. The treatment of ML171 showed improvement of serum BUN and Cr levels in the IRI group, suggesting significant amelioration of the ischemic injury. Therefore, this is the first study to demonstrate the renoprotective effect of NOX1 selective inhibition through the IRI animal model.

The expression of NOX1, NOX2, and NOX4 is closely related to each other [43]. Angiotensin II increases oxidative stress by upregulating the kidney cortical gene product for NOX1 and $p22^{phox}$, a catalytic core of the NOX [38]. Rats with the silenced $p22^{phox}$ gene reduced NOX1, NOX2, and NOX4 expression in the kidney cortex during infusion of angiotensin II [40]. Aoyama et al. showed that angiotensin II-induced NOX4 expression was inhibited by NOX1 knock-out hepatocytes, suggesting that NOX1 could induce NOX4 upregulation [44]. Our results are consistent with the previous study in that NOX4 expression was downregulated after transfection with siRNA against NOX1 into $H_2O_2$-treated MDCK cells. The reduced expression of NOX4 by ML171 treatment might be associated with the causal interaction between NOX1 and NOX4, which could also be explained by the downregulation after reduced oxidative stress by NOX1 inhibition or a partial inhibitory effect of ML171 on NOX4 [45].

$H_2O_2$ is a major marker of oxidative stress, giving rise to tissue injury after IRI [46,47]. In the present study, $H_2O_2$ increased significantly in the kidney after IRI. DCFDA, a compound used to measure generalized oxidative stress including intracellular $H_2O_2$ production, also significantly increased in the tubular cells treated with $H_2O_2$. Therefore, the injury with $H_2O_2$ in the MDCK cells is comparable to the injury induced by IRI in the kidney. SOD2 and GPX are two important components of the defensive mechanisms against oxidative stress by preventing the reactive free radical formation [48–51]. ML171 reduced $H_2O_2$ in the IRI mouse, and the effect was manifested as a subsequent increase in SOD2 and GPX in MDCK cells, suggesting the prevention of kidney damage with oxidative stress by selective NOX1 inhibition.

MAPK is associated with the activation of NOX1 [52]. ERK and p38 as well as JNK are members of MAPK that have proline-directed kinase activity. However, a certain stimulus selectively activates a specific member of the MAPK pathway [53]. Among them, ERK signaling pathway was involved in the present study. Only phosphorylation of ERK increased after ischemia and $H_2O_2$ exposure. ERK phosphorylates $p47^{phox}$ and contributes to NOX1 complex assembly [53]. Our results are consistent with the previous report that suggested the association of ERK with the cellular survival of the kidney with IRI [54].

We also investigated the possible mechanisms by which NOX1 inhibition prevented tubular injury. ROS generated by ischemia or oxidative stress are well-known inducers of apoptosis by activating caspase-3 in kidney tubular cells [6]. It was supported by TUNEL-positive kidney tubular epithelial cells and decreased Bcl-2/Bax ratios [55,56]. ML171 treatment before IRI significantly decreased caspase-3 activity, decreased the number of TUNEL-positive cells, and increased Bcl-2/Bax ratios compared with the IRI group. This suggests that the renoprotective effects of NOX1 inhibition are mediated via modulating kidney tubular cell apoptosis after IRI.

Our study has several limitations. First, our results were not validated with the other oxidative stress injury models such as cisplatin nephrotoxicity or contrast-induced nephropathy. However, the IRI model is a prototype of oxidative stress injury to kidney, and, although other models may show slight differences, we tried to determine NOX1's role in the basic injury model. Second, further experiments with a more specific way to inhibit NOX1 expression are needed to find NOX1's effect in IRI. GKT771, a highly selective NOX1 inhibitor [57] or NOXA1ds, a peptide NOX1 inhibitor with greater specificity and isoform selectivity [58], might reveal the specific effect of NOX1-selective inhibition. Third, our experiment was not performed on murine or human kidney epithelial cell lines. An animal toxicity test and further experiment with human kidney epithelial cells must be accompanied to apply the present results to human medicine. Nevertheless, this is the first study to investigate the renoprotective effect of NOX1 inhibition on the kidneys and kidney tubule cells, which makes it a candidate for treatment of acute kidney injury.

## 5. Conclusions

NOX1-selective inhibition by ML171 attenuated kidney IRI via inhibition of ROS-mediated ERK signaling. NOX1 inhibition by ML171 and siRNA against NOX1 reduced the oxidative stress-induced apoptosis in MDCK cells, indicating NOX1 selective inhibition's potential as a therapeutic target for acute kidney injury associated with ROS generation and subsequent apoptosis.

## 6. Patent

The results of this paper were patented under the name "Composition for preventing or treating ischemia-reperfusion injury comprising NADPH oxidase 1" on 20 April 2020 (Number: 10-2020-0047663).

**Author Contributions:** Conceptualization, H.-Y.J., S.-H.O., and J.-H.C.; Methodology, H.-Y.J., S.-H.O., J.-S.A., E.-J.O., Y.-J.K, and J.-H.C.; Formal Analysis, H.-Y.J., S.-H.O., J.-S.A., E.-J.O., Y.-J.K., and J.-H.C.; Investigation, H.-Y.J., S.-H.O., C.-D.K., S.-H.P., Y.-L.K., and J.-H.C.; Data Curation, H.-Y.J., S.-H.O., J.-S.A., E.-J.O., Y.-J.K., and J.-H.C.; Writing—Original Draft Preparation, H.-Y.J., S.-H.O., and J.-H.C.; Writing—Review and Editing, H.-Y.J. and J.-H.C. All authors have read and agreed to the published version of the manuscript.

**Funding:** This research was supported by the Korea Health Technology R&D Project grant through the Korea Health Industry Development Institute (KHIDI), funded by the Ministry of Health and Welfare, Republic of Korea (grant number: HI15C0001), supported by Medi-Start Up Program funded by the Daegu Metropolitan City (Project Name: Development of the candidate agents for acute kidney injury through the reduction of oxidative stress), and supported by Basic Science Research Program through the National Research Foundation of Korea (NRF) funded by the Ministry of Education (2020R1I1A3068253).

**Conflicts of Interest:** The authors declare no conflict of interest.

## Abbreviations

| | |
|---|---|
| BUN | Blood urea nitrogen |
| Cr | Creatinine |
| IRI | Ischemia-reperfusion injury |
| KHIDI | Korea Health Industry Development Institute |
| MAPK | Mitogen-activated protein kinase |
| MDCK | Madin–Darby Canine Kidney |
| NADPH | Nicotinamide adenine dinucleotide phosphate |
| PAS | Periodic acid-Schiff |
| ROS | Reactive oxygen species |
| TdT | Terminal deoxynucleotidyl transferase |

## References

1. Kalogeris, T.; Baines, C.P.; Krenz, M.; Korthuis, R.J. Cell biology of ischemia/reperfusion injury. *Int. Rev. Cell Mol. Biol.* **2012**, *298*, 229–317. [CrossRef] [PubMed]
2. Noiri, E.; Nakao, A.; Uchida, K.; Tsukahara, H.; Ohno, M.; Fujita, T.; Brodsky, S.; Goligorsky, M.S. Oxidative and nitrosative stress in acute renal ischemia. *Am. J. Physiol. Renal Physiol.* **2001**, *281*, F948–F957. [CrossRef] [PubMed]
3. Han, S.J.; Lee, H.T. Mechanisms and therapeutic targets of ischemic acute kidney injury. *Kidney Res. Clin. Pract.* **2019**, *38*, 427–440. [CrossRef] [PubMed]
4. Kennedy, S.E.; Erlich, J.H. Murine renal ischaemia-reperfusion injury. *Nephrology (Carlton)* **2008**, *13*, 390–396. [CrossRef]
5. Lien, Y.H.; Lai, L.W.; Silva, A.L. Pathogenesis of renal ischemia/reperfusion injury: Lessons from knockout mice. *Life Sci.* **2003**, *74*, 543–552. [CrossRef]
6. Dobashi, K.; Ghosh, B.; Orak, J.K.; Singh, I.; Singh, A.K. Kidney ischemia-reperfusion: Modulation of antioxidant defenses. *Mol. Cell. Biochem.* **2000**, *205*, 1–11. [CrossRef]
7. Kim, J.; Seok, Y.M.; Jung, K.J.; Park, K.M. Reactive oxygen species/oxidative stress contributes to progression of kidney fibrosis following transient ischemic injury in mice. *Am. J. Physiol. Renal Physiol.* **2009**, *297*, F461–F470. [CrossRef]
8. Kim, J.; Jang, H.S.; Park, K.M. Reactive oxygen species generated by renal ischemia and reperfusion trigger protection against subsequent renal ischemia and reperfusion injury in mice. *Am. J. Physiol. Renal Physiol.* **2010**, *298*, F158–F166. [CrossRef]
9. Sedeek, M.; Nasrallah, R.; Touyz, R.M.; Hebert, R.L. NADPH oxidases, reactive oxygen species, and the kidney: Friend and foe. *J. Am. Soc. Nephrol.* **2013**, *24*, 1512–1518. [CrossRef]

10. Arbiser, J.L.; Petros, J.; Klafter, R.; Govindajaran, B.; McLaughlin, E.R.; Brown, L.F.; Cohen, C.; Moses, M.; Kilroy, S.; Arnold, R.S.; et al. Reactive oxygen generated by Nox1 triggers the angiogenic switch. *Proc. Natl. Acad. Sci. USA* **2002**, *99*, 715–720. [CrossRef]
11. Gavazzi, G.; Banfi, B.; Deffert, C.; Fiette, L.; Schappi, M.; Herrmann, F.; Krause, K.H. Decreased blood pressure in NOX1-deficient mice. *FEBS Lett.* **2006**, *580*, 497–504. [CrossRef] [PubMed]
12. Sadok, A.; Bourgarel-Rey, V.; Gattacceca, F.; Penel, C.; Lehmann, M.; Kovacic, H. Nox1-dependent superoxide production controls colon adenocarcinoma cell migration. *Biochim. Biophys. Acta* **2008**, *1783*, 23–33. [CrossRef] [PubMed]
13. El-Naga, R.N. Pre-treatment with cardamonin protects against cisplatin-induced nephrotoxicity in rats: Impact on NOX-1, inflammation and apoptosis. *Toxicol. Appl. Pharmacol.* **2014**, *274*, 87–95. [CrossRef] [PubMed]
14. Cui, Y.; Wang, Y.; Li, G.; Ma, W.; Zhou, X.S.; Wang, J.; Liu, B. The Nox1/Nox4 inhibitor attenuates acute lung injury induced by ischemia-reperfusion in mice. *PLoS ONE* **2018**, *13*, e0209444. [CrossRef] [PubMed]
15. Hosseini, F.; Naseri, M.K.; Badavi, M.; Ghaffari, M.A.; Shahbazian, H.; Rashidi, I. Effect of beta carotene on lipid peroxidation and antioxidant status following renal ischemia/reperfusion injury in rat. *Scand. J. Clin. Lab. Investig.* **2010**, *70*, 259–263. [CrossRef] [PubMed]
16. Beytur, A.; Binbay, M.; Sarihan, M.E.; Parlakpinar, H.; Polat, A.; Gunaydin, M.O.; Acet, A. Dose-dependent protective effect of ivabradine against ischemia-reperfusion-induced renal injury in rats. *Kidney Blood Press. Res.* **2012**, *35*, 114–119. [CrossRef]
17. Alan, C.; Kocoglu, H.; Altintas, R.; Alici, B.; Resit Ersay, A. Protective effect of decorin on acute ischaemia-reperfusion injury in the rat kidney. *Arch. Med. Sci.* **2011**, *7*, 211–216. [CrossRef]
18. Xu, Y.F.; Liu, M.; Peng, B.; Che, J.P.; Zhang, H.M.; Yan, Y.; Wang, G.C.; Wu, Y.C.; Zheng, J.H. Protective effects of SP600125 on renal ischemia-reperfusion injury in rats. *J. Surg. Res.* **2011**, *169*, e77–e84. [CrossRef]
19. Talab, S.S.; Elmi, A.; Emami, H.; Nezami, B.G.; Assa, S.; Ghasemi, M.; Tavangar, S.M.; Dehpour, A.R. Protective effects of acute lithium preconditioning against renal ischemia/reperfusion injury in rat: Role of nitric oxide and cyclooxygenase systems. *Eur. J. Pharmacol.* **2012**, *681*, 94–99. [CrossRef]
20. Jeong, B.Y.; Lee, H.Y.; Park, C.G.; Kang, J.; Yu, S.L.; Choi, D.R.; Han, S.Y.; Park, M.H.; Cho, S.; Lee, S.Y.; et al. Oxidative stress caused by activation of NADPH oxidase 4 promotes contrast-induced acute kidney injury. *PLoS ONE* **2018**, *13*, e0191034. [CrossRef]
21. Gianni, D.; Taulet, N.; Zhang, H.; DerMardirossian, C.; Kister, J.; Martinez, L.; Roush, W.R.; Brown, S.J.; Bokoch, G.M.; Rosen, H. A novel and specific NADPH oxidase-1 (Nox1) small-molecule inhibitor blocks the formation of functional invadopodia in human colon cancer cells. *ACS Chem. Biol.* **2010**, *5*, 981–993. [CrossRef] [PubMed]
22. Bonventre, J.V. Mechanisms of ischemic acute renal failure. *Kidney Int.* **1993**, *43*, 1160–1178. [CrossRef] [PubMed]
23. Sheridan, A.M.; Bonventre, J.V. Cell biology and molecular mechanisms of injury in ischemic acute renal failure. *Curr. Opin. Nephrol. Hypertens.* **2000**, *9*, 427–434. [CrossRef] [PubMed]
24. Droge, W. Free radicals in the physiological control of cell function. *Physiol. Rev.* **2002**, *82*, 47–95. [CrossRef] [PubMed]
25. Nordberg, J.; Arner, E.S. Reactive oxygen species, antioxidants, and the mammalian thioredoxin system. *Free Radic. Biol. Med.* **2001**, *31*, 1287–1312. [CrossRef]
26. Sen, C.K.; Packer, L. Antioxidant and redox regulation of gene transcription. *FASEB J.* **1996**, *10*, 709–720. [CrossRef]
27. Wang, D.; Chen, Y.; Chabrashvili, T.; Aslam, S.; Borrego Conde, L.J.; Umans, J.G.; Wilcox, C.S. Role of oxidative stress in endothelial dysfunction and enhanced responses to angiotensin II of afferent arterioles from rabbits infused with angiotensin II. *J. Am. Soc. Nephrol.* **2003**, *14*, 2783–2789. [CrossRef]
28. Sedeek, M.; Callera, G.; Montezano, A.; Gutsol, A.; Heitz, F.; Szyndralewiez, C.; Page, P.; Kennedy, C.R.; Burns, K.D.; Touyz, R.M.; et al. Critical role of Nox4-based NADPH oxidase in glucose-induced oxidative stress in the kidney: Implications in type 2 diabetic nephropathy. *Am. J. Physiol. Renal Physiol.* **2010**, *299*, F1348–F1358. [CrossRef]
29. Sedeek, M.; Gutsol, A.; Montezano, A.C.; Burger, D.; Nguyen Dinh Cat, A.; Kennedy, C.R.; Burns, K.D.; Cooper, M.E.; Jandeleit-Dahm, K.; Page, P.; et al. Renoprotective effects of a novel Nox1/4 inhibitor in a mouse model of Type 2 diabetes. *Clin. Sci.* **2013**, *124*, 191–202. [CrossRef]

30. Nlandu-Khodo, S.; Dissard, R.; Hasler, U.; Schafer, M.; Pircher, H.; Jansen-Durr, P.; Krause, K.H.; Martin, P.Y.; de Seigneux, S. NADPH oxidase 4 deficiency increases tubular cell death during acute ischemic reperfusion injury. *Sci. Rep.* **2016**, *6*, 38598. [CrossRef]
31. Cho, S.; Yu, S.L.; Kang, J.; Jeong, B.Y.; Lee, H.Y.; Park, C.G.; Yu, Y.B.; Jin, D.C.; Hwang, W.M.; Yun, S.R.; et al. NADPH oxidase 4 mediates TGF-beta1/Smad signaling pathway induced acute kidney injury in hypoxia. *PLoS ONE* **2019**, *14*, e0219483. [CrossRef]
32. Fukuda, M.; Nakamura, T.; Kataoka, K.; Nako, H.; Tokutomi, Y.; Dong, Y.F.; Ogawa, H.; Kim-Mitsuyama, S. Potentiation by candesartan of protective effects of pioglitazone against type 2 diabetic cardiovascular and renal complications in obese mice. *J. Hypertens.* **2010**, *28*, 340–352. [CrossRef] [PubMed]
33. Ohshiro, Y.; Ma, R.C.; Yasuda, Y.; Hiraoka-Yamamoto, J.; Clermont, A.C.; Isshiki, K.; Yagi, K.; Arikawa, E.; Kern, T.S.; King, G.L. Reduction of diabetes-induced oxidative stress, fibrotic cytokine expression, and renal dysfunction in protein kinase Cbeta-null mice. *Diabetes* **2006**, *55*, 3112–3120. [CrossRef] [PubMed]
34. Chew, P.; Yuen, D.Y.; Stefanovic, N.; Pete, J.; Coughlan, M.T.; Jandeleit-Dahm, K.A.; Thomas, M.C.; Rosenfeldt, F.; Cooper, M.E.; de Haan, J.B. Antiatherosclerotic and renoprotective effects of ebselen in the diabetic apolipoprotein E/GPx1-double knockout mouse. *Diabetes* **2010**, *59*, 3198–3207. [CrossRef]
35. Djamali, A.; Vidyasagar, A.; Adulla, M.; Hullett, D.; Reese, S. Nox-2 Is a Modulator of fibrogenesis in kidney allografts. *Am. J. Transplant.* **2009**, *9*, 74–82. [CrossRef]
36. Djamali, A.; Reese, S.; Hafez, O.; Vidyasagar, A.; Jacobson, L.; Swain, W.; Kolehmainen, C.; Huang, L.; Wilson, N.A.; Torrealba, J.R. Nox2 is a mediator of chronic CsA nephrotoxicity. *Am. J. Transplant.* **2012**, *12*, 1997–2007. [CrossRef]
37. Karim, A.S.; Reese, S.R.; Wilson, N.A.; Jacobson, L.M.; Zhong, W.; Djamali, A. Nox2 Is a mediator of ischemia reperfusion injury. *Am. J. Transplant.* **2015**, *15*, 2888–2899. [CrossRef]
38. Chabrashvili, T.; Kitiyakara, C.; Blau, J.; Karber, A.; Aslam, S.; Welch, W.J.; Wilcox, C.S. Effects of ANG II type 1 and 2 receptors on oxidative stress, renal NADPH oxidase, and SOD expression. *Am. J. Physiol. Regul. Integr. Comp. Physiol.* **2003**, *285*, R117–R124. [CrossRef]
39. Kitiyakara, C.; Chabrashvili, T.; Chen, Y.; Blau, J.; Karber, A.; Aslam, S.; Welch, W.J.; Wilcox, C.S. Salt intake, oxidative stress, and renal expression of NADPH oxidase and superoxide dismutase. *J. Am. Soc. Nephrol.* **2003**, *14*, 2775–2782. [CrossRef]
40. Modlinger, P.; Chabrashvili, T.; Gill, P.S.; Mendonca, M.; Harrison, D.G.; Griendling, K.K.; Li, M.; Raggio, J.; Wellstein, A.; Chen, Y.; et al. RNA silencing in vivo reveals role of p22phox in rat angiotensin slow pressor response. *Hypertension* **2006**, *47*, 238–244. [CrossRef]
41. Wilkinson-Berka, J.L.; Deliyanti, D.; Rana, I.; Miller, A.G.; Agrotis, A.; Armani, R.; Szyndralewiez, C.; Wingler, K.; Touyz, R.M.; Cooper, M.E.; et al. NADPH oxidase, NOX1, mediates vascular injury in ischemic retinopathy. *Antioxid. Redox Sign.* **2014**, *20*, 2726–2740. [CrossRef] [PubMed]
42. Braunersreuther, V.; Montecucco, F.; Asrih, M.; Pelli, G.; Galan, K.; Frias, M.; Burger, F.; Quindere, A.L.; Montessuit, C.; Krause, K.H.; et al. Role of NADPH oxidase isoforms NOX1, NOX2 and NOX4 in myocardial ischemia/reperfusion injury. *J. Mol. Cell. Cardiol.* **2013**, *64*, 99–107. [CrossRef] [PubMed]
43. Gill, P.S.; Wilcox, C.S. NADPH oxidases in the kidney. *Antioxid. Redox Sign.* **2006**, *8*, 1597–1607. [CrossRef] [PubMed]
44. Aoyama, T.; Paik, Y.H.; Watanabe, S.; Laleu, B.; Gaggini, F.; Fioraso-Cartier, L.; Molango, S.; Heitz, F.; Merlot, C.; Szyndralewiez, C.; et al. Nicotinamide adenine dinucleotide phosphate oxidase in experimental liver fibrosis: GKT137831 as a novel potential therapeutic agent. *Hepatology* **2012**, *56*, 2316–2327. [CrossRef]
45. Dao, V.T.; Elbatreek, M.H.; Altenhofer, S.; Casas, A.I.; Pachado, M.P.; Neullens, C.T.; Knaus, U.G.; Schmidt, H. Isoform-selective NADPH oxidase inhibitor panel for pharmacological target validation. *Free Radic. Biol. Med.* **2020**, *148*, 60–69. [CrossRef]
46. Choi, H.I.; Kim, H.J.; Park, J.S.; Kim, I.J.; Bae, E.H.; Ma, S.K.; Kim, S.W. PGC-1alpha attenuates hydrogen peroxide-induced apoptotic cell death by upregulating Nrf-2 via GSK3beta inactivation mediated by activated p38 in HK-2 cells. *Sci. Rep.* **2017**, *7*, 4319. [CrossRef]
47. Park, J.S.; Choi, H.I.; Bae, E.H.; Ma, S.K.; Kim, S.W. Small heterodimer partner attenuates hydrogen peroxide-induced expression of cyclooxygenase-2 and inducible nitric oxide synthase by suppression of activator protein-1 and nuclear factor-kappaB in renal proximal tubule epithelial cells. *Int. J. Mol. Med.* **2017**, *39*, 701–710. [CrossRef]

48. Slyshenkov, V.S.; Rakowska, M.; Moiseenok, A.G.; Wojtczak, L. Pantothenic acid and its derivatives protect Ehrlich ascites tumor cells against lipid peroxidation. *Free Radic. Biol. Med.* **1995**, *19*, 767–772. [CrossRef]
49. van Haaften, R.I.; Haenen, G.R.; Evelo, C.T.; Bast, A. Effect of vitamin E on glutathione-dependent enzymes. *Drug Metab. Rev.* **2003**, *35*, 215–253. [CrossRef]
50. Parlakpinar, H.; Olmez, E.; Acet, A.; Ozturk, F.; Tasdemir, S.; Ates, B.; Gul, M.; Otlu, A. Beneficial effects of apricot-feeding on myocardial ischemia-reperfusion injury in rats. *Food Chem. Toxicol.* **2009**, *47*, 802–808. [CrossRef]
51. Walker, E.M., Jr.; Gale, G.R. Methods of reduction of cisplatin nephrotoxicity. *Ann. Clin. Lab. Sci.* **1981**, *11*, 397–410. [PubMed]
52. El Benna, J.; Faust, L.P.; Babior, B.M. The phosphorylation of the respiratory burst oxidase component p47phox during neutrophil activation. Phosphorylation of sites recognized by protein kinase C and by proline-directed kinases. *J. Biol. Chem.* **1994**, *269*, 23431–23436. [PubMed]
53. El Benna, J.; Han, J.; Park, J.W.; Schmid, E.; Ulevitch, R.J.; Babior, B.M. Activation of p38 in stimulated human neutrophils: Phosphorylation of the oxidase component p47phox by p38 and ERK but not by JNK. *Arch. Biochem. Biophys.* **1996**, *334*, 395–400. [CrossRef] [PubMed]
54. Luo, F.; Shi, J.; Shi, Q.; Xu, X.; Xia, Y.; He, X. Mitogen-Activated protein kinases and hypoxic/ischemic nephropathy. *Cell. Physiol. Biochem.* **2016**, *39*, 1051–1067. [CrossRef] [PubMed]
55. Chien, C.T.; Chang, T.C.; Tsai, C.Y.; Shyue, S.K.; Lai, M.K. Adenovirus-mediated bcl-2 gene transfer inhibits renal ischemia/reperfusion induced tubular oxidative stress and apoptosis. *Am. J. Transplant.* **2005**, *5*, 1194–1203. [CrossRef]
56. Havasi, A.; Li, Z.; Wang, Z.; Martin, J.L.; Botla, V.; Ruchalski, K.; Schwartz, J.H.; Borkan, S.C. Hsp27 inhibits Bax activation and apoptosis via a phosphatidylinositol 3-kinase-dependent mechanism. *J. Biol. Chem.* **2008**, *283*, 12305–12313. [CrossRef]
57. Stalin, J.; Garrido-Urbani, S.; Heitz, F.; Szyndralewiez, C.; Jemelin, S.; Coquoz, O.; Ruegg, C.; Imhof, B.A. Inhibition of host NOX1 blocks tumor growth and enhances checkpoint inhibitor-based immunotherapy. *Life Sci. Alliance* **2019**, *2*. [CrossRef]
58. Ranayhossaini, D.J.; Rodriguez, A.I.; Sahoo, S.; Chen, B.B.; Mallampalli, R.K.; Kelley, E.E.; Csanyi, G.; Gladwin, M.T.; Romero, G.; Pagano, P.J. Selective recapitulation of conserved and nonconserved regions of putative NOXA1 protein activation domain confers isoform-specific inhibition of Nox1 oxidase and attenuation of endothelial cell migration. *J. Biol. Chem.* **2013**, *288*, 36437–36450. [CrossRef]

International Journal of
*Molecular Sciences*

*Review*

# Toll-Like Receptor as a Potential Biomarker in Renal Diseases

**Sebastian Mertowski [1,*], Paulina Lipa [2], Izabela Morawska [1], Paulina Niedźwiedzka-Rystwej [3,*], Dominika Bębnowska [3], Rafał Hrynkiewicz [3], Ewelina Grywalska [1,*], Jacek Roliński [1] and Wojciech Załuska [4]**

1 Department of Clinical Immunology and Immunotherapy, Medical University of Lublin, 20-093 Lublin, Poland; izabelamorawska19@gmail.com (I.M.); jacek.rolinski@gmail.com (J.R.)
2 Department of Genetics and Microbiology, Institute of Microbiology and Biotechnology, Faculty of Biology and Biotechnology, Maria Curie-Skłodowska University, Akademicka 19 St., 20-033 Lublin, Poland; paulina.lipa56@gmail.com
3 Institute of Biology, University of Szczecin, Felczaka 3c, 71-412 Szczecin, Poland; bebnowska.d@wp.pl (D.B.); rafal.hrynkiewicz@gmail.com (R.H.)
4 Department of Nephrology, Medical University of Lublin, 20-954 Lublin, Poland; wojciech.zaluska@umlub.pl
* Correspondence: mertowskisebastian@gmail.com (S.M.); paulina.niedzwiedzka-rystwej@usz.edu.pl (P.N.-R.); ewelina.grywalska@gmail.com (E.G.)

Received: 30 August 2020; Accepted: 11 September 2020; Published: 13 September 2020

**Abstract:** One of the major challenges faced by modern nephrology is the identification of biomarkers associated with histopathological patterns or defined pathogenic mechanisms that may assist in the non-invasive diagnosis of kidney disease, particularly glomerulopathy. The identification of such molecules may allow prognostic subgroups to be established based on the type of disease, thereby predicting response to treatment or disease relapse. Advances in understanding the pathogenesis of diseases, such as membranous nephropathy, minimal change disease, focal segmental glomerulosclerosis, IgA (immunoglobulin A) nephropathy, and diabetic nephropathy, along with the progressive development and standardization of plasma and urine proteomics techniques, have facilitated the identification of an increasing number of molecules that may be useful for these purposes. The growing number of studies on the role of TLR (toll-like receptor) receptors in the pathogenesis of kidney disease forces contemporary researchers to reflect on these molecules, which may soon join the group of renal biomarkers and become a helpful tool in the diagnosis of glomerulopathy. In this article, we conducted a thorough review of the literature on the role of TLRs in the pathogenesis of glomerulopathy. The role of TLR receptors as potential marker molecules for the development of neoplastic diseases is emphasized more and more often, as prognostic factors in diseases on several epidemiological backgrounds.

**Keywords:** acute kidney injury; biomarker; diabetic nephropathy; focal segmental glomerulosclerosis; innate immunity; membranous nephropathy; minimal change diseases; TLR

## 1. Introduction

The term "biological marker" in the literature refers to the objective health status of the patient, which can be observed from the outside, i.e., in a way that can be measured in an extremely accurate and, most importantly, repeatable manner. Various medical symptoms can often contrast with each other, or, on the contrary, correlations between them are observed, which may contribute to a better and faster diagnosis of the disease or the effectiveness of the treatment process. A joint project of the World Health Organization together with the United Nations under the name of the International Program on Chemical Safety has attempted to standardize the term biomarker used in the literature.

Currently, a biomarker is defined as "any substance, structure or process that can be measured in the body or its products and that can influence or predict the occurrence of an outcome or disease" [1], which means that the modern definition of biomarkers covers every response of the body, whether functional, physiological, or biochemical, to the occurrence of a potential threat (physical, chemical, or biological) that may modify the body's reactions at the cellular or molecular level. Usually, biomarker is used with two meanings: (1) A biomarker is a component (analyte) of a human biological system (i.e., plasma, urine, etc.); or (2) a biomarker is a biological property (i.e., mass concentration of X in plasma) [2]. Currently, examples of biomarkers can be both simple parameters of heart rate and blood pressure, as well as the determination of complex constituent molecules present in our blood or tissues, which are indicative of health. Types and applications of biomarkers are constantly changing as it evaluates our knowledge about them. Thus, it has recently been shown that counts of urinary T-cell, renal tubular epithelial cells, and podocalyxin-positive cells provide an excellent biomarker for the detection of renal transplant rejection in routine clinical trials [3]. Currently, the role of TLR receptors as potential marker molecules for the development of neoplastic diseases is emphasized more and more often, e.g., TLR5 as a prognostic marker for gastric cancer [4]. It was also shown that the activity of TLR receptor is correlated with the state of injury of post-surgical patients who have a disorder of the immune response related to the interaction of TLR receptors with DAMP (damage-associated molecular pattern). Moreover, the analyses led to conclusions regarding the role of TLR receptors in predicting pathological conditions, including tissue damage, in these patients [5]. One of the increasing threats in today's world is chronic kidney disease, the cause of which may be both primary processes related to the kidneys, and secondary processes observed in the course of rheumatic, cardiological, or diabetic diseases. As indicated in the literature, one of the largest causes of the development of chronic kidney disease in highly developed countries as well as in developing countries is hypertension and type 2 diabetes, currently classified as diseases of civilization [6]. As far as type 2 diabetes and renal disorders are concerned, it was shown that polypharmacy has a great impact on the occurrence, course, and treatment of the disease [7].

Genetic, epigenetic, or environmental factors that play a more or less important role in different regions of the world may lead to diseases associated with kidney glomerular damage, which leads to their chronic hypofunction and subsequent renal failure. Research conducted by O'Shaughnessy et al. [6], aimed to analyze the data from centers dealing with chronic kidney diseases, where several types of nephropathy were considered. Analysis shows that there is a difference in the incidence of individual nephropathy depending on the region. It turned out that focal segmental glomerulosclerosis (FSGS) and diabetic nephropathy are the most numerous in the USA because it occurred in 19% of diagnosed patients; the second type that dominated was IgA nephropathy (12%), another was membranous nephropathy (12%) and lupus nephritis (10%). Furthermore, FSGS was also common in Latin America (16%), although lupus nephritis strongly dominated the region (38%), while diabetic nephropathy (DN) (4%) and IgA nephropathy (IgAN) (6%) were relatively rare. A reverse dependence than in the USA has been observed in Europe and Asia. In Europe, IgA nephropathy dominated the diagnosis, and the second most common diagnosis was FSGS (15%), while in Asia, IgA glomerulopathy included 40% of diagnoses and the second most common diagnosis was lupus nephritis (17%) [8].

All of these diseases are the subject of intensive research by many scientists around the world. The following review of the literature focuses on the problems of diseases associated with glomerular dysfunction, in which there are answers to questions about the participation in the pathogenesis of diseases on TLR, which may become a potential marker molecule.

## 2. Classification of Biomarkers

There are many different ways to classify biological molecules as biomarkers in the literature. One of the basic methods is division according to the type of marker molecule. These are DNA, mitochondrial DNA, RNA, or mRNA molecules that belong to the genomic biomarker category, but also proteins, peptides, or antibodies that are classified as proteomic biomarkers. The third group is metabolic markers (metabolomics), which includes lipids, carbohydrates, enzymes, and products of metabolism (metabolites). Our attention was drawn to a slightly different classification of these unusual molecules, i.e., classification based on genetics and molecular biology, due to the usefulness of biomarkers in diagnostic processes and due to their application (Figure 1). The first group includes three types of biomarkers. Type 0 are biomarkers that correlate over time with known clinical indications and show the natural course and history of the disease. Type I relates to biomarkers of drug activity, which can be divided into biomarkers of efficacy (taking into account the therapeutic effect of a given drug), mechanism (providing information about the drug's mechanism of action), and toxicity (including the toxic effect of a given drug). Type II is known as surrogate biomarkers to help evaluate and predict the effect of therapy [9].

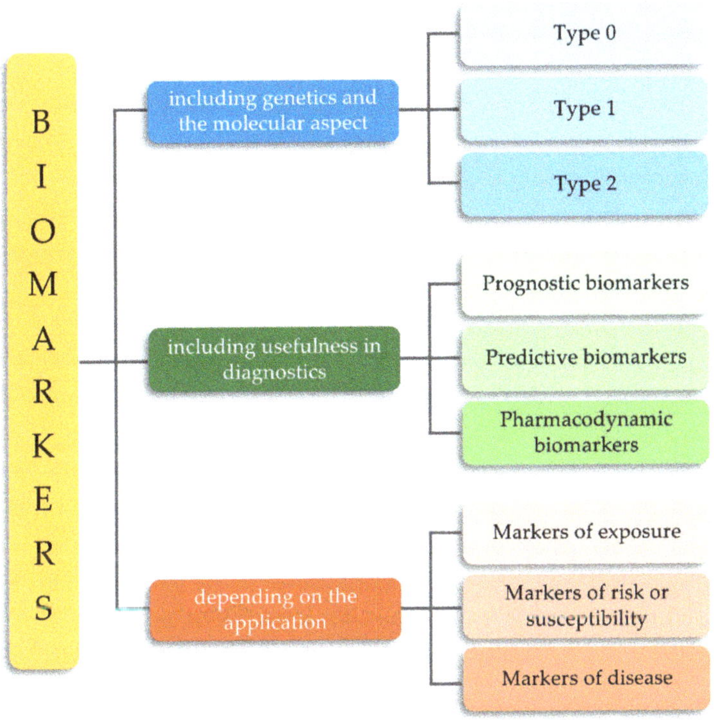


**Figure 1.** Classification of biomarkers due to the genetic and molecular aspect, the usefulness of biomarkers in diagnostic processes, and application.

Due to the usefulness of biomarkers in diagnostics, we can distinguish prognostic biomarkers; in other words, those that suggest the probable outcome of the disease in an untreated individual, and predictive biomarkers, the purpose of which is to identify patients for whom a specific therapy is most effective. Lastly, we can distinguish pharmacodynamic biomarkers that determine the pharmacological action of a given drug [10]. Another classification is based on the use of biomarkers. We distinguish here exposure markers and doses that are used to reconstruct and predict past accidental or occupational exposures. Risk or vulnerability markers, which relate to the identification of vulnerable individuals (or future patients) at increased risk of developing a disease, and disease markers represent the initial cellular or molecular changes that occur during the development of a particular disease entity. It is the latter group that includes TLR receptors [11,12]. However, what characteristics does an ideal biomarker need to meet? Is there an "ideal biomarker"? What features should a biomarker have to be close to the ideal? Well, according to the FDA, an ideal biomarker must meet the following six characteristics (Figure 2). First, it must be specific in the course of a particular disease entity and easy to differentiate between different physiological conditions of the patient. Secondly, such a biomarker must above all be easy to measure and safe. Then, the speed of its detection is also important, as it enables a quick diagnosis as well as the repeatability and accuracy of the results obtained. Attention is also paid to the cost of detecting such biomarkers, which must be relatively cheap. The advantage of such a biomarker is also the consistency between ethnic groups and genders of patients [13].

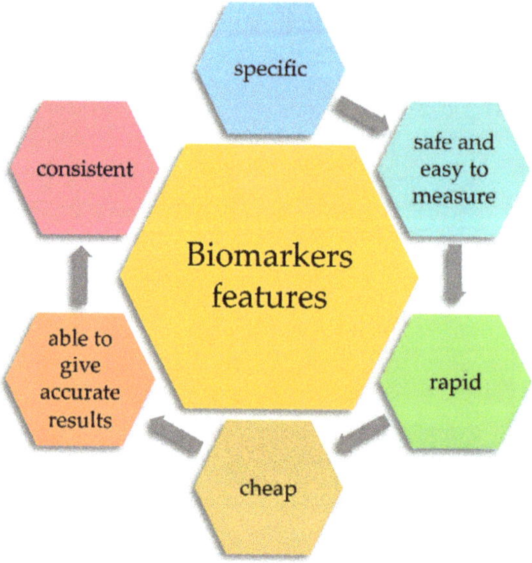


**Figure 2.** Classification of biomarkers due to the genetic and molecular aspect, the usefulness of biomarkers in diagnostic processes, and application.

## 3. Characteristic of the TLR Receptors

Glomerulonephritis is a heterogeneous group of diseases whose common denominator is inflammation, ongoing in the glomerulus, resulting from systemic (secondary glomerulonephritis) or only glomerulonephritis (primary glomerulonephritis) [14–19]. The etiopathogenesis and the cause of the variable course of glomerulopathy is the subject of numerous studies but remains unknown. Although the pathogenesis is not unequivocally elucidated, the literature data clearly indicate the involvement of various immune mechanisms in the etiopathogenesis of glomerulopathy. Researchers indicate the role of the immune system in the development of chronic kidney disease on the basis of primary and secondary disorders of the glomerular functions, and AKI (acute kidney injury) resulting from the above-mentioned entities and other disease states, e.g., sepsis [20]. The main elements involved in promoting kidney damage are dendritic cells, NK (natural killer) cells, macrophages, and proinflammatory cytokines. A critical role is played by the complement system, which can both protect and promote damage to the glomeruli [21].

Literature data suggest the contribution of innate immunity to TLRs in these processes. These receptors are a classic example of pattern recognition receptors (PRRs). Signals received by these receptors by recruiting specific molecules lead to activation of the transcription factors NF-κB (nuclear factor kappa-light-chain-enhancer of activated B cells) and IRF (interferon regulatory factor) and affect various elements of the host's innate immune response [22]. TLR mechanisms are based on the ability to recognize twofold signals. The first one is based on the detection of pathogen-associated molecular patterns (PAMPs), while the second reads molecules related to damage to the body's own cells (DAMPs; danger-associated molecular patterns) [23]. However, the origin of the signal, in the case of PAMP, is compounds of exogenous origin, while DAMP receives endogenous information. The result of receiving signals from both pathways is the effector reaction in which the production of costimulatory molecules and cytokines takes place. The location of TLRs is the cell surface or intracellular compartments, including ER (endoplasmic reticulum), lysosomes, and endosomes. It is pointed out that intracellular localization is important not only for ligand recognition but also for avoiding TLR contact with self-nucleic acids, which could cause autoimmunity. A high number of TLR receptors on cells of the immune system, such as monocytes, macrophages, dendritic cells, or lymphocytes, enables the thesis that they constitute a network allowing rapid cooperation of leukocytes and cells present at the site of infection or in the immediate vicinity of damaged host cells [23,24]. TLR synthesis begins in the rough endoplasmic reticulum, from where it goes to the Golgi apparatus and then to its destinations, in other words to the cell surface or to the intercellular compartments [22].

At present, there are 10 types of TLR receptors in humans and three additional types in mice, whereas others species may have more of these receptors (Table 1). Based on the amino acid sequence homology, TLRs occurring in vertebrates were divided into six subfamilies: TLR 1/2/6/10, TLR3, TLR4, TLR5, followed by TLR 7/8/9, and TLR 11 to the last 12/13 (Table 2). However, not all vertebrates have all types of receptors. PRRs have a specific structure in the form of transmembrane proteins, being an integral component of the cell membrane, in which the N-terminal part is responsible for ligand binding, whereas the C-terminal end is equipped with a signaling domain for IL-1 (TIR; toll IL-1 receptor), being part of the signal induction cascade for the production of anti-inflammatory mediators [23]. The transmembrane domain of TLRs contains about 20, mostly hydrophobic, amino acid residues. The N-terminal end (ECDs (extracellular domain) N-terminal ectodomains) is a glycoprotein of 500–800 amino acid residues. In their structure, we distinguish the presence of leucine-rich tandem repeats (LRRs), the number of which depends on the receptor type and ranges from 20–29 repeats (Table 1).

**Table 1.** Characteristics of individual TLRs (toll-like receptors).

| Name | Location of Coding Genes | Location in the Cell | The Number of Amino Acids | Molecular Weight (kDa) | Number of LLR | Reference |
|---|---|---|---|---|---|---|
| TLR1 | Chromosome 4 | Golgi apparatus, Phagosome, Cell membrane | 786aa | 90.31 | 19 | [25–27] |
| TLR2 | Chromosome 4 | Phagosome | 784aa | 89.83 | 19 | [25,28,29] |
| TLR3 | Chromosome 4 | Early endosome, ER | 904aa | 103.82 | 23 | [25,30,31] |
| TLR4 | Chromosome 9 | Cell membrane, Early endosome | 839aa | 95.68 | 21 | [25,32,33] |
| TLR5 | Chromosome 1 | No data | 858aa | 97.83 | 20 | [25,34,35] |
| TLR6 | Chromosome 4 | Golgi apparatus, Cell membrane, Phagosome | 796aa | 91.88 | 19 | [25,36,37] |
| TLR7 | Chromosome X | Endosomes, Lysosomes, ER, Phagosome | 1049aa | 120.92 | 25 | [25,38] |
| TLR8 | Chromosome X | No data | 1041aa | 119.82 | 25 | [25,39,40] |
| TLR9 | Chromosome 3 | Endosomes, Lysosomes, ER, Phagosome | 1032aa | 115.86 | 25 | [25,41] |
| TLR10 | Chromosome 4 | No data | 811aa | 94.56 | 19 | [25,42,43] |

**Table 1.** *Cont.*

| Name | Location of Coding Genes | Location in the Cell | The Number of Amino Acids | Molecular Weight (kDa) | Number of LLR | Reference |
|---|---|---|---|---|---|---|
| TLR11 | Expression in mice | No data | 926aa | 105.83 | 10 | [44] |
| TLR12 | Expression in mice | No data | 906aa | 99.94 | 17 | [45] |
| TLR13 | Expression in mice | Endosomes | 991aa | 114.44 | 25 | [46] |

TLRs also differ in the cell site. TLR 1/2/4/5/6/10/11/12 receptors are located on the outer membrane of cells, while 3/7/8/9 receptors are located inside of them. Several literature reports have identified specific PAMP and DAMP ligands, which are bound by particular TLRs (Table 2).

**Table 2.** Location and ligands bound by TLR.

| Name | Occurrence | Ligand PAMP | The Origin of PAMP | Ligand DAMP | Reference |
|---|---|---|---|---|---|
| | | **Extracellular** | | | |
| TLR1 | Macrophages<br>Neutrophils<br>B lymphocytes<br>Dendritic cells | Lipopeptides<br>Soluble factors (lipoproteins) | Bacteria | No data | [47,48] |
| TLR2 | Macrophages<br>Neutrophils<br>B lymphocytes<br>Dendritic cells<br>NK cells | Bacterial lipopeptides<br>Teichoic acids,<br>LAM<br>Moduline,<br>Glycolipids of bacteria,<br>Porins, LPS, | Bacteria | Apolipoprotein CIII,<br>Heparin sulphate,<br>Hyaluronic acid,<br>Hsp60, Hsp70,<br>Peroxiredoxin | [47–50] |
| | | Glycosinositolphospholipids | Protozoa, e.g., Trypanosoma cruzi | | |
| | | Zymosan | Fungi | | |
| | | Hemagglutinin | Measles virus | | |
| | | Protein | Herpesvirus | | |
| | | Hsp70 proteins | Host organism | | |
| TLR4 | Macrophages<br>Neutrophils<br>B lymphocytes<br>Dendritic cells<br>NK cells<br>Treg cells | LPS | Bacteria | C-reactive protein,<br>Fibronectin,<br>Fibrinogen,<br>Heparin sulphate,<br>Neutrophil, Elastase,<br>Angiotensin II,<br>Hsp60 | [48–51] |
| | | Fusion proteins,<br>Proteins present in the coating | Viruses, e.g., RSV virus | | |
| | | Taxol | Plants | | |
| | | Hsp60 protein<br>Hsp70 protein<br>A fragment of the A domain of fibronectin<br>Hyaluronic acid oligosaccharide<br>Fibrinogen<br>Heparan sulphate | Host organism | | |
| TLR5 | Macrophages<br>B lymphocytes<br>Dendritic cells<br>Treg cells | Flagellin | Bacteria (Gram-negative) | No data | [48,52] |
| TLR6 | Macrophages<br>Neutrophils<br>Dendritic cells | Diacyl lipopeptides<br>Lipoteichoic acids<br>Zymosan | Bacteria<br>Fungi | Versican | [47–50,53] |
| TLR10 | Dendritic cells | No data | No data | No data | [54] |
| TLR11 | Macrophages<br>Dendritic cells | Flagellin<br>Profilin | Bacteria<br>Protozoa, e.g., Toxoplasma gondii | No data | [55,56] |
| TLR12 | Dendritic cells | Profilin | Protozoa, e.g., Toxoplasma gondii | No data | [55] |

**Table 2.** *Cont.*

| Name | Occurrence | Ligand PAMP | The Origin of PAMP | Ligand DAMP | Reference |
|---|---|---|---|---|---|
| | | **Intracellular** | | | |
| TLR3 | Macrophages<br>Neutrophils<br>B lymphocytes<br>Dendritic cells | Double-stranded RNA | Viruses | Own double-stranded RNA | [57,58] |
| TLR7 | Macrophages<br>Neutrophils<br>Dendritic cells<br>Treg cells | Single-stranded RNA<br>Antiviral and anticancer compounds | Viruses<br>Synthetic | Own single-stranded RNA | [48,59] |
| TLR8 | Dendritic cells<br>Treg cells | Single-stranded RNA<br>Antiviral compounds | Viruses<br>Synthetic | Own single-stranded RNA | [48,60] |
| TLR9 | Macrophages<br>Neutrophils<br>Dendritic cells | Double-stranded DNA (containing unmethylated CpG sequences) | Bacteria, viruses and synthetic | HMGB1<br>Mitochondrial DNA | [48–50,61] |

## 4. The Role of TLRs in Glomerulonephritis

Tissue damage glomerulonephritis predisposes many factors and individual characteristics. Most often, the first reveals hereditary predispositions in response to emerging environmental factors that can lead to a nephrogenic immune response. Then, there is a direct exposure to infectious etiological factors occurring in the environment (PAMP and DAMP), which may be subject to specific modification due to many epigenetic factors (such as physical exercise, microbes, environmental toxins, lifestyle, etc.) [62]. As a consequence of these changes, the innate immune system is activated as a result of interaction with TLRs present on circulating inflammatory cells (neutrophils, macrophages, basophils, and NK cells), as well as on resident glomerular cells and the complement system, which triggers a cascade of antigen-specific non-specific reactions [63]. These receptors are displayed on cells found inside the glomerulus (mesangial cells, monocytes, or dendritic cells) as well as in the renal interstitium (tubular epithelial cells, monocytes), where they interfere with potential ligands [63]. Part of the ligands, such as peptides, structural elements, or genetic material of both bacteria and viruses can be transmitted through the bloodstream to the inside of the nephron, in particular to the glomerulus. In the case of interstitial cells, in addition to the ligands of infectious origin, the potential ligands may also be fibrinogen, fibronectin, defensin 2, or necrotic cells (Figure 3).

In order to prevent over-activity of the immune system, TLRs are downregulated by numerous molecules and various mechanisms. Existing negative regulators target specific key molecules in TLR signaling, such as SOCS1 (suppressor of cytokine signaling 1), SOCS3 (suppressor of cytokine signaling 3), SARM (sterile α-and armadillo-motif containing protein), TANK (TRAF family member associated NF-κB activator), A20, and others [64–69]. Additionally, there are molecules that directly influence the inhibition of NF-kB and IRF-3 [70]. In addition, numerous mi-RNAs were discovered that affect the stability of mRNA encoding signaling molecules and mRNA for cytokines [69,71].

Activation of TLR releases the NF-κB transcription factor, which results in the production of inflammatory mediators (such as IL-1, IL-2, IL-6, IL-12, TNF-α (tumor necrosis factor alpha)), [72,73], and can cause glomerular damage. The next step is the conversion of the innate immune response that begins the antigen-specific reaction cycle. The transformation of the immune response includes several possible mechanisms, such as regulation of natural autoimmunity, conformational changes of epitopes, molecular mimicry, or the autoantigen complementarity phenomenon. TLRs are also required to activate the adaptive immune system by antigen-presenting cells that promote CD4 helper cell differentiation, B cell activation, and antibody production. Antibodies lead to the trapping of the circulating complex or the formation of in situ immune complexes that can activate both TLRs and complement components of the innate immune system [74]. CD4 Th1 and Th2 cells cause damage to the glomerular tissues indirectly, mainly through macrophages and basophils, whereas Th17 cells may directly mediate damage to kidney structures in particular diseases (Figure 4).

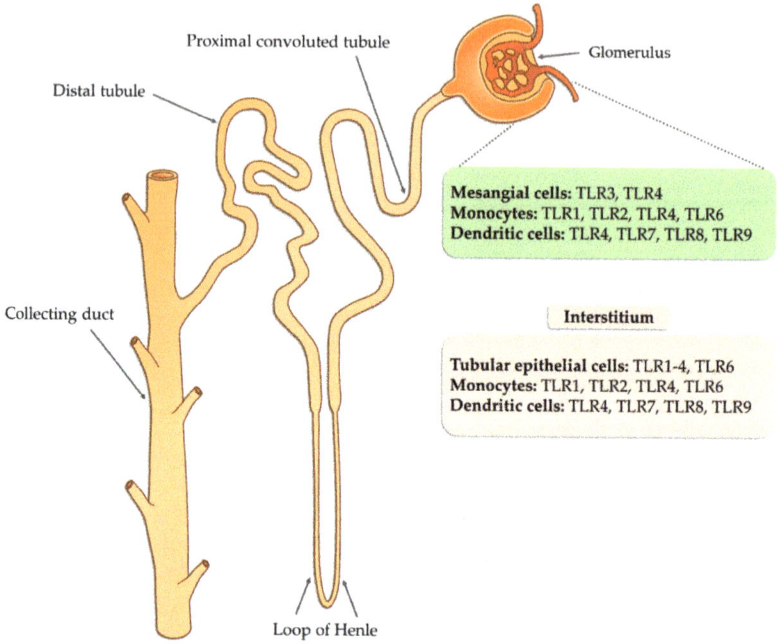


**Figure 3.** The potential occurrence of TLR receptors within the nephron (modified, based on [63]).

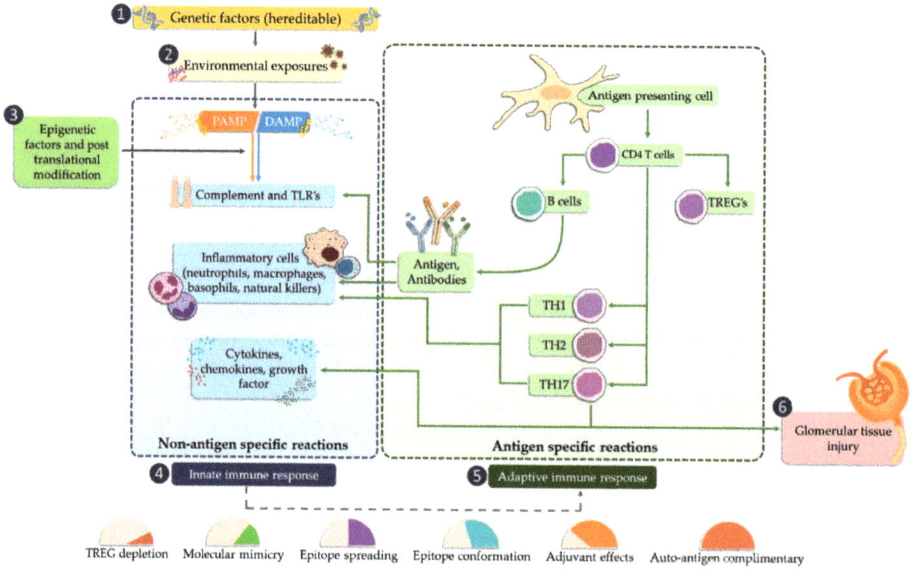


**Figure 4.** The potential occurrence of TLR receptors within the nephron (modified, based on [24]).

Various clinical situations affecting the kidneys, such as ischemic damage, toxic AKI, nephropathies secondary to diabetes mellitus, hypertension, or crystal deposition, are associated with aseptic inflammation caused, among others, by DAMP molecules [75,76]. These molecules can be released from dying parenchyma cells or during remodulation of the extracellular matrix. The presence of cells in the kidney capable of expressing TLR receptors makes it possible to initiate an immune response and inflammation [77,78]. In order to approximate the mode of action of these receptors in the disease state, their involvement in the most frequently diagnosed pathological conditions associated with glomerular dysfunction is presented in the further part of the material [8].

## 5. Biomarkers and Importance of the TLRs in Selected Glomerular Diseases

The literature classification divides the occurring nephropathies into two categories: Primary nephropathies, which are defined as those in which the systemic disease responsible for the condition cannot be established, and secondary nephropathies in which renal lesions appear as a result of other diseases accompanied by characteristic extrarenal symptoms. The first group includes diseases, such as: minimal change nephropathy (MCN), focal segmental glomerulosclerosis (FSGS), and membranous nephropathy (MN), which are also included in the nephrotic syndrome. The second group is primarily diabetic nephropathy and lupus nephropathy. In addition, the studies of our research group have resulted in the finding that the TLR-2 receptor may play an important role as a biomarker of primary non-proliferative nephropathies [79].

## 6. The Role of TLRs in Primary Non-Proliferative Nephropathies

### 6.1. *Focal Segmental Glomerulosclerosis (FSGS)*

FSGS is a diverse syndrome that arises after damage to podocytes for various reasons, some known and unknown. The sources of podocyte injury are diverse (circulating factors (primary FSGS), genetic abnormalities, viral infections, and medications) [80,81]. Most of the mutual interactions between these factors probably result in FSGS. There is a hypothesis about multistage pathogenic activation of autoimmunity in some forms of idiopathic FSGS [81]. Through the interaction of macrophages involved in kidney damage with many chemokines, the migration of monocytes to the site of damage occurs, which initiates the process of fibrosis. These macrophages also have the ability to self-spread and change into myofibroblasts that produce the extracellular matrix. Therefore, it can be assumed that excessive organ infiltration by monocytes and macrophages will cause an intensified fibrosis effect and, consequently, intensification of FSGS symptoms [82,83]. Currently, known biomarkers of FSGS are soluble urokinase-type plasminogen activator receptor (suPAR), soluble IL-2 receptor (sIL-2R), and ATP-binding cassette subfamily B member 1 glycoprotein-P (Figure 5). Damage to podocytes can release molecular patterns of proteins that are recognized by TLR as signals of danger. TLRs stimulate adapter proteins that activate a cascade of kinases, which amplify the signal and transmit it to the transcription factors regulating inflammatory genes. In the inflammatory microenvironment, the podocytes, acting as antigen-presenting cells, have a CD40 and CD80 receptor on their surface, thanks to which they capture antigens and present them to competent T-cells. However, in the case of abnormal expression of CD40 and CD80, they disorganize the cytoskeleton and filtration slit. In addition, CD40 can be identified as a foreign antigen, consequently leading to the production of anti-CD40 auto-antigen. Abnormal expression of CD40, CD80, and autoantibodies may lead to apoptosis of the podocytes, detachment of the podocytes from the glomerular basal membrane, proliferation of parietal epithelial cells, and attack on the glomeruli, and induction of segmental sclerosis [81]. In turn, other literature reports indicate the involvement of fibrinogen (Fg) in an inflammatory process mediated by the toll-like 4 receptor (TLR4) [84]. Fibrinogen is a protein that plays a proinflammatory role in vascular disorders, rheumatoid arthritis, glomerulonephritis, and certain cancers, e.g., myeloproliferative neoplasms [84,85]. Positive correlations have been noted between oxidative stress markers and, among others, fibrinogen, which may impact the course of several disorders [85]. Găman et al. [86] showed that obesity and diabetes are associated with increased levels of ROS (reactive oxygen species), accompanied by a simultaneous deficiency of antioxidants. The authors showed that the results of the free oxygen radical defense (FORT) and free oxygen radical defense (FORD) tests correlated with anthropometric/biochemical parameters in patients with obesity and diabetes. In studies carried out by Wang et al. [84], Fg has been shown to disrupt the actin cytoskeleton and induce apoptosis in podocytes via the TLR4-p38 MAPK-NF-κB p65 pathway in vitro and that co-expression of Fg and TLR4 is elevated in podocytes of Adriamycin-treated mice. It was also indicated that the level of fibrinogen in the urine may reflect the disease activity in patients with FSGS [84]. Literature data show that the use of synthetic small molecules lecinoxoids, which are inhibitors of TLR-2 and TLR-4, affects the activation and recruitment of monocytes in a rat model. The authors indicate [87] that the data demonstrate that targeting TLR-2-TLR-4 and/or monocyte migration directly affects the priming phase of fibrosis and may consequently perturb disease pathogenesis.

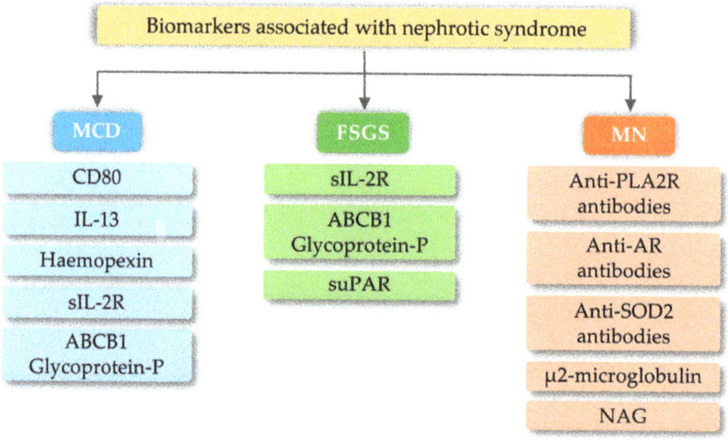


**Figure 5.** Biomarkers associated with nephrotic syndrome based on minimal change disease (MCD), focal segmental glomerulosclerosis (FSGS), and membranous nephropathy (MN) change based on [88]). CD80-Cluster of differentiation 80; IL-13-interleukin 13; sIL-2R-soluble IL-2 receptor; ABCB1 Glycoprotein-P-ATP-binding cassette subfamily B member 1 Glycoprotein-P; suPAR-soluble urokinase-type plasminogen activator receptor; PLA2R-M-type phospholipase A2 receptor; SOD2-manganese superoxide-dismutase 2; AR-Androgen Receptor; NAG-N-Acetyl-β-D Glucosaminidase.

### 6.2. *Minimal Change Disease (MCD)*

MCD is one of the most common glomerular kidney diseases in children and a common cause of nephrotic syndrome in adults. This disease entity is characterized by an outbreak of edema, selective proteinuria, and a clinical response to glucocorticoid therapy, as T-cell mechanisms are involved in the pathogenesis of the disease [89]. The pathogenesis is due to abnormalities in the functioning of podocytes, with the latest literature data suggesting the hypothesis that there are two initiating events. First, there are changes in the cytoskeleton of podocytes and, second, there are regulatory changes in T-cells that exacerbate abnormalities in podocytes [89,90]. Currently known biomarkers in MCD are urine levels and podocyte expression of CD80 (B7.1), interleukin 13, serum levels and protease activity of circulating hemopexin, serum levels of soluble interleukin 2 receptor, and ABCB1 and glycoprotein-P (Figure 5). The development of MCD may be significantly influenced by the body's innate immunity, in which TLRs are involved. Podocytes in the kidney glomeruli, due to their function and place of occurrence, are also equipped with the above receptors. In research conducted by Srivastava et al. [91], the presence of TLR receptors and their potential activity were checked on cell cultures stimulated with LPS (lipopolysaccharides) and the amino nucleoside puromycin (PAN). In the above studies, it was found that cultured human podocytes constitutively express TLR 1-6 and TLR-10 but not TLR 7–9.

Quantitative analysis using the RT-PCR method indicated that LPS at various concentrations and to varying degrees increased the expression of TLR (1–6) genes, the adapter molecule MyD88, and the transcription factor NF-κB within one hour. LPS also caused elevated levels of IL-6, IL-8, and MCP-1 (monocyte chemoattractant protein-1) without exerting any effect on TNF-α, IFN-α, or TGF-β1 after 24 h. It has also been shown that an increase in TLR 1 expression may attenuate the effect of TLR-4 activation, which is thought to be an indirect factor in LPS-induced podocyte damage [91]. Moreover, the increase in TLR-1 expression by LPS suggests that LPS damage to podocytes is associated with an increase in TLR-1 levels and its specific endogenous ligands (heat shock protein, heparin sulphate, and fibronectin). These results allow the conclusion that the main TLR4 ligand, which is LPS, can induce the expression of the genes of many TLR receptors, and thus may lead to changes being induced in podocytes, which may be related to the loss of receptor selectivity and stimulation of receptor interaction in podocytes [91]. An additional possibility indicating the involvement of TLRs in the development of MCD is the increase in the amount of the CD80 receptor in podocytes, after stimulation with ligands for TLR-and TLR-4 receptors. TLR ligands are usually microbial products and can be combined with a well-known association of viral infections as a causative agent of minimal lesion disease [92,93].

### *6.3. Membranous Nephropathy (MN)*

MN is a common cause of nephrotic syndrome in adults. Patients with MN usually develop severe proteinuria, edema, hypoalbuminemia, and hyperlipidemia [94]. It is the most common cause of idiopathic nephrotic syndrome in non-diabetic white adults. About 80% of cases are restricted to the kidneys (primary MN, PMN, idiopathic membranous nephropathy) and 20% are related to other systemic diseases or exposure (secondary MN) [95]. MN is associated with a pathological alteration of the glomerular basement membrane. This change is due to the build-up of immune complexes that appear as granular immunoglobulin (Ig)G deposits after immunofluorescence imaging and as electron-dense deposits of high electron density. Deposits of these immune complexes between podocytes and the basement membrane have a complex that attacks the complement membrane (C5b-9) [96]. The formation of glomerular sub-epithelial immune complex deposits in the IMN is mediated by specific intrinsic podocyte antigens and their corresponding autoantibodies in humans. These include compounds, such as neutral endopeptidase (NEP), type M receptor for secretory phospholipase A2 (PLA2R1), and type 1 7A thrombospondin (THSD7A) (containing domain 8–10) [94–96]. The above-mentioned markers constitute the core of the research into the pathogenesis of membranous nephropathy. However, there are reports of a genetic susceptibility to idiopathic membranous nephropathy. This type of study was conducted in a high-prevalence area in Taiwan [97]. In these studies, the association of the *IL-6, NPHS1 (nephrin), TLR-4, TLR-9, STAT4 (signal transducer and activator of transcription)* and *MYH (mutY DNA glycosylase)*, genes with susceptibility to primary membranous nephropathy in Taiwan was established. In the case of the TLR4 receptor gene, the gene polymorphism indicated a significant single nucleotide difference in the rs10983755 A/G region ($p < 0.001$) and rs1927914 A/G ($p < 0.05$) between the control group and MN patients. In addition, the distributions of rs10759932 C/T and rs11536889 C/T polymorphisms differed significantly [97].

### *6.4. IgA Nephropathy (IgAN)*

The development of IgA nephropathy consists of many mechanisms not yet fully understood. Literature data breaks down biomarkers for IgA nephropathy into a diagnostic and prognostic marker. The first group includes biomarkers detected in serum and urine, such as uromodulin, CD71, IL-6, complement components, and serum BAFF (B-cell activating factor) [98]. However, the group of prognostic markers includes urine kidney injury molecule-1, fractional excretion of IgG, soluble CD89, urinary angiotensinogen, and inflammatory cytokines (Figure 6). The above markers may indicate or predict the main cause of nephropathy development, which is the overproduction of anti-IgA complexes. One of the reasons for stimulating the body to produce IgA-related complexes may be signaling disorders associated with TLRs [99–101]. Ligands of bacterial or viral origin are recognized by toll-like receptors that trigger the process of chemokine release and recruitment of macrophages and neutrophils at the site of infection [102]. In numerous studies on IgAN pathogenesis, various types of receptors that could influence the development of this disease have been analyzed. These receptors were TLR3, mainly recognizing viral dsDNA [103]; TLR7 receptor [104]; binding to ssRNA viruses and TLR4 [105,106]; and binding of a variety of ligands, including LPS Gram-negative bacteria and DAMP (Table 2). Numerous observations of patients with diagnosed IgAN suggest the involvement of pathogens of viral origin, which is also confirmed by experimental models. There is an unexpected increase in the level of TLR4 activation, which is involved in the diagnosis of exogenous bacterial factors (LPS from Gram-negative bacteria, *Chlamydia pneumoniae*, HSP (heat shock proteins) proteins) and endogenous origin (HSP-60, additional fibronectin A domain, low-molecular LDL fractions, acid oligosaccharides hyaluronic acid, heparan sulphate), as well as factors derived from the breakdown of host cells [107–113]. To fully explain kidney damage in IgAN, it is necessary to fully understand the effects of TLR4 in the development of glomerulopathy, involving both glomerular cells and circulating leukocytes. Studies have shown that the administration of LPS activates TLR4 receptors on mesangial cells, and causes the release of chemokines (CXCs), which promotes neutrophil infusion and the development of glomerulonephritis [114–116]. In addition, the IFN-$\gamma$ and IFN-$\alpha$ responses induced by TLR activation induce overexpression of the B-cell activation factor (BAFF) in dendritic cells, favoring the expansion of B-cells and increasing IgA synthesis [117–121]. It was also shown that in kidney biopsies of patients with IgAN, CD19+/CD5+ B cell infiltration is present, which in the progressive forms of this disease produce significant amounts of IFN-$\gamma$ and IgA and are more resistant to apoptosis compared to cells obtained from healthy donors [122,123]. Moreover, Hitoshi Suzuki et al. [101] showed that there is an association between gene polymorphisms for TLR-9 and disease progression. Stimulation with ligands for TLR-9 led to the deterioration of kidney function in mice and influenced the shift of the balance towards Th1 lymphocytes. These findings led to the conclusion that activation of pathways related to this particular type of receptor may influence the severity of IgA nephropathy [101]. Moreover, Coppo et al. [124] showed that in patients diagnosed with IgA nephropathy, higher levels of TLR-4 in mononuclear cells and transcriptional mRNA were observed than in the control group. An important fact is that there is a statistical difference in the level of the above markers in patients with severe disease and those who do not have proteinuria and hematuria [124]. TLR-4 can be activated by many ligands, such as HLPs and LPS and DAMPs [106].

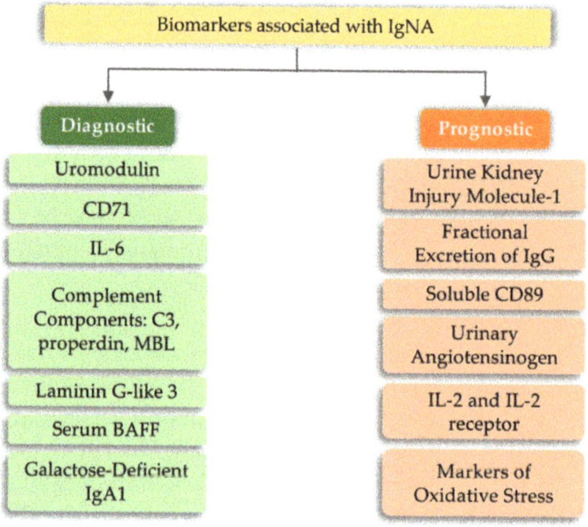


**Figure 6.** Biomarkers in IgA (immunoglobulin A) nephropathy.

## 7. The Role of TLR Receptors in Secondary Nephropathies

### 7.1. Lupus Nephritis

Systemic lupus erythematosus (SLE) is one example of systemic autoimmune diseases. SLE relies on the loss of tolerance to autoantigens, which is caused by the malfunctioning of acquired immunity cells [109,125–127]. In the case of SLE, clinical studies indicate that the most common source of biomarker searches is a urine sample. Due to this, numerous proteins, such as cytokines, chemokines, complement proteins, adhesive molecules, and autoantibodies, have been identified as potential biomarkers of disease activity in cross-sectional studies (Figure 7) [128].

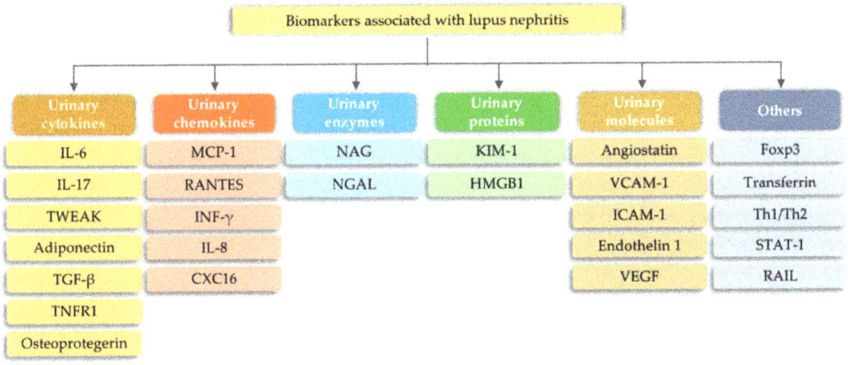


**Figure 7.** Biomarkers associated with lupus nephritis [128]; CXC16—C-X-C motif chemokine 16; FOXP3—forkhead box protein P3; HMGB1—High mobility group box 1; ICAM—Intercellular Adhesion Molecule 1; IL-6—Urinary Interleukin 6; IL-8—Interleukin 8; IL-17—Urinary Interleukin 17; KIM-1—Urinary kidney injury molecule-1; MCP-1—Monocyte chemoattractant protein-1; NAG—N-Acetyl-β-D Glucosaminidase; NGAL—neutrophil gelatinase-associated lipocalin; RAIL—Renal Activity Index for Lupus; RANTES—Regulated upon Activation, Normal T-cell Expressed, and Secreted; STAT-1—Signal transducer and activator of transcription 1; TGF-β—transforming growth factor beta; Th1—T helper 1; Th2—T helper 2; TNFR1—Tumor necrosis factor receptor 1; TWEAK—Urinary TNF-like weak inducer of apoptosis; VCAM—vascular cell adhesion molecule 1; VEGF—Vascular Endothelial Growth Factor.

Literature data of recent years indicate a special contribution to the etiopathogenesis of this disease of innate immunity elements, mainly TLR. External and endogenous ligands may interact with TLRs present on monocytes, dendritic cells, and B lymphocytes, infiltrating the glomeruli, and resulting in increased cytokine secretion [129,130]. In addition, mesangial cells and other cells of the parenchyma express TLR1-4 and TLR6 receptors and secrete interleukins and chemokines [15,129,131–134]. Studies show that most deposits of immune complexes contain TLR agonists that have the ability to activate mesangial cells and contribute to the development of lupus nephropathy [135]. Pawar et al. [136] summarized the literature data, indicating that microbial nucleic acids can constitute a universal PAMP. As a result, it is possible to activate various mechanisms, such as lymphoproliferation, production of autoantibodies, type I interferon, secretion of numerous cytokines, and promotion of lupus development, in genetically predisposed individuals [136].

TLR2 and TLR4 are expressed not only in parenchymal cells but also in infiltrating neutrophils and mononuclear phagocytes, including macrophages and dendritic cells [137]. The HMGB1 (high mobility group box 1) protein, which binds DNA and the lupus autoantigen released under inflammation, can induce the activation of NF-κB in a TLR2-dependent and TLR4-RAGE-dependent manner in mononuclear phagocytes and neutrophils [138–143] as well as in mesangial cells [144]. Mesangial cells and podocytes in humans are characterized by the expression of TLR4 [145]. Mesangial cells isolated from mice with autoimmune diseases have significantly higher TLR4 expression and produce much more proinflammatory chemokines both after LPS stimulation and spontaneously [146]. Other studies also indicate that the necrotic cell debris-enhanced endogenous TLR ligands stimulate cytokine release by TLR2/MyD88 from mesangial cells, which implies the expression of TLR2 in different cell populations, and kidney-building structure [147–150]. Intracellular expression of TLR2 and TLR4 is multiplied in the kidneys of CD32b receptor-deficient mice suffering from glomerulonephritis associated with cryoglobulinemia [145,151,152].

### 7.2. *Diabetic Nephropathy (DN)*

One of the most serious complications for patients diagnosed with type I or II diabetes is diabetic nephropathy, which can be caused by both environmental and genetic factors [18,153]. The diabetic nephropathy is important to the inflammatory process in which, besides an increase in the activity of macrophages and overproduction of adhesion molecules of leukocyte cells, the proximal tubular kidney releases cytokine chemoattractant protein matrix to the interstitium, thereby contributing to the development of the disease [154–156]. Literature studies indicate that the greatest risk of diabetic nephropathy is the occurrence of hyperglycemia, which disrupts the proper functioning of the human body. On the molecular level, hyperglycemia is responsible for promoting the mitochondrial electron transport chain, which causes the formation of excessive amounts of reactive oxygen species (ROS) (through formation of the advanced glycation end products (AGEs) and activation of the polyol pathway, hexosamine pathway, protein kinase C (PKC), and angiotensin II). ROS occurring in the cell initiate or also intensify the formation of oxidative stress, which causes the intensification of inflammation and formation of fibrosis. Abnormalities in the lipid metabolism pathway, activation of the renin-angiotensin-aldosterone system (RAAS), as well as systemic and glomerular hypertension are also involved in the progression of this disease. Impairment of insulin signaling, an increase in growth factors and proinflammatory cytokines, and activation of the intracellular signaling pathway also play a role in the development of this disease [157]. Therefore, the currently known DN biomarkers focus on three areas: Detection of oxidative stress, the occurrence of inflammation, and activation of the RAAS system (Figure 8).

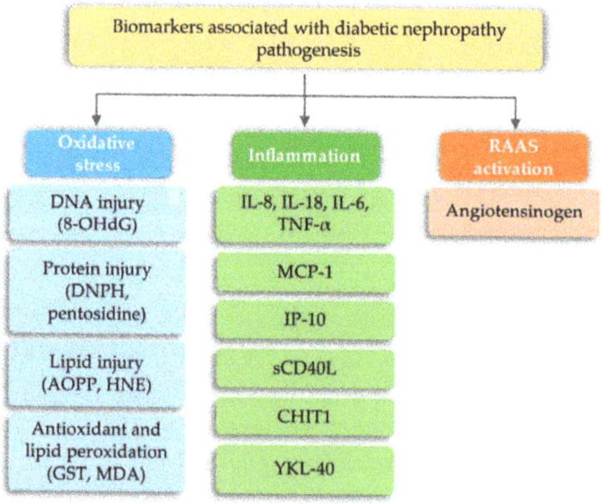


**Figure 8.** Biomarkers associated with diabetic nephropathy pathogenesis (based on [157]). 8-OHdG—8-hydroxy-2′-deoxyguanine; AOPP—advanced oxidation protein product; CHIT1—chitotriosidase; DNPH—2,4-dinitrophenylhydrazine; GS—Glutathione s-transferase; HNE—4-hydroxy-nonenal; IL-6—interleukin 6; IL-8—interleukin 8; IL-18—interleukin 18; IP-10—interferon-inducible protein-10; MCP-1—Monocyte chemoattractant protein-1; MDA—malondialdehyde; sCD40L—soluble CD40 ligand; TNF-α—Tumor necrosis factor alpha; YKL-40—cartilage glycoprotein 40.

Literature data from recent years indicate that an important role in diabetic nephropathy etiopathogenesis may be played by signal transduction pathways that are dependent on TLR2, TLR9, and TLR4 receptors. However, it is not clear which receptor is more pathogenic [154,158–160]. Studies of many research teams indicate increased expression of TLR2 and the presence of endogenous ligands HMGB1 [161,162] and HSP70 [107,122,163], detected on the basis of research conducted on diabetic-induced rats. In addition, the expression of MyD88 and MCP-1, NF-κB, and infiltration of macrophages has been demonstrated [164–167]. High TLR2 expression was also observed in the glomeruli and renal tubules of people with diabetes. The results were confirmed in vitro in cultures of NRK-52E cell lines in which a high glucose concentration induced TLR2 mRNA expression [168–170]. The pathogenic role of TLR4 in diabetic nephropathy has also been found. In vitro studies have shown that activation of NF-κB and the expression of proinflammatory cytokines was reduced when TLR4 expression was silenced or its signaling was inhibited. During mouse studies, higher TLR4 activity and expression of the NF-κB p65 subunit in the kidney cortex of mice with experimental diabetes was demonstrated [171]. In vitro, researchers also observed increased TLR4 expression and proinflammatory cytokine synthesis when podocytes and adipocytes were exposed to both high glucose and NEFA (non-esterified "free" fatty acids), suggesting a key role of TLR4 in supporting inflammation in diabetic nephropathy [171–173]. In addition, another research team [174] showed an increase in the expression of TLR4 and signaling proteins for this receptor along with the activation of NF-κB, but not TLR2, in a mouse mesangium that was exposed to high glucose concentrations. It was also observed that hyperglycemia stimulated the expression of TLR4 in glomerular renal endothelial cells in a mouse model of type 1 and type 2 diabetes, which underlines the relationship of the discussed receptor with diabetic nephropathy [174,175]. In addition, clinical data indicate that in patients with type 1 diabetes, ligands, endotoxins, heat shock proteins 60 (Hsp60), and high mobility groups 1 (HMGB1) of both TLR2 and TLR4 [176,177] are increased. Increased expression of mRNA was also observed. TLR2, MyD88, and proinflammatory cytokines in leukocytes of patients with type 1 diabetes mellitus suggests that the inflammatory process is mediated by TLR2 [176]. However, in patients with type 2 diabetes and confirmed biopsy, diabetic kidney disease has been found to increase TLR4 expression on renal tubules as opposed to TLR2. In addition, in patients with type II diabetes and confirmed diabetic kidney disease, microalbuminuria, mRNA, and TLR4 protein were overexpressed 4 to 10 times more in glomeruli and tubules compared to the control group. However, both TLR2 and TLR4 expression was increased on monocytes in patients with type II diabetes [176]. Although the literature data indicate a key role of TLR2 and TLR4 in the pathophysiology of diabetic nephropathy, the participation of other receptors is not excluded. There is evidence to suggest the involvement of TLR3, TLR7, and TLR9 receptors in the pathogenesis of type 1 diabetes by destroying pancreatic islets induced by viral infection [114,178,179].

### *7.3. Acute Kidney Injury (AKI) to Chronic Kidney Disease (CKD) Development*

The 2019 definition published by Ronco in The Lancet says that AKI: "is defined by a rapid increase in serum creatinine, decrease in urine output, or both". The authors indicate that acute kidney injury accounts for up to 15% of the reasons for admission to hospital and occurs in as much as 50% of patients treated in intensive care units [180]. Therefore, it is argued that AKI is still associated with high morbidity and mortality [181]. There are many causes of AKI, including acute ischemia, analgesic nephropathy, sepsis, and severe glomerulopathies. Meta-analyses and cohort studies confirm the role of acute kidney injury in the development of chronic kidney disease and, as a complication of AKI, the more frequent need for chronic renal replacement therapy in the form of dialysis therapy [182–184]. The literature does not indicate clear causes and markers of the transition of acute kidney injury to chronic kidney disease, although it is known that this process involves numerous immune mechanisms. Inflammation, induced death, and fibrosis are likely contributors to the progression of AKI to CKD [185]. The renal epithelium plays an important role in promoting inflammation after damage by attracting leukocytes to the site of damage, which is seen as a strong role for TLR-4 [186]. The role of TLR2 and TLR4 in reperfusion after ischemic kidney injury is significant, where their expression increases significantly and enhances the proinflammatory response of tissues, with the participation of numerous cytokines and chemokines [187,188]. It is also noteworthy that the TLR-3 receptor system is involved in ischemia/reperfusion injury in the kidney. Studies have been carried out that showed rapid activation of these receptors, resulting in significant kidney damage, which was associated with elevated rates of apoptosis and necrosis in the renal tubes of mice [189]. Both TLR2 and TLR4 are also involved in sepsis-induced kidney damage [190], caused by Gram-positive and G-negative bacteria; nevertheless, the roles of single TLRs are differing [191]. There is also the TLR4-IL-22 pathway, which probably has regenerative functions in opposition to the above, and more research is needed on this topic [192]. After the action of a harmful factor, the repair process takes place, the element of which is sterile ignition [193]. In the first stage of inflammation, neutrophilic exudate appears, which over time is replaced by a monocytic-lymphocytic infiltrate [194,195]. The presence of monocytes is regarded as a mechanism promoting fibrosis and fibroblast proliferation [196]. The influx of cells of the immune system leads to cell apoptosis and the formation of a large amount of breakdown products and other substances that act as DAMPs, which can activate receptors, including TLRs [78,197]. It then promotes and strengthens the inflammatory response, attracting more cells of the immune system and subsequent fibrosis. Kidney infiltration by monocytes is recognized as a feature of chronic kidney disease [198] and the degree of monocyte infiltration correlates with the severity of kidney damage [199]. The above data indicate that it is the intensified process of fibrosis, mediated largely by the elements of the immune system, that can lead to permanent damage to the kidney function and the progression of AKI to CKD.

## 8. Conclusions

The innate immunity system in which TLRs participate, among others, cells, such as monocytes, macrophages, and NK (natural killer) cells, expressing TLR and lectin receptors are the body's first line of defense. TLRs identify the pathogen based on the specific pattern of the molecule and therefore stimulate the immune system acquired, including T and B lymphocytes to fight pathogens [15]. Long-term continuous antigenic stimulation, increasing the work of TLRs, can lead to the development of serious diseases, organ specific or systemic. In an increasing number of studies, the role of TLRs has become more important. Recognition receptors are certainly of importance in the pathogenesis of diseases associated with nephropathy, for example, glomerulopathy, diabetic, lupus IgA, or FSGS [1,16]. However, further research is necessary to clarify the possible involvement of TLR in the development of other disease entities associated with kidney damage.

**Author Contributions:** S.M., P.L., E.G., W.Z.; conceptualization, S.M., P.L., D.B., I.M., P.N.-R., E.G., R.H.; writing—original draft preparation; S.M., P.L., D.B., I.M., P.N.-R., E.G., R.H., W.Z., J.R.; writing—review and editing. All authors have read and agreed to the published version of the manuscript.

**Funding:** This work was supported by Research Grant No. UMO-2016/23/B/NZ6/02844 of the Polish National Science Centre (NCN) and Research Grant No. DS460 of the Medical University of Lublin.

**Conflicts of Interest:** The authors declare no conflict of interest. The funders had no role in the design of the study; in the collection, analyses, or interpretation of data; in the writing of the manuscript, or in the decision to publish the results.

## Abbreviations

| | |
|---|---|
| 8-OHdG | 8-hydroxy-2′-deoxyguanine |
| ABCB1 Glycoprotein-P | ATP-binding cassette subfamily B member 1 Glycoprotein-P |
| AKI | Acute kidney injury |
| AOPP | Advanced oxidation protein product |
| AR | Androgen Receptor |
| BAFF | B-cell activation factor |
| CD80 | Cluster of differentiation 80 |
| CHIT1 | Chitotriosidase; DNPH-2,4-dinitrophenylhydrazine |
| CKD | Chronic kidney disease |

| | |
|---|---|
| CXC16 | C-X-C motif chemokine 16 |
| DAMP | Damage-associated molecular patterns |
| DN | Diabetic nephropathy |
| FOXP3 | Forkhead box protein P3 |
| FSGS | Focal segmental glomerulosclerosis |
| GST | Glutathione s-transferase |
| HMGB1 | High mobility group box 1 |
| HNE | 4-hydroxy-nonenal |
| HSP70 | Heat shock proteins 70 |
| ICAM | Intercellular Adhesion Molecule 1 |
| IFN-α | Interferon alpha |
| IFN-γ | Interferon gamma |
| IgAN | IgA nephropathy |
| IL-17 | Interleukin 13 |
| IL-13 | Interleukin 13 |
| IL-2 | Interleukin 2 |
| IL-6 | Interleukin 6 |
| IL-7 | Interleukin 7 |
| IL-8 | Interleukin 8 |
| IP-10 | Interferon-inducible protein-10 |
| KIM-1 | Urinary kidney injury molecule-1 |
| LPS | Lipopolysaccharides |
| LRRs | Leucine-rich tandem repeats |
| MCN | Minimal change nephropathy |
| MCP-1 | Monocyte chemoattractant protein-1 |
| MDA | Malondialdehyde |
| MN | Membranous nephropathy |
| NAG | N-Acetyl-β-D Glucosaminidase |
| NAG | N-Acetyl-β-D Glucosaminidase |
| NF-κB | Nuclear factor kappa-light-chain-enhancer of activated B cells |
| NGAL | Neutrophil gelatinase-associated lipocalin |
| NK cells | Natural killer cells |
| PAMP | Pathogen-associated molecular patterns |
| PKC | Protein kinase C |
| PLA2R | M-type phospholipase A2 receptor |
| PRRs | Pattern recognition receptors |
| RAAS | Renin-angiotensin-aldosterone system |
| RAIL | Renal Activity Index for Lupus |
| RANTES | Regulated upon Activation, Normal T cell Expressed, and Secreted |
| ROS | Reactive oxygen species |
| sCD40L | Soluble CD40 ligand |
| sIL-2R | Soluble IL-2 receptor |
| SLE | Systemic lupus erythematosus |
| SOD2 | manganese superoxide-dismutase 2 |
| STAT-1 | Signal transducer and activator of transcription 1 |
| suPAR | Soluble urokinase-type plasminogen activator receptor |
| TGF-β1 | Transforming growth factor beta 1 |
| TLR | Toll-like receptor |
| TNF-a | Tumor necrosis factor alpha |
| TNFR1 | Tumor necrosis factor receptor 1 |
| TWEAK | Urinary TNF-like weak inducer of apoptosis |
| VCAM | Vascular cell adhesion molecule 1 |
| VEGF | Vascular Endothelial Growth Factor |
| YKL-40 | Cartilage glycoprotein 40 |

## References


1. World Health Organization; International Programme on Chemical Safety. *Biomarkers in Risk Assessment: Validity and Validation*; World Health Organization: Geneva, Switzerland, 2001; ISBN 978-92-4-157222-4.
2. Fuentes-Arderiu, X. What is a biomarker? It's time for a renewed definition. *Clin. Chem. Lab. Med.* **2013**, *51*, 1689–1690. [CrossRef] [PubMed]
3. Goerlich, N.; Brand, H.A.; Langhans, V.; Tesch, S.; Schachtner, T.; Koch, B.; Paliege, A.; Schneider, W.; Grützkau, A.; Reinke, P.; et al. Kidney transplant monitoring by urinary flow cytometry: Biomarker combination of T cells, renal tubular epithelial cells, and podocalyxin-positive cells detects rejection. *Sci. Rep.* **2020**, *10*, 796. [CrossRef] [PubMed]
4. Kasurinen, A.; Hagström, J.; Laitinen, A.; Kokkola, A.; Böckelman, C.; Haglund, C. Evaluation of toll-like receptors as prognostic biomarkers in gastric cancer: High tissue TLR5 predicts a better outcome. *Sci. Rep.* **2019**, *9*, 12553. [CrossRef] [PubMed]
5. Darrabie, M.D.; Cheeseman, J.; Limkakeng, A.T.; Borawski, J.; Sullenger, B.A.; Elster, E.A.; Kirk, A.D.; Lee, J. Toll-like receptor activation as a biomarker in traumatically injured patients. *J. Surg. Res.* **2018**, *231*, 270–277. [CrossRef]
6. Webster, A.C.; Nagler, E.V.; Morton, R.L.; Masson, P. Chronic Kidney Disease. *Lancet* **2017**, *389*, 1238–1252. [CrossRef]
7. Dobrică, E.-C.; Găman, M.-A.; Cozma, M.-A.; Bratu, O.G.; Pantea Stoian, A.; Diaconu, C.C. Polypharmacy in Type 2 Diabetes Mellitus: Insights from an Internal Medicine Department. *Medicina* **2019**, *55*, 436. [CrossRef]
8. O'Shaughnessy, M.M.; Hogan, S.L.; Thompson, B.D.; Coppo, R.; Fogo, A.B.; Jennette, J.C. Glomerular disease frequencies by race, sex and region: Results from the International Kidney Biopsy Survey. *Nephrol. Dial. Transplant.* **2018**, *33*, 661–669. [CrossRef]
9. Naylor, S. Biomarkers: Current perspectives and future prospects. *Expert Rev. Mol. Diagn.* **2003**, *3*, 525–529. [CrossRef]
10. Sahu, P.; Pinkalwar, N.; Dubey, R.D.; Paroha, S.; Chatterjee, S.; Chatterjee, T. Biomarkers: An Emerging Tool for Diagnosis of a Disease and Drug Development. *Asian J. Res. Pharm. Sci.* **2011**, *1*, 9–16.
11. Drucker, E.; Krapfenbauer, K. Pitfalls and limitations in translation from biomarker discovery to clinical utility in predictive and personalised medicine. *EPMA J.* **2013**, *4*, 7. [CrossRef]
12. Mayeux, R. Biomarkers: Potential Uses and Limitations. *NeuroRx* **2004**, *1*, 182–188. [CrossRef] [PubMed]
13. FDA. About Biomarkers and Qualification. Available online: https://www.fda.gov/drugs/cder-biomarker-qualification-program/about-biomarkers-and-qualification (accessed on 10 August 2020).
14. Levin, A.; Tonelli, M.; Bonventre, J.; Coresh, J.; Donner, J.-A.; Fogo, A.B.; Fox, C.S.; Gansevoort, R.T.; Heerspink, H.J.L.; Jardine, M.; et al. Global kidney health 2017 and beyond: A roadmap for closing gaps in care, research, and policy. *Lancet* **2017**, *390*, 1888–1917. [CrossRef]
15. Devarapu, S.K.; Anders, H. Toll-like receptors in lupus nephritis. *J. Biomed. Sci.* **2018**, *25*, 35. [CrossRef]
16. Luyckx, V.A.; Tonelli, M.; Stanifer, J.W. The global burden of kidney disease and the sustainable development goals. *Bull. World Health Organ.* **2018**, *96*, 414–422D. [CrossRef] [PubMed]
17. Yeo, S.C.; Cheung, C.K.; Barratt, J. New insights into the pathogenesis of IgA nephropathy. *Pediatr. Nephrol.* **2018**, *33*, 763–777. [CrossRef] [PubMed]
18. Zheng, Z.; Zheng, F. Immune Cells and Inflammation in Diabetic Nephropathy. *J. Diabetes Res.* **2016**, *2016*, 1841690. [CrossRef]
19. Mohammad Hosseini, A.; Majidi, J.; Baradaran, B.; Yousefi, M. Toll-Like Receptors in the Pathogenesis of Autoimmune Diseases. *Adv. Pharm. Bull.* **2015**, *5*, 605–614. [CrossRef] [PubMed]
20. Imig, J.D.; Ryan, M.J. Immune and Inflammatory Role in Renal Disease. *Compr. Physiol.* **2013**, *3*, 957–976. [CrossRef]
21. Berger, S.P.; Daha, M.R. Complement in glomerular injury. *Semin. Immunopathol.* **2007**, *29*, 375–384. [CrossRef]
22. Kawasaki, T.; Kawai, T. Toll-Like Receptor Signaling Pathways. *Front. Immunol.* **2014**, *5*, 461. [CrossRef]
23. Eleftheriadis, T.; Lawson, B.R. Toll-like receptors and kidney diseases. *Inflamm. Allergy Drug Targets* **2009**, *8*, 191–201. [CrossRef] [PubMed]
24. Liu, Y.; Xue, G.; Li, S.; Fu, Y.; Yin, J.; Zhang, R.; Li, J. Effect of Intermittent and Mild Cold Stimulation on the Immune Function of Bursa in Broilers. *Animals* **2020**, *10*, 1275. [CrossRef] [PubMed]

25. Botos, I.; Segal, D.M.; Davies, D.R. The Structural Biology of Toll-Like Receptors. *Structure* **2011**, *19*, 447–459. [CrossRef] [PubMed]
26. UniProt. Toll-Like Receptor 1. Available online: https://www.uniprot.org/uniprot/Q15399 (accessed on 10 August 2020).
27. Protein Data Bank in Europe. Crystal Structure of the TLR1-TLR2 Heterodimer Induced by Binding of a tri-Acylatedlipopeptide. Available online: https://www.ebi.ac.uk/pdbe/entry/pdb/2z7x (accessed on 10 August 2020).
28. UniProt. Toll-Like Receptor 2. Available online: https://www.uniprot.org/uniprot/O60603 (accessed on 10 August 2020).
29. Protein Data Bank in Europe. Crystal Structure of TLR2-TLR6-Pam2CSK4 Complex. Available online: https://www.ebi.ac.uk/pdbe/entry/pdb/3a79 (accessed on 10 August 2020).
30. UniProt. Toll-Like Receptor 3. Available online: https://www.uniprot.org/uniprot/O15455 (accessed on 10 August 2020).
31. Protein Data Bank in Europe. Crystal Structure of the Complex of TLR3 and bi-Specific Diabody. Available online: https://www.ebi.ac.uk/pdbe/entry/pdb/5gs0 (accessed on 10 August 2020).
32. UniProt. Toll-Like Receptor 4. Available online: https://www.uniprot.org/uniprot/O00206 (accessed on 10 August 2020).
33. Protein Data Bank in Europe. The Crystal Structure of Mouse TLR4/MD-2/neoseptin-3. Available online: https://www.ebi.ac.uk/pdbe/entry/pdb/5ijc (accessed on 10 August 2020).
34. UniProt. Toll-Like Receptor 5. Available online: https://www.uniprot.org/uniprot/O60602 (accessed on 10 August 2020).
35. Protein Data Bank in Europe. Homology Model of Human Toll-Like Receptor 5 Fitted into an Electron Microscopy Single Particle Reconstruction. Available online: https://www.ebi.ac.uk/pdbe/entry/pdb/3j0a (accessed on 10 August 2020).
36. UniProt. Toll-Like Receptor 6. Available online: https://www.uniprot.org/uniprot/Q9Y2C9 (accessed on 10 August 2020).
37. Protein Data Bank in Europe. Crystal Structure of TIR Domain TLR6. Available online: https://www.ebi.ac.uk/pdbe/entry/pdb/4om7 (accessed on 10 August 2020).
38. UniProt. Toll-Like Receptor 7. Available online: https://www.uniprot.org/uniprot/Q9NYK1 (accessed on 10 August 2020).
39. UniProt. Toll-Like Receptor 8. Available online: https://www.uniprot.org/uniprot/Q9NR97 (accessed on 10 August 2020).
40. Protein Data Bank in Europe. Crystal Structure of Human TLR8 in Complex with XG-1-236. Available online: https://www.ebi.ac.uk/pdbe/entry/pdb/4qc0 (accessed on 10 August 2020).
41. UniProt. Toll-Like Receptor 9. Available online: https://www.uniprot.org/uniprot/Q9NR96 (accessed on 10 August 2020).
42. UniProt. Toll-Like Receptor 10. Available online: https://www.uniprot.org/uniprot/Q9BXR5 (accessed on 10 August 2020).
43. Protein Data Bank in Europe. The TIR Domain of Human Toll-Like Receptor 10 (TLR10). Available online: https://www.ebi.ac.uk/pdbe/entry/pdb/2j67 (accessed on 10 August 2020).
44. UniProt. Toll-Like Receptor 11. Available online: https://www.uniprot.org/uniprot/Q6R5P0 (accessed on 10 August 2020).
45. UniProt. Toll-Like Receptor 12. Available online: https://www.uniprot.org/uniprot/Q6QNU9 (accessed on 10 August 2020).
46. UniProt. Toll-Like Receptor 13. Available online: https://www.uniprot.org/uniprot/Q6R5N8 (accessed on 10 August 2020).
47. Farhat, K.; Riekenberg, S.; Heine, H.; Debarry, J.; Lang, R.; Mages, J.; Buwitt-Beckmann, U.; Röschmann, K.; Jung, G.; Wiesmüller, K.-H.; et al. Heterodimerization of TLR2 with TLR1 or TLR6 expands the ligand spectrum but does not lead to differential signaling. *J. Leukoc. Biol.* **2008**, *83*, 692–701. [CrossRef] [PubMed]
48. Zhao, S.; Zhang, Y.; Zhang, Q.; Wang, F.; Zhang, D. Toll-like receptors and prostate cancer. *Front. Immunol.* **2014**, *5*, 352. [CrossRef]
49. Goulopoulou, S.; McCarthy, C.G.; Clinton Webb, R. Toll-like receptors in the vascular system: Sensing the dangers within. *Pharmacol. Rev.* **2016**, *68*, 142–167. [CrossRef]

50. Schaefer, L. Complexity of danger: The diverse nature of damage-associated molecular patterns. *J. Biol. Chem.* **2014**, *289*, 35237–35245. [CrossRef]
51. Brubaker, S.W.; Bonham, K.S.; Zanoni, I.; Kagan, J.C. Innate immune pattern recognition: A cell biological perspective. *Annu. Rev. Immunol.* **2015**, *33*, 257–290. [CrossRef]
52. Miao, E.A.; Andersen-Nissen, E.; Warren, S.E.; Aderem, A. TLR5 and Ipaf: Dual sensors of bacterial flagellin in the innate immune system. *Semin. Immunopathol.* **2007**, *29*, 275–288. [CrossRef]
53. Takeuchi, O.; Kawai, T.; Sanjo, H.; Copeland, N.G.; Gilbert, D.J.; Jenkins, N.A.; Takeda, K.; Akira, S. TLR6: A novel member of an expanding Toll-like receptor family. *Gene* **1999**, *231*, 59–65. [CrossRef]
54. Oosting, M.; Cheng, S.C.; Bolscher, J.M.; Vestering-Stenger, R.; Plantinga, T.S.; Verschueren, I.C.; Arts, P.; Garritsen, A.; van Eenennaam, H.; Sturm, P.; et al. Human TLR10 is an anti-inflammatory pattern-recognition receptor. *Proc. Natl. Acad. Sci. USA* **2014**, *111*, E4478–E4484. [CrossRef] [PubMed]
55. Raetz, M.; Kibardin, A.; Sturge, C.R.; Pifer, R.; Li, H.; Burstein, E.; Ozato, K.; Larin, S.; Yarovinsky, F. Cooperation of TLR12 and TLR11 in the IRF8-Dependent IL-12 Response to Toxoplasma gondii Profilin. *J. Immunol.* **2013**, *191*, 4818–4827. [CrossRef] [PubMed]
56. Yarovinsky, F.; Zhang, D.; Andersen, J.F.; Bannenberg, G.L.; Serhan, C.N.; Hayden, M.S.; Hieny, S.; Sutterwala, F.S.; Flavell, R.A.; Ghosh, S.; et al. Immunology: TLR11 activation of dendritic cells by a protozoan profilin-like protein. *Science* **2005**, *308*, 1626–1629. [CrossRef] [PubMed]
57. Xiao, X.; Zhao, P.; Rodriguez-Pinto, D.; Qi, D.; Henegariu, O.; Alexopoulou, L.; Flavell, R.A.; Wong, F.S.; Wen, L. Inflammatory Regulation by TLR3 in Acute Hepatitis. *J. Immunol.* **2009**, *183*, 3712–3719. [CrossRef] [PubMed]
58. Negishi, H.; Osawa, T.; Ogami, K.; Ouyang, X.; Sakaguchi, S.; Koshiba, R.; Yanai, H.; Seko, Y.; Shitara, H.; Bishop, K.; et al. A critical link between Toll-like receptor 3 and type II interferon signaling pathways in antiviral innate immunity. *Proc. Natl. Acad. Sci. USA* **2008**, *105*, 20446–20451. [CrossRef]
59. Hemmi, H.; Kaisho, T.; Takeuchi, O.; Sato, S.; Sanjo, H.; Hoshino, K.; Horiuchi, T.; Tomizawa, H.; Takeda, K.; Akira, S. Small-antiviral compounds activate immune cells via the TLR7 MyD88-dependent signaling pathway. *Nat. Immunol.* **2002**, *3*, 196–200. [CrossRef] [PubMed]
60. Peng, G.; Guo, Z.; Kiniwa, Y.; Voo, K.S.; Peng, W.; Fu, T.; Wang, D.Y.; Li, Y.; Wang, H.Y.; Wang, R.F. Immunology: Toll-like receptor 8-mediated reversal of CD4+ regulatory T cell function. *Science* **2005**, *309*, 1380–1384. [CrossRef]
61. Notley, C.A.; Jordan, C.K.; McGovern, J.L.; Brown, M.A.; Ehrenstein, M.R. DNA methylation governs the dynamic regulation of inflammation by apoptotic cells during efferocytosis. *Sci. Rep.* **2017**, *7*, 1–10. [CrossRef]
62. Kanherkar, R.R.; Bhatia-Dey, N.; Csoka, A.B. Epigenetics across the human lifespan. *Front. Cell Dev. Biol.* **2014**, *2*, 49. [CrossRef]
63. Anders, H.-J.; Banas, B.; Schlöndorff, D. Signaling Danger: Toll-Like Receptors and their Potential Roles in Kidney Disease. *J. Am. Soc. Nephrol.* **2004**, *15*, 854–867. [CrossRef]
64. Verstak, B.; Stack, J.; Ve, T.; Mangan, M.; Hjerrild, K.; Jeon, J.; Stahl, R.; Latz, E.; Gay, N.; Kobe, B.; et al. The TLR signaling adaptor TRAM interacts with TRAF6 to mediate activation of the inflammatory response by TLR4. *J. Leukoc. Biol.* **2014**, *96*, 427–436. [CrossRef] [PubMed]
65. Kayagaki, N.; Phung, Q.; Chan, S.; Chaudhari, R.; Quan, C.; O'Rourke, K.M.; Eby, M.; Pietras, E.; Cheng, G.; Bazan, J.F.; et al. DUBA: A deubiquitinase that regulates type I interferon production. *Science* **2007**, *318*, 1628–1632. [CrossRef] [PubMed]
66. Han, C.; Jin, J.; Xu, S.; Liu, H.; Li, N.; Cao, X. Integrin CD11b negatively regulates TLR-triggered inflammatory responses by activating Syk and promoting degradation of MyD88 and TRIF via Cbl-b. *Nat. Immunol.* **2010**, *11*, 734–742. [CrossRef] [PubMed]
67. Skaug, B.; Chen, J.; Du, F.; He, J.; Ma, A.; Chen, Z.J. Direct, noncatalytic mechanism of IKK inhibition by A20. *Mol. Cell* **2011**, *44*, 559–571. [CrossRef] [PubMed]
68. Yuk, J.M.; Shin, D.M.; Lee, H.M.; Kim, J.J.; Kim, S.W.; Jin, H.S.; Yang, C.S.; Park, K.A.; Chanda, D.; Kim, D.K.; et al. The orphan nuclear receptor SHP acts as a negative regulator in inflammatory signaling triggered by Toll-like receptors. *Nat. Immunol.* **2011**, *12*, 742–751. [CrossRef] [PubMed]
69. Kondo, T.; Kawai, T.; Akira, S. Dissecting negative regulation of Toll-like receptor signaling. *Trends Immunol.* **2012**, *33*, 449–458. [CrossRef] [PubMed]

70. Saitoh, T.; Tun-Kyi, A.; Ryo, A.; Yamamoto, M.; Finn, G.; Fujita, T.; Akira, S.; Yamamoto, N.; Lu, K.P.; Yamaoka, S. Negative regulation of interferon-regulatory factor 3-dependent innate antiviral response by the prolyl isomerase Pin1. *Nat. Immunol.* **2006**, *7*, 598–605. [CrossRef]
71. Kawai, T.; Akira, S. The role of pattern-recognition receptors in innate immunity: Update on Toll-like receptors. *Nat. Immunol.* **2010**, *11*, 373–384. [CrossRef]
72. Kawai, T.; Akira, S. Signaling to NF-kappaB by Toll-like receptors. *Trends Mol. Med.* **2007**, *13*, 460–469. [CrossRef]
73. Liu, T.; Zhang, L.; Joo, D.; Sun, S.C. NF-κB signaling in inflammation. *Signal Transduct. Target. Ther.* **2017**, *2*, 1–9. [CrossRef]
74. Couser, W.G.; Johnson, R.J. The etiology of glomerulonephritis: Roles of infection and autoimmunity. *Kidney Int.* **2014**, *86*, 905–914. [CrossRef] [PubMed]
75. Rock, K.L.; Latz, E.; Ontiveros, F.; Kono, H. The sterile inflammatory response. *Annu. Rev. Immunol.* **2010**, *28*, 321–342. [CrossRef] [PubMed]
76. Yamanishi, Y.; Kitaura, J.; Izawa, K.; Kaitani, A.; Komeno, Y.; Nakamura, M.; Yamazaki, S.; Enomoto, Y.; Oki, T.; Akiba, H.; et al. TIM1 is an endogenous ligand for LMIR5/CD300b: LMIR5 deficiency ameliorates mouse kidney ischemia/reperfusion injury. *J. Exp. Med.* **2010**, *207*, 1501–1511. [CrossRef] [PubMed]
77. Anders, H.J. Toll-Like Receptors and Danger Signaling in Kidney Injury. *J. Am. Soc. Nephrol.* **2010**, *21*, 1270–1274. [CrossRef]
78. Rosin, D.L.; Okusa, M.D. Dangers Within: DAMP Responses to Damage and Cell Death in Kidney Disease. *J. Am. Soc. Nephrol.* **2011**, *22*, 416–425. [CrossRef] [PubMed]
79. Mertowski, S.; Grywalska, E.; Gosik, K.; Smarz-Widelska, I.; Hymos, A.; Dworacki, G.; Niedźwiedzka-Rystwej, P.; Drop, B.; Roliński, J.; Załuska, W. TLR2 Expression on Select Lymphocyte Subsets as a New Marker in Glomerulonephritis. *J. Clin. Med.* **2020**, *9*, 541. [CrossRef]
80. Rosenberg, A.Z.; Kopp, J.B. Focal Segmental Glomerulosclerosis. *Clin. J. Am. Soc. Nephrol.* **2017**, *12*, 502–517. [CrossRef]
81. Reggiani, F.; Ponticelli, C. Focal segmental glomerular sclerosis: Do not overlook the role of immune response. *J. Nephrol.* **2016**, *29*, 525–534. [CrossRef]
82. Eardley, K.S.; Kubal, C.; Zehnder, D.; Quinkler, M.; Lepenies, J.; Savage, C.O.; Howie, A.J.; Kaur, K.; Cooper, M.S.; Adu, D.; et al. The role of capillary density, macrophage infiltration and interstitial scarring in the pathogenesis of human chronic kidney disease. *Kidney Int.* **2008**, *74*, 495–504. [CrossRef]
83. Wu, X.; Dolecki, G.J.; Sherry, B.; Zagorski, J.; Lefkowith, J.B. Chemokines are expressed in a myeloid cell-dependent fashion and mediate distinct functions in immune complex glomerulonephritis in rat. *J. Immunol.* **1997**, *158*, 3917–3924.
84. Wang, H.; Zheng, C.; Xu, X.; Zhao, Y.; Lu, Y.; Liu, Z. Fibrinogen links podocyte injury with Toll-like receptor 4 and is associated with disease activity in FSGS patients. *Nephrology* **2018**, *23*, 418–429. [CrossRef] [PubMed]
85. Gaman, A.M.; Moisa, C.; Diaconu, C.C.; Gaman, M.A. Crosstalk between Oxidative Stress, Chronic Inflammation and Disease Progression in Essential Thrombocythemia. *Rev. Chim.* **2019**, *70*, 3486–3489. [CrossRef]
86. Găman, M.A.; Epîngeac, M.E.; Diaconu, C.C.; Găman, A.M. Evaluation of oxidative stress levels in obesity and diabetes by the free oxygen radical test and free oxygen radical defence assays and correlations with anthropometric and laboratory parameters. *World J. Diabetes* **2020**, *11*, 193–201. [CrossRef] [PubMed]
87. Yacov, N.; Feldman, B.; Volkov, A.; Ishai, E.; Breitbart, E.; Mendel, I. Treatment with lecinoxoids attenuates focal and segmental glomerulosclerosis development in nephrectomized rats. *Basic Clin. Pharmacol. Toxicol.* **2019**, *124*, 131–143. [CrossRef]
88. Segarra-Medrano, A.; Carnicer-Cáceres, C.; Arbós-Via, M.A.; Quiles-Pérez, M.T.; Agraz-Pamplona, I.; Ostos-Roldán, E. Biological markers of nephrotic syndrome: A few steps forward in the long way. *Nefrología* **2012**, *32*, 558–572. [CrossRef] [PubMed]
89. Shah, S.R.; Choi, M. Minimal Change Disease in Adults. In *Glomerulonephritis*; Trachtman, H., Herlitz, L.C., Lerma, E.V., Hogan, J.J., Eds.; Springer International Publishing: Cham, Switzerland, 2019; pp. 97–114. ISBN 978-3-319-49379-4.
90. Uwaezuoke, S.N. Biomarkers of Common Childhood Renal Diseases. In *Biomarker—Indicator of Abnormal Physiological Process*; IntechOpen: London, UK, 2018. [CrossRef]

91. Srivastava, T.; Sharma, M.; Yew, K.H.; Sharma, R.; Duncan, R.S.; Saleem, M.A.; McCarthy, E.T.; Kats, A.; Cudmore, P.A.; Alon, U.S.; et al. LPS and PAN-induced podocyte injury in an in vitro model of minimal change disease: Changes in TLR profile. *J. Cell Commun. Signal.* **2013**, *7*, 49–60. [CrossRef]
92. Mishra, O.P.; Kumar, R.; Narayan, G.; Srivastava, P.; Abhinay, A.; Prasad, R.; Singh, A.; Batra, V.V. Toll-like receptor 3 (TLR-3), TLR-4 and CD80 expression in peripheral blood mononuclear cells and urinary CD80 levels in children with idiopathic nephrotic syndrome. *Pediatr. Nephrol.* **2017**, *32*, 1355–1361. [CrossRef] [PubMed]
93. Ishimoto, T.; Shimada, M.; Araya, C.E.; Huskey, J.; Garin, E.H.; Johnson, R.J. Minimal Change Disease: A CD80 podocytopathy? *Semin. Nephrol.* **2011**, *31*, 320–325. [CrossRef]
94. Lai, W.L.; Yeh, T.H.; Chen, P.M.; Chan, C.K.; Chiang, W.C.; Chen, Y.M.; Wu, K.D.; Tsai, T.J. Membranous nephropathy: A review on the pathogenesis, diagnosis, and treatment. *J. Formos. Med. Assoc.* **2015**, *114*, 102–111. [CrossRef]
95. Couser, W.G. Primary Membranous Nephropathy. *Clin. J. Am. Soc. Nephrol.* **2017**, *12*, 983–997. [CrossRef]
96. Liu, W.; Gao, C.; Dai, H.; Zheng, Y.; Dong, Z.; Gao, Y.; Liu, F.; Zhang, Z.; Liu, Z.; Liu, W.; et al. Immunological Pathogenesis of Membranous Nephropathy: Focus on PLA2R1 and Its Role. *Front. Immunol.* **2019**, *10*, 1809. [CrossRef] [PubMed]
97. Chen, S.Y.; Chen, C.H.; Huang, Y.C.; Chan, C.J.; Chen, D.C.; Tsai, F.J. Genetic susceptibility to idiopathic membranous nephropathy in high-prevalence Area, Taiwan. *Biomedicine* **2014**, *4*, 9. [CrossRef] [PubMed]
98. Nafar, M.; Samavat, S. Biomarkers in IgA Nephropathy. In *Biomarkers in Kidney Disease*; Patel, V.B., Ed.; Springer: Dordrecht, The Netherlands, 2015; pp. 1–29. ISBN 978-94-007-7743-9.
99. Liu, Y.; Ma, X.; Lv, J.; Shi, S.; Liu, L.; Chen, Y.; Zhang, H. Risk factors for pregnancy outcomes in patients with IgA nephropathy: A matched cohort study. *Am. J. Kidney Dis.* **2014**, *64*, 730–736. [CrossRef] [PubMed]
100. Coppo, R.; Camilla, R.; Amore, A.; Peruzzi, L. Oxidative Stress in IgA Nephropathy. *Nephron Clin. Pract.* **2010**, *116*, c196–c199. [CrossRef]
101. Suzuki, H.; Suzuki, Y.; Narita, I.; Aizawa, M.; Kihara, M.; Yamanaka, T.; Kanou, T.; Tsukaguchi, H.; Novak, J.; Horikoshi, S.; et al. Toll-Like Receptor 9 Affects Severity of IgA Nephropathy. *J. Am. Soc. Nephrol.* **2008**, *19*, 2384–2395. [CrossRef]
102. Rollino, C.; Vischini, G.; Coppo, R. IgA nephropathy and infections. *J. Nephrol.* **2016**, *29*, 463–468. [CrossRef]
103. Merkle, M.; Ribeiro, A.; Köppel, S.; Pircher, J.; Mannell, H.; Roeder, M.; Wörnle, M. TLR3-dependent immune regulatory functions of human mesangial cells. *Cell. Mol. Immunol.* **2012**, *9*, 334–340. [CrossRef]
104. Coppo, R.; Amore, A.; Peruzzi, L.; Vergano, L.; Camilla, R. Innate immunity and IgA nephropathy. *J. Nephrol.* **2010**, *23*, 626–632.
105. Sheng, X.; Zuo, X.; Liu, X.; Zhou, Y.; Sun, X. Crosstalk between TLR4 and Notch1 signaling in the IgA nephropathy during inflammatory response. *Int. Urol. Nephrol.* **2018**, *50*, 779–785. [CrossRef]
106. Lim, B.J.; Lee, D.; Hong, S.W.; Jeong, H.J. Toll-Like Receptor 4 Signaling is Involved in IgA-Stimulated Mesangial Cell Activation. *Yonsei Med. J.* **2011**, *52*, 610–615. [CrossRef]
107. Chebotareva, N.; Bobkova, I.; Shilov, E. Heat shock proteins and kidney disease: Perspectives of HSP therapy. *Cell Stress Chaperones* **2017**, *22*, 319–343. [CrossRef] [PubMed]
108. Kaneko, T.; Mii, A.; Fukui, M.; Nagahama, K.; Shimizu, A.; Tsuruoka, S. IgA Nephropathy and Psoriatic Arthritis that Improved with Steroid Pulse Therapy and Mizoribine in Combination with Treatment for Chronic Tonsillitis and Epipharyngitis. *Intern. Med.* **2015**, *54*, 1085–1090. [CrossRef] [PubMed]
109. Brown, H.J.; Lock, H.R.; Wolfs, T.G.A.M.; Buurman, W.A.; Sacks, S.H.; Robson, M.G. Toll-like receptor 4 ligation on intrinsic renal cells contributes to the induction of antibody-mediated glomerulonephritis via CXCL1 and CXCL2. *J. Am. Soc. Nephrol.* **2007**, *18*, 1732–1739. [CrossRef] [PubMed]
110. Myllymäki, J.; Syrjänen, J.; Helin, H.; Pasternack, A.; Kattainen, A.; Mustonen, J. Vascular diseases and their risk factors in IgA nephropathy. *Nephrol. Dial. Transplant.* **2006**, *21*, 1876–1882. [CrossRef] [PubMed]
111. Feehally, J.; Barratt, J. The Genetics of IgA Nephropathy: An Overview from Western Countries. *Kidney Dis.* **2015**, *1*, 33–41. [CrossRef]
112. Takeda, K.; Kaisho, T.; Akira, S. Toll-Like Receptors. *Annu. Rev. Immunol.* **2003**, *21*, 335–376. [CrossRef] [PubMed]
113. Sano, N.; Kitazawa, K.; Sugisaki, T. Localization and roles of CD44, hyaluronic acid and osteopontin in IgA nephropathy. *Nephron* **2001**, *89*, 416–421. [CrossRef]

114. Zhang, Y.-M.; Zhou, X.-J.; Zhang, H. What Genetics Tells Us About the Pathogenesis of IgA Nephropathy: The Role of Immune Factors and Infection. *Kidney Int. Rep.* **2017**, *2*, 318–331. [CrossRef]
115. Cui, Y.; Liu, S.; Cui, W.; Gao, D.; Zhou, W.; Luo, P. Identification of potential biomarkers and therapeutic targets for human IgA nephropathy and hypertensive nephropathy by bioinformatics analysis. *Mol. Med. Rep.* **2017**, *16*, 3087–3094. [CrossRef]
116. Tycová, I.; Hrubá, P.; Maixnerová, D.; Girmanová, E.; Mrázová, P.; Straňavová, L.; Zachoval, R.; Merta, M.; Slatinská, J.; Kollár, M.; et al. Molecular profiling in IgA nephropathy and focal and segmental glomerulosclerosis. *Physiol. Res.* **2018**, *67*, 93–105. [CrossRef]
117. Wardle, E.N. B Lymphocyte Stimulator and Autoimmune Disease. *Saudi J. Kidney Dis. Transplant.* **2004**, *15*, 155.
118. Li, W.; Peng, X.; Liu, Y.; Liu, H.; Liu, F.; He, L.; Liu, Y.; Zhang, F.; Guo, C.; Chen, G.; et al. TLR9 and BAFF: Their expression in patients with IgA nephropathy. *Mol. Med. Rep.* **2014**, *10*, 1469–1474. [CrossRef] [PubMed]
119. Gao, R.; Wu, W.; Wen, Y.; Li, X. Hydroxychloroquine alleviates persistent proteinuria in IgA nephropathy. *Int. Urol. Nephrol.* **2017**, *49*, 1233–1241. [CrossRef] [PubMed]
120. Wu, M.Y.; Chen, C.S.; Yiang, G.T.; Cheng, P.W.; Chen, Y.L.; Chiu, H.C.; Liu, K.H.; Lee, W.C.; Li, C.J. The Emerging Role of Pathogenesis of IgA Nephropathy. *J. Clin. Med.* **2018**, *7*, 225. [CrossRef] [PubMed]
121. Coppo, R. Treatment of IgA nephropathy: Recent advances and prospects. *Nephrol. Ther.* **2018**, *14*, S13–S21. [CrossRef]
122. Yuling, H.; Ruijing, X.; Xiang, J.; Yanping, J.; Lang, C.; Li, L.; Dingping, Y.; Xinti, T.; Jingyi, L.; Zhiqing, T.; et al. CD19+CD5+ B Cells in Primary IgA Nephropathy. *J. Am. Soc. Nephrol.* **2008**, *19*, 2130–2139. [CrossRef]
123. Wang, Y.Y.; Zhang, L.; Zhao, P.W.; Ma, L.; Li, C.; Zou, H.B.; Jiang, Y.F. Functional implications of regulatory B cells in human IgA nephropathy. *Scand. J. Immunol.* **2014**, *79*, 51–60. [CrossRef]
124. Coppo, R.; Camilla, R.; Amore, A.; Peruzzi, L.; Daprà, V.; Loiacono, E.; Vatrano, S.; Rollino, C.; Sepe, V.; Rampino, T.; et al. Toll-like receptor 4 expression is increased in circulating mononuclear cells of patients with immunoglobulin A nephropathy. *Clin. Exp. Immunol.* **2010**, *159*, 73–81. [CrossRef]
125. Almaani, S.; Meara, A.; Rovin, B.H. Update on Lupus Nephritis. *Clin. J. Am. Soc. Nephrol.* **2017**, *12*, 825–835. [CrossRef]
126. Ruiz Irastorza, G.; Espinosa, G.; Frutos, M.A.; Jiménez Alonso, J.; Praga, M.; Pallarés, L.; Rivera, F.; Robles Marhuenda, A.; Segarra, A.; Quereda, C.; et al. Diagnosis and treatment of lupus nephritis. Consensus document from the systemic auto-immune disease group (GEAS) of the Spanish Society of Internal Medicine (SEMI) and Spanish Society of Nephrology (S.E.N.). *Nefrologia* **2012**, *32* (Suppl. 1), 1–35. [CrossRef]
127. Klonowska-Szymczyk, A.; Kulczycka-Siennicka, L.; Robak, T.; Smolewski, P.; Cebula-Obrzut, B.; Robak, E. The impact of agonists and antagonists of TLR3 and TLR9 on concentrations of IL-6, IL10 and sIL-2R in culture supernatants of peripheral blood mononuclear cells derived from patients with systemic lupus erythematosus. *Adv. Hyg. Exp. Med.* **2017**, *71*, 867–875. [CrossRef] [PubMed]
128. Aragón, C.C.; Tafúr, R.A.; Suárez-Avellaneda, A.; Martínez, M.D.T.; de las Salas, A.; Tobón, G.J. Urinary biomarkers in lupus nephritis. *J. Transl. Autoimmun.* **2020**, *3*, 100042. [CrossRef] [PubMed]
129. Patole, P.S.; Pawar, R.D.; Lech, M.; Zecher, D.; Schmidt, H.; Segerer, S.; Ellwart, A.; Henger, A.; Kretzler, M.; Anders, H.-J. Expression and regulation of Toll-like receptors in lupus-like immune complex glomerulonephritis of MRL-Fas(lpr) mice. *Nephrol. Dial. Transplant.* **2006**, *21*, 3062–3073. [CrossRef] [PubMed]
130. Pawar, R.D.; Patole, P.S.; Zecher, D.; Segerer, S.; Kretzler, M.; Schlöndorff, D.; Anders, H.J. Toll-Like Receptor-7 Modulates Immune Complex Glomerulonephritis. *J. Am. Soc. Nephrol.* **2006**, *17*, 141–149. [CrossRef] [PubMed]
131. Gao, R.; Yu, W.; Wen, Y.; Li, H. Beta2-glycoprotein I Expression in Lupus Nephritis Patients with Antiphospholipid-associated Nephropathy. *J. Rheumatol.* **2016**, *43*, 2026–2032. [CrossRef]
132. Kwok, S.K.; Tsokos, G.C. New insights into the role of renal resident cells in the pathogenesis of lupus nephritis. *Korean J. Intern. Med.* **2018**, *33*, 284–289. [CrossRef]
133. Urbonaviciute, V.; Starke, C.; Pirschel, W.; Pohle, S.; Frey, S.; Daniel, C.; Amann, K.; Schett, G.; Herrmann, M.; Voll, R.E. Toll-like Receptor 2 Is Required for Autoantibody Production and Development of Renal Disease in Pristane-Induced Lupus. *Arthritis Rheum.* **2013**, *65*, 1612–1623. [CrossRef]

134. Conti, F.; Spinelli, F.R.; Truglia, S.; Miranda, F.; Alessandri, C.; Ceccarelli, F.; Bombardieri, M.; Giannakakis, K.; Valesini, G. Kidney Expression of Toll Like Receptors in Lupus Nephritis: Quantification and Clinicopathological Correlations. *Mediat. Inflamm.* **2016**, *2016*, 7697592. [CrossRef]
135. Lorenz, G.; Lech, M.; Anders, H.J. Toll-like receptor activation in the pathogenesis of lupus nephritis. *Clin. Immunol.* **2017**, *185*, 86–94. [CrossRef]
136. Pawar, R.D.; Patole, P.S.; Ellwart, A.; Lech, M.; Segerer, S.; Schlondorff, D.; Anders, H.J. Ligands to Nucleic Acid–Specific Toll-Like Receptors and the Onset of Lupus Nephritis. *J. Am. Soc. Nephrol.* **2006**, *17*, 3365–3373. [CrossRef]
137. Lorenz, G.; Anders, H.J. Neutrophils, Dendritic Cells, Toll-Like Receptors, and Interferon-α in Lupus Nephritis. *Semin. Nephrol.* **2015**, *35*, 410–426. [CrossRef]
138. Chen, D.N.; Fan, L.; Wu, Y.X.; Zhou, Q.; Chen, W.; Yu, X.Q. A Predictive Model for Estimation Risk of Proliferative Lupus Nephritis. *Chin. Med. J.* **2018**, *131*, 1275–1281. [CrossRef] [PubMed]
139. Pisetsky, D.S. HMGB1: A smoking gun in lupus nephritis? *Arthritis Res. Ther.* **2012**, *14*, 112. [CrossRef] [PubMed]
140. Sun, F.; Teng, J.; Yu, P.; Li, W.; Chang, J.; Xu, H. Involvement of TWEAK and the NF-κB signaling pathway in lupus nephritis. *Exp. Ther. Med.* **2018**, *15*, 2611–2619. [CrossRef] [PubMed]
141. Watanabe, H.; Watanabe, K.S.; Liu, K.; Hiramatsu, S.; Zeggar, S.; Katsuyama, E.; Tatebe, N.; Akahoshi, A.; Takenaka, F.; Hanada, T.; et al. Anti-high Mobility Group Box 1 Antibody Ameliorates Albuminuria in MRL/lpr Lupus-Prone Mice. *Mol. Ther. Meth. Clin. Dev.* **2017**, *6*, 31–39. [CrossRef]
142. Ma, K.; Li, J.; Fang, Y.; Lu, L. Roles of B Cell-Intrinsic TLR Signals in Systemic Lupus Erythematosus. *Int. J. Mol. Sci.* **2015**, *16*, 13084–13105. [CrossRef] [PubMed]
143. Wirestam, L.; Schierbeck, H.; Skogh, T.; Gunnarsson, I.; Ottosson, L.; Erlandsson-Harris, H.; Wetterö, J.; Sjöwall, C. Antibodies against High Mobility Group Box protein-1 (HMGB1) versus other anti-nuclear antibody fine-specificities and disease activity in systemic lupus erythematosus. *Arthritis Res. Ther.* **2015**, *17*, 338. [CrossRef]
144. Qing, X.; Pitashny, M.; Thomas, D.B.; Barrat, F.J.; Hogarth, M.P.; Putterman, C. Pathogenic anti-DNA antibodies modulate gene expression in mesangial cells: Involvement of HMGB1 in anti-DNA antibody-induced renal injury. *Immunol. Lett.* **2008**, *121*, 61–73. [CrossRef]
145. Banas, M.C.; Banas, B.; Hudkins, K.L.; Wietecha, T.A.; Iyoda, M.; Bock, E.; Hauser, P.; Pippin, J.W.; Shankland, S.J.; Smith, K.D.; et al. TLR4 Links Podocytes with the Innate Immune System to Mediate Glomerular Injury. *J. Am. Soc. Nephrol.* **2008**, *19*, 704–713. [CrossRef]
146. Jończyk, M.; Kuliczkowska-Płaksej, J.; Mierzwicka, A.; Bolanowski, M. The polycystic ovarian syndrome and chronic inflammation: The role of Toll-like receptors. *Postepy Hig. Med. Dosw.* **2018**, *72*, 1199–1207. [CrossRef]
147. Lartigue, A.; Colliou, N.; Calbo, S.; François, A.; Jacquot, S.; Arnoult, C.; Tron, F.; Gilbert, D.; Musette, P. Critical role of TLR2 and TLR4 in autoantibody production and glomerulonephritis in lpr mutation-induced mouse lupus. *J. Immunol.* **2009**, *183*, 6207–6216. [CrossRef] [PubMed]
148. Horton, C.G.; Pan, Z.; Farris, A.D. Targeting toll-like receptors for treatment of SLE. *Mediat. Inflamm.* **2010**, *2010*, 498980. [CrossRef] [PubMed]
149. Wardle, E.N. Toll-Like Receptors and Glomerulonephritis. *Saudi J. Kidney Dis. Transpl.* **2007**, *18*, 159–172.
150. Lichtnekert, J.; Vielhauer, V.; Zecher, D.; Kulkarni, O.; Clauss, S.; Hornung, V.; Mayadas, T.; Beutler, B.; Akira, S.; Anders, H.-J. Trif is not required for immune complex glomerulonephritis: Dying cells activate mesangial cells via Tlr2/Myd88 rather than Tlr3/Trif. *Am. J. Physiol. Renal. Physiol.* **2009**, *296*, F867–F874. [CrossRef]
151. Pradhan, V.; Patwardhan, M.; Ghosh, K. Fc gamma receptor polymorphisms in systemic lupus erythematosus and their correlation with the clinical severity of the disease. *Indian J. Hum. Genet.* **2008**, *14*, 77–81. [CrossRef] [PubMed]
152. Mackay, M.; Stanevsky, A.; Wang, T.; Aranow, C.; Li, M.; Koenig, S.; Ravetch, J.V.; Diamond, B. Selective dysregulation of the FcγIIB receptor on memory B cells in SLE. *J. Exp. Med.* **2006**, *203*, 2157–2164. [CrossRef] [PubMed]
153. Lim, A.K. Diabetic nephropathy—Complications and treatment. *Int. J. Nephrol. Renovasc. Dis.* **2014**, *7*, 361–381. [CrossRef] [PubMed]

154. Mudaliar, H.; Pollock, C.; Panchapakesan, U. Role of Toll-like receptors in diabetic nephropathy. *Clin. Sci.* **2014**, *126*, 685–694. [CrossRef] [PubMed]
155. Conserva, F.; Gesualdo, L.; Papale, M. A Systems Biology Overview on Human Diabetic Nephropathy: From Genetic Susceptibility to Post-Transcriptional and Post-Translational Modifications. *J. Diabetes Res.* **2016**, *2016*, 7934504. [CrossRef] [PubMed]
156. Umanath, K.; Lewis, J.B. Update on Diabetic Nephropathy: Core Curriculum 2018. *Am. J. Kidney Dis.* **2018**, *71*, 884–895. [CrossRef]
157. Zhang, J.; Liu, J.; Qin, X.; Zhang, J.; Liu, J.; Qin, X. Advances in early biomarkers of diabetic nephropathy. *Rev. Assoc. Med. Bras.* **2018**, *64*, 85–92. [CrossRef] [PubMed]
158. Mansour, I.; Thajudeen, B. Overview of Diabetic Nephropathy. *J. R. Soc. Med.* **2017**, 1–21. [CrossRef]
159. Wifi, M.-N.A.; Assem, M.; Elsherif, R.H.; El-Azab, H.A.-F.; Saif, A. Toll-like receptors-2 and -9 (TLR2 and TLR9) gene polymorphism in patients with type 2 diabetes and diabetic foot. *Medicine* **2017**, *96*, e6760. [CrossRef] [PubMed]
160. Eknoyan, G. A Historical Overview of Diabetic Nephropathy. In *Diabetic Nephropathy*; Springer: Cham, Switzerland, 2019; pp. 3–19. [CrossRef]
161. Chen, X.; Ma, J.; Kwan, T.; Stribos, E.G.D.; Messchendorp, A.L.; Loh, Y.W.; Wang, X.; Paul, M.; Cunningham, E.C.; Habib, M.; et al. Blockade of HMGB1 Attenuates Diabetic Nephropathy in Mice. *Sci. Rep.* **2018**, *8*, 8319. [CrossRef]
162. Shi, H.; Che, Y.; Bai, L.; Zhang, J.; Fan, J.; Mao, H. High mobility group box 1 in diabetic nephropathy (Review). *Exp. Ther. Med.* **2017**, *14*, 2431–2433. [CrossRef]
163. Bellini, S.; Barutta, F.; Mastrocola, R.; Imperatore, L.; Bruno, G.; Gruden, G. Heat Shock Proteins in Vascular Diabetic Complications: Review and Future Perspective. *Int. J. Mol. Sci.* **2017**, *18*, 2709. [CrossRef]
164. Guo, C.; Zhang, L.; Nie, L.; Zhang, N.; Xiao, D.; Ye, X.; Ou, M.; Liu, Y.; Zhang, B.; Wang, M.; et al. Association of polymorphisms in the MyD88, IRAK4 and TRAF6 genes and susceptibility to type 2 diabetes mellitus and diabetic nephropathy in a southern Han Chinese population. *Mol. Cell. Endocrinol.* **2016**, *429*, 114–119. [CrossRef]
165. Wang, Y.; Li, Y.; Zhang, T.; Chi, Y.; Liu, M.; Liu, Y. Genistein and Myd88 Activate Autophagy in High Glucose-Induced Renal Podocytes In Vitro. *Med. Sci. Monit.* **2018**, *24*, 4823–4831. [CrossRef]
166. Murea, M.; Register, T.C.; Divers, J.; Bowden, D.W.; Carr, J.J.; Hightower, C.R.; Xu, J.; Smith, S.C.; Hruska, K.A.; Langefeld, C.D.; et al. Relationships between serum MCP-1 and subclinical kidney disease: African American-Diabetes Heart Study. *BMC Nephrol.* **2012**, *13*, 148. [CrossRef]
167. Suryavanshi, S.V.; Kulkarni, Y.A. NF-κβ: A Potential Target in the Management of Vascular Complications of Diabetes. *Front. Pharmacol.* **2017**, *8*, 798. [CrossRef]
168. Lu, Q.; Wang, W.-W.; Zhang, M.-Z.; Ma, Z.-X.; Qiu, X.-R.; Shen, M.; Yin, X.-X. ROS induces epithelial-mesenchymal transition via the TGF-β1/PI3K/Akt/mTOR pathway in diabetic nephropathy. *Exp. Ther. Med.* **2019**, *17*, 835–846. [CrossRef]
169. Tong, Y.; Chuan, J.; Bai, L.; Shi, J.; Zhong, L.; Duan, X.; Zhu, Y. The protective effect of shikonin on renal tubular epithelial cell injury induced by high glucose. *Biomed. Pharmacother.* **2018**, *98*, 701–708. [CrossRef]
170. Li, F.; Yang, N.; Zhang, L.; Tan, H.; Huang, B.; Liang, Y.; Chen, M.; Yu, X. Increased Expression of Toll-Like Receptor 2 in Rat Diabetic Nephropathy. *Am. J. Nephrol.* **2010**, *32*, 179–186. [CrossRef]
171. Cha, J.J.; Hyun, Y.Y.; Lee, M.H.; Kim, J.E.; Nam, D.H.; Song, H.K.; Kang, Y.S.; Lee, J.E.; Kim, H.W.; Han, J.Y.; et al. Renal protective effects of toll-like receptor 4 signaling blockade in type 2 diabetic mice. *Endocrinology* **2013**, *154*, 2144–2155. [CrossRef]
172. Stadler, K.; Goldberg, I.J.; Susztak, K. The Evolving Understanding of the Contribution of Lipid Metabolism to Diabetic Kidney Disease. *Curr. Diabetes Rep.* **2015**, *15*, 40. [CrossRef]
173. Cao, A.; Wang, L.; Chen, X.; Guo, H.; Chu, S.; Zhang, X.; Peng, W. Ursodeoxycholic Acid Ameliorated Diabetic Nephropathy by Attenuating Hyperglycemia-Mediated Oxidative Stress. *Biol. Pharm. Bull.* **2016**, *39*, 1300–1308. [CrossRef]
174. Kaur, H.; Chien, A.; Jialal, I. Hyperglycemia induces Toll like receptor 4 expression and activity in mouse mesangial cells: Relevance to diabetic nephropathy. *Am. J. Physiol. Renal Physiol.* **2012**, *303*, F1145–F1150. [CrossRef]
175. Takata, S.; Sawa, Y.; Uchiyama, T.; Ishikawa, H. Expression of Toll-Like Receptor 4 in Glomerular Endothelial Cells under Diabetic Conditions. *Acta Histochem. Cytochem.* **2013**, *46*, 35–42. [CrossRef]

176. Panchapakesan, U.; Pollock, C. The role of toll-like receptors in diabetic kidney disease. *Curr. Opin. Nephrol. Hypertens.* **2018**, *27*, 30–34. [CrossRef]
177. Aluksanasuwan, S.; Sueksakit, K.; Fong-Ngern, K.; Thongboonkerd, V. Role of HSP60 (HSPD1) in diabetes-induced renal tubular dysfunction: Regulation of intracellular protein aggregation, ATP production, and oxidative stress. *FASEB J.* **2017**, *31*, 2157–2167. [CrossRef]
178. Zyzak, J.; Matuszyk, J.; Siednienko, J. Multilevel maturation of Toll-like receptor 9. *Postepy Hig. Med. Dosw.* **2013**, *67*, 1034–1046. [CrossRef] [PubMed]
179. Zipris, D. Toll-like receptors and type 1 diabetes. *Adv. Exp. Med. Biol.* **2010**, *654*, 585–610. [CrossRef]
180. Ronco, C.; Bellomo, R.; Kellum, J.A. Acute kidney injury. *Lancet* **2019**, *394*, 1949–1964. [CrossRef]
181. Baer, P.C.; Koch, B.; Geiger, H. Kidney Inflammation, Injury and Regeneration. *Int. J. Mol. Sci.* **2020**, *21*, 1164. [CrossRef] [PubMed]
182. Coca, S.G.; Yusuf, B.; Shlipak, M.G.; Garg, A.X.; Parikh, C.R. Long-term risk of mortality and other adverse outcomes after acute kidney injury: A systematic review and meta-analysis. *Am. J. Kidney Dis.* **2009**, *53*, 961–973. [CrossRef]
183. Hsu, C.; Chertow, G.M.; McCulloch, C.E.; Fan, D.; Ordoñez, J.D.; Go, A.S. Nonrecovery of kidney function and death after acute on chronic renal failure. *Clin. J. Am. Soc. Nephrol.* **2009**, *4*, 891–898. [CrossRef]
184. Wald, R.; Quinn, R.R.; Luo, J.; Li, P.; Scales, D.C.; Mamdani, M.M.; Ray, J.G.; University of Toronto Acute Kidney Injury Research Group. Chronic dialysis and death among survivors of acute kidney injury requiring dialysis. *JAMA* **2009**, *302*, 1179–1185. [CrossRef]
185. Dong, Y.; Zhang, Q.; Wen, J.; Chen, T.; He, L.; Wang, Y.; Yin, J.; Wu, R.; Xue, R.; Li, S.; et al. Ischemic Duration and Frequency Determines AKI-to-CKD Progression Monitored by Dynamic Changes of Tubular Biomarkers in IRI Mice. *Front. Physiol.* **2019**, *10*, 153. [CrossRef]
186. Leemans, J.C.; Stokman, G.; Claessen, N.; Rouschop, K.M.; Teske, G.J.D.; Kirschning, C.J.; Akira, S.; van der Poll, T.; Weening, J.J.; Florquin, S. Renal-associated TLR2 mediates ischemia/reperfusion injury in the kidney. *J. Clin. Investig.* **2005**, *115*, 2894–2903. [CrossRef]
187. Kim, B.S.; Lim, S.W.; Li, C.; Kim, J.S.; Sun, B.K.; Ahn, K.O.; Han, S.W.; Kim, J.; Yang, C.W. Ischemia-reperfusion injury activates innate immunity in rat kidneys. *Transplantation* **2005**, *79*, 1370–1377. [CrossRef]
188. Wolfs, T.G.A.M.; Buurman, W.A.; van Schadewijk, A.; de Vries, B.; Daemen, M.A.R.C.; Hiemstra, P.S.; van't Veer, C. In vivo expression of Toll-like receptor 2 and 4 by renal epithelial cells: IFN-gamma and TNF-alpha mediated up-regulation during inflammation. *J. Immunol.* **2002**, *168*, 1286–1293. [CrossRef]
189. Paulus, P.; Rupprecht, K.; Baer, P.; Obermüller, N.; Penzkofer, D.; Reissig, C.; Scheller, B.; Holfeld, J.; Zacharowski, K.; Dimmeler, S.; et al. The early activation of toll-like receptor (TLR)-3 initiates kidney injury after ischemia and reperfusion. *PLoS ONE* **2014**, *15*, e94366. [CrossRef] [PubMed]
190. Good, D.W.; George, T.; Watts, B.A. Toll-like Receptor 2 Is Required for LPS-induced Toll-like Receptor 4 Signaling and Inhibition of Ion Transport in Renal Thick Ascending Limb. *J. Biol. Chem.* **2012**, *287*, 20208–20220. [CrossRef] [PubMed]
191. Good, D.W.; George, T.; Watts, B.A. Toll-like receptor 2 mediates inhibition of $HCO_3^-$ absorption by bacterial lipoprotein in medullary thick ascending limb. *Am. J. Physiol. Renal Physiol.* **2010**, *299*, F536–F544. [CrossRef] [PubMed]
192. Vallés, P.G.; Lorenzo, A.G.; Bocanegra, V.; Vallés, R. Acute kidney injury: What part do toll-like receptors play? *Int. J. Nephrol. Renovasc. Dis.* **2014**, *7*, 241–251. [CrossRef]
193. Bonventre, J.V.; Yang, L. Cellular pathophysiology of ischemic acute kidney injury. *J. Clin. Investig.* **2011**, *121*, 4210–4221. [CrossRef]
194. Devarajan, P. Update on Mechanisms of Ischemic Acute Kidney Injury. *J. Am. Soc. Nephrol.* **2006**, *17*, 1503–1520. [CrossRef]
195. Kinsey, G.R.; Li, L.; Okusa, M.D. Inflammation in acute kidney injury. *Nephron Exp. Nephrol.* **2008**, *109*, e102–e107. [CrossRef]
196. Venkatachalam, M.A.; Griffin, K.A.; Lan, R.; Geng, H.; Saikumar, P.; Bidani, A.K. Acute kidney injury: A springboard for progression in chronic kidney disease. *Am. J. Physiol. Renal Physiol.* **2010**, *298*, F1078–F1094. [CrossRef]
197. Lee, S.; Huen, S.; Nishio, H.; Nishio, S.; Lee, H.K.; Choi, B.-S.; Ruhrberg, C.; Cantley, L.G. Distinct macrophage phenotypes contribute to kidney injury and repair. *J. Am. Soc. Nephrol.* **2011**, *22*, 317–326. [CrossRef]

198. Wang, Y.; Harris, D.C.H. Macrophages in Renal Disease. *J. Am. Soc. Nephrol.* **2011**, *22*, 21–27. [CrossRef] [PubMed]
199. Lan, H.Y.; Paterson, D.J.; Atkins, R.C. Initiation and evolution of interstitial leukocytic infiltration in experimental glomerulonephritis. *Kidney Int.* **1991**, *40*, 425–433. [CrossRef] [PubMed]

International Journal of
*Molecular Sciences*

MDPI

*Review*

# The Role of Endocan in Selected Kidney Diseases

**Magdalena Nalewajska [1], Klaudia Gurazda [2], Małgorzata Marchelek-Myśliwiec [1], Andrzej Pawlik [3,*] and Violetta Dziedziejko [2]**

1 Department of Nephrology, Transplantology and Internal Medicine, Pomeranian Medical University, Powstańców Wlkp 72 Str, 70-111 Szczecin, Poland; magda_nalewajska@yahoo.co.uk (M.N.); malgorzata.marchelek@gmail.com (M.M.-M.)

2 Department of Biochemistry and Medical Chemistry, Pomeranian Medical University, Powstańców Wlkp 72 Str, 70-111 Szczecin, Poland; gurazdaklaudia@gmail.com (K.G.); viola@pum.edu.pl (V.D.)

3 Department of Physiology, Pomeranian Medical University, Powstańców Wlkp 72 Str, 70-111 Szczecin, Poland

* Correspondence: pawand@poczta.onet.pl; Tel.: +48-91-466-16-11

Received: 1 August 2020; Accepted: 23 August 2020; Published: 25 August 2020

check for updates

**Abstract:** Endocan, previously referred to as an endothelial-cell-specific molecule-1 (ESM-1) is a member of a proteoglycan family that is secreted by vascular endothelial cells of different organs, mainly lungs and kidneys. It is assumed to participate in endothelial activation and the triggering of inflammatory reactions, especially in microvasculatures. Thanks to its solubility in human fluids, i.e., urine and blood plasma, its stability and its low concentrations in physiological conditions, endocan has been proposed as an easily available, non-invasive biomarker for identifying and predicting the course of many diseases. Recently, endocan has been studied in relation to kidney diseases. In general, endocan levels have been linked to worse clinical outcomes of renal dysfunction; however, results are conflicting and require further evaluation. In this review, authors summarize available knowledge regarding the role of endocan in pathogenesis and progression of selected kidney diseases.

**Keywords:** endocan; ESM-1; acute kidney injury; chronic kidney disease; renal replacement therapy; kidney transplantation

## 1. Introduction

Endocan, formerly known as endothelial-cell-specific molecule-1 (ESM-1) is a soluble dermatan sulphate proteoglycan with a molecular mass of 50 kDa that is expressed and secreted into the bloodstream from vascular endothelial cells, mainly of lungs and kidneys [1,2]. Its expression is upregulated either by proangiogenic factors, such as vascular endothelial growth factor (VEGF), fibroblast growth factor 2 (FGF-2) or proinflammatory cytokines, like tumor necrosis factor alfa (TNFalfa), interleukin-1beta, hypoxia-inducible factor-1alfa, and lipopolysaccharide, whereas it is downregulated by interferon gamma [2]. It has been reported that endocan is involved in the rearrangement of endothelial cells, namely cell adhesion, migration, proliferation and angiogenesis, as well as playing a crucial role in inflammatory processes [3]. Nonetheless, studies provide conflicting results regarding the biological role of endocan in pathological processes. Some authors report that endocan upregulates cell adhesion molecules—ICAM-1 (intracellular cell adhesion molecule-1), VCAM-1 (vascular cellular adhesion molecule-1) and E-selectin—or activates the nuclear factor-kappa B pathway, an important mediator in inflammatory processes; therefore, endocan could take part in vascular inflammation and endothelial cell activation [4]. Contrarily, endocan could display anti-inflammatory properties by blocking the recruitment, adhesion and activation of leukocytes through direct binding to LFA-1 (leukocyte function-associated antigen 1) and interference with the LFA-1/ICAM-1 pathway [5].

Despite these conflicting results, the characteristics of endocan—its extremely low concentrations in physiological conditions, its stability, and its easy and non-invasive detection in body fluids—suggest endocan as a possible biomarker of clinical importance [6,7]. Endocan has already been linked to the occurrence and course of various conditions, including inflammatory diseases, cancer, sepsis, cardiovascular events (CVE) and kidney diseases [1,7–9].

So far, endocan has been studied in acute (AKI) and chronic kidney disease (CKD) and renal replacement therapy (RRT). In this paper, authors review available research concerning the role of endocan in the development and progression of selected kidney diseases. The most valuable studies concerning the role of endocan in kidney diseases have been summarized in Table A1.

## 2. Endocan in AKI

AKI is a theoretically reversible condition characterized by a rapid reduction in renal function that could lead to the accumulation of nitrogen-based end-products or a decline in urine output [10]. AKI is diagnosed upon one of the following definitions: an increase in serum creatinine levels by either ≥0.3 mg/dL within 48 h or ≥1.5-fold from a known or assumed baseline, or a reduction in urinary output by less than 0.5 mL/kg/h over 6 h [10]. Since inflammation and endothelial dysfunction play a part in the pathogenesis of AKI, it has been assumed that endocan could reflect renal dysfunction in this group of patients. However, little data is available covering the role of endocan in AKI.

In 2015, Rahmania et al. assessed the predictive value of endocan in relation to acute renal failure and the need for RRT in a group of intensive care unit (ICU) patients admitted due to the diagnosis of acute respiratory distress syndrome (ARDS) [11]. In total, 17% of the 96 subjects required RRT at some point during hospitalization, and these patients displayed higher plasma endocan and creatinine levels than those who did not need RRT. ROC AUC identified combined serum endocan and creatinine levels as the most valuable mean for predicting the need for RRT, in comparison to either creatinine or endocan alone. Gunay et al. published the results of a study evaluating the levels of endocan in the serum of patients diagnosed with AKI [12]. Among other parameters, serum endocan, creatinine and blood urea nitrogen were higher in the AKI group than in healthy subjects. The ROC analysis further displayed the high sensitivity and specificity (59% and 76.3%, respectively) of endocan plasma measurements in the identification of AKI. The authors, however, did not clarify the renal clearance of endocan and, thus, were not able to evaluate whether endocan levels in AKI were increased following its enhanced production or decreased elimination. p14, endocan peptide cleavage of 14 kDa was recently identified as a product of endocan proteolysis by cathepsin G and was evaluated in sepsis [13]. Gaudet et al. conducted a post hoc analysis of the data from previous research of septic patients in relation to p14 and renal function [14,15]. Authors calculated the plasma endocan cleavage ratio (ECR) using the following equation: Plasma p14/(endocan + p14), and the results were expressed in pmol/mL. The ECRs were measured at baseline and 24, 48, and 72 h after admission to the ICU. The results demonstrated that the renal component of the SOFA scale (sequential organ assessment score) was related to an increased ECR at baseline. At 72 h, patients with a SOFA scale >4 at enrolment displayed significantly higher ECR than those with a score <4. The authors suggest that plasmatic levels of p14 could rely upon renal function. Measurements of p14 in urine could be of more value as p14 is supposed to be eliminated through glomerular filtration due to its smaller molecular weight and the lack of a polyanionic glycanic chain.

It has been also hypothesized that examining serum endocan levels could help differentiating between various pathogenesis of intrinsic AKI [6]. Following the considerations of Azimi [6], intrinsic causes of AKI could be divided into two large groups: Tubular and glomeruli/vasculatures injuries. The first group is represented by ischemic/toxic tubular injuries and tubulointerstitial pathologies, whereas the other one by i.e., glomerulonephritis and vasculitis. Endocan as a marker of endothelial disfunction, a disfunction that is an important contributor to glomeruli/vasculatures pathologies, and less to tubular and tubulointerstitial diseases of the kidney could serve as a useful tool in diagnostics of these two entities [6].

## 3. Endocan in CKD

CKD is defined as a decreased glomerular filtration rate (GFR) of less than 60 mL/min/1.73 $m^2$ or damaged kidney structure, identified by imagining studies or renal biopsy, which occurs for more than 3 months. Diabetes mellitus, primary glomerulonephritis and hypertension (HT) are listed as the three main causes of CKD. The course of CKD is associated with a gradual loss of kidney function that can eventually result in the need of RRT or renal transplantation, and end-stage renal disease (ESRD) itself is linked to increased mortality, particularly from cardiovascular diseases [16]. As mentioned previously, endocan has been proven to display a prognostic value in CKD, among other conditions [8], as reduced kidney function is linked to endothelial dysfunction and inflammation [17].

In a study by Yilmaz et al., the serum concentrations of endocan were assessed in stage 1–5 CKD patients in the pre-dialysis period in relation to inflammation, endothelial dysfunction, cardiovascular incidence and overall survival [9]. The results showed that patients with CKD displayed higher plasma endocan levels than controls, and the concentrations of endocan correlated positively with CKD stage and negatively with estimated glomerular filtration rate (eGFR). Plasma endocan levels further correlated positively with inflammatory markers, such as hsCRP (high-sensitivity C-reactive protein) and PTX3 (pentraxin 3), and carotid-intima media thickness. Cox survival analysis also demonstrated the positive association between endocan plasma concentrations and all-cause mortality and CVE in CKD patients. Further analysis also displayed an increased predictive value of endocan in relation to CVE in CKD subjects compared with the usual risk factors. Following the results of other studies, the authors explained that endocan could affect vascular inflammation by interacting with ICAM-1LFA-1 and leukocyte extravasation [5]. Pawlak et al. evaluated the role of endocan in CKD patients with CVE [18]. In their study, serum endocan levels, serum levels of soluble ICAM-1 and VCAM-1 and inflammatory markers were significantly elevated in the CKD group compared to controls. In contrast to a study by Yilmaz et al. [9], the authors did not display correlation between endocan and markers of kidney function, suggesting that decreased clearance does not influence the endocan levels [18]. Furthermore, endocan, sICAM-1, sVCAM-1 and the majority of inflammatory marker concentrations were higher in CKD in the CVE group than in the group of CKD without CVE [18]. Samouilidou et al. recently studied the association between serum endocan levels and lipid profiles of CKD patients with dyslipidemia, dividing patients into non-dialyzed and HD subgroups [19]. Endocan concentrations were also verified in relation to two members of the paraoxonase family, PON1 and PON3, which contribute to HDL-related antiatherogenic properties due to the inhibition of LDL oxidation. The results of the study indicated that endocan serum levels were significantly higher in the HD subgroup compared to others; PON1 levels were decreased in the HD group, whereas PON3 levels were increased in both studied subgroups compared to controls. The endocan levels correlated positively with total cholesterol and LDL-C in both studied groups and inversely with HDL-C in hemodialyzed patients. Furthermore, endocan correlated with PON1 in both CKD groups. The authors suggest that the elevated endocan levels in HD patients may be related to increased endocan production due to the atherosclerotic state, as indicated by the lowered HDL-C levels in this group. Moreover, the decrease in PON1 levels in HD subjects might be the main factor influencing the elevated endocan levels in the mentioned group.

Another research group investigated the role of endocan and another glycoprotein, endoglin, in CKD caused by diabetes mellitus [20]. The study included diabetic patients with and without diabetic nephropathy (DN), and controls. The results indicated that both endocan and endoglin levels were higher in diabetes mellitus patients than in the control group. Moreover, patients with microalbuminuria displayed increased endocan plasma concentrations in comparison to normoalbuminuric diabetic patients and controls, whereas endoglin concentrations in DN patients were higher only compared to healthy subjects. Therefore, the authors concluded that endocan could serve as a potential marker of microvascular complications of diabetes mellitus. In the study conducted by Arman et al., diabetic patients with no other inflammatory diseases displayed higher endocan serum concentrations than the control group [21]. After 3 months of lifestyle modifications and pharmacological treatment of diabetes, the endocan levels and albuminuria decreased in the studied group. Additionally, results showed a positive correlation between the decrease in endocan and albuminuria levels. On the other hand, in a study performed by Cikrikcioglu et al., patients with macroalbuminuria in the course of diabetes mellitus surprisingly showed lower serum endocan levels in comparison to normoalbuminuric and microalbuminuric patients [22]. Moreover, the urine albumin-creatinine ratio (UACR) and urine protein-creatinine ratio (UPCR) displayed negative correlation with endocan levels. No correlation was established between serum endocan levels and duration of diabetes, serum creatinine and eGFR. The authors hypothesized that the obtained results could occur due to the VEGF-related mechanism. In the hyperglycemia state, VEGF is responsible for abnormal angiogenesis and enhanced permeability of blood vessels and is also supposed to stimulate endocan release [23]. Since podocytes and renal tubular cells are responsible for VEGF secretion [23], the increasing renal injury with the clinical manifestation of macroalbuminuria leads to decreased VEGF expression and, therefore, to decreased plasma endocan levels [24,25]. Zheng et al. studied the glomerular transcriptomes from murine strains of different DN susceptibility in order to identify genes that are responsible for DN occurrence [26]. Authors recognized the ESM-1 gene as a DN resistance factor. In the study, the glomerular ESM-1 expression correlated negatively with DN susceptibility and also inhibited leukocyte infiltration, one of the pathophysiological processes that occurs in DN. Moreover, urine ESM-1 significantly increased with diabetes in the DN-resistant strain in vivo, indicating that urine ESM-1 could serve as a non-invasive biomarker of glomerular ESM-1.

Oktar et al. have recently evaluated plasma endocan levels in patients with newly diagnosed HT [27]. Significantly elevated endocan levels in HT have already been reported in previous studies [28,29]. However, the study by Oktar et al. was the first to indicate that microalbuminuria is elevated in patients with newly diagnosed HT and that it positively correlates with endocan concentrations.

In another study, the relevance of endocan levels in IgA nephropathy (IgAN) has been verified [30]. Both plasma and urine concentration have been significantly increased in the IgAN group compared with controls. The levels of plasma endocan did not differ among CKD stage groups; however, the urine endocan levels increased in the advanced CKD groups. Also, both plasma and urine endocan levels were increased in the advanced pathologic grades in kidney biopsies according to the Lee classification, but not the Oxford classification. Furthermore, high plasma endocan concentrations were assessed as an independent risk factor for renal function decline. Authors suggest that elevated plasma endocan levels could be secondary to pathologic changes and endothelial damage, whereas increased urine concentrations may occur due to a damaged glomerular basement membrane.

The role of endocan, among other molecules associated with endothelial function, has also been evaluated in a study of ADPKD (autosomal dominant polycystic kidney disease) patients [31]. The subjects included in the study were divided into the following groups: ADPKD patients with impaired renal function, ADPKD patients with preserved renal function and matched control group. Patients included in the first group had significantly increased levels of endocan in comparison to the second group and the controls. Concomitantly, ADPKD patients with normal renal function displayed higher endocan levels than the control group. The results also showed an inverse correlation of endocan and eGFR. In this study, the authors indicated that ADPKD pathogenesis could also depend upon impaired endothelial function, increased angiogenesis and hypoxia.

## 4. Endocan in RRT

ESRD requires RRT—HD, peritoneal dialysis (PD) or kidney transplantation (KT). KT is the method of choice in the treatment of ESRD; however, progressive graft function still remains a clinical challenge. Identification of new biomarkers that would enable timely diagnosis and management of graft function deterioration is of great importance.

In 2012, Li et al. studied the significance of dynamic monitoring of endocan expression in the serum and renal allograft tissues of kidney transplant recipients diagnosed with an acute rejection (AR) [32]. Despite improved short-term graft function due to advanced immunosuppressants, ARs can still contribute to chronic allograft dysfunction. In the presented study, endocan expression was elevated in the blood and allograft tissues in ARs compared to patients with normal allograft function and allograft dysfunction from other causes. The anti-rejection treatment was able to decrease its expression. As expected, endocan mRNA in peripheral blood was increased in patients with acute vascular rejection in comparison to acute cellular rejection. Authors point out the damaged endothelium of the donor kidney as the source of endocan in AR patients. They further inform that endocan could serve as a sensitive and specific marker for AR detection, and its value could even increase when combined with assessment of urine HLA-DR+ lymphocytes. Lee et al. further evaluated the role of endocan as a diagnostic marker for antibody-mediated rejection (AMBR) in patients after KT [33]. The AMBR manifests as vascular inflammation—glomerulitis and peritubular capillaritis—and is related to endothelial dysfunction. In the mentioned study, endocan levels in the serum and urine were higher in patients with AMBR than with other kidney allograft pathologies (acute tubular necrosis, BK virus associated nephropathy, T-cell mediated rejection). Endocan levels correlated positively with scores of glomerulitis and peritubular capillaritis but neither with tubulitis nor interstitial inflammation severity, indicating the endothelial origin of endocan. Moreover, patients with AMBR and elevated urine and plasma endocan levels displayed worse renal function despite its function at baseline. The main finding of this research is that evaluation of both urine and serum endocan levels could serve as a diagnostic tool for vascular inflammation in kidney transplant recipients and could be convenient in distinguishing between AMBR and other allograft pathologies. Another cross-sectional study has been conducted to assess the relationship between serum endocan levels and severity of chronic graft dysfunction in kidney transplant recipients [8]. Serum endocan levels correlated with CKD stage, and patients with higher endocan levels displayed higher creatinine and lower GFR levels than patients with lower endocan concentrations in the 3-month follow-up. Furthermore, endocan correlated with TNF$\alpha$, a cytokine participating in endothelial activation. In vitro stimulation of endothelial cells with TNF$\alpha$ resulted in increased production of endocan and TGF-$\beta$1, and reduced IL-10 expression. The authors concluded that TNFalfa shows bidirectional properties in maintaining immune balance in kidney transplant recipients—it contributes to elevated leucocyte recruitment at inflammatory sites in endocan-mediated pathways but displays anti-inflammatory properties through TGF-$\beta$1 activity. In a study by Malyszko et al., endocan plasma concentrations were significantly elevated in kidney transplant recipients with stable graft function compared to healthy subjects [34]. Endocan levels correlated positively with other markers of endothelial dysfunction (i.e., ICAM and VCAM), with creatinine levels, and inversely with eGFR. Further analysis indicated creatinine, ICAM and VCAM as predictors of endocan expression. Authors conclude that endocan levels reflect the degree of endothelial damage and, therefore, it may play a role as a marker of graft injury and graft function deterioration. De Souza et al. studied serum endocan concentrations in pediatric patients 6–24 months after KT, in relation to HT and renal graft function [35]. Patients with HT and CKD displayed higher endocan plasma levels than those without HT and CKD, and these levels correlated positively with systolic blood pressure and pulse pressure and negatively with eGFR. The cut-off point of 7.0 ng/mL of endocan concentrations managed to identify children with HT and CKD with 100% sensitivity and 75% specificity.

Endocan has also been studied recently in PD patients. Oka et al. assessed correlation between serum endocan levels and the extent of urine decline in 21 PD patients [36]. Decline in urine volume is one of the main negative consequences of PD, which leads to disrupted fluid control. It mainly results from decreased residual renal function. In the study, the serum endocan levels were increased in PD patients compared to controls. They also positively correlated with proteinuria, serum creatinine, TNFalfa, beta2-macroglobulin level and PD drainage volume; there was no correlation between endocan and urine volume at baseline. However, further analysis identified serum endocan and proteinuria levels at baseline as predictors of the extent of urine decline in the studied group. Poon et al. [37] studied the relationship between endocan levels in the serum of PD patients and clinical outcomes. The authors hypothesized that endothelial injury may influence the vascular physiology and peritoneal transport in PD; therefore, endocan may be useful as a prognostic marker in this group of patients. The results of the study indicated the negative correlation between serum albumin and endocan levels, the progressive decrease in subjective global assessment scale and an increase in comprehensive malnutrition-inflammation score in relation to endocan; thus, it may play a role in the nutritional status of PD patients. The endocan levels also positively correlated with CRP levels and arterial stiffness markers, which is consistent with previous studies. Poon et al. were, however, the first to reveal that higher serum endocan levels are linked to worse cardiovascular event-free survival in PD patients with uncontrolled blood pressure.

## 5. Conclusions

Non-invasive diagnosis of various kidney diseases remains a challenge in clinical practice. Serum creatinine level, blood urea nitrogen and proteinuria are among the commonly practiced diagnostic means to evaluate kidney pathologies; however, they are not specific or immediate, and are imprecise in predicting renal function. There is emerging evidence linking endocan and the identification and outcomes of AKI, CKD and kidney transplantation, thereby bringing hope for a novel, non-invasive diagnostic marker. Nevertheless, the results of the conducted studies are conflicting. Since kidney diseases display high diversity in terms of pathogenesis and clinical course, the exact mechanisms by which endocan could affect kidney functions is yet to be determined. The issue as to whether serum endocan levels are a consequence of increased production or decreased renal clearance, and also whether the origin of urinary endocan lies upon its secretion by damaged renal tubular cells or its leakage from plasma through disrupted glomerular basement membrane is still to be clarified. The hypothesis that proposes endocan as an anti-inflammatory mediator in terms of disruption of lymphocytes adhesion to endothelium, thereby mediating immune balance in kidney diseases, is also of great interest, however, still needs further evaluation. Further analyses are mandatory before endocan could be used as a diagnostic tool in clinical practice.

**Author Contributions:** Conceptualization, project administration and supervision, manuscript revision, A.P. and V.D.; literature search, review and interpretation, manuscript writing, M.N. and K.G.; review and interpretation, helped with manuscript writing, M.M.-M.; final editing, M.M.-M. All authors have read and agreed to the published version of the manuscript.

**Funding:** The project was financed by the Minister of Science and Higher Education in the "Regional Initiative of Excellence" program, in years 2019–2022, No. 002/RID/2018/19.

**Conflicts of Interest:** The authors declare no conflict of interest.

**Ethical Approval:** This article does not contain any studies with human participants performed by any of the authors.

## Appendix A

**Table A1.** Most valuable studies examining the role of endocan in various kidney diseases.

| Condition | Aims | Study Group | Results | References |
|---|---|---|---|---|
| AKI | Correlation between endocan levels and renal function and need for RRT in ARDS patients in ICU | 96 patients with ARDS in ICU department who did not require RRT at baseline | Serum creatinine and endocan together—most valuable in predicting the need for RRT (ROC AUC 0.77) | [11] |
| AKI | serum endocan levels as potential biomarkers for diagnosing AKI and its pathogenesis | 39 patients diagnosed with AKI according to KDIGO definition | Endocan displayed 59% of sensitivity and 76.3% of specificity in the diagnosis of AKI | [12] |
| CKD | Endocan levels in CKD and non-CKD patients; relationship between endocan levels and inflammatory and endothelial dysfunction markers in CKD; endocan as predictive marker of all-cause mortality and CVE in CKD | 251 CKD pre-dialysis patients (23.1% DM; 18.7% HT; 15.9% chronic glomerulonephritis; 27.1% unknow etiology) | CKD patients displayed higher plasma endocan levels than controls; plasma endocan correlated with eGFR, different markers of inflammation and vascular abnormalities (FMV and CIMT); endocan levels were associated with all-cause mortality and CVE independent of traditional risk factors | [9] |
| DN | Predictive role of endocan and endoglin as markers of DN progression | 96 patients with DM2 (40 patients with normoalbuminuria, 56 patients with DN) | Endocan and endoglin serum levels were higher in DM2 patients; endocan, but not endoglin levels were higher in DN compared to normoalbuminuric patients ($p = 0.011$ and $p = 0.822$, respectively) | [20] |
| IgAN | Relevance of plasma and urine endocan levels in IgAN | 64 patients with IgAN diagnosed upon renal biopsy | Urine and plasma endocan levels were significantly higher in IgAN group than controls; urine, but not plasma endocan correlated with CKD stage; high plasma endocan was an independent risk factor for CKD progression | [30] |
| AR after KT | Dynamic monitoring of serum endocan levels in diagnosing ARs | 60 patients after KT (20 with normal renal function, 20 with biopsy-proven AR, 20 with renal allograft dysfunction from other causes) | Elevated blood and tissue expression of endocan in the AR group compared to others | [32] |
| AR after KT | Endocan as marker of microvascular inflammation in KT patients | 203 patients after KT | Increased urine and plasma endocan levels in AMBR patients than others; higher scores of microvascular inflammation in biopsy specimens and worse renal survival in patients with increased endocan levels (urine and/or plasma); serum and urinary endocan were valuable in distinguishing between AMBR and other graft pathologies | [33] |

AKI—acute kidney injury; RRT—renal replacement therapy; ARDS—acute respiratory distress syndrome; ICU—intensive care unit; CKD—chronic kidney disease; CVE—cardiovascular events; DM—diabetes mellitus; HT—hypertension; eGFR -estimated glomerular filtration rate; FMV—flow-mediated vasodilation; CIMT—carotid intima media thickness; DN—diabetic nephropathy; IgAN—IgA nephropathy; AR—acute rejection; KT—kidney transplantation; AMBR—antibody-mediated acute rejection.

## References


1. Kali, A.; Rathan Shetty, K.S. Endocan: A novel circulating proteoglycan. *Indian J. Pharmacol.* **2014**, *46*, 579–583. [CrossRef]
2. Lassalle, P.; Molet, S.; Janin, A.; Van der Heyden, J.; Tavernier, J.; Fiers, W.; Devos, R.; Tonnel, A.B. ESM-1 is a novel human endothelial cell-specific molecule expressed in lung and regulated by cytokines. *J. Biol. Chem.* **1996**, *271*, 20458–20464. [CrossRef] [PubMed]
3. Afsar, B.; Takir, M.; Kostek, O.; Covic, A.; Kanbay, M. Endocan: A new molecule playing a role in the development of hypertension and chronic kidney disease? *J. Clin. Hypertens.* **2014**, *16*, 914–916. [CrossRef] [PubMed]
4. Lee, W.; Ku, S.K.; Kim, S.W.; Bae, J.S. Endocan elicits severe vascular inflammatory responses in vitro and in vivo. *J. Cell. Physiol.* **2014**, *229*, 620–630. [CrossRef] [PubMed]
5. Béchard, D.; Scherpereel, A.; Hammad, H.; Gentina, T.; Tsicopoulos, A.; Aumercier, M.; Pestel, J.; Dessaint, J.P.; Tonnel, A.B.; Lassalle, P. Human endothelial-cell specific molecule-1 binds directly to the integrin CD11a/CD18 (LFA-1) and blocks binding to intercellular adhesion molecule-1. *J. Immunol.* **2001**, *167*, 3099–3106. [CrossRef] [PubMed]
6. Azimi, A. Could "calprotectin" and "endocan" serve as "troponin of nephrologists"? *Med. Hypotheses.* **2017**, *99*, 29–34. [CrossRef]
7. Tsai, J.C.; Zhang, J.; Minami, T.; Voland, C.; Zhao, S.; Yi, X.; Lassale, P.; Oettgen, P.; Aird, W.C. Cloning and characterization of the human lung endothelial-cell-specific molecule-1 promoter. *J. Vasc. Res.* **2002**, *39*, 148–159. [CrossRef]
8. Su, Y.H.; Shu, K.H.; Hu, C.P.; Cheng, C.H.; Wu, M.J.; Yu, T.M.; Chuang, Y.W.; Huang, S.T.; Chen, C.H. Serum endocan correlated with stage of chronic kidney disease and deterioration in renal transplant recipients. *Transplant. Proc.* **2014**, *46*, 323–327. [CrossRef]
9. Yilmaz, M.I.; Siriopol, D.; Saglam, M.; Kurt, Y.G.; Unal, H.U.; Eyileten, T.; Gok, M.; Cetinkaya, H.; Oguz, Y.; Sari, S.; et al. Plasma endocan levels associate with inflammation, vascular abnormalities, cardiovascular events, and survival in chronic kidney disease. *Kidney Int.* **2014**, *86*, 1213–1220. [CrossRef]
10. Kellum, J.A.; Lameire, N.; Aspelin, P.; Barsoum, R.S.; Burdmann, E.A.; Goldstein, S.L.; Herzog, C.A.; Joannidis, M.; Kribben, A.; Levey, A.S.; et al. Kidney disease: Improving global outcomes (KDIGO) acute kidney injury work group. KDIGO clinical practice guideline for acute kidney injury. *Kidney Int. Suppl.* **2012**, *2*, 1–138. [CrossRef]
11. Rahmania, L.; Orbegozo Cortés, D.; Irazabal, M.; Mendoza, M.; Santacruz, C.; De Backer, D.; Creteur, J.; Vincent, J.L. Elevated endocan levels are associated with development of renal failure in ARDS patients. *Intensive Care Med. Exp.* **2015**, *3*, A264. [CrossRef]
12. Gunay, M.; Mertoglu, C. Increase of endocan, a new marker for inflammation and endothelial dysfunction, in acute kidney injury. *North. Clin. Istanb.* **2018**, *6*, 124–128. [CrossRef] [PubMed]
13. De Freitas Caires, N.; Legendre, B.; Parmentier, E.; Scherpereel, A.; Tsicopoulos, A.; Mathieu, D.; Lassalle, P. Identification of a 14kDa endocan fragment generated by cathepsin G, a novel circulating biomarker in patients with sepsis. *J. Pharm. Biomed. Anal.* **2013**, *78–79*, 45–51. [CrossRef] [PubMed]
14. Gaudet, A.; Parmentier, E.; Dubucquoi, S.; Poissy, J.; Duburcq, T.; Lassalle, P.; De Freitas Caires, N.; Mathieu, D. Low endocan levels are predictive of acute respiratory distress Syndrome in severe sepsis and septic shock. *J. Crit. Care* **2018**, *47*, 121–126. [CrossRef]
15. Gaudet, A.; Parmentier, E.; De Freitas Caires, N.; Portier, L.; Dubucquoi, S.; Poissy, J.; Duburcq, T.; Hureau, M.; Lassale, P.; Mathieu, D. Impact of acute renal failure on plasmatic levels of cleaved endocan. *Crit. Care* **2019**, *23*, 55. [CrossRef]
16. Vaidya, S.R.; Aeddula, N.R. Chronic renal failure. In *StatPearls [Internet]*; StatPearls Publishing: Treasure Island, FL, USA, 2020.
17. Go, A.S.; Chertow, G.M.; Fan, D.; McCulloch, C.E.; Hsu, C.Y. Chronic kidney disease and the risks of death, cardiovascular events, and hospitalization. *N. Engl. J. Med.* **2004**, *351*, 1296–1305. [CrossRef]
18. Pawlak, K.; Mysliwiec, M.; Pawlak, D. Endocan—The new endothelial activation marker independently associated with soluble endothelial adhesion molecules in uraemic patients with cardiovascular disease. *Clin. Biochem.* **2015**, *48*, 425–430. [CrossRef]

19. Samouilidou, E.; Bountou, E.; Papandroulaki, F.; Papamanolis, M.; Papakostas, D.; Grapsa, E. Serum Endocan Levels are Associated with Paraoxonase 1 Concentration in Patients With Chronic Kidney Disease. *Ther. Apher. Dial.* **2018**, *22*, 325–331. [CrossRef]
20. Ekiz-Bilir, B.; Bilir, B.; Aydın, M.; Soysal-Atile, N. Evaluation of endocan and endoglin levels in chronic kidney disease due to diabetes mellitus. *Arch. Med. Sci.* **2019**, *15*, 86–91. [CrossRef] [PubMed]
21. Arman, Y.; Akpinar, T.S.; Kose, M.; Emet, S.; Yuruyen, G.; Akarsu, M.; Ozcan, M.; Yegit, O.; Cakmak, R.; Altun, O.; et al. Effect of glycemic regulation on endocan levels in patients with diabetes. *Angiology* **2016**, *67*, 239–244. [CrossRef]
22. Cikrikcioglu, M.A.; Erturk, Z.; Kilic, E.; Celik, K.; Ekinci, I.; Yasin Cetin, A.I.; Ozkan, T.; Cetin, G.; Dae, S.A.; Kazancioglu, R. Endocan and albuminuria in type 2 diabetes mellitus. *Ren. Fail.* **2016**, *38*, 1647–1653. [CrossRef] [PubMed]
23. Wakelin, S.J.; Marson, L.; Howie, S.E.M.; Garden, J.; Lamb, J.R.; Forsythe, J.L.R. The role of vascular endothelial growth factor in the kidney in health and disease. *Nephron Physiol.* **2004**, *98*, 73–79. [CrossRef] [PubMed]
24. Nakagawa, T.; Kosugi, T.; Haneda, M.; Rivard, C.J.; Long, D.A. Abnormal angiogenesis in diabetic nephropathy. *Diabetes* **2009**, *58*, 1471–1478. [CrossRef] [PubMed]
25. Maezawa, Y.; Takemoto, M.; Yokote, K. Cell biology of diabetic nephropathy: Roles of endothelial cells, tubulointerstitial cells and podocytes. *J. Diabetes Investig.* **2015**, *6*, 3–15. [CrossRef]
26. Zheng, X.; Soroush, F.; Long, J.; Hall, E.T.; Adishesha, P.K.; Bhattacharya, S.; Kiani, M.F.; Bhalla, V. Murine glomerular transcriptome links endothelial cell-specific molecule-1 deficiency with susceptibility to diabetic nephropathy. *PLoS ONE* **2017**, *12*, e0185250. [CrossRef] [PubMed]
27. Oktar, S.F.; Guney, I.; Eren, S.A.; Oktar, L.; Kosar, K.; Buyukterzi, Z.; Alkan, E.; Biyik, Z.; Erdem, S.S. Serum endocan levels, carotid intima-media thickness and microalbuminuria in patients with newly diagnosed hypertension. *Clin. Exp. Hypertens.* **2019**, *41*, 787–794. [CrossRef] [PubMed]
28. Balta, S.; Mikhailidis, D.P.; Demirkol, S.; Ozturk, C.; Kurtoglu, E.; Demir, M.; Celik, T.; Turker, T.; Iyisoy, A. Endocan—A novel inflammatory indicator in newly diagnosed patients with hypertension: A pilot study. *Angiology* **2014**, *65*, 773–777. [CrossRef] [PubMed]
29. Çimen, T.; Bilgin, M.; Akyel, A.; Felekoglu, M.A.; Nallbani, A.; Özdemir, S.; Erden, G.; Ozturk, A.; Dogan, M.; Yeter, E. Endocan and non-dipping circadian pattern in newly diagnosed essential hypertension. *Korean Circ. J.* **2016**, *46*, 827–833. [CrossRef] [PubMed]
30. Lee, Y.H.; Kim, J.S.; Kim, S.Y.; Kim, Y.G.; Moon, J.Y.; Jeong, K.H.; Lee, T.W.; Ihm, C.G.; Lee, S.H. Plasma endocan level and prognosis of immunoglobulin A nephropathy. *Kidney Res. Clin. Pract.* **2016**, *35*, 152–159. [CrossRef]
31. Raptis, V.; Bakogiannis, C.; Loutradis, C.; Boutou, A.K.; Lampropoulou, I.; Intzevidou, E.; Sioulis, A.; Elias, B.; Sarafidis, P.A. Levels of Endocan, Angiopoietin-2, and Hypoxia-Inducible Factor-1a in Patients with Autosomal Dominant Polycystic Kidney Disease and Different Levels of Renal Function. *Am. J. Nephrol.* **2018**, *47*, 231–238. [CrossRef]
32. Li, S.; Wang, L.; Wang, C.; Wang, Q.; Yang, H.; Liang, P.; Jin, F. Detection on dynamic changes of endothelial cell specific molecule1 in acute rejection after renal transplantation. *Urology* **2012**, *80*, 738.e1–738.e8. [CrossRef] [PubMed]
33. Lee, Y.H.; Kim, S.Y.; Moon, H.; Seo, J.W.; Kim, D.J.; Park, S.H.; Kim, Y.G.; Moon, J.Y.; Kim, J.S.; Jeong, K.H. Endocan as a marker of microvascular inflammation in kidney transplant recipients. *Sci. Rep.* **2019**, *9*, 1854. [CrossRef] [PubMed]
34. Malyszko, J.; Koc-Żórawska, E.; Malyszko, J.S. Endocan Concentration in Kidney Transplant Recipients. *Transplant. Proc.* **2018**, *50*, 1798–1801. [CrossRef] [PubMed]
35. De Souza, L.V.; Oliveira, V.; Laurindo, A.O.; Huarachi, D.R.G.; Nogueira, P.C.K.; Feltran, L.D.S.; de Santis Feltran, L.; Medina-Pestana, J.O.; do Carmo Franco, M. Serum endocan levels associated with hypertension and loss of renal function in pediatric patients after two years from renal transplant. *Int. J. Nephrol.* **2016**, *2016*, 2180765. [CrossRef] [PubMed]

36. Oka, S.; Obata, Y.; Sato, S.; Torigoe, K.; Sawa, M.; Abe, S.; Muta, K.; Ota, Y.; Kitamura, M.; Kwasaki, S.; et al. Serum endocan as a predictive marker for decreased urine volume in peritoneal dialysis patients. *Med. Sci. Monit.* **2017**, *23*, 1464–1470. [CrossRef] [PubMed]
37. Poon, P.Y.K.; Ng, J.K.C.; Fung, W.W.S.; Chow, K.M.; Kwan, B.C.H.; Li, P.K.T.; Szeto, C.C. Relationship between Plasma Endocan Level and Clinical Outcome of Chinese Peritoneal Dialysis Patients. *Kidney Blood Press. Res.* **2019**, *44*, 1259–1270. [CrossRef]

International Journal of
*Molecular Sciences*

MDPI

*Review*

# Podocytes—The Most Vulnerable Renal Cells in Preeclampsia

**Ewa Kwiatkowska [1,†], Katarzyna Stefańska [2,†,*], Maciej Zieliński [3,†], Justyna Sakowska [3], Martyna Jankowiak [3], Piotr Trzonkowski [3], Natalia Marek-Trzonkowska [4,5] and Sebastian Kwiatkowski [6]**

1 Clinical Department of Nephrology, Transplantology and Internal Medicine, Pomeranian Medical University, 70-111 Szczecin, Poland; ewakwiat@gmail.com
2 Department of Obstetrics, Medical University of Gdańsk, 80-210 Gdańsk, Poland
3 Department of Medical Immunology, Medical University of Gdańsk, 80-210 Gdańsk, Poland; mzielinski@gumed.edu.pl (M.Z.); justynas@gumed.edu.pl (J.S.); martyna830@gumed.edu.pl (M.J.); ptrzon@gumed.edu.pl (P.T.)
4 International Centre for Cancer Vaccine Science Cancer Immunology Group, University of Gdansk, 80-822 Gdańsk, Poland; natalia.marek@gumed.edu.pl
5 Laboratory of Immunoregulation and Cellular Therapies, Department of Family Medicine, Medical University of Gdańsk, 80-210 Gdańsk, Poland
6 Department of Obstetrics and Gynecology, Pomeranian Medical University, 70-111 Szczecin, Poland; kwiatkowskiseba@gmail.com
* Correspondence: kciach@wp.pl
† These authors equally contributed to the study.

Received: 22 June 2020; Accepted: 14 July 2020; Published: 17 July 2020

**Abstract:** Preeclampsia (PE) is a disorder that affects 3–5% of normal pregnancies. It was believed for a long time that the kidney, similarly to all vessels in the whole system, only sustained endothelial damage. The current knowledge gives rise to a presumption that the main role in the development of proteinuria is played by damage to the podocytes and their slit diaphragm. The podocyte damage mechanism in preeclampsia is connected to free VEGF and nitric oxide (NO) deficiency, and an increased concentration of endothelin-1 and oxidative stress. From national cohort studies, we know that women who had preeclampsia in at least one pregnancy carried five times the risk of developing end-stage renal disease (ESRD) when compared to women with physiological pregnancies. The focal segmental glomerulosclerosis (FSGS) is the dominant histopathological lesion in women with a history of PE. The kidney's podocytes are not subject to replacement or proliferation. Podocyte depletion exceeding 20% resulted in FSGS, which is a reason for the later development of ESRD. In this review, we present the mechanism of kidney (especially podocytes) injury in preeclampsia. We try to explain how this damage affects further changes in the morphology and function of the kidneys after pregnancy.

**Keywords:** preeclampsia; podocytes; VEGF; FSGS; proteinuria

## 1. Preeclampsia

According to state-of-the-art research and current knowledge, generalized endothelial damage caused by factors excreted by the placenta into the maternal circulation is the cause of preeclampsia (PE). Angiogenic imbalance leads to epithelial dysfunction. In turn, the imbalance is caused by decreased concentrations of vascular endothelial growth factor (VEGF) and placental growth factor (PlGF), and increased concentrations of soluble fms-like tyrosine kinase-1 (sFlt-1)—a VEGF receptor, and endoglin [1]. The development of preeclampsia is associated with arterial hypertension, proteinuria—usually nephrotic, and decreased glomerular filtration often meeting the criteria for acute kidney injury.

## 2. Glomerular Lesions Secondary to Preeclampsia

The most characteristic histopathological lesion observed in the kidneys of preeclamptic patients is glomerular endotheliosis, which is known to include swollen epithelial cells showing fenestration loss, and fibrin deposits in the subendothelial regions, with both lesions leading to the narrowing or even closing of the glomerular capillaries, and the appearance is that of a "bloodless glomerulus" [2]. Based on the histopathological appearance, it was believed for a long time that the kidney, similarly to all vessels in the whole system, only sustained endothelial damage. Proteinuria was thought to be caused by damage to this part of the filtration barrier. In the glomerulus, the filtration membrane has a unique three-layer structure. Its luminal surface consists of the endothelium, the basement membrane constitutes the inner layer, and the third layer is made of podocytes, with the slit diaphragm sealing the spaces between them. In preeclampsia, two of the filtration membrane components—the endothelium and the podocytes—are damaged, thus leading to proteinuria. Podocytes, with their well-developed contractile apparatus, are capable of regulating the filtration area and the hydraulic resistance of the entire filtration barrier [3]. By contracting their processes, they counter the pressure that inflates the capillaries and thus stabilize the structure of the glomerulus [4]. In a mature glomerulus, podocytes are the only cells participating in the metabolic turnover of the basement membrane, synthesizing its components and producing the proteinases that degrade it [4,5]. Additionally, they produce proteins modulating the properties of the capillary endothelium and are thus regulators of both the expression and function of all the filtration barrier elements [6]. The currently accepted knowledge gives rise to a presumption that the main role in the development of proteinuria is played by damage to the podocytes and their slit diaphragm.

## 3. Podocytes

As mentioned before, podocytes line the external surface of the glomerular basement membrane. Each podocyte is associated with more than one arteriole, and each arteriole is covered by more than one podocyte. Podocytes are composed of the cellular body, primary processes, and foot processes (or pedicels). The foot processes contain a contractile apparatus including actin, myosin, actinin, talin, vinculin, and vimentin, which opposes the hemodynamic forces of the glomerular capillaries. [7,8] Podocytes' main task is to participate in glomerular filtration. The glomerular filtrate flows through endothelial fenestrae, the basement membrane, and the slit diaphragms in the spaces between the foot processes. The slit diaphragms are the most important functional elements of the three-layer filtration membrane. They are anchored in the basolateral region of the foot processes. The pedicels are composed of many proteins that form an interacting complex. Damage to one of its elements disorders the function of the slit diaphragms. One of the main proteins of the complex is nephrin, which has an extracellular domain, a transmembrane domain, and an intracellular domain. The extracellular domain forms a network of connections, thus creating the structure for the slit diaphragm, while the intracellular fragment interacts with other proteins, such as CD2AP and CD2-associated protein, podocin, and kinases, passing information from the slit diaphragms on to the podocyte. [9,10] Neph1, a protein similar to nephrin, joins forces with nephrin in building the slit diaphragm structure. Another membrane protein—podocin—binds with the cytoplasmic domain of nephrin and two other proteins—CD2AP and Neph1 [11]. Podocin stabilizes the interacting complex of nephrin, Neph1, and CD2AP. CD2AP is an adaptor protein. It contains five parts, one of which binds with actin. CD2AP is found in all human tissues, although experiments on murine models have shown that normal function only requires its presence in the kidneys [12,13]. Proper interaction of the nephrin-podocin-CD2AP complex is believed to be essential for the flow of fluids, electrolytes, and proteins through the filtration slit to occur [8]. Neph1 also interacts with the protein zonula occludens-1 (ZO-1) [11]. $\alpha$-actinin that binds actin is another slit diaphragm protein [14]. It is responsible for the contractility of the podocyte processes and the adhesion of pedicels to the basement membrane. Nephrin is believed to bind with α-actinin through podocin. A genetic defect of the proteins forming the slit diaphragm structure—nephrin and Neph1—leads to massive proteinuria. Defects to the intracellular proteins (CD2AP, podocin, and α-actinin-4) cause less pronounced proteinuria, often in later life [15]. Disordered cooperation between the slit diaphragm structure proteins and the contractile element—actin—of the pedicels leads to atrophy of the pedicels, their detachment from the basement membrane, and proteinuria [11]. Podocytes are damaged by detachment from the basement membrane that is associated with the presence of podocytes and their proteins in the urine, or mitotic catastrophe—podocytes may enter the cell cycle, but they rarely undergo mitosis and cannot complete cytokinesis and may undergo apoptosis for variety of reasons. Such damage to the filtration membrane cause proteinuria [6,16,17]. Understandingly, podocytes include other proteins, as well, such as synaptopodin that cooperates with the contractile apparatus, podocalyxin that covers the surface of podocytes giving them negative electric charge, and integrins that attach the pedicels to the basement membrane. Figure 1 shows the scheme of podocytes foot process and slit diaphragm proteins.

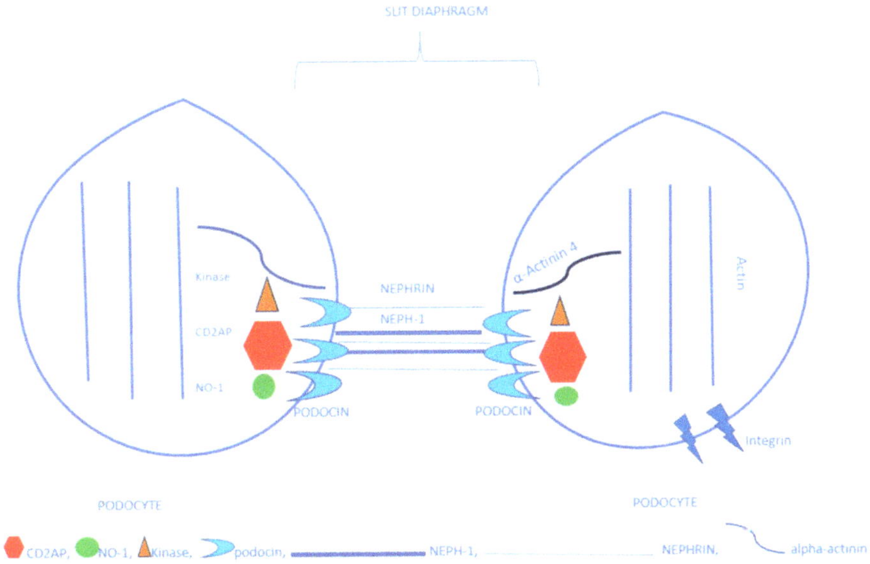


**Figure 1.** The simplified picture of the construction of a slit diaphragm.

## 4. Urinary Excretion of Podocytes and Their Proteins Secondary to Preeclampsia

Many reports are pointing to damage to individual elements of podocytes and slit diaphragms in preeclampsia. As mentioned above, the principal building blocks of the slit diaphragm include nephrin, another job of which is to pass the information on to the pedicels. Ozdemir et al. have found increased concentrations of nephrin in the blood and the urine of patients with severe preeclampsia and intrauterine growth restriction (IUGR). In their study, nephrin levels correlated negatively with fetal weight and age, and positively with creatinine concentration and systolic and diastolic pressure [18]. Wang has found that urine nephrin levels correlate with the severity of proteinuria—in other words, the more severe podocyte and slit diaphragm damage the more pronounced the proteinuria [19]. Jung has noticed that increased urine concentrations of nephrin predate the signs of preeclampsia by an average of nine days [20]. Additionally, other authors have observed that urinary levels of nephrin are higher in PE patients than both in control group women and patients with gestational hypertension [21]. Many reports indicate, as well, the presence of podocytes in the urine, which suggests they have lost attachment to the basement membrane and the filtration membrane has been ruptured. The urinary amounts of podocytes correlate with the severity of preeclampsia [19]. Wang et al. have observed decreased nephrin expression in the excreted podocytes. In their study, they encouraged oxidative stress in the incubated healthy podocyte environment and found that nephrin expression went down. In the same podocytes, they also found downregulated expression of superoxide dismutase—an antioxidant enzyme (CuZn-SOD) [22]. Biopsy specimens from PE patients revealed decreased expression of nephrin compared with the control group [23]. In an experiment in which sFlt and anti-VEGF antibodies were administered intraperitoneally to mice, a similar biopsy specimen appearance was observed. Collino et al. noticed that podocyte incubation with plasma from PE patients did not lead to nephrin depletion. In their study, they subsequently incubated glomerular endothelial cells in PE patient plasma and used the resulting environment to incubate podocytes. They found that nephrin was lost as a result of cleavage of its extracellular domain by proteases and its redistribution. Further on, they established that in response to the PE patient serum, the endothelium produced endothelin 1 (ET-1), which, in addition to being the main cause of activation of the proteases that cleaved nephrin's extracellular domain, which is the main protein of slit diaphragm [24,25]. The application of recombinant endothelin on cultured podocytes caused the shedding of nephrin from these cells [24]. The same author blocked the activity of VEGF on the glomerular endothelium to find increased endothelin production [25]. Kerlay has analyzed the available clinical studies that assessed urinary podocyte proteins as markers for the development of preeclampsia [26]. In his study, he found that urinary nephrin had the highest sensitivity (0.81) and specificity (0.84) as a marker for the development of preeclampsia [26]. Podocin stabilizes the nephrin-Neph1-CD2AP complex and binds nephrin to $\alpha$-actinin. This is a key protein in transmitting information from the slit diaphragm to the inside of the podocyte. In his study, Martineau found that preeclamptic patients had higher urinary podocin concentrations than the control group [27]. These concentrations correlated positively with the severity of albuminuria, proteinuria, and arterial pressure, and negatively with gestational age [27]. In his study, Gialni examined podocin-positive extracellular vesicles in the urine and found there were higher levels in PE patients than in the control group. In his paper, he presented the concept that damage to the podocytes is associated with nephrinuria related to nephrin shedding from these cells. According to his claim, this phenomenon causes decreased expression of nephrin in the renal biopsy specimens and in the urine podocytes. Podocin stays bound to the podocytes and its presence in the urine is associated with podocyturia [28]. In his experiment on murine models in which preeclampsia was caused by the administration of a nitric oxide analog, Baijnath identified the mRNA of podocin and nephrin in the urine [29]. As mentioned above, the adaptor protein CD2AP is part of the nephrin-Neph1-Podocin complex. In his study, Henao experimented with podocytes placed in PE patient sera [30]. He found that the distribution of two proteins—podocin and CD2AP—changed. He also noticed that their changed distribution caused an increase in the tension of the contractile apparatus of the podocyte. Additionally, he studied electrical resistance of the podocyte layer and found that, if increased, it suggested low permeability of the filtration membrane, especially for proteins. Podocytes placed in PE pregnant patient serum had lower electrical resistance. The author believed that the changed podocin and CD2AP distribution disordered the entire complex composed of the slit diaphragm and the inside of the foot process containing the contractile apparatus [30].

## 5. The Podocyte Damage Mechanism in Preeclampsia

### *Free VEGF Deficiency*

sFlt-1 that is present in preeclampsia binds with the receptor for VEGF and inhibits its impact on various cells in the system. In the podocytes, especially their foot processes, the expression of all the VEGF-A isoforms is observed. Podocytes are the main sources of VEGF in the glomerulus [31]. A study using the electron microscope established the presence of VEGF in the foot process, the basement membrane, and the luminal surface of the endothelium. It was found that VEGF produced by the podocytes moved in the opposite direction to the glomerular filtrate. VEGF receptors were found both on the podocytes and the endothelial cells. VEGF produced by the podocytes has autocrine and paracrine effects on the endothelium [32,33]. In other studies, mice deprived of podocyte-produced VEGF died upon birth due to renal failure. No normally developed filtration membrane was found in the renal specimens. The problem did not only affect the podocytes, though, as the endothelial cells failed to form the fenestration typical of the glomerulus, as well. Such a phenotype is the responsibility of VEGF produced and secreted by podocytes [24]. The lack of VEGF's paracrine effect on the endothelium is believed to be responsible for the typical histopathological appearance of the glomerulus in preeclampsia, i.e., glomerular endotheliosis. This experiment proved the influence of VEGF produced by podocytes on the function of podocytes and the endothelium [34]. Podocyte-produced VEGF is bound by heparan sulfate present in the basement membrane, where it is stored and from where it is transported further on. VEGF is known to be necessary for normal podocyte function. It stimulates phosphorylation of nephrin, which prevents podocyte apoptosis [32]. Moreover, VEGF increases interaction between podocin and CD2AP [35]. Administration of anti-VEGF antibodies or sFlt-1 prevents nephrin expression in the podocytes and damages them [33]. In a study on cancer patients treated with anti-VEGF antibodies, podocyturia was observed [36]. Podocytes have a type 1 receptor for VEGF, i.e., VEGFR1, through which VEGF exerts an autocrine effect. No VEGFR-2 receptor was found on their surface. Preeclampsia is known to be accompanied by increased levels of the soluble form of the VEGF receptor, i.e., fms-like tyrosine kinase-1 (sFlt-1), a compound that competes with VEGFR1 for VEGF, which is why podocytes are so exposed to damage in preeclampsia [37]. Experiments have shown that VEGF is necessary to transmit impulses from nephrin (its extracellular domain) to actin—a component of the contractile elements of the podocyte process [35]. Mature mice deprived of VEGF demonstrated damage to all three layers of the filtration membrane [35].

## 6. Endothelial Damage-Related Disorders

### 6.1. Nitric Oxide (NO) Deficiency

Excess amounts of antiangiogenic factors sFlt-1 and endolgin, and a deficiency of angiogenic factors VEGF and PlGF, lead to generalized endothelial damage. This is associated with reduced activity of nitric oxide synthase and decreased levels of this vasodilating factor [38]. In his experiment on murine models, Baijnath administered an analog of L-arginine that inhibited nitric oxide synthesis and caused preeclampsia-like symptoms, including podocyturia, defined as the urinary presence of the mRNA of podocin and nephrin. The histopathological appearance mainly included endothelial damage in the form of swelling, loss of fenestration, and the closing of the vascular walls. This experiment proves the interdependence of the endothelium and the podocytes. The lack of endothelial synthesis of NO causes damage to the podocytes. This mechanism is not yet fully understood. In the same experiment, sildenafil citrate, known to increase cGMP levels (the same result as that of NO), eliminated podocyturia, and prevented histopathological lesions in the glomerulus [29]. It was found that the administration of sildenafil citrate decreased the level of sFlt-1 and increased VEGF synthesis.

### 6.2. Endothelin-1

Collino's experiment indicating that the decreased nephrin expression was not caused by the PE patient plasma itself but by endothelin-1, produced by the endothelium under the influence of that plasma, was mentioned above. The application of recombinant endothelin on cultured podocytes caused the shedding of nephrin from the podocytes [24,25]. Preeclamptic patients are observed to have significantly increased plasma concentrations of endothelin-1 [39]. In one study, the administration of blockers of receptors for endothelin-1 before the infusion of sFlt-1 prevented the development of hypertension in murine experiments [40].

### 6.3. Oxidative Stress

The abnormal placenta of a PE patient is the source of reactive oxygen species, as well as compounds that damage the endothelium, which itself becomes the source of reactive oxygen species [41]. Wang's experiment proved that oxidative stress causes damage to podocytes [22]. The podocytes singled out from PE patient urine were shown to demonstrate no expression of nephrin, and none of the superoxide dismutase (SOD) that is normally present on the surface of the foot processes. The author theorized that at this location the job for superoxide dismutase was to protect nephrin (its extracellular domain) against oxidative stress. To prove his thesis, he subjected cultured podocytes to oxidative stress. He achieved the loss of expression of nephrin and superoxide dismutase. He could not prove the direct interdependence of SOD and nephrin but showed that oxidative stress caused nephrin shedding, which had a damaging effect on the filtration membrane [22]. Another author, Zao, studied biopsy specimens from preeclamptic patients to find their decreased expression of nephrin, which proved damage to the podocytes. He also examined a marker of oxidative stress. He found an increased expression of nitrotyrosine and a decreased expression of CuZn-SOD in the biopsy specimens collected from preeclamptic patients when compared with the control group. Nitrotyrosine is a marker of increased oxidative stress and it is formed when a protein molecule is nitrated by peroxynitrite. Superoxide dismutase is the only antioxidant enzyme to dismutate superoxide radicals generated by living cells [42].

## 7. Preeclampsia and the Risk of Developing End-Stage Renal Disease (ESRD)

The effect of past preeclampsia on the women's health in later life has long been the subject of much debate. Many authors implicate that a history of PE increases the risk of cardiovascular and renal diseases [43,44]. Other studies have shown a higher incidence of microalbuminuria 5 years after preeclampsia [45]. As it was not certain whether that was the result of PE or perhaps co-morbidities that contributed to PE, national cohort studies were carried out. One such study was a Norwegian research paper published in 2008 that was based on the birth registry for 1967–1991, and the ESRD diagnosis registry for 1980 to date. The research showed a higher incidence of ESRD in former preeclamptic patients [43]. Similarly, Swedish national cohort study results published in 2019 confirmed that women who had preeclampsia in at least one pregnancy carried five-times the risk of developing ESRD when compared to women with physiological pregnancies. This correlation was independent of other factors such as co-morbidities, socioeconomic status, or age [46]. Thought needs to be given as to why this happens. In the above work, it was shown that preeclampsia was associated with damage to the podocytes. Podocytes are terminally differentiated cells that do not proliferate or renew. Their damage decreases their number in the glomerulus and leaves a void instead. Podocytes injury is depicted in the following scheme (Figure 2).

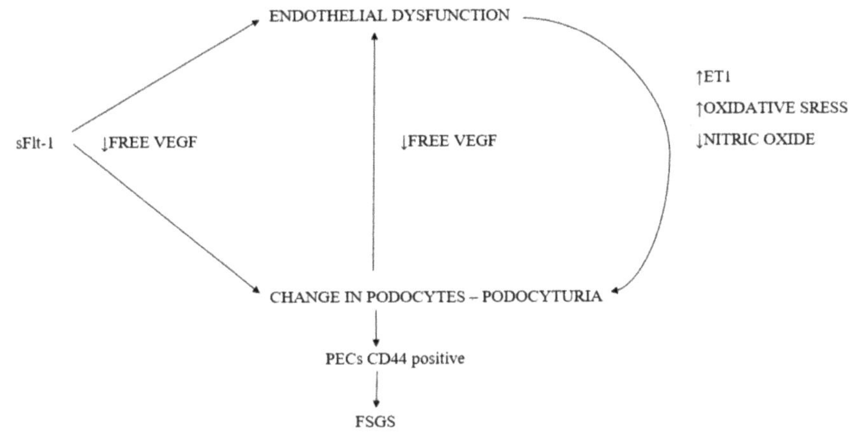


**Figure 2.** The scheme of podocytes injury in preeclampsia.

## 8. The Mechanism behind Focal Segmental Glomerulosclerosis (FSGS)

There are very few reports on histopathological lesions in the kidneys of patients with a history of PE, which is linked to the ethical contraindications for such studies. However, even those few existing ones suggest that focal segmental glomerulosclerosis (FSGS) is the dominant histopathological lesion [47–50]. The development of FSGS begins with the loss of podocytes. The kidney of an adult person has approx. 500–600 podocytes per glomerulus, which are not subject to replacement or proliferation. In their study on murine models, Wharram et al. found that podocyte depletion exceeding 20% resulted in FSGS [51]. The development of FSGS because of podocyte depletion has been proven in experimental and clinical studies [52,53]. Podocyte depletion results in a mismatch between the vascular basement membrane area requiring coverage by podocytes and the actual area of the podocytes. The capillaries with the uncovered basement membrane move towards Bowman's capsule to establish a sort of connection (a cell bridge) with its epithelium Parietal Epithelial Cells (PECs) (lining Bowman's capsule). Between these bridges, an extracellular matrix gathers that forms fibrous connections with Bowman's capsule (tuft adhesion). Additionally, after cell bridge formation, PECs de novo express the marker of activation CD44 and start to deposit the Bowman's-type matrix leading in the tuft adhesion. The CD44-positive PECs are found only in the sclerotic region. [54] Recently are more and more information about the role of PECs in the sclerotic process in secondary FSGS even in PE. [55] Instead of moving to the proximal tubule, the filtrate produced here moves—under Bowman's capsule epithelial cells—to the peritubular space thus causing tubular atrophy, which then inflicts irreversible damage on the glomerulus. This filtrate has a large protein content as it is not filtrated by the podocyte layer. A further gathering of the extracellular matrix and hyaline substance at the site of the connection with Bowman's capsule leads to obliteration of the glomerular capillaries. This is where mesangial expansion often occurs [56]. A typical appearance of focal segmental glomerulosclerosis develops. It should be added that proteinuria is not only a sign of filtration membrane damage, as the appearance of proteins in the so-called Bowman's space causes further damage to the podocytes and Bowman's capsule epithelial cells and stimulates their apoptosis. In this way, the segmental lesion leads with time to the development of generalized glomerulosclerosis [57]. Additionally, research on children with idiopathic FSGS has shown that proteinuria stimulates the apoptosis of proximal and distal tubular epithelial cells [58]. This provokes the spread of the lesions beyond the glomerulus and across the entire nephron. Moreover, Matsusaka has proven that damage to one podocyte is carried over to the neighboring healthy podocytes, thus causing the domino effect [59]. As a result of the mismatch between the podocyte area and the glomerular basement membrane area, some endothelial cells are not affected by the paracrine effect of VEGF (which is secreted by the podocyte under normal circumstances). This leads to damage to the endothelium—its typical fenestrated phenotype. The changed endothelium may produce compounds that exacerbate podocyte damage [60]. The process, initiated by primary damage to the podocytes secondary to preeclampsia, continues to develop postpartum when the original damaging factors are no longer present. Initially, this causes FSGS-type lesions, and in the long-term leads to the sclerosis of the entire glomerulus and damage to the entire nephron.

## 9. Conclusions

In preeclampsia, the angiogenic imbalance leads mainly to podocyte damage. The disordered structure of the podocytes leads to their detachment from the basement membrane and urinary excretion (podocyturia). As podocytes do not undergo replacement or proliferation, their numbers are reduced. If the percentage of the damaged podocytes exceeds 20, FSGS-type lesions set in and, being irreversible and progressive, lead with time to the deterioration of renal function.

A history of preeclampsia is known to be associated with a higher (by five times) probability of developing ESRD, but despite the increased probability, the condition does not affect a large percentage of patients. It is our job as physicians to inform our patients of the need for long-term follow-up monitoring. This should include an albuminuria test, urinalysis, renal function assessment, and arterial pressure measurement on a yearly basis, at least. Patients must be made aware that a past preeclampsia increases the risk of cardiovascular diseases, as well. Apart from reporting for follow-up tests, they could be stimulated to also adopt a healthy lifestyle and avoid any additional risk factors for cardiovascular and renal diseases. The importance of the right diet, exercise, and body weight control, and the need to avoid smoking and alcohol, should be highlighted.

**Funding:** This study was supported with funds from the Polish National Science Center based on Decision no. 2014/15/B/NZ5/03499.

**Conflicts of Interest:** The authors declare no conflict of interest

## References

1. Tomimatsu, T.; Mimura, K.; Endo, M.; Kumasawa, K.; Kimura, T. Pathophysiology of Preeclampsia: An Angiogenic Imbalance and Long-Lasting Systemic Vascular Dysfunction. *Hypertens. Res.* **2017**, *40*, 305–310. [CrossRef] [PubMed]
2. Hussein, W.; Lafayette, R.A. Renal Function in Normal and Disordered Pregnancy. *Curr. Opin. Nephrol. Hypertens.* **2014**, *23*, 46–53. [CrossRef] [PubMed]
3. Morton, M.J.; Hutchinson, K.; Mathieson, P.W.; Witherden, I.R.; Saleem, M.A.; Hunter, M. Human podocytes possess a stretch-sensitive, $Ca_2$+-activated K+ channel: Potential implications for the control of glomerular filtration. *J. Am. Soc. Nephrol.* **2004**, *15*, 2981–2987. [CrossRef]
4. Mundel, P.; Kriz, W. Structure and function of podocytes: An update. *Anat. Embryol.* **1995**, *192*, 385–397. [CrossRef]
5. Asanuma, K.; Shirato, I.; Ishidoh, K.; Kominami, E.; Tomino, Y. Selective modulation of the secretion of proteinases and their inhibitors by growth factors in cultured differentiated podocytes. *Kidney Int.* **2002**, *62*, 822–831. [CrossRef]
6. Armaly, Z.; Jadaon, J.E.; Jabbour, A.; Abassi, Z.A. Preeclampsia: Novel Mechanisms and Potential Therapeutic Approaches. *Front. Physiol.* **2018**, *259*, 973. [CrossRef]
7. Humphries, J.D.; Wang, P.; Streuli, C.; Geiger, B.; Humphries, M.J.; Ballestrem, C. Vinculin controls focal adhesion formation by direct interactions with talin and actin. *J. Cell Biol.* **2007**, *179*, 1043–1057. [CrossRef]
8. Ichimura, K.; Kurihara, H.; Sakai, T. Actin filament organization of foot processes in rat podocytes. *J. Histochem. Cytochem.* **2003**, *51*, 1589–1600. [CrossRef]

9. Philippe, A.; Nevo, F.; Esquivel, E.L.; Reklaityte, D.; Gribouval, O.; Tete, M.J.; Loirat, C.; Dantal, J.; Fischbach, M.; Pouteil-Noble, C.; et al. Nephrin mutations can cause childhood-onset steroid-resistant nephrotic syndrome. *J. Am. Soc. Nephrol.* **2008**, *19*, 1871–1878. [CrossRef]
10. Garg, P.; Verma, R.; Nihalani, D.; Johnstone, D.B.; Holzman, L.B. Neph1 cooperates with nephrin to transduce a signal that induces actin polymerization. *Mol. Cell Biol.* **2007**, *27*, 8698–8712. [CrossRef]
11. Jalanko, H. Pathogenesis of proteinuria: Lessons learned from nephrin and podocin. *Pediatr. Nephrol.* **2003**, *18*, 487–491. [CrossRef] [PubMed]
12. Grunkemeyer, J.A.; Kwoh, C.; Huber, T.B.; Shaw, A.S. CD2-associated Protein (CD2AP) Expression in Podocytes Rescues Lethality of CD2AP Deficiency. *J. Biol. Chem.* **2005**, *19*, 29677–29681. [CrossRef] [PubMed]
13. Grahammer, F.; Schell, C.; Huber, T.B. The podocyte slit diaphragm—From a thin grey line to a complex signalling hub. *Nat. Rev. Nephrol.* **2013**, *9*, 587–598. [CrossRef] [PubMed]
14. Kaplan, J.M.; Kim, S.H.; North, K.N.; Rennke, H.; Correia, L.A.; Tong, H.Q.; Mathis, B.J.; Rodríguez-Pérez, J.C.; Allen, P.G.; Beggs, A.H.; et al. Mutations in ACTN4, Encoding alpha-actinin-4, Cause Familial Focal Segmental Glomerulosclerosis. *Nat. Genet.* **2000**, *24*, 251–256. [CrossRef] [PubMed]
15. Meyrier, A. Mechanisms of Disease: Focal Segmental Glomerulosclerosis. *Nat. Clin. Pract. Nephrol.* **2005**, *1*, 44–54. [CrossRef] [PubMed]
16. Craici, I.M.; Wagner, S.J.; Bailey, K.R.; Fitz-Gibbon, P.D.; Wood-Wentz, C.M.; Turner, S.T.; Hayman, S.R.; White, W.M.; Brost, B.C.; Rose, C.H.; et al. Podocyturia predates proteinuria and clinical features of preeclampsia: Longitudinal prospective study. *Hypertension* **2013**, *61*, 1289–1296. [CrossRef] [PubMed]
17. Liapis, H.; Romagnani, P.; Anders, H.J. New Insights into the Pathology of Podocyte Loss: Mitotic catastrophe. *Am. J. Pathol.* **2013**, *183*, 1364–1374. [CrossRef]
18. Ozdemir, F.; Tayyar, A.T.; Acmaz, G.; Aksoy, H.; Erturk, G.; Muhtaroglu, S.; Tayyar, M. Comparison of blood and urine nephrin levels in preeclampsia and intrauterine growth retardation. *Pak. J. Med. Sci.* **2016**, *32*, 40–43. [CrossRef]
19. Wang, Y.; Gu, Y.; Loyd, S.; Jia, X.; Groome, L.J. Increased urinary levels of podocyte glycoproteins, matrix metallopeptidases, inflammatory cytokines, and kidney injury biomarkers in women with preeclampsia. *Am. J. Physiol. Renal Physiol.* **2015**, *309*, 1009–1017. [CrossRef]
20. Jung, Y.J.; Cho, H.Y.; Cho, S.; Kim, Y.H.; Jeon, J.D.; Kim, Y.J.; Lee, S.; Park, J.; Kim, H.Y.; Park, Y.W.; et al. The Level of Serum and Urinary Nephrin in Normal Pregnancy and Pregnancy with Subsequent Preeclampsia. *Yonsei Med. J.* **2017**, *58*, 401–406. [CrossRef]
21. Garovic, V.D.; Wagner, S.J.; Turner, S.T.; Rosenthal, D.W.; Watson, W.J.; Brost, B.C.; Rose, C.H.; Gavrilova, L.; Craigo, P.; Bailey, K.R.; et al. Urinary podocyte excretion as a marker for preeclampsia. *Am. J. Obstet. Gynecol.* **2007**, *196*, 320. [CrossRef] [PubMed]
22. Wang, Y.; Zhao, S.; Gu, Y.; Lewis, D.F. Loss of slit protein nephrin is associated with reduced antioxidant superoxide dismutase expression in podocytes shed from women with preeclampsia. *Physiol. Rep.* **2018**, *6*, 13785. [CrossRef] [PubMed]
23. Konieczny, A.; Ryba, M.; Wartacz, J.; Czyżewska-Buczyńska, A.; Hruby, Z.; Witkiewicz, W. Podocytes in Urine, a Novel Biomarker of Preeclampsia? *Adv. Clin. Exp. Med.* **2013**, *22*, 145–149. [PubMed]
24. Hauser, P.V.; Collino, F.; Bussolati, B.; Camussi, G. Nephrin and endothelial injury. *Curr. Opin. Nephrol. Hypertens.* **2009**, *18*, 3–8. [CrossRef] [PubMed]
25. Collino, F.; Bussolati, B.; Gerbaudo, E.; Marozio, L.; Pelissetto, S.; Benedetto, C.; Camussi, G. Preeclamptic sera induce nephrin shedding from podocytes through endothelin-1 release by endothelial glomerular cells. *Am. J. Physiol. Renal Physiol.* **2008**, *294*, 1185–1194. [CrossRef] [PubMed]
26. Kerley, R.N.; McCarthy, C. Biomarkers of Glomerular Dysfunction in Pre-Eclampsia—A Systematic Review. *Pregnancy Hypertens.* **2018**, *14*, 265–272. [CrossRef]
27. Martineau, T.; Boutin, M.; Côté, A.M.; Maranda, B.; Bichet, D.G.; Auray-Blais, C. Tandem Mass Spectrometry Analysis of Urinary Podocalyxin and Podocin in the Investigation of Podocyturia in Women with Preeclampsia and Fabry Disease Patients. *Clin. Chim. Acta* **2019**, *495*, 67–75. [CrossRef]
28. Gilani, S.I.; Anderson, U.D.; Jayachandran, M.; Weissgerber, T.L.; Zand, L.; White, W.M.; Milic, N.; Gonzalez Suarez, M.L.; Vallapureddy, R.R.; Nääv, A.; et al. Urinary Extracellular Vesicles of Podocyte Origin and Renal Injury in Preeclampsia. *J. Am. Soc. Nephrol.* **2017**, *28*, 3363–3372. [CrossRef]

29. Baijnath, S.; Murugesan, S.; Mackraj, I.; Gathiram, P.; Moodley, J. The effects of sildenafil citrate on urinary podocin and nephrin mRNA expression in an L-NAME model of pre-eclampsia. *Mol. Cell. Biochem.* **2016**, *427*, 59–67. [CrossRef]
30. Henao, D.E.; Arias, L.F.; Mathieson Ni, L.; Welsh, G.I.; Bueno, J.C.; Agudelo, B.; Cadavid, A.P.; Saleem, M.A. Preeclamptic Sera Directly Induce Slit-Diaphragm Protein Redistribution and Alter Podocyte Barrier-Forming Capacity. *Nephron. Exp. Nephrol.* **2008**, *110*, 73–81. [CrossRef]
31. Guan, F.; Villegas, G.; Teichman, J.; Mundel, P.; Tufro, A. Autocrine VEGF-A System in Podocytes Regulates Podocin and Its Interaction with CD2AP. *Am. J. Physiol. Renal Physiol.* **2006**, *291*, 422–428. [CrossRef] [PubMed]
32. Eremina, V.; Quaggin, S.E. The Role of VEGF-A in Glomerular Development and Function. *Curr. Opin. Nephrol. Hypertens.* **2004**, *13*, 9–15. [CrossRef] [PubMed]
33. Wagner, S.J.; Craici, I.M.; Grande, J.P.; Garovic, V.D. From Placenta to Podocyte: Vascular and Podocyte Pathophysiology in Preeclampsia. *Clin. Nephrol.* **2012**, *78*, 241–249. [CrossRef]
34. Eremina, V.; Sood, M.; Haigh, J.; Nagy, A.; Lajoie, G.; Ferrara, N.; Gerber, H.P.; Kikkawa, Y.; Miner, J.H.; Quaggin, S.E. Glomerular-specific alterations of VEGF-A expression lead to distinct congenital and acquired renal diseases. *J. Clin. Invest.* **2003**, *111*, 707–716. [CrossRef] [PubMed]
35. Tufro, A.; Veron, D. VEGF and Podocytes in Diabetic Nephropathy. *Semin. Nephrol.* **2012**, *32*, 385–393. [CrossRef] [PubMed]
36. Müller-Deile, J.; Bröcker, V.; Grünwald, V.; Hiss, M.; Bertram, A.; Kubicka, S.; Ganser, A.; Haller, H.; Schiffer, M. Renal side effects of VEGF-blocking therapy. *NDT Plus* **2010**, *3*, 172–175. [CrossRef]
37. Kwiatkowski, S.; Kwiatkowska, E.; Torbe, A. The role of disordered angiogenesis tissue markers (sflt-1, Plgf) in present day diagnosis of preeclampsia. *Ginekol. Pol.* **2019**, *90*, 173–176. [CrossRef] [PubMed]
38. Sharma, D.; Trivedi, S.S.; Bhattacharjee, J. Oxidative Stress and eNOS (Glu298Asp) Gene Polymorphism in Preeclampsia in Indian Population. *Mol. Cell Biochem.* **2011**, *353*, 189–193. [CrossRef]
39. Saleh, L.; Verdonk, K.; Visser, W.; Meiracker, A.H.; Danser, A.H.J. The Emerging Role of endothelin-1 in the Pathogenesis of Pre-Eclampsia. *Ther. Adv. Cardiovasc. Dis.* **2016**, *10*, 282–293. [CrossRef]
40. Murphy, S.R.; LaMarca, B.B.D.; Cockrell, K.; Granger, J.P. Role of Endothelin in Mediating Soluble Fms-Like Tyrosine Kinase 1-induced Hypertension in Pregnant Rats. *Hypertension* **2010**, *55*, 394–398. [CrossRef]
41. Aouache, R.; Biquard, L.; Vaiman, D.; Miralles, F. Oxidative Stress in Preeclampsia and Placental Diseases. *Int. J. Mol. Sci.* **2018**, *19*, 1496. [CrossRef] [PubMed]
42. Zhao, S.; Gu, X.; Groome, L.J.; Wang, Y. Decreased Nephrin and GLEPP-1, But Increased VEGF, Flt-1, and Nitrotyrosine, Expressions in Kidney Tissue Sections from Women with Preeclampsia. *Reprod. Sci.* **2009**, *16*, 970–979. [CrossRef] [PubMed]
43. Vikse, B.E.; Irgens, M.; Leivestad, T.; Skjaerven, R.; Iversen, B.M. Preeclampsia and the Risk of End-Stage Renal Disease. *N. Engl. J. Med.* **2008**, *359*, 800–809. [CrossRef] [PubMed]
44. Smith, G.C.; Pell, J.P.; Walsh, D. Pregnancy Complications and Maternal Risk of Ischaemic Heart Disease: A Retrospective Cohort Study of 129,290 Births. *Lancet* **2001**, *357*, 2002–2006. [CrossRef]
45. Bar, J.; Kaplan, B.; Wittenberg, C.; Erman, A.; Boner, G.; Ben-Rafael, Z.; Hod, M. Microalbuminuria After Pregnancy Complicated by Pre-Eclampsia. *Nephrol. Dial. Transplant.* **1999**, *14*, 1129–1132. [CrossRef] [PubMed]
46. Khashan, A.S.; Evans, M.; Kublickas, M.; McCarthy, F.P.; Kenny, L.C.; Stenvinkel, P.; Fitzgerald, T.; Kublickiene, K. Preeclampsia and Risk of End Stage Kidney Disease: A Swedish Nationwide Cohort Study. *PLoS Med.* **2019**, *16*, 1002875. [CrossRef]
47. Webster, P.; Webster, L.M.; Cook, H.T.; Horsfield, C.; Seed, P.T.; Vaz, R.; Santos, C.; Lydon, I.; Homsy, M.; Lightstone, L.; et al. A Multicenter Cohort Study of Histologic Findings and Long-Term Outcomes of Kidney Disease in Women Who Have Been Pregnant. *Clin. J. Am. Soc. Nephrol.* **2017**, *12*, 408–416. [CrossRef]
48. Kida, H.; Takeda, S.; Yokoyama, H.; Tomosugi, N.; Abe, T.; Hattori, N. Focal glomerular sclerosis in pre-eclampsia. *Clin. Nephrol.* **1985**, *24*, 221–227. [PubMed]
49. Nochy, D.; Hinglais, N.; Jacquot, C.; Gaudry, C.; Remy, P.; Bariety, J. De novo focal glomerular sclerosis in preeclampsia. *Clin. Nephrol.* **1986**, *25*, 116–121.
50. Nagai, Y.; Arai, H.; Washizawa, Y.; Ger, Y.; Tanaka, M.; Maeda, M.; Kawamura, S. FSGS-like lesions in pre-eclampsia. *Clin. Nephrol.* **1991**, *36*, 134–140.

51. Wharram, B.L.; Goyal, M.; Wiggins, J.E.; Sanden, S.K.; Hussain, S.; Filipiak, W.E.; Saunders, T.L.; Dysko, R.C.; Kohno, K.; Holzman, L.B.; et al. Podocyte Depletion Causes Glomerulosclerosis: Diphtheria Toxin-Induced Podocyte Depletion in Rats Expressing Human Diphtheria Toxin Receptor Transgene. *J. Am. Soc. Nephrol.* **2005**, *16*, 2941–2952. [CrossRef] [PubMed]
52. Fukuda, A.; Wickman, L.T.; Venkatareddy, M.P.; Sato, Y.; Chowdhury, M.A.; Wang, S.Q.; Shedden, K.A.; Dysko, R.C.; Wiggins, J.E.; Wiggins, R.C. Angiotensin II-dependent Persistent Podocyte Loss From Destabilized Glomeruli Causes Progression of End Stage Kidney Disease. *Kidney Int.* **2012**, *81*, 40–55. [CrossRef] [PubMed]
53. Matsusaka, T.; Xin, J.; Niwa, S.; Kobayashi, K.; Akatsuka, A.; Hashizume Wang, Q.C.; Pastan, I.; Fogo, A.G.; Ichikawa, L. Genetic Engineering of Glomerular Sclerosis in the Mouse via Control of Onset and Severity of Podocyte-Specific Injury. *J. Am. Soc. Nephrol.* **2005**, *16*, 1013–1023. [CrossRef] [PubMed]
54. Smeets, B.; Kuppe, C.; Sicking, E.M.; Fuss, A.; Jirak, P.; Kuppevelt, T.H.; Endlich, K.; Wetzels, J.F.M.; Gröne, H.J.; Floege, J.; et al. Parietal Epithelial Cells Participate in the Formation of Sclerotic Lesions in Focal Segmental Glomerulosclerosis. *J. Am. Soc. Nephrol.* **2011**, *22*, 1262–1274. [CrossRef]
55. Saritas, T.; Moeller, M.J. Glomerular Disease: Pre-Eclampsia, Podocyturia and the Role of Parietal Epithelial Cells. *Nat. Rev. Nephrol.* **2014**, *10*, 615–616. [CrossRef]
56. Jefferson, J.A.; Shankland, S.J. The Pathogenesis of Focal Segmental Glomerulosclerosis. *Adv. Chronic Kidney Dis.* **2014**, *21*, 408–416. [CrossRef]
57. Chang, A.M.; Ohse, T.; Krofft, R.D.; Wu, J.S.; Eddy, A.A.; Pippin, J.W.; Shankland, S.J. Albumin-induced Apoptosis of Glomerular Parietal Epithelial Cells Is Modulated by Extracellular Signal-Regulated Kinase $^{1/2}$. *Nephrol. Dial. Transplant.* **2012**, *27*, 1330–1343. [CrossRef]
58. Erkan, E.; Garcia, C.D.; Patterson, L.T.; Mishra, J.; Mitsnefes, M.; Kaskel, F.J.; Devarajan, P. Induction of Renal Tubular Cell Apoptosis in Focal Segmental Glomerulosclerosis: Roles of Proteinuria and Fas-Dependent Pathways. *J. Am. Soc. Nephrol.* **2005**, *16*, 398–407. [CrossRef]
59. Matsusaka, T.; Sandgren, E.; Shintani, A.; Kon, V.; Pastan, I.; Fogo, A.G.; Ichikawa, I. Podocyte Injury Damages Other Podocytes. *J. Am. Soc. Nephrol.* **2011**, *22*, 1275–1285. [CrossRef]
60. Eremina, V.; Jefferson, J.A.; Kowalewska, J.; Hochster, H.; Haas, M.; Weisstuch, J.; Richardson, C.; Kopp, J.B.; Kabir, M.G.; Backx, P.H.; et al. VEGF Inhibition and Renal Thrombotic Microangiopathy. *N. Engl. J. Med.* **2008**, *358*, 1129–1136. [CrossRef]

International Journal of
*Molecular Sciences*

MDPI

*Article*

# Cyclophilin A Promotes Inflammation in Acute Kidney Injury but Not in Renal Fibrosis

**Khai Gene Leong [1,2], Elyce Ozols [1,2], John Kanellis [1,2], David J. Nikolic-Paterson [1,2,*] and Frank Y. Ma [1,2]**

1 Department of Nephrology, Monash Health, Monash Medical Centre, Clayton, Victoria 3168, Australia; khaigeneleong@gmail.com (K.G.L.); elyce.ozols@monash.edu (E.O.); john.kanellis@monash.edu (J.K.); frank.ma@monash.edu (F.Y.M.)

2 Monash University Centre for Inflammatory Diseases, Monash Medical Centre, Clayton, Victoria 3168, Australia

* Correspondence: david.nikolic-paterson@monash.edu

Received: 4 May 2020; Accepted: 20 May 2020; Published: 22 May 2020

**Abstract:** Cyclophilin A (CypA) is a highly abundant protein in the cytoplasm of most mammalian cells. Beyond its homeostatic role in protein folding, CypA is a Damage-Associated Molecular Pattern which can promote inflammation during tissue injury. However, the role of CypA in kidney disease is largely unknown. This study investigates the contribution of CypA in two different types of kidney injury: acute tubular necrosis and progressive interstitial fibrosis. *CypA (Ppia)* gene deficient and wild type (WT) littermate controls underwent bilateral renal ischaemia/reperfusion injury (IRI) and were killed 24 h later or underwent left unilateral ureteric obstruction (UUO) and were killed 7 days later. In the IRI model, *CypA*$^{-/-}$ mice showed substantial protection against the loss of renal function and from tubular cell damage and death. This was attributed to a significant reduction in neutrophil and macrophage infiltration since *CypA*$^{-/-}$ tubular cells were not protected from oxidant-induced cell death in vitro. In the UUO model, *CypA*$^{-/-}$ mice were not protected from leukocyte infiltration or renal interstitial fibrosis. In conclusion, CypA promotes inflammation and acute kidney injury in renal IRI, but does not contribute to inflammation or interstitial fibrosis in a model of progressive kidney fibrosis.

**Keywords:** acute kidney injury; chronic kidney disease; cyclophilin A; fibrosis; inflammation; renal fibrosis; tubular necrosis

## 1. Introduction

Cyclophilins are ubiquitously expressed proteins which belong to the immunophilin family [1,2]. All cyclophilins possess the "peptidyl-prolyl isomerase" (PPIase) activity that catalyses the interconversion of *cis* and *trans* isomers of proline to facilitate protein folding [2,3]. Cyclophilin A (CypA) is a highly abundant cytoplasmic protein that is expressed by virtually all mammalian cells [1,2]. Beyond its homeostatic role, CypA can contribute to the inflammatory response. CypA can be released from cells via active secretion, or passively during necrotic cell death, and bind to CD147 on the surface of leukocytes, including neutrophils, monocyte/macrophages and T cells. In vitro studies have demonstrated that CypA can promote monocyte and neutrophil migration, and macrophage activation [4–6]. Indeed, *CypA* gene-deficient mice are protected from acetaminophen-induced liver toxicity and inflammation, leading to the description of CypA as a Damage-Associated Molecular Pattern [7]. Indeed, the administration of supraphysiologic doses of recombinant CypA to mice can induce systemic inflammation [8]. CD147, the only known CypA receptor, is also expressed by many non-leukocyte populations, including tubular epithelial cells of the kidney [1,9,10]. Furthermore,

CD147 is a scavenger receptor which can bind many other ligands, including leukocyte integrins, Selectin E, CD44 and S100A9 [11]. Indeed, *Cd147* gene-deficient mice are sterile with a variety of abnormalities, consistent with CD147 being a receptor for multiple ligands [12,13].

Acute kidney injury (AKI) is clinically defined as an acute increase in serum creatinine (>27 mmol/L within 48 h or >1.5-fold over a week) or loss of urine output. AKI is commonly seen in the emergency department where a variety of pre-renal causes (e.g., severe blood loss, major cardiac or abdominal surgery, sepsis, severe dehydration) result in low blood pressure and hypo-perfusion of the kidney [14,15]. In addition, acute kidney injury can result from acute tubular necrosis induced by nephrotoxic agents, including chemotherapeutic drugs, environmental toxins, contrast media and drug overdose [16]. Severe AKI is associated with high mortality rates and necessitates immediate dialysis [14,17], while those recovering from AKI are at increased risk of developing, or exacerbating, chronic kidney disease [18].

CypA levels have been examined as potential biomarkers of kidney injury. Lee et al. [19], found that elevated serum and urine CypA levels correlated with subsequent development of acute kidney injury in patients undergoing cardiac surgery. In addition, increased urine and plasma levels of CypA correlate with the progression of diabetic kidney disease [20,21], and urine CypA levels can predict microalbuminuria in children with type 1 diabetes [22]. Despite these encouraging clinical studies, the pathological role of CypA in acute kidney injury or progressive renal fibrosis has not been investigated. Therefore, the aim of this study was to determine whether CypA contributes to inflammation and kidney injury in models of acute kidney injury and of progressive renal fibrosis. To achieve this, we investigated mice lacking CypA ($CypA^{-/-}$) in two disease models: acute kidney failure due to IRI, and progressive renal interstitial fibrosis following unilateral ureteric obstruction (UUO).

## 2. Results

### 2.1. CypA Deletion Protects against Acute Renal Failure, Tubular Damage and Cell Death in Renal IRI

In wild type (WT) mice, CypA mRNA levels showed a small, but significant, increase at 24 h after renal IRI (Figure 1A). Renal IRI caused an acute and severe loss of renal function in WT mice as shown by an 8-fold rise in serum creatinine levels compared to sham controls (Figure 1B). This was associated with extensive tubular damage in the inner cortex and outer medulla consisting of dilated tubules, loss of brush border, tubular cell loss/sloughing, and cast formation (Figure 1C,D). Consistent with the marked histologic damage, there was a significant increase in mRNA levels of the tubular damage marker KIM-1/HAVCR1 and a reduction in mRNA levels of the reno-protective molecule, Klotho (Figure 2A,B). A significant induction of tubular cell death was also shown by TUNEL staining (Figure 2C).

$CypA^{-/-}$ mice were substantially protected from acute renal failure in the IRI model with 50% lower serum creatinine levels (Figure 1B). This protection was associated with a significant reduction in the percentage of damaged tubules (Figure 1C,D), a reduction in KIM-1/HAVCR2 mRNA levels (Figure 2A), a reduction in the number of TUNEL+ tubular cells (Figure 2C), and a significantly lesser reduction in Klotho mRNA levels (Figure 2B).

To investigate whether CypA plays a direct role in protecting tubular cells from oxidant-induced cell death, we analysed primary cultures of tubular epithelial cells from WT and $CypA^{-/-}$ mice. In a dose-response study, WT and $CypA^{-/-}$ tubular cells showed a comparable susceptibility to $H_2O_2$-induced cell death (Figure 2D).

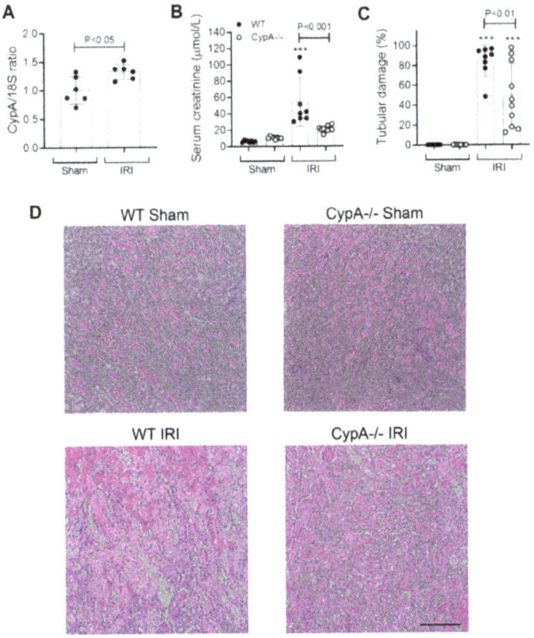


**Figure 1.** Renal function and tubular damage at 24 h in renal ischaemia/reperfusion injury (IRI) and sham controls for wild type (WT; closed circles) and *CypA*$^{-/-}$ (open circles) mice. (**A**) RT-PCR analysis of CypA mRNA levels in WT mice. (**B**) Serum creatinine levels. (**C**) Graph of tubular damage. (**D**) Periodic acid-Schiff stained kidney sections from each group. Bar = 200 μm. Data are mean ± SD. *** $p < 0.001$ versus WT sham control.

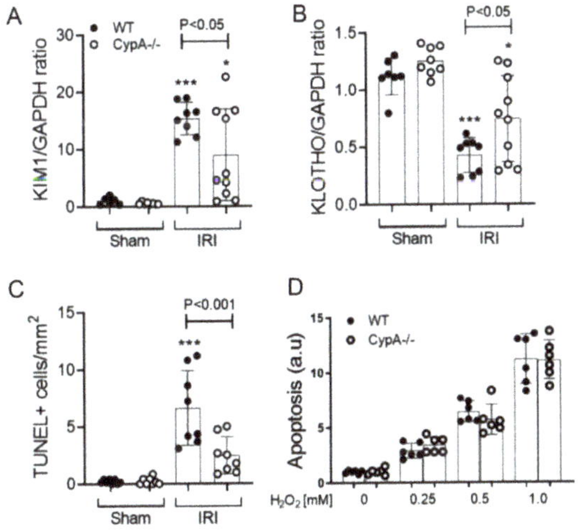


**Figure 2.** Tubular damage and cell death at 24 h in renal IRI and sham controls for WT (closed circles) and *CypA*$^{-/-}$ (open circles) mice. RT-PCR for mRNA levels of (**A**) KIM1, and (**B**) Kotho. (**C**) Quantification of the number of TUNEL+ tubular cells. (**D**) A dose-response of $H_2O_2$ induced cell death in primary cultures of tubular epithelial cells from WT and *CypA*$^{-/-}$ mice. Data are mean ± SD. * $p < 0.05$, *** $p < 0.0001$ versus WT sham control.

## 2.2. CypA Deletion Protects against Leukocyte Infiltration in Renal IRI

Neutrophil infiltration is a prominent response to renal IRI and plays a significant role in the induction of tubular necrosis [23–25]. In this study, WT mice exhibited a marked neutrophil infiltrate in the area of tubular damage (Figure 3A,B). In addition, a significant macrophage infiltrate was evident at 24 h after renal IRI, as shown by the increased CD68 mRNA levels (Figure 3C), although no significant T cell infiltrate was evident based upon CD3 mRNA levels (Figure 3D). *CypA*$^{-/-}$ mice exhibited a 73% reduction in neutrophil infiltration and a 40% reduction in CD68 mRNA levels (Figure 3A–C).

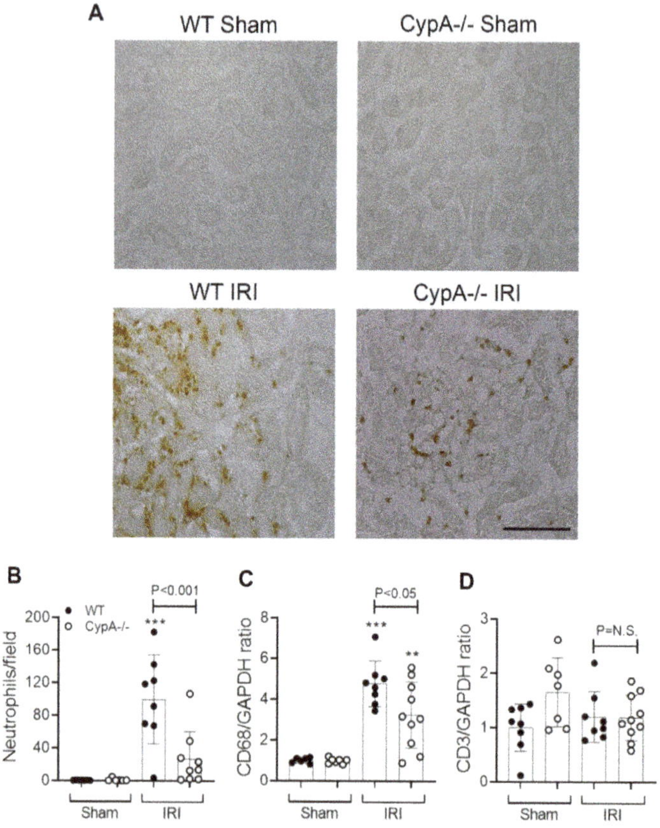


**Figure 3.** Neutrophil and macrophage infiltration at 24 h in renal IRI and sham controls for WT (closed circles) and *CypA*$^{-/-}$ (open circles) mice. (**A**) Immunoperoxidase staining for infiltrating neutrophils. Bar = 100 µm. (**B**) Quantification of neutrophil infiltration. RT-PCR analysis of (**C**) CD68, and (**D**) CD3 mRNA levels. Data are mean ± SD. ** $p < 0.05$, *** $p < 0.0001$ versus WT sham control. NS, not significant.

## 2.3. CypA Deletion Does Not Protect against Tubular Damage in UUO

WT mice showed a small but significant increase in CypA mRNA levels on day 7 after UUO (Figure 4A). We also demonstrated that angiotensin II and TNF, two factors implicated in the pathogenesis of renal fibrosis in the UUO model [26], can induce CypA secretion by cultured WT tubular epithelial cells (Figure 4B).

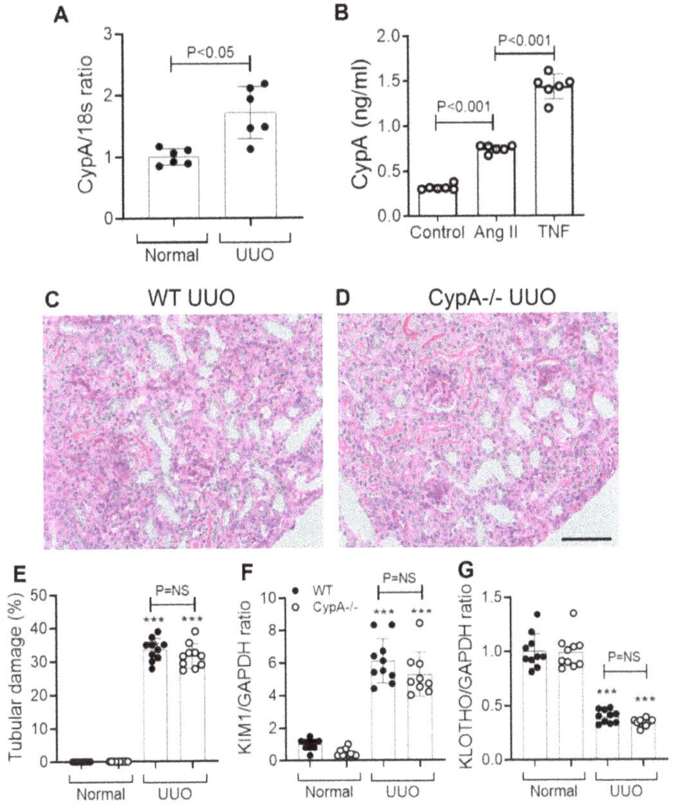


**Figure 4.** Tubular damage in day 7 unilateral ureteric obstruction (UUO) kidney compared to normal controls for WT (closed circles) and *CypA*$^{-/-}$ (open circles) mice. (**A**) RT-PCR analysis of CypA mRNA levels in WT mice. (**B**) Secretion of CypA in response to stimulation by angiotensin II or TNF in primary cultures of WT tubular epithelial cells. Periodic acid-Schiff stained kidney sections of (**C**) WT UUO and (**D**) CypA$^{-/-}$ UUO. Bar = 100 μm. (**E**) Tubular damage score. RT-PCR for mRNA levels of: (**F**) KIM1, and (**G**) Klotho. Data are mean ± SD. **** $p < 0.0001$ versus WT sham control; NS, not significant.

WT mice showed tubular dilation and atrophy, an expansion of the interstitial space and an interstitial cell infiltrate on day 7 UUO in WT mice (Figure 4C,E). Tubular damage in WT mice was also evident by the increased KIM-1 mRNA levels and reduced Klotho mRNA levels (Figure 4F,G).

*CypA*$^{-/-}$ mice showed a similar histologic pattern of tubular damage, interstitial expansion and cellular infiltration to that seen in WT mice on day 7 UUO (Figure 4D). The degree of tubular damage, shown by histology and by changes in KIM-1 and Klotho mRNA levels, was not different between *CypA*$^{-/-}$ and WT day 7 UUO (Figure 4E–G).

### *2.4. CypA Deletion Does Not Protect against Inflammation or Fibrosis in UUO*

Infiltrating macrophages promote interstitial fibrosis in the UUO model [27–30]. A substantial macrophage infiltrate was evident on day 7 UUO in WT mice as shown by F4/80 immunostaining and CD68 mRNA levels (Figure 5A–C). The increase in both NOS2 and CD206 mRNA levels on day 7 UUO indicates the presence of both M1- and M2-type macrophage phenotypes (Figure 5D,E). In addition, immunostaining identified a significant CD3$^{+}$ T cell infiltrate, with T cell activation indicated by increased IL-2 mRNA levels (Figure 6A,B). There was also a minor neutrophil infiltrate on day 7 UUO in WT mice (Figure 6C).

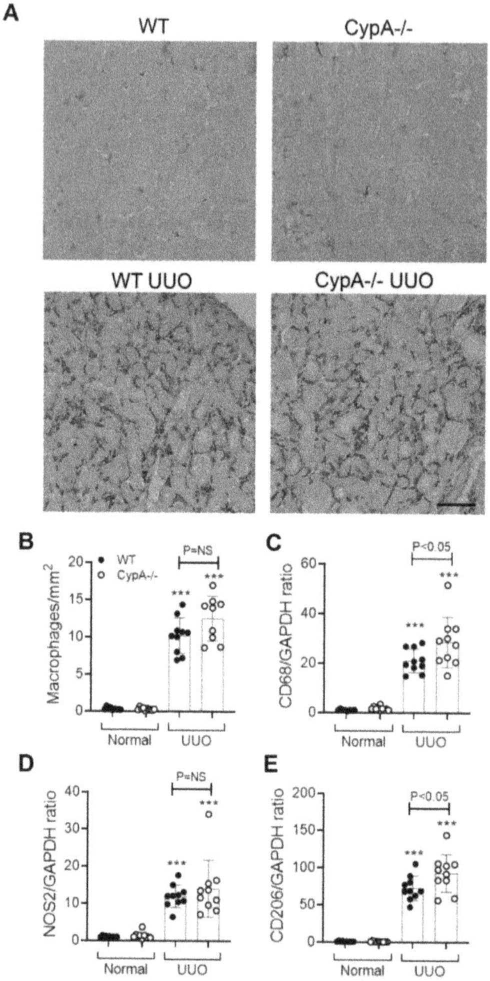


**Figure 5.** Macrophage infiltration and activation in day 7 UUO kidney compared to normal controls for WT (closed circles) and *CypA*$^{-/-}$ (open circles) mice. (**A**) Immunoperoxidase staining for F4/80$^{+}$ macrophages in the different groups. Bar = 100 µm. (**B**) Quantification of the number of stained F4/80$^{+}$ macrophages. RT-PCR for mRNA levels of: (**C**) CD68; (**D**) NOS2, and (**E**) CD206. Data are mean ± SD. *** $p < 0.0001$ versus WT sham control; NS, not significant.

Immunostaining showed a prominent infiltrate of F4/80+ macrophages in the day 7 UUO kidney in *CypA*$^{-/-}$ mice (Figure 5A), and this was not different compared to the WT UUO kidney (Figure 5B). An estimation of macrophage infiltration by CD68 mRNA levels showed a small, but significant, increase in *CypA*$^{-/-}$ compared to WT mice on day 7 UUO (Figure 5C). Levels of NOS2 mRNA were not different between *CypA*$^{-/-}$ and WT day 7 UUO kidney, although there was a small increase in CD206 mRNA levels in *CypA*$^{-/-}$ day 7 UUO (Figure 5D,E). T cell infiltration and activation and neutrophil infiltration were not different between *CypA*$^{-/-}$ and WT day 7 UUO kidney (Figure 6A–C).

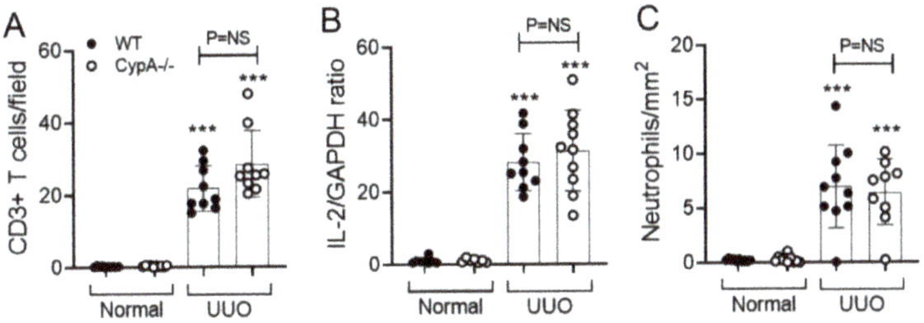


**Figure 6.** T cell and neutrophil infiltration in day 7 UUO kidney compared to normal controls for WT (closed circles) and *CypA*$^{-/-}$ (open circles) mice. (**A**) Quantification of the number of stained CD3$^{+}$ T cells. (**B**) RT-PCR for IL-2 mRNA levels. (**C**) Quantification of the number of stained neutrophils. Data are mean ± SD. *** $p < 0.0001$ versus WT sham control; NS, not significant.

The day 7 WT UUO kidney exhibited marked fibrosis, as illustrated by the interstitial deposition of collagen IV and an increase in mRNA levels for collagen I and α-SMA/ACTA2 (Figure 7A–D). The pattern and degree of collagen IV deposition on day 7 UUO was not altered in *CypA*$^{-/-}$ mice (Figure 7A,B). Similarly, the increase in α-SMA mRNA levels was not different to that in the WT UUO kidney; however, there was a small, but significant, increase in collagen I mRNA levels in *CypA*$^{-/-}$ UUO (Figure 7C,D).

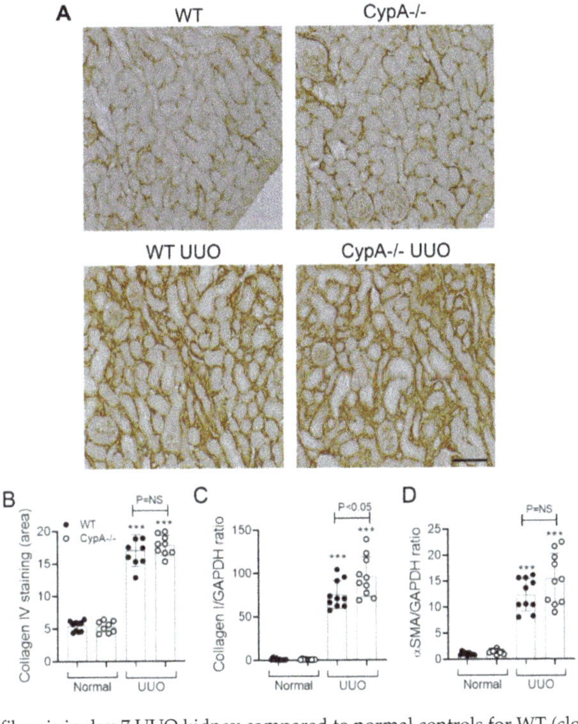


**Figure 7.** Renal fibrosis in day 7 UUO kidney compared to normal controls for WT (closed circles) and *CypA*$^{-/-}$ (open circles) mice. (**A**) Immunoperoxidase staining for collagen IV in the different groups. Bar = 100 μm. (**B**) Quantification of the area of interstitial collagen IV staining. RT-PCR for mRNA levels of: (**C**) collagen I and (**D**) α-SMA/ACTA2. Data are mean ± SD. *** $p < 0.0001$ versus WT sham control; NS, not significant.

## 3. Discussion

This study found CypA to be important in leukocyte accumulation and acute renal injury in the IRI model, but to be redundant in leukocyte accumulation and renal fibrosis in the UUO model.

Necrosis is the main form of tubular cell death occurring after renal IRI, which is most prominent in the S3 segment of the proximal tubule due to its high energy requirements and disproportionate reduction in blood flow [31]. We found clear protection from IRI-induced acute renal failure and tubular cell death and damage in *CypA*$^{-/-}$ mice. This could be due to two potential mechanisms. Firstly, CypA may act directly within tubular cells to promote cell death. However, this mechanism was not supported by the finding that cultured *CypA*$^{-/-}$ tubular epithelial cells were not protected from oxidant-induced cell death. This contrasts with the significant protection against oxidant-induced cell death seen in cultured *CypD*$^{-/-}$ tubular cells and with pan-cyclophilin inhibitors such as cyclosporine [32,33]. Secondly, CypA released from damaged cells may promote the recruitment of neutrophils and macrophages to promote tubular cell necrosis and impaired kidney function. This mechanism is supported by the marked reduction in neutrophil accumulation seen in the *CypA*$^{-/-}$ mice, and by studies identifying the extracellular release of CypA during the early stages of necroptosis [34]. A role for neutrophils in promoting tubular cell necrosis in the IRI model is well-established through neutrophil depletion studies and strategies to block neutrophil recruitment [23–25]. The reduction in macrophage accumulation into the injured kidney in *CypA*$^{-/-}$ mice might also have contributed to protection against tubular necrosis and acute renal failure, although macrophage depletion strategies have produced variable results which are likely to be due to differences in macrophage populations depleted [35].

The ability of cyclosporine treatment to prevent acute renal failure in IRI models has been attributed to blockade of CypD [32,36]. However, our findings demonstrate a specific role for CypA in renal IRI. The contrast between the protection of *CypD*$^{-/-}$ tubular cells from oxidant-induced cell death [33], and our finding that *CypA*$^{-/-}$ tubular cells are not protected in the same assay, suggests that CypA and CypD contribute to acute kidney injury in renal IRI via distinct mechanisms. Our findings are consistent with studies showing that *CypA–/–* mice are protected in cardiac IRI in association with a substantial reduction in neutrophil and macrophage infiltration [37]. In addition, mice lacking CD147 are protected in renal IRI with a marked reduction in neutrophil recruitment, although this was attributed to a CD147/Selectin-E-based mechanism rather than a CD147/CypA mechanism [38].

Macrophages play a prominent role in the rapidly progressive renal interstitial fibrosis seen in the UUO model [27–30]. In addition, there are a small number of studies to support a role for T cells in this model [39–41]. In stark contrast to the findings in the IRI model, *CypA*$^{-/-}$ mice showed no reduction in the infiltration of macrophages, T cells or neutrophils. Furthermore, there was no reduction in macrophage M1 and M2 activation markers, and no reduction in T cell activation based on IL-2 mRNA levels.

This contrast in myeloid cell accumulation between the IRI and UUO models may reflect a much greater extracellular release of CypA in the IRI model due to the substantial necroptosis. Tubular damage caused by ureter obstruction results in small numbers of apoptotic tubular cells with no evidence of necrosis and may result in little or no CypA release. We have shown that angiotensin II and TNF-$\alpha$, two factors that promote macrophage infiltration and renal fibrosis in this model [26], can induce CypA secretion by tubular epithelial cells in culture. However, we were unable to measure extracellular CypA in the obstructed kidney to determine whether significant levels of CypA are released in this model. Myeloid cell infiltration in the UUO model presumably operates via different chemotactic molecules [42].

The lack of an effect of *CypA* gene deletion in the UUO model contrasts with studies examining gene deletion of other cyclophilin members. *CypD*$^{-/-}$ mice showed a reduction in renal fibrosis on day 12, but not on day 7 [33]. This was attributed to indirect effects of reducing tubular cell death and peritubular capillary loss [33]. In a separate study, *CypB*$^{-/-}$ mice showed a reduction in tubular dilation and macrophage accumulation on day 7 UUO, although there was no effect upon renal fibrosis based upon collagen I and *Tgfb1* mRNA levels [43]. This same study described that CypA silencing in the HK-2 tubular cell line triggers a loss of epithelial features and enhances TGF-β1-induced epithelial-mesenchymal transition [43]. However, we did not observe epithelial-mesenchymal transition (i.e., α-SMA expression by tubular epithelial cells) in *CypA*$^{-/-}$ or WT mice in the UUO model.

Our findings in the UUO model are, in part, similar to those reported in *Cd147*$^{-/-}$mice. Kato et al. [44], found that *Cd147*$^{-/-}$ mice were not protected from tubular dilation, tubular cell death or interstitial fibrosis on day 7 UUO, despite a reduction in macrophage infiltration. However, *Cd147*$^{-/-}$ mice did show a reduction in renal fibrosis on day 14 UUO, which was associated with a significant reduction in matrix metalloproteinase activity in the UUO kidney [44].

In summary, we have shown that CypA promotes neutrophil and macrophage accumulation and kidney damage in a model of acute kidney injury, but not in a model of progressive interstitial fibrosis. These findings lend weight to the concept of therapeutic inhibition of cyclophilins in the setting of acute kidney injury.

## 4. Material and Methods

### 4.1. Animals

*CypA*$^{+/-}$ mice (129.Cg-Ppia$^{tm1Lubn}$/J) on the 129S1/SvimJ background were purchased from JAX Mice and Services, Bar Harbor, ME, USA, and a colony maintained at the Monash Animal Research Platform. Littermate *CypA*$^{-/-}$ and *CypA*$^{+/+}$ (WT controls) mice were used. The experiments were approved by the Monash Medical Centre Animal Ethics Committee (MMCB/2015/21, 18 September 2015 to 31 December 2019) and performed according to the 8th Edition of the Australian Code of Practice for the Care and Use of Animals for Scientific Purposes.

### 4.2. Renal Ischaemia-Reperfusion Injury (IRI)

Surgery was performed as previously described [24]. Groups of 10 male mice were anaesthetized with ketamine and xylazine. Body temperature was maintained at 37 °C using a heating blanket connected to a rectal thermometer. A midline abdominal incision was made and both renal pedicles were clamped using non-traumatic vascular clamps for 19 min, during which the abdomen was temporarily sutured to minimize heat and fluid loss. Clamps were removed and reperfusion of the kidneys visually confirmed, abdominal incisions were sutured in 2 layers, and saline provided by subcutaneous injection. Analgesia was provided by subcutaneous injection of 0.05 mg/kg Buprenorphine and 4.4 mg/kg Carprofen at the end of surgery. Control animals were sham operated, having the same procedure performed, except that the renal pedicles were not clamped.

### 4.3. Unilateral Ureteric Obstruction (UUO)

Surgery was performed as previously described [33,45]. Groups of 10 female mice were anaesthetized with ketamine and xyzaline. A midline incision was performed, the left ureter identified and ligated using two 6.0 silk sutures. The midline abdominal incision was sutured in 2 layers and analgesia provided by subcutaneous injection of 0.05 mg/kg Buprenorphine and 4.4 mg/kg Carprofen at the end of surgery. Mice were killed 7 days after UUO surgery. Control mice did not undergo surgery.

### 4.4. Renal Function

Serum creatinine was measured using an ARL Analyzer (Dupont, North Ryde, NSW, Australia), by the Department of Clinical Biochemistry, Monash Health.

### 4.5. Histology

Kidney histology was assessed on Periodic acid-Schiff stained 2 μm sections of formalin-fixed, paraffin embedded tissue. In the IRI model, the outer medulla was viewed at high power (400×). The percentage of tubular cross-sections exhibiting damage was scored; damage was characterized as loss of the brush border, nuclear loss, and sloughing of cells into the lumen. In the UUO model, the percentage of tubules showing dilation or atrophy were scored in the entire cortex. All analysis was performed on blinded slides.

### 4.6. Immunohistochemistry

Immunoperoxidase staining for macrophages (rat anti-mouse F4/80; Bio-Rad, Gladesville, Australia) and collagen IV (goat anti-collagen IV; Southern Biotechnology, Birmingham, AL, USA) was performed on 4 μm sections of methylcarn-fixed tissue as previously described [33]. Immunoperoxidase staining for neutrophils (rat anti-mouse Ly6G; Abcam, Melbourne, Australia) and T cells (rat anti-mouse CD3; Bio-Rad) was performed on 5 μm cryostat sections of tissues fixed in 2% paraformaldehyde as previously described [24].

In the IRI model, the number of neutrophils was counted in high-power fields (400×) covering the entire inner cortex and outer medulla. In the UUO model, the number of macrophages, T cells and neutrophils was counted in high-power fields (400×) covering the entire cortex. The area of interstitial collagen IV staining in the entire cortex (excluding large vessels) was assessed under medium power (200×) by image analysis using cellSens software version 1.18 (Olympus Australia, Notting Hill, Australia).

Cell death was assessed in 4 μm sections of formalin-fixed tissue by TUNEL staining with the ApopTag Peroxidase In Situ Apoptosis Detection Kit (Millipore-Chemicon, Ryde, Australia). The number of TUNEL+ tubular cells in the inner cortex and outer medulla were counted in high-power (400×) fields. All scoring was performed on blinded slides.

### 4.7. Real Time Polymerase Chain Reaction (RT-PCR)

The total RNA was extracted from a kidney slice using the Ambion RiboPure Kit (Thermo Fisher Scientific, Scoresby, Australia) and reverse transcribed into cDNA using random primers with the SuperScript III First-Strand Synthesis System (Thermo Fisher Scientific). PCR was run on the StepOne Real-Time PCR system (Thermo Fisher Scientific) using Taqman probes. The primer/probes for α-SMA, NOS2 and CD206 have been published previously [45,46], and the other primer/probes were purchased from Thermo Fisher Scientific. The relative amount of mRNA was determined using the comparative Ct (ΔΔCt) method. All amplicons were normalized against GAPDH which was analysed in the same reaction as an internal control.

### 4.8. Cell Culture Studies

Cultures of tubular epithelial cells were prepared from normal kidneys of $CypA^{-/-}$ and WT mice as previously described [46]. To examine cell death, cells were starved in 1% FCS for 18 h, and then varying concentrations of $H_2O_2$ were added for 24 h. Cells then were analysed using the Cell Death Detection ELISA Kit (Roche, Mannheim, Germany) according to the manufacturer's instructions, with results normalized to the DNA content in cell lysates using a Quant-iT DNA Assay Kit (Molecular Probes) and expressed as the ratio of optical density to DNA content. In addition, WT tubular cells were starved in 1% FCS for 18 h, and then stimulated with $10^{-6}$ M angiotensin II or 5 ng/mL TNF for 24 h. A CypA section in the culture media was measure by ELISA (USCN Life Science, Wangarra, Australia).

### 4.9. Statistics

All data are shown as mean ± SD. Data were analyzed by one-way ANOVA with Tukey's multiple comparison test, except for the analysis of CypA mRNA levels, which used the Student's t-test. The analysis was performed using GraphPad Prism (GraphPad Prism 8.0 software, San Diego, CA, USA).

**Author Contributions:** Conceptualization, K.G.L., D.J.N.-P. and F.Y.M.; Methodology, K.G.L., E.O., F.Y.M.; Validation, E.O., J.K. and F.Y.M.; Formal Analysis, K.G.L., J.K., D.J.N.-P., F.Y.M.; Investigation, K.G.L., E.O. and F.Y.M.; Data Curation, K.G.L. and D.J.N.-P.; Writing—Original Draft Preparation, K.G.L.; Writing—Review & Editing, D.J.N.-P.; Supervision, J.K. and D.J.N.-P.; Funding Acquisition, K.G.L. and D.J.N.-P. All authors have read and agreed to the published version of the manuscript.

**Funding:** This work was funded by the National Health and Medical Research Council of Australia (1058175) and an Australian Postgraduate Award (K.G.L.).

**Conflicts of Interest:** The authors declare no conflict of interest.

## References

1. Qu, X.; Wang, C.; Zhang, J.; Qie, G.; Zhou, J. The roles of CD147 and/or cyclophilin A in kidney diseases. *Mediat. Inflamm.* **2014**, *2014*, 728673. [CrossRef]
2. Nigro, P.; Pompilio, G.; Capogrossi, M.C. Cyclophilin A: A key player for human disease. *Cell Death Dis.* **2013**, *4*, e888. [CrossRef]
3. Bukrinsky, M. Extracellular cyclophilins in health and disease. *Biochim. Et Biophys. Acta* **2015**, *1850*, 2087–2095. [CrossRef] [PubMed]
4. Heine, S.J.; Olive, D.; Gao, J.L.; Murphy, P.M.; Bukrinsky, M.I.; Constant, S.L. Cyclophilin A cooperates with MIP-2 to augment neutrophil migration. *J. Inflamm. Res.* **2011**, *4*, 93–104. [PubMed]
5. Kim, H.; Kim, W.J.; Jeon, S.T.; Koh, E.M.; Cha, H.S.; Ahn, K.S.; Lee, W.H. Cyclophilin A may contribute to the inflammatory processes in rheumatoid arthritis through induction of matrix degrading enzymes and inflammatory cytokines from macrophages. *Clin. Immunol.* **2005**, *116*, 217–224. [CrossRef] [PubMed]
6. Yuan, W.; Ge, H.; He, B. Pro-inflammatory activities induced by CyPA-EMMPRIN interaction in monocytes. *Atherosclerosis* **2010**, *213*, 415–421. [CrossRef]
7. Dear, J.W.; Simpson, K.J.; Nicolai, M.P.J.; Catterson, J.H.; Street, J.; Huizinga, T.; Craig, D.G.; Dhaliwal, K.; Webb, S.; Bateman, D.N.; et al. Cyclophilin A Is a Damage-Associated Molecular Pattern Molecule That Mediates Acetaminophen-Induced Liver Injury. *J. Immunol.* **2011**, *187*, 3347. [CrossRef]
8. Kalinina, A.; Zamkova, M.; Antoshina, E.; Trukhanova, L.; Gorkova, T.; Kazansky, D.; Khromykh, L. Analyses of the toxic properties of recombinant human Cyclophilin A in mice. *J. Immunotoxicol.* **2019**, *16*, 182–190. [CrossRef]
9. Fossum, S.; Mallett, S.; Barclay, A.N. The MRC OX-47 antigen is a member of the immunoglobulin superfamily with an unusual transmembrane sequence. *Eur. J. Immunol.* **1991**, *21*, 671–679. [CrossRef]
10. Paterson, D.J.; Jefferies, W.A.; Green, J.R.; Brandon, M.R.; Corthesy, P.; Puklavec, M.; Williams, A.F. Antigens of activated rat T lymphocytes including a molecule of 50,000 Mr detected only on CD4 positive T blasts. *Mol. Immunol.* **1987**, *24*, 1281–1290. [CrossRef]
11. Muramatsu, T. Basigin (CD147), a multifunctional transmembrane glycoprotein with various binding partners. *J. Biochem.* **2016**, *159*, 481–490. [CrossRef] [PubMed]
12. Igakura, T.; Kadomatsu, K.; Kaname, T.; Muramatsu, H.; Fan, Q.W.; Miyauchi, T.; Toyama, Y.; Kuno, N.; Yuasa, S.; Takahashi, M.; et al. A null mutation in basigin, an immunoglobulin superfamily member, indicates its important roles in peri-implantation development and spermatogenesis. *Dev. Biol.* **1998**, *194*, 152–165. [CrossRef] [PubMed]
13. Igakura, T.; Kadomatsu, K.; Taguchi, O.; Muramatsu, H.; Kaname, T.; Miyauchi, T.; Yamamura, K.; Arimura, K.; Muramatsu, T. Roles of basigin, a member of the immunoglobulin superfamily, in behavior as to an irritating odor, lymphocyte response, and blood-brain barrier. *Biochem. Biophys. Res. Commun.* **1996**, *224*, 33–36. [CrossRef] [PubMed]
14. O'Neal, J.B.; Shaw, A.D.; Billings, F.T. Acute kidney injury following cardiac surgery: Current understanding and future directions. *Crit. Care* **2016**, *20*, 187. [CrossRef]
15. Peerapornratana, S.; Manrique-Caballero, C.L.; Gomez, H.; Kellum, J.A. Acute kidney injury from sepsis: Current concepts, epidemiology, pathophysiology, prevention and treatment. *Kidney Int.* **2019**, *96*, 1083–1099. [CrossRef]
16. Uber, A.M.; Sutherland, S.M. Nephrotoxins and nephrotoxic acute kidney injury. *Pediatr. Nephrol.* E-pub 24 Oct 2019. [CrossRef]
17. Acedillo, R.R.; Wald, R.; McArthur, E.; Nash, D.M.; Silver, S.A.; James, M.T.; Schull, M.J.; Siew, E.D.; Matheny, M.E.; House, A.A.; et al. Characteristics and Outcomes of Patients Discharged Home from an Emergency Department with AKI. *Clin. J. Am. Soc. Nephrol.* **2017**, *12*, 1215–1225. [CrossRef]
18. Noble, R.A.; Lucas, B.J.; Selby, N.M. Long-Term Outcomes in Patients with Acute Kidney Injury. *Clin. J. Am. Soc. Nephrol.* **2020**, *15*, 423–429. [CrossRef]

19. Lee, C.C.; Chang, C.H.; Cheng, Y.L.; Kuo, G.; Chen, S.W.; Li, Y.J.; Chen, Y.T.; Tian, Y.C. Diagnostic Performance of Cyclophilin A in Cardiac Surgery-Associated Acute Kidney Injury. *J. Clin. Med.* **2019**, *9*, 108. [CrossRef]
20. Chiu, P.F.; Su, S.L.; Tsai, C.C.; Wu, C.L.; Kuo, C.L.; Kor, C.T.; Chang, C.C.; Liu, C.S. Cyclophilin A and CD147 associate with progression of diabetic nephropathy. *Free Radic. Res.* **2018**, *52*, 1456–1463. [CrossRef]
21. Tsai, S.F.; Su, C.W.; Wu, M.J.; Chen, C.H.; Fu, C.P.; Liu, C.S.; Hsieh, M. Urinary Cyclophilin A as a New Marker for Diabetic Nephropathy: A Cross-Sectional Analysis of Diabetes Mellitus. *Medicine* **2015**, *94*, e1802. [CrossRef] [PubMed]
22. Salem, N.A.; El Helaly, R.M.; Ali, I.M.; Ebrahim, H.A.A.; Alayooti, M.M.; El Domiaty, H.A.; Aboelenin, H.M. Urinary Cyclophilin A and serum Cystatin C as biomarkers for diabetic nephropathy in children with type 1 diabetes. *Pediatr. Diabetes* **2020**. [CrossRef] [PubMed]
23. Klausner, J.M.; Paterson, I.S.; Goldman, G.; Kobzik, L.; Rodzen, C.; Lawrence, R.; Valeri, C.R.; Shepro, D.; Hechtman, H.B. Postischemic renal injury is mediated by neutrophils and leukotrienes. *Am. J. Physiol.* **1989**, *256*, F794–F802. [CrossRef]
24. Ryan, J.; Kanellis, J.; Blease, K.; Ma, F.Y.; Nikolic-Paterson, D.J. Spleen Tyrosine Kinase Signaling Promotes Myeloid Cell Recruitment and Kidney Damage after Renal Ischemia/Reperfusion Injury. *Am. J. Pathol.* **2016**, *186*, 2032–2042. [CrossRef] [PubMed]
25. Singbartl, K.; Ley, K. Protection from ischemia-reperfusion induced severe acute renal failure by blocking E-selectin. *Crit. Care Med.* **2000**, *28*, 2507–2514. [CrossRef] [PubMed]
26. Guo, G.; Morrissey, J.; McCracken, R.; Tolley, T.; Liapis, H.; Klahr, S. Contributions of angiotensin II and tumor necrosis factor-alpha to the development of renal fibrosis. *Am. J. Physiol. Ren. Physiol.* **2001**, *280*, F777–F785. [CrossRef]
27. Buchtler, S.; Grill, A.; Hofmarksrichter, S.; Stockert, P.; Schiechl-Brachner, G.; Rodriguez Gomez, M.; Neumayer, S.; Schmidbauer, K.; Talke, Y.; Klinkhammer, B.M.; et al. Cellular Origin and Functional Relevance of Collagen I Production in the Kidney. *J. Am. Soc. Nephrol.* **2018**, *29*, 1859–1873. [CrossRef]
28. Henderson, N.C.; Mackinnon, A.C.; Farnworth, S.L.; Kipari, T.; Haslett, C.; Iredale, J.P.; Liu, F.T.; Hughes, J.; Sethi, T. Galectin-3 expression and secretion links macrophages to the promotion of renal fibrosis. *Am. J. Pathol.* **2008**, *172*, 288–298. [CrossRef]
29. Kitagawa, K.; Wada, T.; Furuichi, K.; Hashimoto, H.; Ishiwata, Y.; Asano, M.; Takeya, M.; Kuziel, W.A.; Matsushima, K.; Mukaida, N.; et al. Blockade of CCR2 ameliorates progressive fibrosis in kidney. *Am. J. Pathol.* **2004**, *165*, 237–246. [CrossRef]
30. Sung, S.A.; Jo, S.K.; Cho, W.Y.; Won, N.H.; Kim, H.K. Reduction of renal fibrosis as a result of liposome encapsulated clodronate induced macrophage depletion after unilateral ureteral obstruction in rats. *Nephron Exp. Nephrol.* **2007**, *105*, e1–e9. [CrossRef]
31. Pefanis, A.; Ierino, F.L.; Murphy, J.M.; Cowan, P.J. Regulated necrosis in kidney ischemia-reperfusion injury. *Kidney Int.* **2019**, *96*, 291–301. [CrossRef] [PubMed]
32. Devalaraja-Narashimha, K.; Diener, A.M.; Padanilam, B.J. Cyclophilin D gene ablation protects mice from ischemic renal injury. *Am. J. Physiol. Ren. Physiol.* **2009**, *297*, F749–F759. [CrossRef] [PubMed]
33. Hou, W.; Leong, K.G.; Ozols, E.; Tesch, G.H.; Nikolic-Paterson, D.J.; Ma, F.Y. Cyclophilin D promotes tubular cell damage and the development of interstitial fibrosis in the obstructed kidney. *Clin. Exp. Pharm. Physiol.* **2018**, *45*, 250–260. [CrossRef] [PubMed]
34. Christofferson, D.E.; Yuan, J. Cyclophilin A release as a biomarker of necrotic cell death. *Cell Death Differ.* **2010**, *17*, 1942–1943. [CrossRef]
35. Ferenbach, D.A.; Sheldrake, T.A.; Dhaliwal, K.; Kipari, T.M.; Marson, L.P.; Kluth, D.C.; Hughes, J. Macrophage/monocyte depletion by clodronate, but not diphtheria toxin, improves renal ischemia/reperfusion injury in mice. *Kidney Int.* **2012**, *82*, 928–933. [CrossRef]
36. Singh, D.; Chander, V.; Chopra, K. Cyclosporine protects against ischemia/reperfusion injury in rat kidneys. *Toxicology* **2005**, *207*, 339–347. [CrossRef]
37. Seizer, P.; Ochmann, C.; Schonberger, T.; Zach, S.; Rose, M.; Borst, O.; Klingel, K.; Kandolf, R.; MacDonald, H.R.; Nowak, R.A.; et al. Disrupting the EMMPRIN (CD147)-cyclophilin A interaction reduces infarct size and preserves systolic function after myocardial ischemia and reperfusion. *Arterioscler. Thromb. Vasc. Biol.* **2011**, *31*, 1377–1386. [CrossRef]

38. Kato, N.; Yuzawa, Y.; Kosugi, T.; Hobo, A.; Sato, W.; Miwa, Y.; Sakamoto, K.; Matsuo, S.; Kadomatsu, K. The E-selectin ligand basigin/CD147 is responsible for neutrophil recruitment in renal ischemia/reperfusion. *J. Am. Soc. Nephrol.* **2009**, *20*, 1565–1576. [CrossRef]
39. Liu, L.; Kou, P.; Zeng, Q.; Pei, G.; Li, Y.; Liang, H.; Xu, G.; Chen, S. CD4+ T Lymphocytes, especially Th2 cells, contribute to the progress of renal fibrosis. *Am. J. Nephrol.* **2012**, *36*, 386–396. [CrossRef]
40. Nikolic-Paterson, D.J. CD4+ T cells: A potential player in renal fibrosis. *Kidney Int.* **2010**, *78*, 333–335. [CrossRef]
41. Tapmeier, T.T.; Fearn, A.; Brown, K.; Chowdhury, P.; Sacks, S.H.; Sheerin, N.S.; Wong, W. Pivotal role of CD4+ T cells in renal fibrosis following ureteric obstruction. *Kidney Int.* **2010**, *78*, 351–362. [CrossRef] [PubMed]
42. Anders, H.J.; Vielhauer, V.; Frink, M.; Linde, Y.; Cohen, C.D.; Blattner, S.M.; Kretzler, M.; Strutz, F.; Mack, M.; Grone, H.J.; et al. A chemokine receptor CCR-1 antagonist reduces renal fibrosis after unilateral ureter ligation. *J. Clin. Investig.* **2002**, *109*, 251–259. [CrossRef]
43. Sarro, E.; Duran, M.; Rico, A.; Bou-Teen, D.; Fernandez-Majada, V.; Croatt, A.J.; Nath, K.A.; Salcedo, M.T.; Gundelach, J.H.; Batlle, D.; et al. Cyclophilins A and B Oppositely Regulate Renal Tubular Epithelial Cell Phenotype. *J. Mol. Cell Biol.* E-pub 12 March 2020. [CrossRef] [PubMed]
44. Kato, N.; Kosugi, T.; Sato, W.; Ishimoto, T.; Kojima, H.; Sato, Y.; Sakamoto, K.; Maruyama, S.; Yuzawa, Y.; Matsuo, S.; et al. Basigin/CD147 promotes renal fibrosis after unilateral ureteral obstruction. *Am. J. Pathol.* **2011**, *178*, 572–579. [CrossRef] [PubMed]
45. Ma, F.Y.; Tesch, G.H.; Nikolic-Paterson, D.J. ASK1/p38 signaling in renal tubular epithelial cells promotes renal fibrosis in the mouse obstructed kidney. *Am. J. Physiol. Ren. Physiol.* **2014**, *307*, F1263–F1273. [CrossRef]
46. Ma, F.Y.; Tesch, G.H.; Ozols, E.; Xie, M.; Schneider, M.D.; Nikolic-Paterson, D.J. TGF-beta1-activated kinase-1 regulates inflammation and fibrosis in the obstructed kidney. *Am. J. Physiol. Ren. Physiol.* **2011**, *300*, F1410–F1421. [CrossRef]

International Journal of
*Molecular Sciences*

MDPI

*Article*

# Cilastatin Preconditioning Attenuates Renal Ischemia-Reperfusion Injury via Hypoxia Inducible Factor-1α Activation

**Yu Ah Hong [1], So Young Jung [2], Keum Jin Yang [2], Dai Sig Im [3,4], Kyung Hwan Jeong [5], Cheol Whee Park [1] and Hyeon Seok Hwang [5,*]**

1 Division of Nephrology, Department of Internal Medicine, The Catholic University of Korea, Seoul 06591, Korea; amorfati@catholic.ac.kr (Y.A.H.); cheolwhee@catholic.ac.kr (C.W.P.)
2 Clinical Research Institute, Daejeon St. Mary's Hospital, Daejeon 34943, Korea; syzzim84@gmail.com (S.Y.J.); nadia@cnu.ac.kr (K.J.Y.)
3 Department of Chemistry, College of Natural Sciences, Soonchunhyang University, Asan 31538, Korea; dsim@sch.ac.kr
4 SH Company, 507, SCH BIT Business Incubator B/D, 22 Soonchunhyang-ro, Shinchang, Asan, Chungnam 31538, Korea
5 Division of Nephrology, Department of Internal Medicine, College of Medicine, Kyung Hee University, Seoul 02447, Korea; khjeong@khu.ac.kr
* Correspondence: hwanghsne@gmail.com; Tel.: +82-2-958-8114

Received: 17 April 2020; Accepted: 16 May 2020; Published: 19 May 2020

check for updates

**Abstract:** Cilastatin is a specific inhibitor of renal dehydrodipeptidase-1. We investigated whether cilastatin preconditioning attenuates renal ischemia-reperfusion (IR) injury via hypoxia inducible factor-1α (HIF-1α) activation. Human proximal tubular cell line (HK-2) was exposed to ischemia, and male C57BL/6 mice were subjected to bilateral kidney ischemia and reperfusion. The effects of cilastatin preconditioning were investigated both in vitro and in vivo. In HK-2 cells, cilastatin upregulated HIF-1α expression in a time- and dose-dependent manner. Cilastatin enhanced HIF-1α translation via the phosphorylation of Akt and mTOR was followed by the upregulation of erythropoietin (EPO) and vascular endothelial growth factor (VEGF). Cilastatin did not affect the expressions of PHD and VHL. However, HIF-1α ubiquitination was significantly decreased after cilastatin treatment. Cilastatin prevented the IR-induced cell death. These cilastatin effects were reversed by co-treatment of HIF-1α inhibitor or HIF-1α small interfering RNA. Similarly, HIF-1α expression and its upstream and downstream signaling were significantly enhanced in cilastatin-treated kidney. In mouse kidney with IR injury, cilastatin treatment decreased HIF-1α ubiquitination independent of PHD and VHL expression. Serum creatinine level and tubular necrosis, and apoptosis were reduced in cilastatin-treated kidney with IR injury, and co-treatment of cilastatin with an HIF-1α inhibitor reversed these effects. Thus, cilastatin preconditioning attenuated renal IR injury via HIF-1α activation.

**Keywords:** cilastatin; hypoxia inducible factor-1-α; ischemia-reperfusion injury

## 1. Introduction

Renal ischemia-reperfusion (IR) injury is a major cause of acute kidney injury [1]. Acute ischemic injury produces excessive apoptotic cell death, and several studies have explored various stimuli to reduce injury processes [2,3]. Hypoxia-inducible factor-1α (HIF-1α) is the master regulator of cell response to hypoxia [4]. It increases the expression of several genes, including angiogenic growth factors, erythropoietin, and nitric oxide synthases [5–7]. Activation of these genes enhances adaptation to hypoxia and improves cell survival. Therefore, it is reasonable that HIF-1α activation before IR injury might exhibit protective effects.

Cilastatin is a molecule designed to inhibit brush border–sorted dehydrogenase peptide-1 (DHP-1). In current clinical settings, cilastatin is used to prevent the hydrolysis of antibiotics and decrease antibiotic-induced nephrotoxicity [8]. Previous in vitro and in vivo experimental studies have demonstrated that cilastatin has antioxidant and anti-apoptotic effects in drug-induced nephropathy, such as cisplatin, calcineurin inhibitor, and vancomycin [9–12]. These effects of cilastatin were associated with reduced accumulation of drug within the kidney and renal proximal tubular epithelial cells. However, the cilastatin effect is rarely investigated in the non-pharmacological renal injury. Moreover, it is unclear that cilastatin exhibits protective effects on kidney injuries.

Cilastatin binds to lipid raft in which DHP-1 is embedded. The lipid raft acts as a major platform for signaling regulation and controls Akt signaling pathways [13,14]. The Akt/mammalian target of rapamycin (mTOR) pathway is potent regulator of HIF-1α expression at translational or transcriptional level [15,16]. Therefore, cilastatin treatment can modulate the HIF-1α activity via lipid raft-related signaling pathway. However, it is less known that the cilastatin as a preconditioning stimulus activates HIF-1α pathway and the underlying mechanism of cilastatin treatment is not evaluated in the renal IR injury.

Therefore, we investigated whether preconditioning with cilastatin exhibits renoprotective effects in a mouse model of IR injury, and whether cilastatin is effective in preventing proximal tubular cell death after IR injury. We hypothesized that cilastatin treatment activates HIF-1α signaling pathway, which leads to protective effects against renal IR injury.

## 2. Results

### 2.1. Cilastatin Upregulates HIF-1α and Its Downstream Effector in HK-2 Cells

Figure 1 shows the effects of cilastatin on HIF-1α expression in HK-2 cells. The expression of HIF-1α was significantly increased after cilastatin treatment in a dose- and time-dependent manner (Figure 1A,B). However, the HIF-1α mRNA level was not affected in cilastatin-treated HK-2 cells (Figure S1). Downstream effectors of HIF-1α, such as erythropoietin (EPO) and vascular endothelial growth factor (VEGF), were significantly upregulated after cilastatin treatment, respectively (Figure 1C).

### 2.2. Cilastatin Upregulates HIF-1α and Its Downstream Effector in HK-2 Cells

We studied the involved phase of protein synthesis for HIF-1α in HK-2 cells. The Akt/mTOR pathway was evaluated to assess the upstream signaling of HIF-1α, which translated the HIF-1α protein. The phosphorylation of Akt was significantly increased with maximal expression occurring at 6 h after cilastatin treatment. The phosphorylation of mTOR was also enhanced in a time-dependent manner (Figure 2A). To confirm whether HIF-1α upregulation was dependent on Akt/mTOR pathway, we exposed the cells to cilastatin in the presence of rapamycin, an mTOR inhibitor. Cilastatin increased HIF-1α expression, and co-treatment of rapamycin with cilastatin significantly reversed the HIF-1α upregulation (Figure 2B).

We conducted further experiments to investigate whether HIF-1α upregulation is dependent on lipid raft, because lipid raft modulates p-Akt/Akt signaling pathways [13,14]. The disruption of lipid raft with methyl-β-cyclodextrin (MβCD) significantly suppressed the HIF-1α expression when cilastatin increased HIF-1α expression (Figure 2C).

### 2.3. PHD/VHL-Independent Ubiquitination Pathway is Involved in Cilastatin-Mediated HIF-1α Upregulation in HK-2 cells

To identify whether cilastatin preconditioning activates HIF-1α by impairing its degradation pathway, the expression levels of prolyl hydroxylase domain (PHD) and von Hippel-Lindau (VHL) protein were evaluated. Cilastatin did not significantly alter the expression of PHD and VHL (Figure 3) compared to control. Therefore, cilastatin did not activate HIF-1α through the canonical HIF-1α degradation pathway. We further evaluated the interaction between HIF-1α and ubiquitin. In contrast to previous results, HIF-1α/ubiquitin complex formation was decreased after cilastatin preconditioning compared to control cells. These results suggested that cilastatin-induced HIF-1α activation was closely associated with decreased ubiquitination independent of PHD and VHL expression.

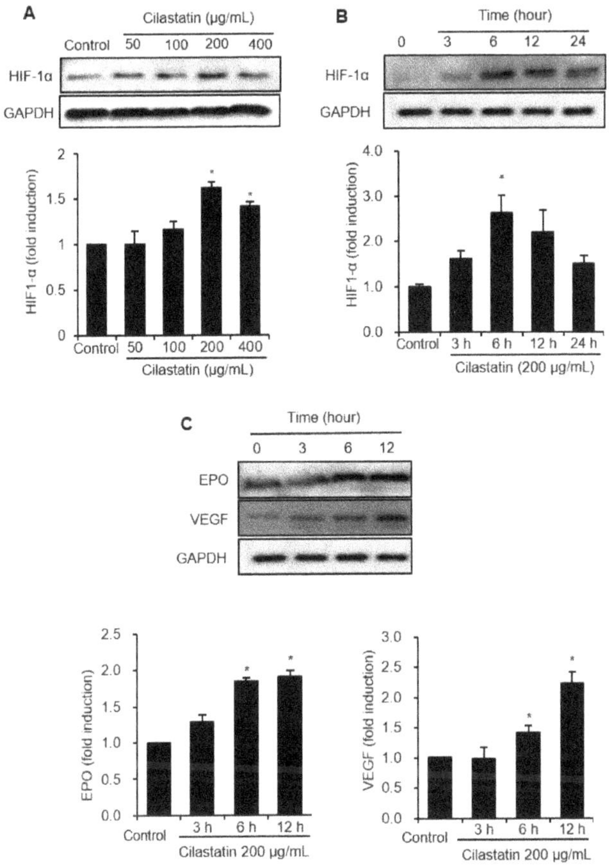


**Figure 1.** Cilastatin treatment upregulated the expressions of HIF-1α and its downstream pathway in HK-2 cells. (**A**) Semiquantitative immunoblotting revealed upregulation of HIF-1α expression by cilastatin treatment in a dose-dependent manner. (**B**) Semiquantitative immunoblotting revealed upregulation of HIF-1α expression by treatment with 200 μg/mL cilastatin in a time-dependent manner. (**C**) The expressions of VEGF and EPO proteins, determined by semiquantitative immunoblotting, were significantly elevated by treatment with 200 μg/mL cilastatin in a time-dependent manner as compared to untreated control. The data are presented as means ± SEM. * $p < 0.05$ vs. control.

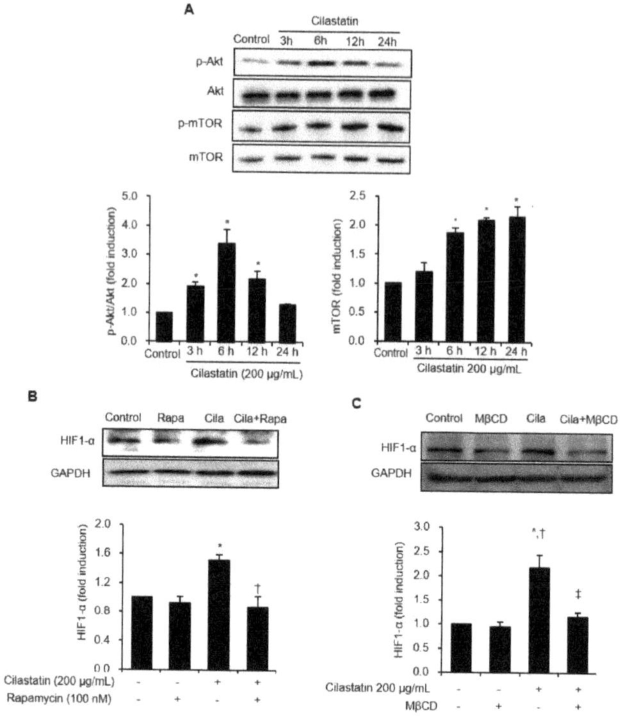


**Figure 2.** Cilastatin treatment induced HIF-1α expression via Akt/mTOR dependent pathway in HK-2 cells. (**A**) Semiquantitative immunoblotting revealed increase in Akt and mTOR expression by treatment with 200 μg/mL cilastatin in a time-dependent manner. The data are presented as means ± SEM. $^{*}p < 0.05$ vs. control. (**B**) Cilastatin pretreatment increased HIF-1α expression and the treatment of rapamycin, an mTOR inhibitor, significantly decreased HIF-1α expression despite cilastatin pretreatment. The data are presented as means ± SEM. * $p < 0.05$ vs. control, † $p < 0.05$ vs. rapamycin, and ‡$p < 0.05$ vs. cilastatin. (**C**) Cilastatin treatment increased HIF-1α expression and the destruction of lipid raft by MβCD significantly decreased HIF-1α expression despite cilastatin treatment. The data are presented as means ± SEM. * $p < 0.05$ vs. control, † $p < 0.05$ vs. MβCD, and ‡ $p < 0.05$ vs. cilastatin.

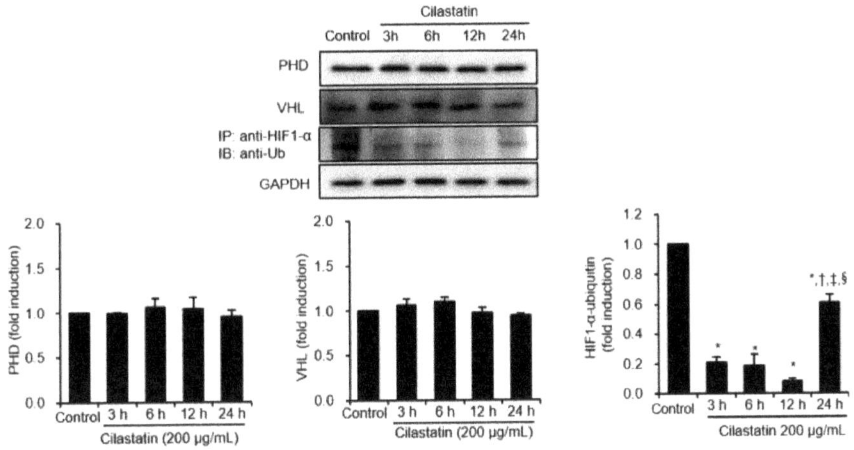


**Figure 3.** Cilastatin preconditioning upregulated HIF-1α expression via the inhibition of ubiquitination in HK-2 cells. Semiquantitative immunoblotting showed that cilastatin pretreatment did not affect the levels of VHL and PHD expressions. Immunoprecipitation showed that HIF-1α/ubiquitin complex formation was significantly suppressed in cilastatin-treated HK-2 cells compared to control in a time-dependent manner, but it was significantly increased at 24 h after cilastatin pretreatment. The data are presented as means ± SEM. *$p < 0.05$ vs. control, †,‡,§ $p < 0.05$ vs. 3 h, 6 h, and 12 h after cilastatin treatment.

### 2.4. Cilastatin Preconditioning Enhances HIF-1α-Mediated Cell Survival in IR-Exposed HK-2 Cells

We evaluated whether cilastatin preconditioning provided protection against IR injury in HK-2 cells and whether HIF-1α mediated its protective effects. Cilastatin preconditioning and IR exposure increased HIF-1α level compared with control group (Figure 4A). Cilastatin preconditioning further enhanced the HIF-1α expression in IR-exposed cells than in non-exposed cells. IR exposure significantly reduced cell viability compared to the control group and cilastatin prevented this IR-induced cell death. The protective effect of cilastatin in IR-exposed cells was reversed by the co-treatment of YC-1, which downregulated HIF-1α at the post-translational level (Figure 4B). To evaluate whether the enhanced cell survival was associated with the specific activation of HIF-1α, we performed further experiments using HIF-1α small interfering (si) RNA. The viability of cells treated with HIF-1α siRNA was similar to that of control cells and HIF-1α siRNA treatment blocked the protective effects of cilastatin (Figure 4C).

### 2.5. Cilastatin Upregulates HIF-1α Expression Via Akt/mTOR Pathway in Mouse Kidney

Next, we investigated the effect of cilastatin treatment in mouse kidney. The expression of HIF-1α was significantly increased after cilastatin treatment in a time-dependent pattern (Figure 5A). The effect of cilastatin treatment on the ubiquitination pathway was evaluated in mouse kidney, and it was found that cilastatin did not affect the expressions of PHD and VHL. The expression of VEGF, which is downstream of HIF-1α, was also increased in mouse kidney. Similar to in vitro study, cilastatin treatment significantly increased the phosphorylation of both Akt and mTOR (Figure 5B).

### 2.6. Cilastatin Preconditioning Activates HIF-1α Signaling Pathway in Renal IR Injury

As shown in Figure 6, HIF-1α/ubiquitin complex formation was significantly suppressed in mice with IR injury, and cilastatin preconditioning further inhibited this complex formation. HIF-1α expression in immunoblot was significantly increased in mice with IR injury, and it was further increased after cilastatin preconditioning. The expression of EPO, a downstream effector of HIF-1α, was significantly increased in sham-operated mice with cilastatin preconditioning. IR injury reduced the EPO expression in mouse kidney, which recovered in cilastatin-treated mice with IR injury.

### 2.7. *Cilastatin Preconditioning Protects Against Renal IR Injury*

Serum creatinine levels were significantly increased at 24 h after IR injury compared with those in sham-operated mice (Figure 7A). Cilastatin preconditioning improved serum creatinine levels compared with the mice without cilastatin preconditioning. Histologic examination of tissue sections indicated extensive tubular necrosis in the kidneys of ischemic mice compared with those of sham-operated mice (Figure 7B). Tubular necrosis was improved in the cilastatin-treated mice with IR injury compared with those not treated with cilastatin.

### 2.8. *Cilastatin Preconditioning Attenuates Apoptosis in Renal IR Injury*

The number of terminal deoxynucleotidyl transferase-mediated dUTP nick end-labeling (TUNEL)-positive cells was increased in mice with IR injury compared to those of sham-operated mice, and it was decreased in cilastatin-treated mice with IR injury (Figure 8A). IR injury increased the expression of the proapoptotic protein Bcl-2-associated X (Bax) and decreased the expression of the antiapoptotic protein B-cell lymphoma 2 (Bcl-2). Cilastatin preconditioning significantly attenuated Bax levels and increased Bcl-2 expression in ischemic mouse kidney (Figure 8B).

### 2.9. *Cilastatin Protects Against Renal IR Injury Via HIF-1α Pathway*

Cilastatin attenuates renal dysfunction in mouse kidney with IR injury, and co-treatment with YC-1 restored IR injury to a great extent (Figure 9A). The quantitative tubular necrosis score of YC-1 co-treated ischemic mouse kidney was significantly higher than that of the mouse kidney treated with only cilastatin (Figure 9B).

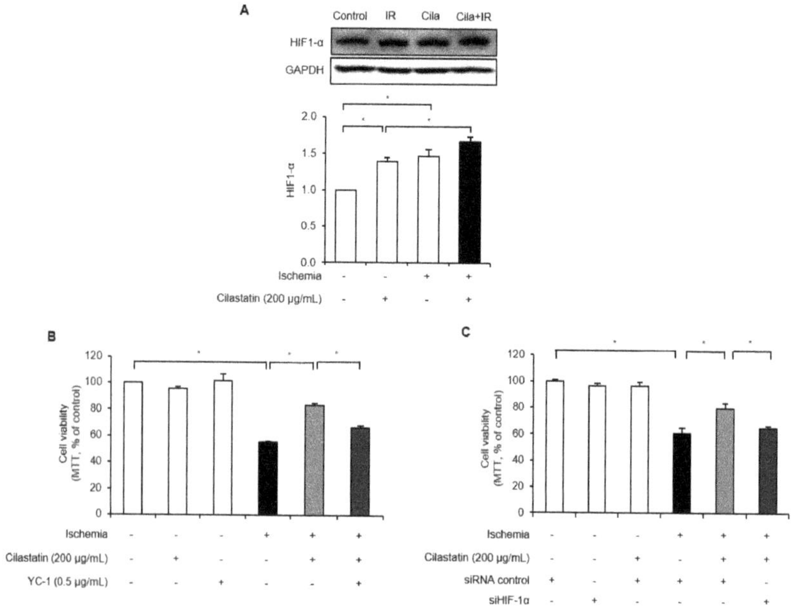


**Figure 4.** Cilastatin preconditioning protected IR-induced cell death via the activation of HIF-1α in HK-2 cells. (**A**) Semiquantitative immunoblotting of HIF-1α expression revealed that IR injury upregulated HIF-1α expression and cilastatin pretreatment further enhanced HIF-1α expression in IR-exposed cells. Cilastatin treatment also prevented IR-induced cell death. Co-treatment with cilastatin and (**B**) HIF-1α inhibitor, YC-1, or (**C**) HIF-1α siRNA restored cell death similar to those of IR-exposed cells without cilastatin treatment. The data are presented as means ± SEM. * $p < 0.05$.

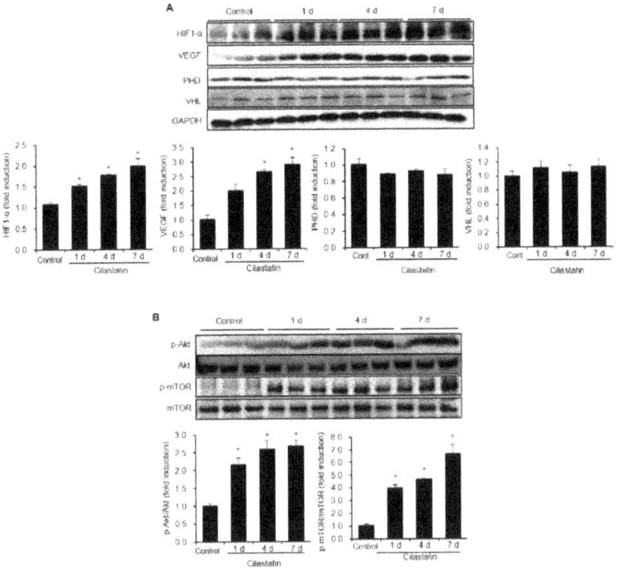


**Figure 5.** Cilastatin treatment upregulated HIF-1α expression and its upstream and downstream signaling pathways in mouse kidney. (**A**) Cilastatin treatment enhanced HIF-1α and VEGF expression in a time-dependent manner in mouse kidney, but it did not affect VHL and PHD expression. (**B**) Cilastatin treatment enhanced Akt and mt Or phosphorylation in a time-dependent manner in mouse kidney. The data are presented as means ± SEM. * $p < 0.05$.

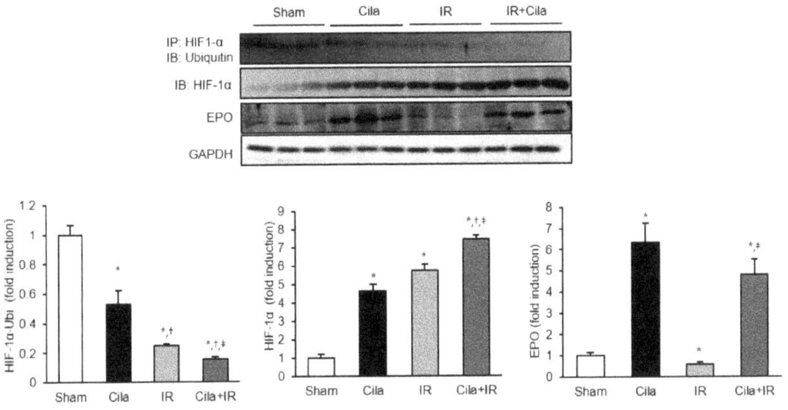


**Figure 6.** Cilastatin preconditioning upregulated HIF-1α expression and its downstream signaling pathway and decreased the ubiquitination of HIF-1α in mouse kidney with IR injury. Immunoprecipitation showed that HIF-1α/ubiquitin complex formation was significantly decreased in mouse kidney with IR injury compared to sham-operated mice; however, it more significantly decreased in cilastatin-treated mouse kidney with IR injury. Therefore, semiquantitative immunoblotting revealed that HIF-1α expression markedly increased in cilastatin-treated mouse kidney with IR injury compared to other groups. EPO expression was significantly increased in cilastatin-treated mouse kidney and was decreased in mouse kidney with IR injury; however, it increased in cilastatin-treated mouse kidney with IR injury. The data are presented as means ± SEM.* $p < 0.05$ vs. sham group; † $p < 0.05$ vs. Cila group; ‡ $p < 0.05$ vs. IR group.

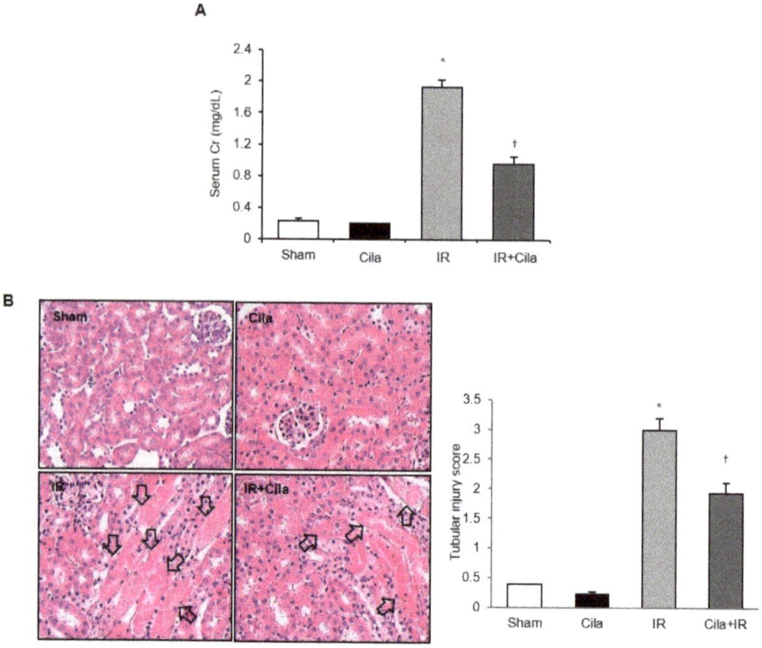


**Figure 7.** Cilastatin preconditioning improved renal function and tubular necrosis in mouse kidney with IR injury. (**A**) Serum creatinine levels were significantly increased at 24 h after IR injury compared with serum creatinine levels in sham-operated mice. Cilastatin pretreatment improved serum creatinine level in mouse kidney with IR injury. (**B**) The representative staining with hematoxylin and eosin showed a decreased tubular necrosis (arrows) in the cilastatin-treated mouse kidney with IR injury compared with mouse kidney with IR injury not treated with cilastatin (original magnification, × 200). The data are presented as means ± SEM. * $p < 0.05$ vs. sham and Cila group; † $p < 0.05$ vs. IR group.

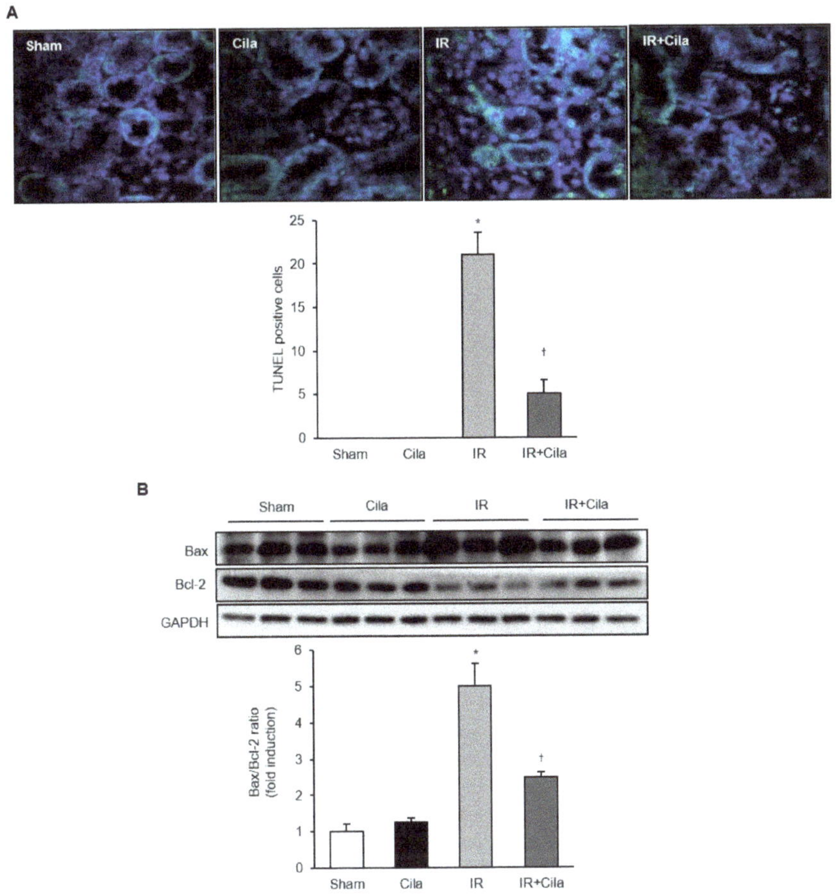


**Figure 8.** Cilastatin preconditioning attenuates apoptosis in mouse kidney with IR injury. (**A**) TUNEL assay revealed that cilastatin pretreatment significantly attenuated number of TUNEL-positive cells in mouse kidney with IR injury (original magnification, ×400). (**B**) Semiquantitative immunoblotting indicated that the level of pro-apoptotic marker, Bax, decreased in cilastatin-treated mouse kidney with IR injury, compared with mouse kidney with IR injury alone. Significant increase in levels of anti-apoptotic marker protein, Bcl-2, was noted after cilastatin pretreatment in mouse kidney with IR injury. The data are presented as means ± SEM. * $p < 0.05$ vs. sham and cila group; † $p < 0.05$ vs. IR group.

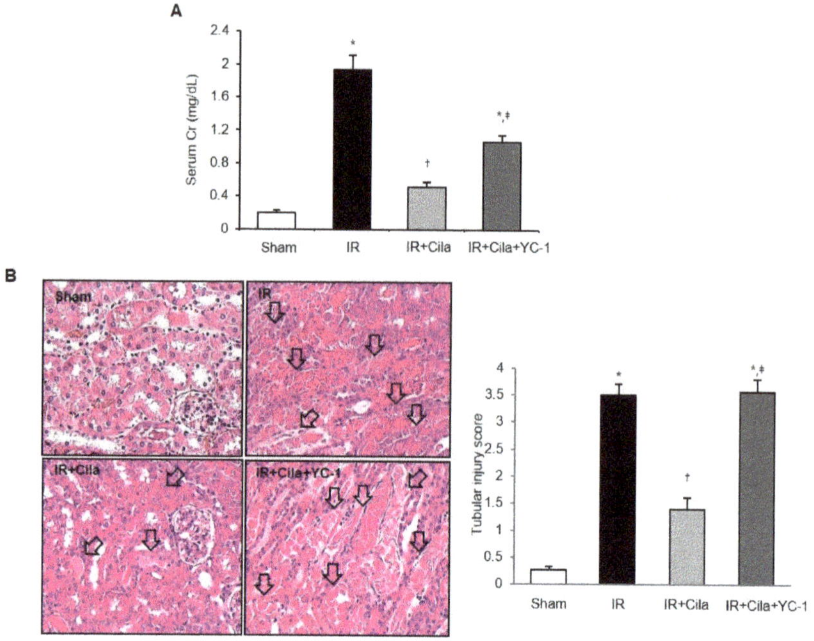


**Figure 9.** The co-treatment of YC-1, an HIF-1α inhibitor, with cilastatin worsened renal function and tubular necrosis in mouse kidney with IR injury. (**A**) Serum creatinine levels were significantly increased at 24 h after IR injury and decreased in mouse kidney with IR injury with cilastatin pretreatment. Co-treatment with cilastatin and YC-1 exacerbated renal function in mouse kidney with IR injury. (**B**) The representative staining with hematoxylin and eosin showed a decreased tubular necrosis (arrows) in the cilastatin-treated mouse kidney with IR injury, and aggravated tubular necrosis in mouse kidney with IR injury co-treated with cilastatin and YC-1 (original magnification, × 200). The data are presented as means ± SEM. * $p < 0.05$ vs. sham; † $p < 0.05$ vs. IR group; ‡ $p < 0.05$ vs. IR + Cila group.

## 3. Discussion

Our study demonstrated that cilastatin preconditioning induced the upregulation of HIF-1α via activation of Akt/mTOR pathway and inhibition of PHD/VHL-independent ubiquitination pathway. The cilastatin-induced HIF-1α upregulation prevented proximal tubular cell death during IR injury. In mouse kidney, cilastatin preconditioning again upregulated HIF-1α expression in the same fashion and the activated HIF-1α pathway suppressed renal dysfunction, tubular damage, and apoptotic cell death after IR injury. These findings suggested that cilastatin preconditioning exhibits protective effects against renal IR injury via HIF-1α activation.

Preconditioning refers to exposure to a stimulus to protect organs or tissues before subjection to ischemic injury, and HIF-1α has been implicated as an attractive target pathway for ischemic preconditioning for prevention against acute kidney injury [17,18]. Our study demonstrated that cilastatin preconditioning increased the expression of HIF-1α protein and enhanced its downstream pathway. In addition, the destruction of lipid raft blocked cilastatin-induced HIF-1α expression. These findings suggested that cilastatin effectively activates HIF-1α signaling pathway and that cell membrane structure having an affinity with cilastatin is important to activate a preconditioning target.

HIF-1α is mainly located in proximal tubular cells and can be upregulated at transcriptional or translational level [17,19]. Therefore, we investigated the mRNA level of HIF-1α and Akt/mTOR pathway. We found that phosphorylated Akt/mTOR level was abundant after cilastatin preconditioning and the inhibition of mTOR pathway reduced the HIF-1α expression in cilastatin-treated HK-2 cells.

However, cilastatin preconditioning did not increase the HIF-1α mRNA level in HK-2 cells. These findings demonstrated that cilastatin induces the expression of HIF-1α at the translational level, not at the transcriptional level.

HIF-1α expression can be enhanced via the enhanced Akt/mTOR pathway or by impairment of ubiquitin-proteasome degradation pathway [20,21]. Under normoxic conditions, PHD enzymes hydroxylated a subunit of HIF-1α and VHL captured them to undergo ubiquitin-protease pathway resulting in HIF-1α degradation [21,22]. However, ubiquitination of HIF-1α is also modulated via an oxygen/PHD/VHL-independent pathway involving the p53, glycogen synthase kinase 3, and the molecular chaperone 90 kDa heat-shock proteins [23–25]. In the present study, we demonstrated that the expressions of PHD and VHL were not altered in both HK-2 cells and mouse kidney after cilastatin preconditioning. On the other hand, immunoprecipitation analysis showed that the interactive binding between HIF-1α and ubiquitin was significantly decreased in cilastatin-treated cells under normoxic condition. Furthermore, the interaction between HIF-1α and ubiquitin was significantly decreased in mouse kidney with IR injury, and was further suppressed in cilastatin-treated mouse kidney with IR injury. These findings suggested that cilastatin may suppress HIF-1α degradation via the PHD and VHL-independent ubiquitin pathway in both normoxic and hypoxic condition.

Upregulation of renal HIF-1α plays an important role in the protection against IR injury and several studies reported HIF-1α as a potential therapeutic target [26,27]. Our study demonstrated that IR injury increased the expression of HIF-1α in proximal tubular cells and mouse kidney, and cilastatin preconditioning further increased the expression of HIF-1α. In addition, HIF-1α siRNA transfection or co-treatment with an YC-1 significantly reversed the protective effects of cilastatin in terms of proximal tubular cell death, renal dysfunction, and tubular necrosis. These data suggested that activation of HIF-1α signaling pathway plays a pivotal role in the renoprotective effect of cilastatin in IR injury.

HIF-1α regulates the adaptive response to hypoxia and other stresses by orchestrating the transcription of protective genes [17]. EPO, a representative downstream effector of HIF-1α, prevents apoptotic cell death, and promotes tubular cell regeneration during renal IR injury [28,29]. HIF-1α activation also activates the anti-apoptotic protein, bcl-2 in renal IR injury [30,31]. Our study showed that cilastatin preconditioning upregulated the expression of EPO and decreased apoptosis in mouse kidney with IR injury. These findings suggested that cilastatin-induced HIF-1α upregulation activates downstream effectors to reduce apoptosis during renal IR injury.

There are some interesting points and limitation in this study. Nuclear factor-erythroid-2-related factor 2 (Nrf2) is a transcription factor that regulates genes encoding antioxidant and detoxifying molecules [32,33]. It is known that Nrf2 has preventive effects against drug nephrotoxicity and ischemia reperfusion injury [34,35]. Therefore, cilastatin effects on Nrf2 is the attractive target as potential protective mechanism. Furthermore, we found Akt phosphorylation was decreased at 12 and 24 hours in cilastatin preconditioning. The reduced Akt activity was simply associated with limited working time of cilastatin. Otherwise, feedback from mTOR activation might negatively regulate the Akt activity [36,37]. The phosphorylation of mTOR at 12 h and 24 h in this experiment also supports this hypothesis. Finally, preconditioning effect of cilastatin has limitation in the clinical setting, because renal damage is already underway without preconditioning patients. Therefore, further experiments on the rescue effect of cilastatin after IR injury are required to increase the clinical usefulness.

In conclusion, cilastatin preconditioning protects against renal IR injury via the HIF-1α dependent pathway. Cilastatin preconditioning upregulated the HIF-1α expression by enhancing translational efficiency involving the Akt/mTOR pathway and by suppressing PHD/VHL-independent ubiquitination pathway. Our study provided evidence of the protective effects of cilastatin in non-pharmacological renal injury and demonstrated that the wide clinical application of cilastatin could be expected to prevent acute kidney injury.

## 4. Materials and Methods

### 4.1. Human Proximal Tubular Cell Culturing

HK-2 cells were purchased from American Type Culture Collection (Manassas, VA, USA). The cells were grown and passaged in Dulbecco's modified Eagle's medium (DMEM) supplemented with 10% fetal bovine serum, 50 U/mL penicillin, and 50 μg/mL streptomycin. The cells were cultivated in a humidified 5% CO2 environment at 37 °C. HK-2 cells were plated and cultured to 80% confluence.

HK-2 cells were treated with different doses of cilastatin for different times. The control cells were treated with distilled water. We also harvested the cells 24 h after co-treatment of cilastatin and MβCD (Sigma-Aldrich, St Louis, MO, USA), or mTOR inhibitor (rapamycin, Sigma-Aldrich, St Louis, MO, USA).

HK-2 cells were placed in serum-free media for 16 h at 80% confluence and were pretreated with cilastatin, HIF-1α inhibitor, YC-1 [38], or HIF-1α siRNA (Bioneer, Daejeon, Korea) for 1 h. Scrambled siRNA were complexed with a transfection reagent (Invitrogen, Carlsbad, CA, USA). After washing with phosphate-buffered saline (PBS), they were exposed to ischemia by immersing the cellular monolayer in mineral oil (Sigma-Aldrich, St Louis, MO, USA) for 90 min [39]. Then, the cells were washed twice and then received the same treatment.

### 4.2. Cell Viability

A commercially available MTT assay kit (EZ-Cytox; Daeil Lab Service, Seoul, Korea) determined cell viability. After exposure to ischemia and 24 h reperfusion, 10 μL of cell viability assay reagent was added. The optical densities of the samples were determined at 450 nm in a microplate reader (Bio-Rad Laboratories, Hercules, CA, USA).

### 4.3. Animal Model of Renal IR Injury

Seven- to eight-week-old male C57BL/6J mice were housed under a 12 h light–dark cycle, and food and water were freely available. Crystalline cilastatin was kindly provided by Im DS (Department of Chemistry, Soonchunhyang University, Cheonan, Korea). The experimental protocol was approved by the animal experiments' ethics committee of Daejeon St. Mary's Hospital (1st February 2016, CMCDJ-AP-2016-009).

Mice were divided into five groups (sham, sham + cilastatin, IR, IR + cilastatin, and IR + cilastatin + YC-1) and each group consisted of six mice. Cilastatin was diluted in saline, and 300 mg/kg of cilastatin, with or without YC-1 (5 mg/kg/day), was intraperitoneally injected daily for seven consecutive days before ischemia induction. The sham and IR groups of mice received the same volume of saline. Renal IR injury was performed under tiletamine–zolazepam (30 mg/kg) and xylazine (10 mg/kg) anesthesia. The mice were subjected to renal IR injury using previously described methods [40–42]. The bilateral renal pedicles were occluded for 23 min using microvascular clamps. A homoeothermic pad maintained the core body temperature of mice. The mice were sacrificed 24 h after ischemia and tissue and blood samples were collected.

### 4.4. Functional and Morphological Changes due to Kidney Injury

Serum creatinine level was measured by an IDEXX VetTest® Chemistry Analyzer (IDEXX Laboratories, Inc., Westbrook, ME, USA). The kidney tissues were fixed in 10% formalin buffer, embedded in paraffin, and then, cut into 3.5 mm-thick sections. Hematoxylin and eosin staining was performed to evaluate the degree of tubular damage. Markers of tubular damage were scored by calculating the percentage of tubules in the corticomedullary junction that displayed cell necrosis, loss of brush border, cast formation, and tubular dilation, as follows: 0, none; 1, ≤10%; 2, 11–25%; 3, 26–50%; 4, 51–75% and 5, ≥76%. The tubular necrosis score was quantified per high power field of each kidney and at least 20 fields were reviewed from each slide.

### 4.5. Immunofluorescence Staining

The number of apoptotic HK-2 cells was counted by TUNEL using a TUNEL Apoptosis Detection kit (Intergen, Purchase, NY, USA). The immunofluorescence images for TUNEL assay were captured by confocal microscopy (LSM5 Live Configuration Variotwo VRGB; Zeiss, Oberkochen, Germany). The number of positive cells was quantified per high-power field (HPF) of each kidney, and at least 20 fields were reviewed for each slide.

### 4.6. Immunoblotting Analyses of HK-2 Cells And Kidney Tissue

We performed the immunoblotting analyses for mouse kidneys and HK-2 cell lysates as described previously [42]. Kidney tissues were homogenized and resolved by SDS-polyacrylamide gel electrophoresis (SDS-PAGE) after centrifugation. HK-2 cells were harvested, washed with cold PBS, and resuspended in lysis buffer. Equal amounts of protein were electroblotted onto a nitrocellulose membrane. The membrane was blocked and incubated with primary antibodies directed against HIF-1α (Abcam, Cambridge, UK), Akt (Cell Signaling Technology, Beverly, MA, USA), pS473 Akt (Cell Signaling Technology), mTOR (Cell Signaling Technology), pSer2448 mTOR (Cell Signaling Technology), PHD (Cell Signaling Technology), VHL (von Hippel-Lindau, Santa Cruz Biotechnology), EPO (Abcam), VEGF (Abcam, Cambridge, UK), Bax (Cell Signaling Technology), Bcl-2 (Cell Signaling Technology), and glyceraldehyde-3-phosphate dehydrogenase (GAPDH, Cell Signaling Technology). They were then incubated with horseradish peroxidase-conjugated anti-rabbit IgG or anti-mouse IgG antibody (Invitrogen, Carlsbad, CA, USA). Positive bands were detected and analyzed using the ChemiDoc XRS Image system (Bio-Rad Laboratories, Hercules, CA, USA).

### 4.7. Real-Time Reverse Transcription PCR

Total RNA was isolated from kidney tissues and HK-2 cells using a NucleoSpin® RNA II kit (Macherey-Nagel, Düren, Germany). cDNA was synthesized using Reverse Transcriptase Premix (Elpis Biotech, Daejeon, Korea) and amplified in a Power SYBR®Green polymerase chain reaction (PCR) Master Mix (Applied Biosystems, Warrington, UK) with gene-specific primer pairs (HIF-1α: F; 5′-TGCCCCAGATTCAAGATCAGC-3′, R; 5′-GGCTGGGAAAAGT TAGGAGTGT-3′) Quantitative real-time PCR was performed on an ABI 7500 FAST instrument (Applied Biosystems, Warrington, UK). The expression levels of mRNAs were normalized to the expression of GAPDH.

### 4.8. Immunoprecipitation

Cultured HK-2 cells and kidney tissues were lysed with kinase buffer and then 1 mg of lysate was immunoprecipitated using 1 μg of anti-ubiquitin antibody (Santa Cruz Biotechnology) and protein G Sepharose 4 Fast Flow (GE Healthcare, Danderyd, Sweden). After washing with KB without 1% NO40, immunoblotting was performed using HIF-1α antibody (Biorbyt Ltd., Cambridge, UK).

### 4.9. Statistical Analysis

Data are expressed as the mean ± standard error of the mean (SEM) of ≥3 independent experiments. Differences between the two groups were determined using Student's t test or the Mann–Whitney U test. Multiple comparisons were performed using one-way analysis of variance and Tukey's post hoc test. Statistical analysis was performed using SPSS software (version 22.0; IBM, Armonk, NY). Results were considered significant when $p < 0.05$.

**Supplementary Materials:** Supplementary materials can be found at http://www.mdpi.com/1422-0067/21/10/3583/s1.

**Author Contributions:** Conceptualization, Y.A.H., C.W.P. and H.S.H.; methodology, S.Y.J. and K.J.Y.; software, H.S.H.; validation, K.H.J. and C.W.P.; formal analysis, Y.A.H.; investigation, S.Y.J. and K.J.Y.; resources, D.S.I. and H.S.H.; data curation, S.Y.J.; writing—original draft preparation, Y.A.H.; writing—review and editing, H.S.H.; visualization, K.H.J.; supervision, K.H.J. and C.W.P.; project administration, D.S.I.; funding acquisition, Y.A.H., D.S.I. and H.S.H. All authors have read and agreed to the published version of the manuscript.

**Funding:** This research was supported by the Basic Science Research Program through the National Research Foundation of Korea (NRF) funded by the Ministry of Education, Science and Technology (2015R1A1A1A05001599) and by the Ministry of Science and ICT, Republic of Korea (2018R1C1B5045006). The authors also wish to acknowledge the financial support of the Korean Society of Nephrology (Chong Kun Dang, 2016) and Soonchunhyang University Research Fund.

**Conflicts of Interest:** The authors declare no conflict of interest.

## Abbreviations

| | |
|---|---|
| IR | Ischemia–reperfusion |
| HIF-1α | Hypoxia-inducible factor-1α |
| DHP-1 | Dehydrogenase peptide-1 |
| mTOR | Mammalian target of rapamycin |
| EPO | Erythropoietin |
| VEGF | Vascular endothelial growth factor |
| MβCD | Methyl-β-cyclodextrin |
| PHD | Prolyl hydroxylase |
| VHL | Von Hippel-Lindau |
| si | Small interfering |
| TUNEL | terminal deoxynucleotidyl transferase-mediated dUTP nick end-labeling |
| Nrf2 | nuclear factor-erythroid-2-related factor 2 |
| Bax | Bcl-2-associated X protein |
| Bcl-2 | B-cell lymphoma 2 |
| GAPDH | glyceraldehyde-3-phosphate dehydrogenase |
| PCR | polymerase chain reaction |

## References

1. Liano, F.; Pascual, J. Epidemiology of acute renal failure: A prospective, multicenter, community-based study. Madrid Acute Renal Failure Study Group. *Kidney Int.* **1996**, *50*, 811–818. [CrossRef] [PubMed]
2. Smith, S.F.; Hosgood, S.A.; Nicholson, M.L. Ischemia-reperfusion injury in renal transplantation: 3 key signaling pathways in tubular epithelial cells. *Kidney Int.* **2019**, *95*, 50–56. [CrossRef] [PubMed]
3. Baer, P.C.; Koch, B.; Geiger, H. Kidney Inflammation, Injury and Regeneration. *Int. J. Mol. Sci.* **2020**, *21*, 1164. [CrossRef] [PubMed]
4. Semenza, G.L. Hypoxia-inducible factor 1: Oxygen homeostasis and disease pathophysiology. *Trends Mol. Med.* **2001**, *7*, 345–350. [CrossRef]
5. Haase, V.H. Hypoxic regulation of erythropoiesis and iron metabolism. *Am. J. Physiol. Renal Physiol.* **2010**, *299*, F1–F13. [CrossRef]
6. Sethi, K.; Rao, K.; Bolton, D.; Patel, O.; Ischia, J. Targeting HIF-1α to Prevent Renal Ischemia-Reperfusion Injury: Does It Work? *Int. J. Cell Biol.* **2018**, *2018*, 9852791. [CrossRef]
7. Kaelin, W.G.; Ratcliffe, P.J., Jr. Oxygen sensing by metazoans: The central role of the HIF hydroxylase pathway. *Mol. Cell* **2008**, *30*, 393–402. [CrossRef]
8. Buckley, M.M.; Brogden, R.N.; Barradell, L.B.; Goa, K.L. Imipenem/Cilastatin: A Reappraisal of its Antibacterial Activity, Pharmacokinetic Properties and Therapeutic Efficacy. *Drugs* **1992**, *44*, 408–444. [CrossRef]
9. Perez, M.; Castilla, M.; Torres, A.M.; Lázaro, J.A.; Sarmiento, E.; Tejedor, A. Inhibition of brush border dipeptidase with cilastatin reduces toxic accumulation of cyclosporin A in kidney proximal tubule epithelial cells. *Nephrol. Dial. Transplant.* **2004**, *19*, 2445–2455. [CrossRef]
10. Camano, S.; Lazaro, A.; Moreno-Gordaliza, E.; Torres, A.M.; de Lucas, C.; Humanes, B.; Lazaro, J.A.; Milagros Gomez-Gomez, M.; Bosca, L.; Tejedor, A. Cilastatin attenuates cisplatin-induced proximal tubular cell damage. *J. Pharmacol. Exp. Ther.* **2010**, *334*, 419–429. [CrossRef]
11. Luo, K.; Lim, S.W.; Jin, J.; Jin, L.; Gil, H.W.; Im, D.S.; Hwang, H.S.; Yang, C.W. Cilastatin protects against tacrolimus-induced nephrotoxicity via anti-oxidative and anti-apoptotic properties. *BMC Nephrol.* **2019**, *20*, 221. [CrossRef] [PubMed]

12. Im, D.S.; Shin, H.J.; Yang, K.J.; Jung, S.Y.; Song, H.Y.; Hwang, H.S.; Gil, H.W. Cilastatin attenuates vancomycin-induced nephrotoxicity via P-glycoprotein. *Toxicol. Lett.* **2017**, *277*, 9–17. [CrossRef] [PubMed]
13. Reis-Sobreiro, M.; Roué, G.; Moros, A.; Gajate, C.; de la Iglesia-Vicente, J.; Colomer, D.; Mollinedo, F. Lipid raft-mediated Akt signaling as a therapeutic target in mantle cell lymphoma. *Blood Cancer J.* **2013**, *3*, e118. [CrossRef] [PubMed]
14. Parkin, E.T.; Turner, A.J.; Hooper, N.M. Differential effects of glycosphingolipids on the detergent-insolubility of the glycosylphosphatidylinositol-anchored membrane dipeptidase. *Biochem. J.* **2001**, *358*, 209–216. [CrossRef]
15. Harada, H.; Itasaka, S.; Kizaka-Kondoh, S.; Shibuya, K.; Morinibu, A.; Shinomiya, K.; Hiraoka, M. The Akt/mTOR pathway assures the synthesis of HIF-1alpha protein in a glucose- and reoxygenation-dependent manner in irradiated tumors. *J. Biol. Chem.* **2009**, *284*, 5332–5342. [CrossRef]
16. Pore, N.; Jiang, Z.; Shu, H.K.; Bernhard, E.; Kao, G.D.; Maity, A. Akt1 activation can augment hypoxia-inducible factor-1alpha expression by increasing protein translation through a mammalian target of rapamycin-independent pathway. *Mol. Cancer Res.* **2006**, *4*, 471–479. [CrossRef]
17. Bernhardt, W.M.; Campean, V.; Kany, S.; Jürgensen, J.S.; Weidemann, A.; Warnecke, C.; Arend, M.; Klaus, S.; Günzler, V.; Amann, K.; et al. Preconditional activation of hypoxia-inducible factors ameliorates ischemic acute renal failure. *J. Am. Soc. Nephrol.* **2006**, *17*, 1970–1978. [CrossRef]
18. Kapitsinou, P.P.; Haase, V.H. Molecular mechanisms of ischemic preconditioning in the kidney. *Am. J. Physiol. Renal Physiol.* **2015**, *309*, F821–F834. [CrossRef]
19. Rosenberger, C.; Mandriota, S.; Jürgensen, J.S.; Wiesener, M.S.; Hörstrup, J.H.; Frei, U.; Ratcliffe, P.J.; Maxwell, P.H.; Bachmann, S.; Eckardt, K.U. Expression of hypoxia-inducible factor-1alpha and -2alpha in hypoxic and ischemic rat kidneys. *J. Am. Soc. Nephrol.* **2002**, *13*, 1721–1732. [CrossRef]
20. Lee, J.W.; Bae, S.H.; Jeong, J.W.; Kim, S.H.; Kim, K.W. Hypoxia-inducible factor (HIF-1)alpha: Its protein stability and biological functions. *Exp. Mol. Med.* **2004**, *36*, 1–12. [CrossRef]
21. Salceda, S.; Caro, J. Hypoxia-inducible factor 1alpha (HIF-1alpha) protein is rapidly degraded by the ubiquitin-proteasome system under normoxic conditions. Its stabilization by hypoxia depends on redox-induced changes. *J. Biol. Chem.* **1997**, *272*, 22642–22647. [CrossRef] [PubMed]
22. Schofield, C.J.; Ratcliffe, P.J. Oxygen sensing by HIF hydroxylases. *Nat. Rev. Mol. Cell Biol.* **2004**, *5*, 343–354. [CrossRef] [PubMed]
23. Chen, D.; Li, M.; Luo, J.; Gu, W. Direct interactions between HIF-1 alpha and Mdm2 modulate p53 function. *J. Biol. Chem.* **2003**, *278*, 13595–13598. [CrossRef] [PubMed]
24. Flugel, D.; Gorlach, A.; Michiels, C.; Kietzmann, T. Glycogen synthase kinase 3 phosphorylates hypoxia-inducible factor 1alpha and mediates its destabilization in a VHL-independent manner. *Mol. Cell Biol.* **2007**, *27*, 3253–3265. [CrossRef] [PubMed]
25. Van de Sluis, B.; Groot, A.J.; Vermeulen, J.; van der Wall, E.; van Diest, P.J.; Wijmenga, C.; Klomp, L.W.; Vooijs, M. COMMD1 Promotes pVHL and O2-Independent Proteolysis of HIF-1alpha via HSP90/70. *PLoS ONE* **2009**, *4*, e7332. [CrossRef] [PubMed]
26. Hill, P.; Shukla, D.; Tran, M.G.; Aragones, J.; Cook, H.T.; Carmeliet, P.; Maxwell, P.H. Inhibition of hypoxia inducible factor hydroxylases protects against renal ischemia-reperfusion injury. *J. Am. Soc. Nephrol.* **2008**, *19*, 39–46. [CrossRef]
27. Ong, S.G.; Hausenloy, D.J. Hypoxia-inducible factor as a therapeutic target for cardioprotection. *Pharmacol. Ther.* **2012**, *136*, 69–81. [CrossRef]
28. Zhang, Y.B.; Wang, X.; Meister, E.A.; Gong, K.R.; Yan, S.C.; Lu, G.W.; Ji, X.M.; Shao, G. The effects of CoCl2 on HIF-1$\alpha$ protein under experimental conditions of autoprogressive hypoxia using mouse models. *Int. J. Mol. Sci.* **2014**, *18*, 10999–11012. [CrossRef]
29. Imamura, R.; Moriyama, T.; Isaka, Y.; Namba, Y.; Ichimaru, N.; Takahara, S.; Okuyama, A. Erythropoietin protects the kidneys against ischemia reperfusion injury by activating hypoxia inducible factor-1alpha. *Transplantation* **2007**, *83*, 1371–1379. [CrossRef]
30. Yang, C.C.; Lin, L.C.; Wu, M.S.; Chien, C.T.; Lai, M.K. Repetitive hypoxic preconditioning attenuates renal ischemia/reperfusion induced oxidative injury via upregulating HIF-1 alpha-dependent bcl-2 signaling. *Transplantation* **2009**, *88*, 1251–1260. [CrossRef]

31. Jamadarkhana, P.; Chaudhary, A.; Chhipa, L.; Dubey, A.; Mohanan, A.; Gupta, R.; Deshpande, S. Treatment with a novel hypoxia-inducible factor hydroxylase inhibitor (TRC160334) ameliorates ischemic acute kidney injury. *Am. J. Nephrol.* **2012**, *36*, 208–218. [CrossRef] [PubMed]
32. Ruiz, S.; Pergola, P.E.; Zager, R.A.; Vaziri, N.D. Targeting the transcription factor Nrf2 to ameliorate oxidative stress and inflammation in chronic kidney disease. *Kidney Int.* **2013**, *83*, 1029–1041. [CrossRef] [PubMed]
33. Nezu, M.; Suzuki, N. Roles of Nrf2 in Protecting the Kidney from Oxidative Damage. *Int. J. Mol. Sci.* **2020**, *21*, 2951. [CrossRef] [PubMed]
34. Jakobs, P.; Serbulea, V.; Leitinger, N.; Eckers, A.; Haendeler, J. Nuclear Factor (Erythroid-Derived 2)-Like 2 and Thioredoxin-1 in Atherosclerosis and Ischemia/Reperfusion Injury in the Heart. *Antioxid. Redox Signal.* **2017**, *26*, 630–644. [CrossRef]
35. Limonciel, A.; Jennings, P. A review of the evidence that ochratoxin A is an Nrf2 inhibitor: Implications for nephrotoxicity and renal carcinogenicity. *Toxins* **2014**, *6*, 371–379. [CrossRef]
36. Manning, B.D.; Toker, A. AKT/PKB Signaling: Navigating the Network. *Cell* **2017**, *169*, 381–405. [CrossRef]
37. Hsu, P.P.; Kang, S.A.; Rameseder, J.; Zhang, Y.; Ottina, K.A.; Lim, D.; Peterson, T.R.; Choi, Y.; Gray, N.S.; Yaffe, M.B.; et al. The mTOR-regulated phosphoproteome reveals a mechanism of mTORC1-mediated inhibition of growth factor signaling. *Science* **2011**, *332*, 1317–1322. [CrossRef]
38. Yeo, E.J.; Chun, Y.S.; Cho, Y.S.; Kim, J.; Lee, J.C.; Kim, M.S.; Park, J.W. YC-1: A potential anticancer drug targeting hypoxia-inducible factor 1. *J. Natl. Cancer Inst.* **2003**, *95*, 516–525. [CrossRef]
39. Meldrum, K.K.; Meldrum, D.R.; Hile, K.L.; Burnett, A.L.; Harken, A.H. A novel model of ischemia in renal tubular cells which closely parallels in vivo injury. *J. Surg. Res.* **2001**, *99*, 288–293. [CrossRef]
40. Hwang, H.S.; Yang, K.J.; Park, K.C.; Choi, H.S.; Kim, S.H.; Hong, S.Y.; Jeon, B.H.; Chang, Y.K.; Park, C.W.; Kim, S.Y.; et al. Pretreatment with paricalcitol attenuates inflammation in ischemia-reperfusion injury via the up-regulation of cyclooxygenase-2 and prostaglandin E2. *Nephrol. Dial. Transplant.* **2013**, *28*, 1156–1166. [CrossRef]
41. Imtiazul, I.M.; Asma, R.; Lee, J.H.; Cho, N.J.; Park, S.; Song, H.Y.; Gil, H.W. Change of surfactant protein D and A after renal ischemia reperfusion injury. *PLoS ONE* **2019**, *14*, e0227097. [CrossRef] [PubMed]
42. Hong, Y.A.; Yang, K.J.; Jung, S.Y.; Park, K.C.; Choi, H.; Oh, J.M.; Lee, S.J.; Chang, Y.K.; Park, C.W.; Yang, C.W.; et al. Paricalcitol Pretreatment Attenuates Renal Ischemia-Reperfusion Injury via Prostaglandin E2 Receptor EP4 Pathway. *Oxid. Med. Cell. Longev.* **2017**, *2017*, 5031926. [PubMed]

International Journal of
*Molecular Sciences*

MDPI

*Article*

# Macrophage-Secreted Lipocalin-2 Promotes Regeneration of Injured Primary Murine Renal Tubular Epithelial Cells

**Anja Urbschat [1], Anne-Kathrin Thiemens [2], Christina Mertens [3], Claudia Rehwald [3], Julia K. Meier [3], Patrick C. Baer [2,†] and Michaela Jung [3,*,†]**

1 Department of Biomedicine, Aarhus University, 8000 Aarhus, Denmark; anja.urbschat@biomed.au.dk
2 Division of Nephrology, Department of Internal Medicine III, Goethe-University Frankfurt, 60323 Frankfurt am Main, Germany; Anne-Kathrin.Thiemens@web.de (A.-K.T.); p.baer@em.uni-frankfurt.de (P.C.B.)
3 Institute of Biochemistry I, Goethe-University Frankfurt, Faculty of Medicine, 60323 Frankfurt am Main, Germany; Christina.Mertens@med.uni-heidelberg.de (C.M.); rehwald@biochem.uni-frankfurt.de (C.R.); meier@biochem.uni-frankfurt.de (J.K.M.)
* Correspondence: m.jung@biochem.uni-frankfurt.de
† Theses authors contributed equally to this work.

Received: 11 February 2020; Accepted: 13 March 2020; Published: 16 March 2020

**Abstract:** Lipocalin-2 (Lcn-2) is rapidly upregulated in macrophages after renal tubular injury and acts as renoprotective and pro-regenerative agent. Lcn-2 possesses the ability to bind and transport iron with high affinity. Therefore, the present study focuses on the decisive role of the Lcn-2 iron-load for its pro-regenerative function. Primary mouse tubular epithelial cells were isolated from kidney tissue of wildtype mice and incubated with 5 μM Cisplatin for 24 h to induce injury. Bone marrow-derived macrophages of wildtype and Lcn-2$^{-/-}$ mice were isolated and polarized with IL-10 towards an anti-inflammatory, iron-release phenotype. Their supernatants as well as recombinant iron-loaded holo-Lcn-2 was used for stimulation of Cisplatin-injured tubular epithelial cells. Incubation of tubular epithelial cells with wildtype supernatants resulted in less damage and induced cellular proliferation, whereas in absence of Lcn-2 no protective effect was observed. Epithelial integrity as well as cellular proliferation showed a clear protection upon rescue experiments applying holo-Lcn-2. Notably, we detected a positive correlation between total iron amounts in tubular epithelial cells and cellular proliferation, which, in turn, reinforced the assumed link between availability of Lcn-2-bound iron and recovery. We hypothesize that macrophage-released Lcn-2-bound iron is provided to tubular epithelial cells during toxic cell damage, whereby injury is limited and recovery is favored.

**Keywords:** renal tubular epithelial cells; macrophages; lipocalin-2; iron

## 1. Introduction

Despite enormous advances in treatment of patients suffering from acute kidney injury, we still encounter a high morbidity and mortality rate. Hence, effective approaches for prevention and treatment are still lacking [1,2], with only limited and unsatisfactory therapeutic options. Fortunately, the kidney has the intrinsic capacity to recover from ischemic or toxic insults that cause renal cell death [3]. Therefore, timely rescue of affected renal tubules may arrest progression of injury and pave the way for recovery. The response to acute kidney injury involves a complex network of interconnected and orchestrated mechanisms. Herein, macrophages (MΦ) constitutes one of the major infiltrating cell populations in acute renal injury [4,5]. Moreover, MΦ-infiltration was recognized as a crucial feature of both the initial severity of injury and progression of renal failure, but also following regeneration and repair phase [6]. In this regard, MΦ shows a remarkable repertoire of functional and phenotypic activation states [7,8]. In particular, during the acute phase of tissue injury, MΦ shows a pro-inflammatory phenotype, whereas they adopt an anti-inflammatory phenotype during later phases of tissue recovery [9–12]. This enables them to determine the fine balance of injury versus regeneration of damaged renal tissue. Accordingly, we found that MΦ genetically modified ex vivo in order to express a predetermined anti-inflammatory phenotype showed a clearly protective role upon re-infusion into ischemic kidneys [10]. Therefore, it might be speculated that the control of the local MΦ phenotype plays a decisive role for the inflammatory outcome and, thus, disease progression.

We recently described lipocalin-2 (Lcn-2) as a potent determent of MΦ polarization in the context of kidney injury [9]. Lcn-2 itself is a 25 kDa protein of the lipocalin superfamily that is rapidly upregulated after renal tubular injury [13,14]. It represents both a biomarker of renal ischemic injury [15] including Cisplatin injury [16] and a renoprotective agent when exogenously administered [17–19]. Lcn-2 is expressed in MΦ upon contact to apoptotic cells [11,20,21]. Mechanistically, the induction of Lcn-2 was stimulated by apoptotic cell-secreted sphingosine-1-phophate (S1P) and the downstream activation of the STAT3 signaling pathway [20].

Though, using a neutralizing antibody approach, we previously were able to show that Lcn-2 plays a pivotal role during injury, but also in the reparative phases of ischemia reperfusion injury. Intriguingly, Lcn-2-mediated cell regeneration was dependent on the inflammatory micromilieu of the tissue [22]. Moreover, the infusion of Lcn-2-overexpressing macrophages significantly increased renal epithelial cell proliferation. This effect was blocked by Lcn-2 neutralizing antibodies or the infusion of MΦ with a knockdown of Lcn-2 [9]. However, it was previously described that exclusively iron-loaded Lcn-2 triggers cell survival upon internalization [23]. Thus, the functional outcome of Lcn-2 seems to largely depend on its iron-load. It was already speculated that the beneficial effect of Lcn-2 against ischemia reperfusion injury to the kidney may be a result of its ability to bind and transport iron to viable cells, thereby limiting cell death, promoting proliferation, and enhancing recovery [17,18,24,25]. Although its ability to transport and donate iron to cells seems to determine the pro-survival and/or anti-apoptotic function of Lcn-2, the decisive role of the iron-load of Lcn-2 has not been investigated so far in a Cisplatin-dependent nephrotoxicity model.

Given the pivotal role of Lcn-2 as well as MΦ for iron homeostasis and the fact that the presence of both was associated with increased renal regeneration upon injury, the current study aimed at investigating their interconnection. Considering that we previously observed that the administration of Interleukin (IL)-10-overexpressing MΦ induces Lcn-2 and its receptors in the kidney [10] and as Cisplatin is known to affect mainly the proximal tubular cells of the kidney [26–28], we performed a cell culture study with isolated primary murine renal tubular epithelial cells injured by various doses of Cisplatin. In order to better understand renal damage and repair mechanisms as well as for testing potential therapeutic options, post-injury recovery was favored through exposure to conditioned medium from either murine wildtype (wt) C57BL/6 or Lcn-2$^{-/-}$ C57BL/6 bone marrow-derived MΦ (BMDM).

## 2. Results

### 2.1. *Dose-Dependent Injury of Primary Mouse Tubular Epithelial Cells (mTECs) upon Incubation with Cisplatin*

Isolated primary mTECs of wt C57BL/6 mice displaying the morphology of renal tubular epithelial cells (Figure 1B, left) and were first stained with cytokeratin to prove their epithelial origin (Figure 1B, right). qPCR analysis of epithelial cell markers cytokeratin 18 (CK18), E-Cadherin, and zona occludens (ZO)-1 confirmed the tubular epithelial origin of isolated mTECs (Figure 1C). In order to evaluate the appropriate Cisplatin concentration, which injured the cells, but still allowed cellular recovery, we measured cell vitality via XTT assay using increasing Cisplatin concentrations: 0.1 µM, 1 µM, 5 µM, 10 µM, 20 µM, and 50 µM compared to untreated controls (ctrl) for 24 h and 48 h, respectively (Figure 1D). This has been performed twice with in total 9 technical replicates with 5% FCS and confirmed once with 6 technical replicates without FCS. As expected, vitality significantly decreased with increasing Cisplatin concentrations. mTECs cultured with FCS (Figure 1D, left) represented overall higher levels of mTEC vitality than mTECs cultured without FCS (Figure 1D, right). A significant difference between 24 h or 48 h of Cisplatin treatment was not observed for none of the experimental groups. Based on these results, we used 5 μM Cisplatin without FCS for all following experiments, as this turned out to represent the most adequate dosage, displaying measurable injury parameters, but moderate cell injury.

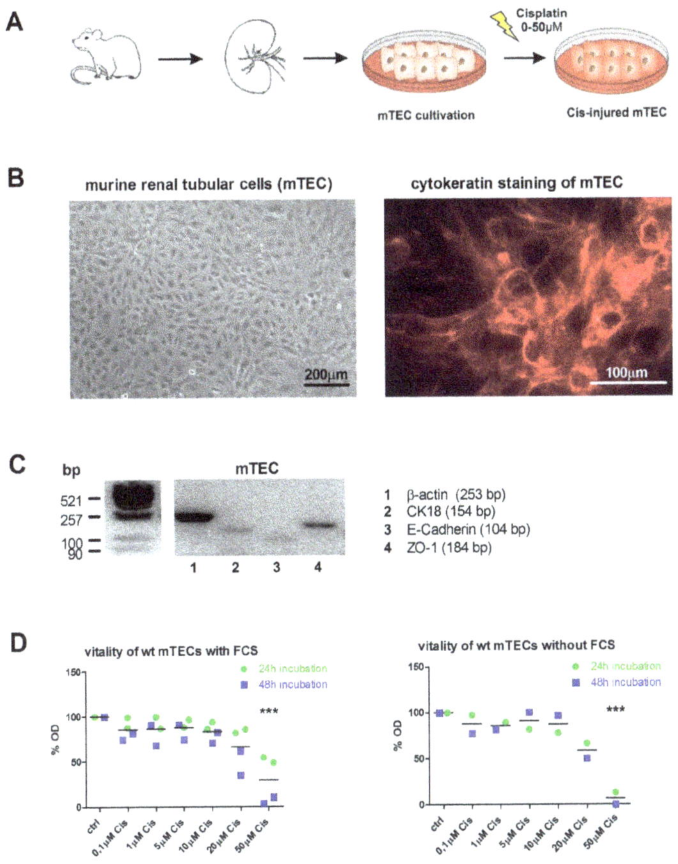


**Figure 1.** Primary murine tubular epithelial cells respond to Cisplatin-induced injury. (**A**) Schematic overview of experimental setup. (**B**) Cultured murine renal tubular epithelial cells (mTEC) in vitro displaying an epithelial morphology in culture (left) and stained positive for the epithelial cell marker cytokeratin 18 (right). (**C**) qPCR-analysis of epithelial cell markers cytokeratin 18 (CK18), E-Cadherin, and ZO-1 confirmed the epithelial origin of isolated primary mTEC. (**D**) Measurement of cell vitality via XTT assay using increasing Cisplatin concentrations: 0.1 μM, 1 μM, 5 μM, 10 μM, 20 μM, 50 μM, and untreated control (ctrl) for 24 h and 48 h, respectively. The untreated ctrl has been set on 100% of optical density (OD), and treated cells are given in percentage in relation to ctrl. *** $p < 0.001$ ($n = 3$, one-way ANOVA followed by Tukey's Multiple Comparison Test).

### 2.2. Establishment of Conditioned Media and Macrophage Polarization

We next isolated primary murine MΦ from wt and Lcn-2$^{-/-}$ mice and stimulated them with IL-10 (20 ng/mL) for 24 h to induce an anti-inflammatory activated as well as iron-releasing phenotype.

The resulting conditioned medium (cm) was collected for further analysis and subsequent stimulation of mTEC. A schematic representation of the experimental set-up is given in Figure 2A. qRT-PCR analyses of polarized MΦ show low expression of pro-inflammatory markers IL-1β (Interleukin 1β) ($p < 0.01$; $n = 5$), TNF-α (tumor necrosis factor) ($p < 0.01$; $n = 5$), and iNOS (inducible nitric oxide synthase) ($p < 0.05$; $n = 5$), whereas the anti-inflammatory markers MRC (macrophage mannose receptor) (ns), Ym1 (chitinase 3-like 3), CD163, and MARCO (macrophage receptor with collagenous structure) were elevated compared to untreated control MΦ (Figure 2B). In order to verify the iron-releasing MΦ phenotype, we determined the iron amount in the supernatant via atomic absorption spectroscopy (AAS) relative to the total protein content, showing a significant increase in relative iron levels in IL-10-treated MΦ supernatants (Figure 2C, $p < 0.01$; $n = 5$). As previously observed for human MΦ [29], we also observed an increased release of Lcn-2 to the supernatant of IL-10-stimulated murine MΦ (Figure 2D). In order to determine the amount of iron bound to Lcn-2 in MΦ supernatants, we performed an immunoprecipitation for Lcn-2 with subsequent measurement of the Lcn-2-bound iron applying AAS of immunoprecipitated samples. Interestingly, Lcn-2-bound iron was significantly elevated in IL-10-treated MΦ supernatants (Figure 2E, $p < 0.05$; $n = 5$).

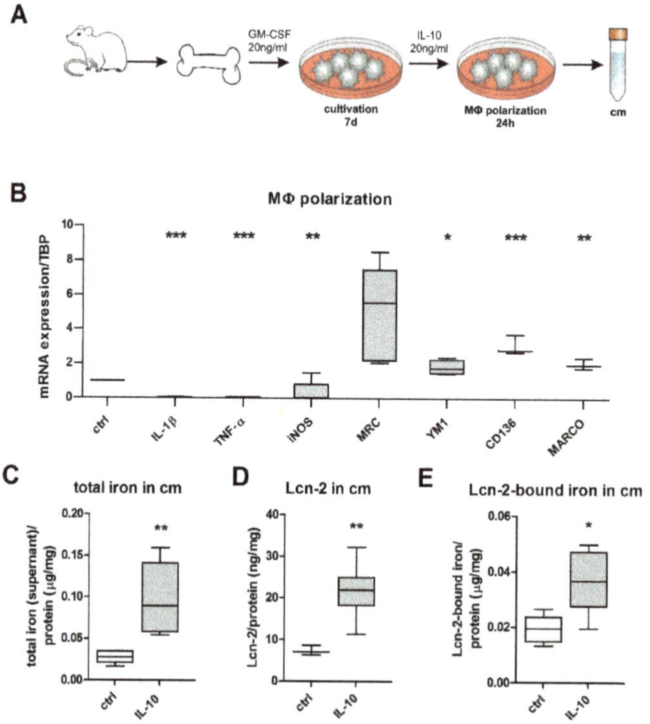


**Figure 2.** Primary bone marrow-derived macrophages (BMDM) release Lcn-2-bound iron upon IL-10 treatment. (**A**) Schematic representation for the generation of conditioned media from BMDMs. (**B**) qRT-PCR analysis of IL-10-stimulated macrophages compared to untreated control relative to the housekeeping gene TBP ($n = 5$; *t*-test). (**C**) Total iron amount in the supernatant of both wt and Lcn-2$^{-/-}$ BMDM measured by atomic absorption spectrometry (AAS). (**D**) Measurement of Lcn-2 protein in macrophage conditioned media via ELISA. (E) Immunoprecipitation of Lcn-2 with subsequent iron measurements via AAS to determine the amount of Lcn-2-bound iron in macrophage conditioned media. * $p < 0.05$, ** $p < 0.01$, *** $p < 0.001$ ($n = 5$; *t*-test).

### 2.3. Conditioned Medium From wt MΦ or the Supply of Holo-Lcn-2 Tends to Promote Epithelial Viability upon Cisplatin Treatment

We next aimed at determining the influence of MΦ-released Lcn-2, especially in its iron-loaded form, on mTEC recovery after Cisplatin-induced injury. In Figure 3A, the experimental set-up is visualized. mTECs were either cultured with standard medium without FCS (ctrl) or injured with 5 μM Cisplatin both for 24 h and left without further treatment (Cis) or treated with cm for an additional 24 h, deriving either from IL-10-treated wt (wt cm) or Lcn-$2^{-/-}$ MΦ (cm Lcn-$2^{-/-}$). We then measured the expression of kidney injury molecule 1 (KIM-1), a well-accepted acute injury marker of the proximal tubule system, also in Cisplatin-induced renal injury both in vitro and in vivo [30]. KIM-1 protein expression increased upon Cisplatin treatment and was lowered to control levels upon incubation of mTEC with the supernatant of wt MΦ, showing a trend towards the recovery of mTECs (ns). In contrast, the addition of Lcn-$2^{-/-}$ cm did not decrease KIM-1 expression of mTECs. However, the addition of recombinant, iron-loaded Lcn-2 (holo-Lcn-2) to Lcn-2 lacking cm appeared to reduce KIM-1 expression (Figure 3B, $n = 3$, ns). We next analyzed the expression of Klotho, as it is highly expressed in the healthy kidney and known to significantly decline upon kidney injury but rises gradually to control level during recovery [31–33]. Accordingly, we observed a conversely trajectory compared to KIM-1, with a decrease of Klotho protein expression upon cisplatin treatment (ns). However, we observed no changes of Klotho expression upon cm treatment, neither from wt nor from Lcn-$2^{-/-}$ MΦ (Figure 3C, $n = 3$, ns). We obtained similar results as for Klotho expression for viability test via XTT, again lacking statistical significance (ns; $n = 3$) (Figure 3D).

Furthermore, we analyzed the expression of epithelial cell markers ZO-1 (Figure 4A), β-catenin (Figure 4B), and E-Cadherin (Figure 4C) via qRT-PCR. Upon Cisplatin treatment, all three markers decreased, which could be rescued by the addition of wt cm, whereas Lcn-$2^{-/-}$ cm did not induce recovery of mTECs. The addition of iron-loaded Lcn-2 induced the expression of epithelial markers, thereby rescuing the deleterious effect of Lcn-$2^{-/-}$ cm on mTECs recovery profile ($n = 6$). This is further visualized by cytoskeletal integrity of mTECs applying phalloidin staining. Cisplatin-treated mTECs showed marked rarefaction of the cytoskeleton and junctional ring formation of F-actin fibers close to the surface. Upon incubation of Cisplatin-injured mTECs with wt cm, we observed a significant recovery of the cytoskeletal distribution across the cell, which was not observed upon stimulation with Lcn-$2^{-/-}$ cm. Again, the addition of iron-loaded Lcn-2 significantly improved cytoskeletal integrity of damaged mTECs (Figure 4D).

### 2.4. Lcn-2-Mediated Iron Uptake Promote Proliferation of Cisplatin-Injured mTECs

To investigate regenerative and proliferative parameters, we performed gene expression analyses on stathmin and proliferating-cell-nuclear-antigen (PCNA) gene expression, which are well-described markers in recovery from acute kidney injury [34,35]. Both stathmin (Figure 5A) and PCNA (Figure 5B) displayed decreased mRNA expression upon Cisplatin treatment and significantly increased upon treatment with wt cm treatment. In contrast, Lcn-$2^{-/-}$ cm did not induce stathmin and PCNA expression in Cisplatin-injured mTECs, which could be rescued by the addition of recombinant holo-Lcn-2 protein. These observations were confirmed by proliferation measurements in real time up to 72 h (Figure 5C). Finally, we checked if mTEC take up MΦ-released iron and performed AAS-measurements of mTEC cellular lysates after cm-stimulation (Figure 5D, $n = 6$; $p < 0.001$). We observed a significant increase in intracellular iron amount upon treatment with wt cm, whereas the treatment with Lcn-$2^{-/-}$ cm remained without effect. The addition of holo-Lcn-2 showed significantly enhanced intracellular iron levels in mTECs. The relevance of our findings could be reinforced by analyzing the correlation of intracellular iron amount and cellular proliferation (Figure 5E). Notably, the total iron content correlated with mTEC proliferation measured via xCELLigence (all values included; Spearman $r = 0.862$, $p < 0.001$).

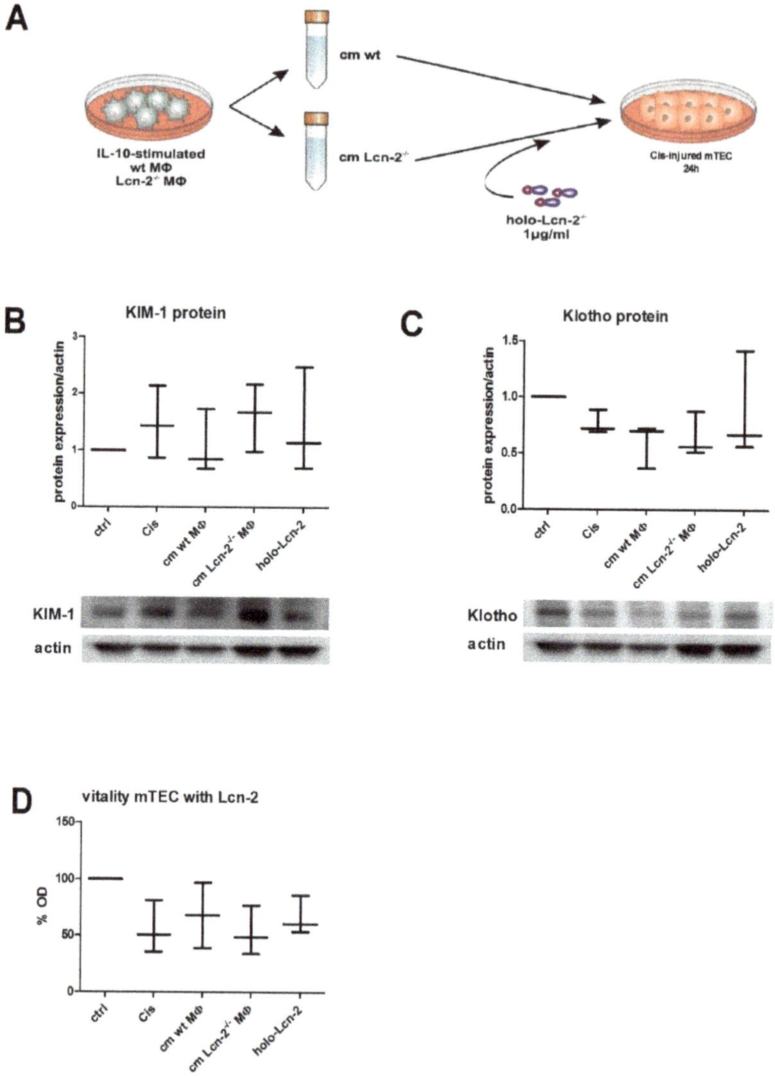


**Figure 3.** Cellular vitality depends on the presence of Lcn-2-bound iron in macrophage supernatants. (**A**) Visualization of the experimental set up. mTECs were either cultivated with standard medium without FCS (ctrl) or injured by 24 h incubation with 5 μM Cisplatin (Cis). Hereafter, Cisplatin-injured mTECs were cultured 24 h further in conditioned medium from IL-10-stimulated MΦ from wt mice (wt cm) or Lcn-$2^{-/-}$ mice (Lcn-$2^{-/-}$ cm). The latter group was further cultivated with supplementation of iron-containing holo-Lcn-2 (designated as Lcn-$2^{-/-}$ cm + holo-Lcn-2). (**B**) Kidney injury molecule 1 (KIM-1) (44kDA) and (**C**) Klotho (130kDA) protein expression relative to β-actin (ns; $n$ = 3). (**D**) Measurement of cellular vitality after cm-treatments via XTT (ns; $n$ = 3).

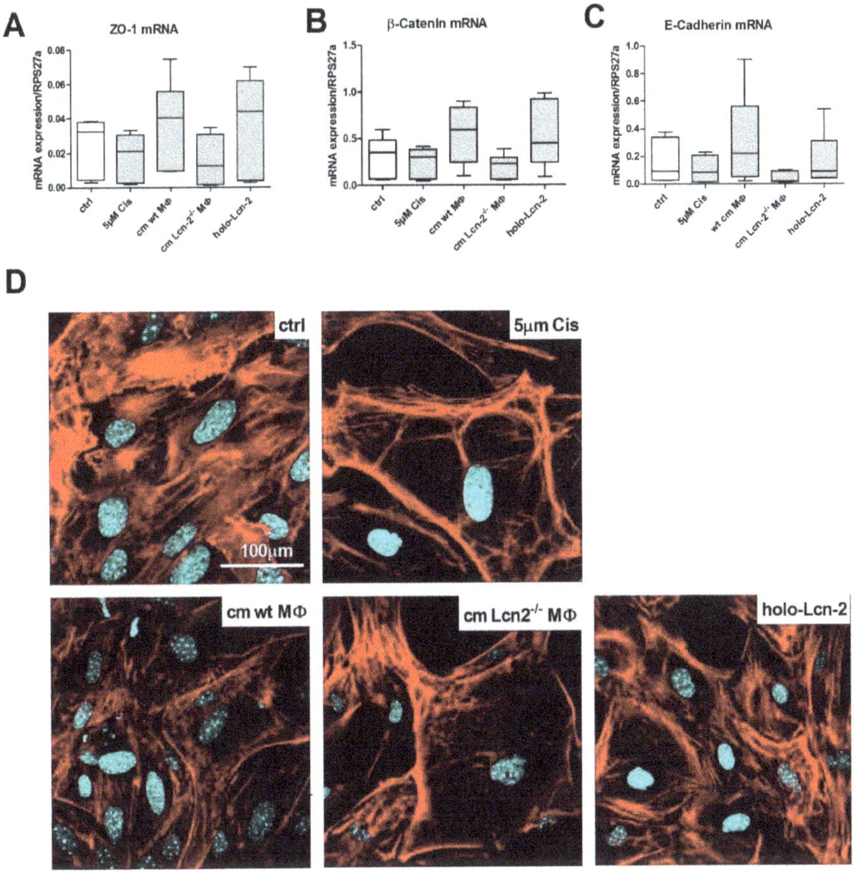


**Figure 4.** The epithelial phenotype is rescued by Lcn-2. mRNA expression relative to the housekeeping gene RPS27a of the epithelial phenotype markers (**A**) Zonula occludens-1 (ZO-1), (**B**) β-catenin, and (**C**) E-Cadherin (ns; $n = 6$). (**D**) Phalloidin staining visualizing the cytoskeleton and the F-actin stress fibers in red and nuclei in blue.

As proof of concept that the delivery of iron supports mTEC recovery, we first measured the expression of KIM-1 as an injury marker (Figure S1A). Results show that the addition of the iron chelator 2′2 DPD (dipyridyl; 100 μM, 24 h) to wt cm treated mTEC increased the mRNA expression of KIM-1 (ns), indicating increased tubular damage. On the contrary, by measuring the epithelial markers E-Cadherin, β-catenin, and ZO-1, we observed a significant decrease (except for E-Cadherin) upon 2′2 DPD addition (Figure S1B). Moreover, proliferation markers PCNA and stathmin corroborated these observations (Figure S1C), showing significantly reduced expression.

We therefore postulate that MΦ-released Lcn-2 binds and transports iron to damaged mTEC. In turn, the uptake of iron-Lcn-2 complexes facilitates tissue regeneration and promotes cellular proliferation. This hypothesis is depicted in Figure 6.

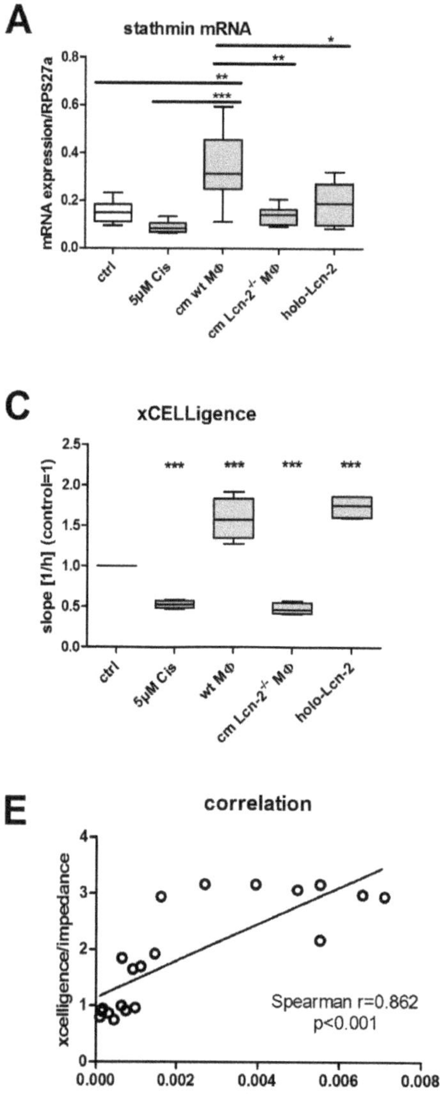

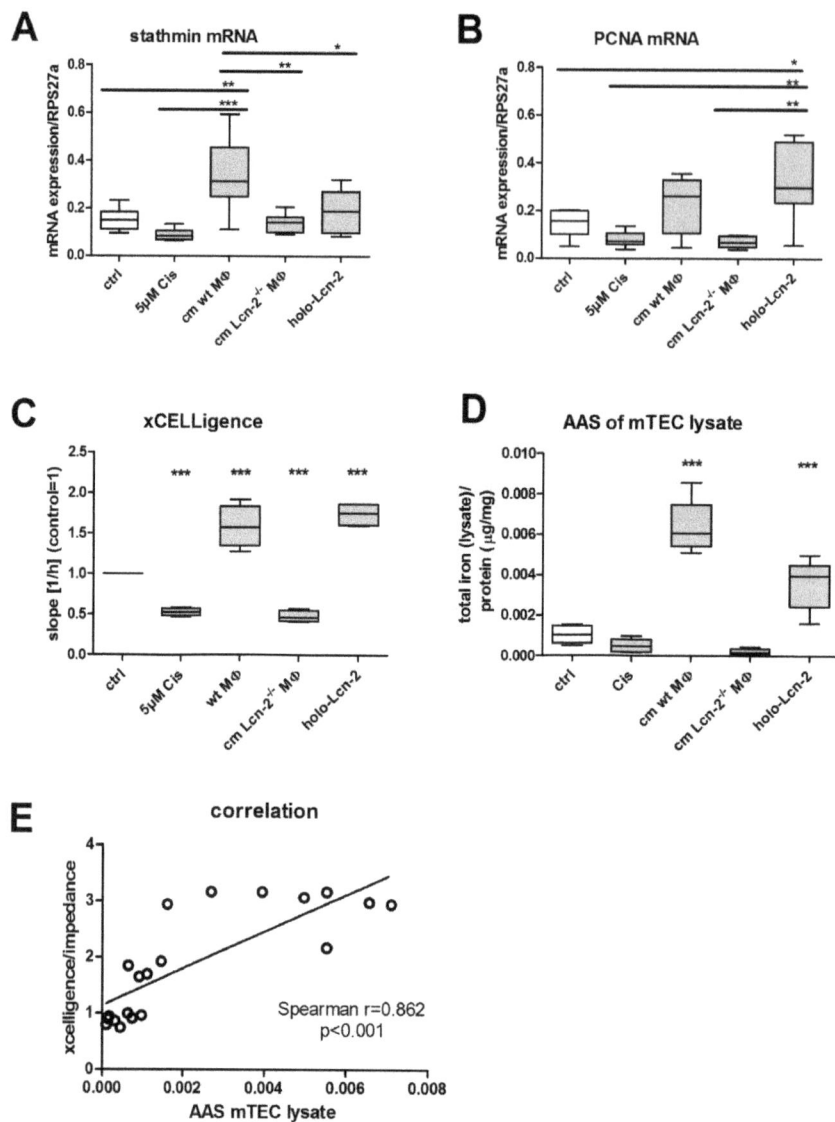


**Figure 5.** mTEC take up Lcn-2-bound iron that correlates with cellular proliferation. mRNA expression of (**A**) stathmin and (**B**) PCNA expression relative to the housekeeping gene RPS27a ($n = 6$). (**C**) Measurement of real-time proliferation via xCELLigence ($p < 0.001$; $n = 5$; one-way ANOVA followed by Tukey's Multiple Comparison Test). (**D**) Measurement of total iron content in lysates of differently treated mTEC via AAS ($n = 6$). * $p < 0.05$, ** $p < 0.01$, *** $p < 0.001$. (**E**) Correlation between total iron amount in mTEC lysates and proliferation (all values included; Spearman r = 0.862, $p < 0.001$).

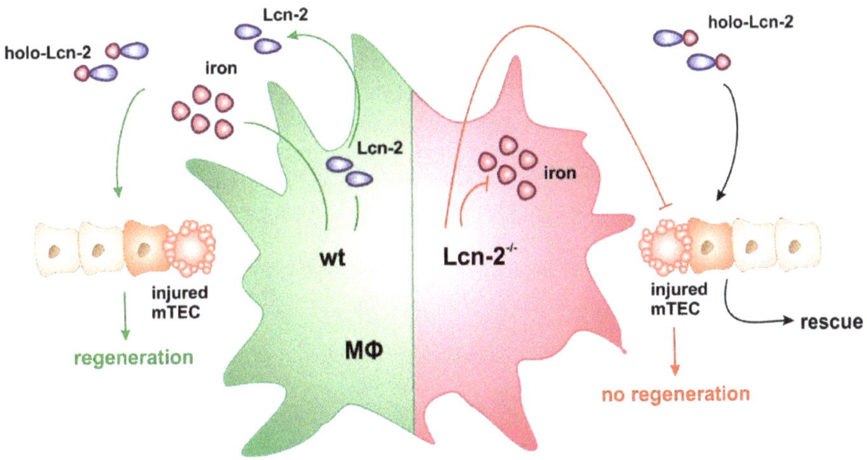


**Figure 6.** Results summary. Schematic overview of the hypothesis. After the stimulation of wt macrophages (MΦ) with IL-10, they adopt an iron-releasing phenotype, whereas Lcn-$2^{-/-}$ macrophages do not release iron to the extracellular space. Wt MΦ also produce Lcn-2 in high numbers that chelates iron and donates these complexes to injured tubular epithelial cells (TEC), where recovery and regeneration are promoted. The addition of iron-containing holo-Lcn-2 rescues the negative effect of Lcn-$2^{-/-}$ MΦ supernatants.

## 3. Discussion

The present study unravels a previously underappreciated function of MΦ-derived Lcn-2 in renal epithelial cell regeneration. Evidently, iron-loaded Lcn-2 promotes an epithelial phenotype integrity as well as cellular proliferation after Cisplatin-induced injury in vitro. A number of studies previously acknowledged the protective role of Lcn-2 in kidney injury, both in acute and chronic pathologies. Our current study adds to the emerging role of iron in determining the pro-regenerative function of Lcn-2 after renal injury, including ischemia/reperfusion injury (IRI) as well as nephrotoxic Cisplatin-induced damage.

Following kidney injury, renal tubular epithelial cells regenerate depending on the degree of damage or microenvironmental conditions [3]. Previous studies from our and other groups delineated a pivotal role for the MΦ phenotype influencing the inflammatory environment and determining kidney repair [10,11,36]. Besides, data from our group suggest that renal cell regeneration after mouse kidney IRI depends on endogenously generated MΦ-derived Lcn-2, whose expression is mainly affected by inflammatory cytokines [6,11]. Moreover, in a Cisplatin-induced rat renal injury model, Lcn-2 was found to be expressed in epithelial cells of the affected proximal renal tubules, whereby regeneration was promoted [37]. It is well established that the expression of Lcn-2 in renal tubular epithelial cells correlates to the degree of damage induced by either Cisplatin or IRI, whereby Lcn-2 serves as a biomarker and an acute phase protein. With regard to our previous observations as well as the results of the present study, it is therefore very important to distinguish the source of Lcn-2 as well as its iron-load in the kidney to determine its biological activity.

The infusion of exogenous Lcn-2 not only enhanced cellular proliferation, but also induced the expression of early progenitor markers in the kidney, thus suggesting that Lcn-2 might act as a growth and differentiation marker [19]. These observations are in line with results from the present study, showing that Lcn-2 enhanced epithelial integrity and polarity by inducing the expression of ZO-1, β-catenin, and E-Cadherin after Cisplatin-induced injury in primary mTEC. In line, it was previously appreciated that kidney injury results in loss of epithelial cell polarity, disruption of the actin cytoskeleton, and disassembly of junctional complexes [38,39]. In addition, one of our previous studies as well as Krudering et al. demonstrated that Cisplatin affects directly the cytoskeleton structure and causes apoptosis and cell detachment, resulting in a loss of F-actin fibers within a few hours of exposure [40,41]. We were able to confirm these morphological alterations in the present in vitro experiments: Cisplatin exposure clearly induced the rarefication and congestion of F-actin stress fibers. Yet, application of holo-Lcn2 led to recovery of F-actin fiber distribution across the cells and, thus, cellular integrity. In order to sustain these findings, we analyzed PCNA and stathmin as accepted regenerative markers in kidney injury [22,42,43]. Furthermore, the expression of both stathmin and PCNA mRNA is known to decrease following Cisplatin application in vivo [34], which is in line with our results in vitro. Previous own investigations showed that the proliferative markers Ki-67 and PCNA markedly increased in Lcn-2-overexpressing MΦ-treated rats after IRI [9]. However, blocking Lcn-2 production reduced the potency of a MΦ-based cell therapy approach, thereby substantiating the pro-proliferative and anti-inflammatory role of Lcn-2. In this regard, Kashiwagi et al. defined in their in vivo Cisplatin-induced rat kidney injury study that immunohistochemical expressions of Lcn-2 was mainly observed in regenerating renal tubules in the affected cortico-medullary junction and that the number of PCNA-positive cells significantly correlated with Lcn-2 scoring [37]. Taking these observations into account, the interplay between Lcn-2 and pro-regenerative MΦ holds potential in renal epithelial cell regeneration and hence, may define injury outcome.

Along these lines of evidence, it was previously recognized that anti-inflammatory polarized MΦ plays a crucial role during tissue repair, which is mainly achieved through phagocytosis of apoptotic cells and the subsequent production of anti-inflammatory mediators. Previous studies from our group indicate that sphingosine-1-phosphate (S1P) is released during apoptotic cell death and participates in coordinating anti-inflammatory responses in macrophages through the induction of Lcn-2 [11]. Bone-marrow-derived MΦ, engineered ex vivo to overexpress the anti-inflammatory cytokine IL-10, accumulated in IRI-damaged kidney tissue and promoted tissue regeneration. Interestingly, these infused cells showed enhanced iron levels as well as Lcn-2, which, at least in part, explained the pro-regenerative capacity of these cells in vivo [10]. Moreover, we and others observed that IL-10-treated primary human MΦ adopted an iron-releasing phenotype with consequences for tumor cell proliferation in vitro [44,45]. In the present study, we not only confirmed the anti-inflammatory and iron-releasing phenotype in primary murine MΦ but could also determine enhanced iron-loaded Lcn-2 in the MΦ-supernatant. Considering that both the release of iron as well as the production and secretion of Lcn-2 is a biological response of IL-10-treatment in MΦ, we hypothesized that MΦ-delivered iron-bound Lcn-2 accounts for mTEC recovery from Cisplatin-induced injury in vitro. The application of MΦ-conditioned media from both wt and Lcn-$2^{-/-}$ mice to injured primary mTEC as well as rescue experiments applying iron-loaded recombinant Lcn-2 protein confirmed this speculation. Notably, we could detect a positive correlation between total intracellular iron amount in mTEC lysates and their proliferation, which, in turn, reinforced this assumed link between availability of iron-bound Lcn-2 and its release by anti-inflammatory MΦ. These findings suggest a direct implication of MΦ-Lcn-2 in main cytoprotective mechanisms during Cisplatin-induced renal injury. The above findings match with recent evidences implying that Lcn-2 functions as an additional alternative iron transporter within the tissue microenvironment [46,47].

In sum, we could show that mTEC are able to increase their intracellular iron pool by taking up MΦ-secreted iron-loaded Lcn-2, whereby proliferation and epithelial cell polarity is promoted. Still, not only mechanistic insights regarding Lcn-2 downstream signaling in renal epithelial cells is lacking, but also how iron is recycled and used in renal cells to promote recovery. Therefore, the understanding of molecular and genetic mechanisms that control Lcn-2 signaling and recycling of iron could offer new perspectives for future therapeutic avenues in acute kidney injury and progressive interstitial fibrosis.

## 4. Materials and Methods

### 4.1. Animals

C57BL/6 wt and Lcn-$2^{-/-}$ mice with C57BL/6 background (both bred at mfd diagnostics, Wendelsheim, Germany) were kept in the central research facility of the university hospital Frankfurt. They were housed with water and food ad libitum in rooms with a 12h light cycle. Organ removal and animal care were performed in accordance with the "Guide for the care and use of laboratory animals" (National Institutes of Health, volume 25, no. 28, revised 1996), EU Directive 86/609 EEC, and German Protection of Animals Act. No additional animal ethics approval is needed for organ removal for subsequent isolation of primary murine cells.

### 4.2. Isolation and Culture of Murine Proximal Tubular Epithelial Cells

Murine primary tubular epithelial cells (mTECs) were isolated from above described wt and Lcn-$2^{-/-}$ mice as previously described [48,49]. In brief, after kidney removal, the tissue was minced and digested with a collagenase/dispase suspension. The digested fragments were passed through a 100 and 70 μm mesh. Subsequently cells caught with a 40 μm mesh were isolated and grown in DMEM/HAM's F12 (1:1) with GlutaMAX (31331-028, Gibco, obtained from Thermo Fisher, Dreieich, Germany), supplemented with 10% FCS and 1% Penicillin/Streptomycin at 37 °C and 5% $CO_2$ in a humidified atmosphere.

### 4.3. Establishment of Cisplatin Injury in mTECs Model

Cisplatin (cis-diamminedichloroplatinum II) is commonly used for chemotherapy in a wide variety of tumors [50]. However, it nonetheless has nephrotoxicity as a major side effect and limiting factor in clinical practice [51]. Mechanistically, Cisplatin causes primarily tubular necrosis and apoptosis [26–28] in a dose-and duration-dependent manner in both in vitro and in vivo [26,52]. Therefore, we established an in vitro cell culture model using cisplatin as a well-accepted clinically relevant model (Figure 1A). Viability of mTECs was determined by a photometric assay using 2,3-Bis-(2-Methoxy-4-Nitro-5-Sulfophenyl)-2H-Tetrazolium-5-Carboxanilide (XTT). In brief, subconfluent cells in 96-well plates were exposed to Cisplatin (Teva®, Ulm, Germany (stock solution 1 mg/mL (3.3 mM)) for 24 h or 48 h. Hereafter, XTT reagent was added to each well as described by the manufacturer (A8088, Applichem, Darmstadt, Germany) and incubated at 37 °C. Absorbance was measured in a microplate reader (ELx808, Bio-TEC Instruments Inc., Bad Friedrichshall, Germany) at 450 nm vs. 630 nm. Experiments were conducted in triplicate, sixfold, or ninefold in one to three independent experimental settings and are represented as mean ± SEM. The value of viability is expressed as percentage of viability of untreated control cells set as 100%.

### 4.4. Generation of Murine BMDM and Generation of Conditioned Media

Murine BMDM were generated by isolating the bone marrow of above described wt and Lcn-$2^{-/-}$ mice. Cells were differentiated directly in 6-well plates (6 × 106 cells/well) in the presence of 20 ng/mL macrophage colony-stimulating factor (M-CSF) (Peprotech, Hamburg, Germany) for up to 7 days. At day 3, fresh M-CSF was added. For 24 h prior to stimulation cells were serum-starved. BMDM were stimulated for 24 h in RPMI medium supplemented with 20 ng/mL IL-10 (Peprotech, Hamburg, Germany) for the induction of an anti-inflammatory, iron-release phenotype as previously published [36]. The conditioned media of polarized BMDM were collected, centrifuged at 1000× $g$ for 5 min, and aliquots were stored at −80 °C until further use. Supernatant of unstimulated MΦ served as control. Where indicated, iron chelator 2′2 DPD was added to wt cm at a concentration of 100 μM for 24 h.

### 4.5. Generation of Recombinant Lcn-2

Recombinant mouse Lcn-2 was produced by transformation of *E. coli* with a pGEX-4T-3-NGAL plasmid as already described for human recombinant Lcn-2 [21]. In order to test efficient Lcn-2-catechol-iron complex formation, UV-visible spectroscopy (UV-vis) was used as previously described [44]. To generate the holo-Lcn-2 protein equimolar amounts of 10 μM Lcn-2 were incubated with 10 μM catechol (Sigma-Aldrich, Steinheim, Germany) and 10 μM iron (Sigma).

### 4.6. Lcn-2 Immunoprecipitation

For immunoprecipitation (IP), supernatants of stimulated BMDMs were collected as described above. Dynabeads (Thermo Fisher, Dreieich, Germany) were added, and 1mg protein was incubated overnight at 4 °C in the presence of a specific antibody against Lcn-2 (MAB1857, R&D, Wiesbaden, Germany). Beads were precipitated using the DynaMag-2 magnet (Thermo Fisher, Dreieich, Germany) and washed three times with IP buffer. Protein was eluted by addition of 2× loading buffer and incubated at 95 °C for 5 min.

### 4.7. Atomic Absorption Spectrometry

Wt or Lcn-$2^{-/-}$ MΦ were stimulated with IL-10 (20 ng/mL) for 24 h. Afterwards, mTEC were stimulated for 24 h with cm from either wt or Lcn-$2^{-/-}$ MΦ. Where indicated, holo-Lcn-2 (1 μg/mL) was added to Lcn-$2^{-/-}$ media for rescue experiments. The iron content of MΦ supernatants as well as the intracellular iron amount of stimulated mTECs was determined by graphite furnace atomic absorption spectrometry (AAS). Samples were measured as triplicates with a PinAAcleTM 900 T Atomic Absorption Spectrometer (PerkinElmer, Rodgau, Germany). Slit 0.2 nm and wavelength 248.33 nm were used as spectrometer parameters. A hollow cathode iron lamp (30 mA maximum operating current) was run at 100% maximum current. The calibration solutions (10 μg/L to 90 μg/L) were prepared by adequate dilution of iron standard for AAS (Sigma-Aldrich, Steinheim, Germany) stock solution. A pyrolysis temperature of 1400 °C and an atomization temperature of 2100 °C were used.

### 4.8. Establishment of Rescue Model Following Cisplatin Injury in mTECs

mTECs were either cultured in standard medium without FCS (designated as ctrl) or injured with 5 μM Cisplatin (designated as Cis) for 24 h. Hereafter, Cisplatin-injured mTECs were cultured for a further 24 h in cm from IL-10-stimulated MΦ from wt (designated as cm wt MΦ) or Lcn-$2^{-/-}$ mice (designated as cm Lcn-$2^{-/-}$ MΦ). For rescue experiments, cm from Lcn-$2^{-/-}$ was supplemented with holo-Lcn-2 (designated as holo-Lcn-2).

### 4.9. RNA Extraction and Quantitative Real-Time PCR (qPCR)

RNA isolation cDNA synthesis and qPCR were performed as previously described [46]. Briefly, RNA was isolated (30-1010, peqlab, Erlangen, Germany) and transcribed into cDNA (K1642, Thermo Fisher), serving as template in qPCR mix (1725006CUST, Bio-Rad, Dreieich, Germany). We used TBP (TATA-binding protein) as an internal housekeeping gene control for detection of gene expression in BMDM, while RPS27a (ribosomal protein 27a) mRNA expression served as a housekeeping gene for real-time (RT)-PCR and β-actin for qPCR analysis in mTEC [53]. Primers were bought from Bio-Rad, Biomers (Ulm, Germany), or Thermo Fisher and are listed in Table 1.

### 4.10. Western Blot

Protein samples of 5 μg were dissolved in sample buffer (Laemmli buffer, Bio-Rad) containing DTT (dithiothreitol) and treated for 5 min at 95 °C. Protein samples were separated on a 4–12% CRIT XT BIS-TRIS GEL (Bio-Rad) and transferred to a PVDF membrane (Bio-Rad). Membranes were blocked with 5% fat-free milk in tris-buffered saline containing 0.1% Tween-20 for 1.5 h. Primary antibodies were added and membranes were incubated overnight at 4 °C. Hereafter, an adequate horseradish peroxidase (HRP)-conjugated secondary antibodies were added and incubated for 2 h at room temperature. Visualization was performed using Clarity ECL or Clarity ECL max (Biorad). Primary Antibodies: Klotho (MAB1819, 1:500, R&D), KIM-1 (#3809, 1:1000, ProSci, Poway, CA, USA), Pan-Actin antibody (#4968, dilution, Cell Signaling, Frankfurt am Main, Deutschland).

**Table 1.** Primer sequences.

| Primer | Sequence |
|---|---|
| β-actin | Forward: 5-CCACCATGTACCCAGGCATT-3<br>Reverse: 5-AGGGTGTAAAACGCAGCTCA-3 |
| β-Catenin | Forward: 5-TCTGAGGACAAGCCACAGGATTACA-3<br>Reverse: 5-GGGCACCAATGTCCAGTCCAA-3 |
| CK18 | Forward: 5-TTGTCACCACCAAGTCTGCC-3<br>Reverse: 5-TTGTATCGGGCCTCCACATC-3 |
| E-Cadherin (real-time) | Forward: 5-TGAAGAAGGAAGAAGA-3<br>Reverse: 5-TGGGAGCCACTTTCGA-3 |
| E-Cadherin (qRT) | Forward: CAACGATCCTGACCAGCAGT<br>Reverse: TGTATTGCTGCTTGGCCTCA |
| IL-1β | Forward: 5-AGGCCACAGGTATTTTGTCG-3<br>Reverse: 5-GACCTTCCAGGATGAGGACA-3 |
| iNOS | Forward: 5-ACCCTAAGAGTCACAAAATGGC-3<br>Reverse: 5-TTGATCCTCACATACTGTGGACG-3 |
| Lcn-2 | qHsaCED0045408 |
| MRC | Forward: 5-GGAGTGATGGAACCCCAGTG-3<br>Reverse: 5-CTGTCCGCCCAGTATCCATC-3 |
| PCNA | Forward: 5-AATGGGGTGAAGTTTTCTGC-3<br>Reverse: 5-CAGTGGAGTGGCTTTTGTGA-3 |
| RPS27a | Forward: 5-GACCCTTACGGGGAAAACCAT-3<br>Reverse: 5-AGACAAAGTCCGGCCATCTTC-3 |
| Stathmin | Forward: 5-CTTGCGAGAGAAGGACAAGC-3<br>Reverse: 5-CGGTCCTACATCGGCTTCTA-3 |
| TBP | Forward: 5-GGGCCGCCGGTTAACT-3<br>Reverse: 5-AGCCCTGAGCGTGGCA-3 |
| TNFα | Forward: 5-CCATTCCTGAGTTCTGCAAAGG-3<br>Reverse: 5-AGGTAGGAAGGCCTGAGATCTTATC-3 |
| YM-1 | Forward: 5-GGGCATACCTTTATCCTGAG-3<br>Reverse: 5-CCACTGAAGTCATCCATGTC-3 |
| ZO-1 (real-time) | Forward: 5-GCCATTACACGGTCCTCTGA-3<br>Reverse: 5-GCGAAAGGTAAGGGACTGG-3 |
| ZO-1 (qPCR) | Forward: GCCATTACACGGTCCTCTGA<br>Reverse: GCGAAAGGTAAGGGACTGGA |

### 4.11. *Lcn-2 ELISA*

Supernatants were collected from cultured MΦ. A volume of 100 μL of each sample was applied to an ELISA well-plate previously covered with the anti-Lcn-2 (MAB1857, R&D) and blocked for 1 h. After sample incubation, the detection anti-Lcn-2 antibody was added. HRP-conjugated avidin (Invitrogen, obtained from Thermo Fisher) was incubated for 1h, the color reagent (OPD tablets; Dako, obtained from Agilent, Waldbronn, Germany) was added, and the color development was assessed.

### 4.12. *Phalloidin-Staining*

Changes in the cytoskeleton and the F-actin stress fibers were visualized by phalloidin staining. Briefly, cells were fixed in 4% buffered formaldehyde for 10 min and then permeabilized with PBS containing 0.1% Triton X-100 and 1% BSA for 30 min. The slides were then incubated with Alexa Fluor 568 phalloidin (00027, dilution 1:40, Molecular Probes Inc.) in PBS with 1% BSA for 30 min, counterstained with DAPI (D9542, Sigma-Aldrich, Steinheim, Germany), washed three times with PBS, and finally mounted using mowiol (Calbiochem, Darmstadt, Germany). Images were acquired on an LSM 800 (Zeiss, Wetzlar, Germany) confocal microscope.

### 4.13. Immunofluoresecence Cytokeratin Stain

Confluent monolayers were rinsed three times with PBS and fixed with ice-cold methanol/acetone (1:1) for 5 min. The fixed cells were washed twice. Unspecific binding sites were blocked by PBS containing 5% normal goat serum for 20 min. Primary antibody (anti-Pan Cytokeratin C2931, 1:400, Sigma-Aldrich, Steinheim, Germany) was applied and incubated for 30 min at 37 °C with gentle shaking. After washing, cells were incubated with a Cy3-conjugated goat-anti-mouse IgG mAb for 30 min at 37 °C. Slides were mounted with mounting medium and examined using Zeiss fluorescence microscope equipment.

### 4.14. xCELLigence Proliferation Assay

Proliferation of mTECs was measured using the RTCA DP xCELLigence instrument (OLS, Bremen, Germany) as described previously [20]. Data are presented as the slope per hour (slope 1/h) of the normalized cell index as a measure for the time-dependent changes in impedance.

### 4.15. Statistical Analyses

Statistical analyses were performed applying GraphPad Prism® 5.02 software (GraphPad Software, San Diego, CA, USA). The distribution of variables was tested for normality using the Kolmogorov–Smirnov test. Accordingly, statistical significance was calculated using one-way ANOVA followed by Tukey's multiple comparison test or Kruskal–Wallis test followed by Dunn's posthoc test, where applicable. Significance of correlations was determined by Spearman's test including all investigated groups. $p$-values $\leq 0.05$ were assumed as statistically significant. In the figures, horizontal lines within the boxes represent the medians, boxes represent the interquartile range (25–75%). Whiskers above and below the box indicate the 90th and 10th percentiles. The individual points that are plotted beyond the whiskers represent outliers, which were included in the statistical analyses.

**Supplementary Materials:** Supplementary materials can be found at http://www.mdpi.com/1422-0067/21/6/2038/s1.

**Author Contributions:** Conceptualization: A.U. and M.J.; Investigation and data interpretation: A.U., A.-K.T., C.M., C.R., P.C.B., J.K.M., M.J.; Writing—Original Draft Preparation: A.U. and M.J.; Writing—Review & Editing: A.U., A.-K.T., C.M., C.R., P.C.B., J.K.M., M.J. All authors have read and agreed to the published version of the manuscript.

**Funding:** The study was financed by the Wilhelm Sander-Stiftung. The foundation had no influence on design of the study, data collection and interpretation, or the decision to publish.

**Acknowledgments:** We especially thank Petra Metzler and Christine von Hayn for their technical support.

**Conflicts of Interest:** The authors declare no conflict of interest.

## Abbreviations

| | |
|---|---|
| AAS | Atomic absorption spectrometry |
| BMDM | Bone marrow-derived macrophages |
| Cis | Cisplatin |
| Cm | Conditioned medium |
| ctrl | Control |
| IL-10 | Interleukin 10 |
| IRI | Ischemia-reperfusion injury |
| KIM-1 | Kidney injury molecule 1 |
| Lcn-2 | Lipocalin-2 |
| mTEC | Murine tubular epithelial cells |
| MΦ | Macrophages |
| wt | Wildtype |

## References


1. Urbschat, A.; Obermuller, N.; Haferkamp, A. Biomarkers of kidney injury. *Biomarkers* **2011**, *16*, S22–S30. [CrossRef] [PubMed]
2. Ronco, C.; Bellomo, R.; Kellum, J.A. Acute kidney injury. *Lancet* **2019**, *394*, 1949–1964. [CrossRef]
3. Bonventre, J.V. Dedifferentiation and proliferation of surviving epithelial cells in acute renal failure. *J. Am. Soc. Nephrol.* **2003**, *14*, S55–S61. [CrossRef] [PubMed]
4. Huen, S.C.; Cantley, L.G. Macrophages in Renal Injury and Repair. *Annu. Rev. Physiol.* **2017**, *79*, 449–469. [CrossRef] [PubMed]
5. Ysebaert, D.K.; De Greef, K.E.; Vercauteren, S.R.; Ghielli, M.; Verpooten, G.A.; Eyskens, E.J.; De Broe, M.E. Identification and kinetics of leukocytes after severe ischaemia/reperfusion renal injury. *Nephrol. Dial. Transpl.* **2000**, *15*, 1562–1574. [CrossRef] [PubMed]
6. Vinuesa, E.; Hotter, G.; Jung, M.; Herrero-Fresneda, I.; Torras, J.; Sola, A. Macrophage involvement in the kidney repair phase after ischaemia/reperfusion injury. *J. Pathol.* **2008**, *214*, 104–113. [CrossRef]
7. Mosser, D.M.; Edwards, J.P. Exploring the full spectrum of macrophage activation. *Nat. Rev. Immunol.* **2008**, *8*, 958–969. [CrossRef]
8. Labonte, A.C.; Tosello-Trampont, A.C.; Hahn, Y.S. The role of macrophage polarization in infectious and inflammatory diseases. *Mol. Cells* **2014**, *37*, 275–285. [CrossRef]
9. Jung, M.; Brune, B.; Hotter, G.; Sola, A. Macrophage-derived Lipocalin-2 contributes to ischemic resistance mechanisms by protecting from renal injury. *Sci. Rep.* **2016**, *6*, 21950. [CrossRef]
10. Jung, M.; Sola, A.; Hughes, J.; Kluth, D.C.; Vinuesa, E.; Vinas, J.L.; Perez-Ladaga, A.; Hotter, G. Infusion of IL-10-expressing cells protects against renal ischemia through induction of lipocalin-2. *Kidney Int.* **2012**, *81*, 969–982. [CrossRef]
11. Sola, A.; Weigert, A.; Jung, M.; Vinuesa, E.; Brecht, K.; Weis, N.; Brune, B.; Borregaard, N.; Hotter, G. Sphingosine-1-phosphate signalling induces the production of Lcn-2 by macrophages to promote kidney regeneration. *J. Pathol.* **2011**, *225*, 597–608. [CrossRef] [PubMed]
12. Recalcati, S.; Locati, M.; Cairo, G. Systemic and cellular consequences of macrophage control of iron metabolism. *Semin. Immunol.* **2012**, *24*, 393–398. [CrossRef] [PubMed]
13. Haase, M.; Devarajan, P.; Haase-Fielitz, A.; Bellomo, R.; Cruz, D.N.; Wagener, G.; Krawczeski, C.D.; Koyner, J.L.; Murray, P.; Zappitelli, M.; et al. The outcome of neutrophil gelatinase-associated lipocalin-positive subclinical acute kidney injury: A multicenter pooled analysis of prospective studies. *J. Am. Coll. Cardiol.* **2011**, *57*, 1752–1761. [CrossRef] [PubMed]
14. Paragas, N.; Qiu, A.; Zhang, Q.; Samstein, B.; Deng, S.X.; Schmidt-Ott, K.M.; Viltard, M.; Yu, W.; Forster, C.S.; Gong, G.; et al. The Ngal reporter mouse detects the response of the kidney to injury in real time. *Nat. Med.* **2011**, *17*, 216–222. [CrossRef]
15. Mishra, J.; Ma, Q.; Prada, A.; Mitsnefes, M.; Zahedi, K.; Yang, J.; Barasch, J.; Devarajan, P. Identification of neutrophil gelatinase-associated lipocalin as a novel early urinary biomarker for ischemic renal injury. *J. Am. Soc. Nephrol.* **2003**, *14*, 2534–2543. [CrossRef]
16. Mishra, J.; Mori, K.; Ma, Q.; Kelly, C.; Barasch, J.; Devarajan, P. Neutrophil gelatinase-associated lipocalin: A novel early urinary biomarker for cisplatin nephrotoxicity. *Am. J. Nephrol.* **2004**, *24*, 307–315. [CrossRef]
17. Mishra, J.; Mori, K.; Ma, Q.; Kelly, C.; Yang, J.; Mitsnefes, M.; Barasch, J.; Devarajan, P. Amelioration of ischemic acute renal injury by neutrophil gelatinase-associated lipocalin. *J. Am. Soc. Nephrol.* **2004**, *15*, 3073–3082. [CrossRef]
18. Mori, K.; Lee, H.T.; Rapoport, D.; Drexler, I.R.; Foster, K.; Yang, J.; Schmidt-Ott, K.M.; Chen, X.; Li, J.Y.; Weiss, S.; et al. Endocytic delivery of lipocalin-siderophore-iron complex rescues the kidney from ischemia-reperfusion injury. *J. Clin. Investig.* **2005**, *115*, 610–621. [CrossRef]
19. Gwira, J.A.; Wei, F.; Ishibe, S.; Ueland, J.M.; Barasch, J.; Cantley, L.G. Expression of neutrophil gelatinase-associated lipocalin regulates epithelial morphogenesis in vitro. *J. Biol. Chem.* **2005**, *280*, 7875–7882. [CrossRef]
20. Jung, M.; Oren, B.; Mora, J.; Mertens, C.; Dziumbla, S.; Popp, R.; Weigert, A.; Grossmann, N.; Fleming, I.; Brune, B. Lipocalin 2 from macrophages stimulated by tumor cell-derived sphingosine 1-phosphate promotes lymphangiogenesis and tumor metastasis. *Sci. Signal.* **2016**, *9*, ra64. [CrossRef]

21. Oren, B.; Urosevic, J.; Mertens, C.; Mora, J.; Guiu, M.; Gomis, R.R.; Weigert, A.; Schmid, T.; Grein, S.; Brune, B.; et al. Tumour stroma-derived lipocalin-2 promotes breast cancer metastasis. *J. Pathol.* **2016**, *239*, 274–285. [CrossRef] [PubMed]
22. Vinuesa, E.; Sola, A.; Jung, M.; Alfaro, V.; Hotter, G. Lipocalin-2-induced renal regeneration depends on cytokines. *Am. J. Physiol. Ren. Physiol.* **2008**, *295*, F1554–F1562. [CrossRef] [PubMed]
23. Devireddy, L.R.; Gazin, C.; Zhu, X.; Green, M.R. A cell-surface receptor for lipocalin 24p3 selectively mediates apoptosis and iron uptake. *Cell* **2005**, *123*, 1293–1305. [CrossRef] [PubMed]
24. Paller, M.S.; Hedlund, B.E. Role of iron in postischemic renal injury in the rat. *Kidney Int.* **1988**, *34*, 474–480. [CrossRef] [PubMed]
25. Paller, M.S.; Hedlund, B.E. Extracellular iron chelators protect kidney cells from hypoxia/reoxygenation. *Free Radic. Biol. Med.* **1994**, *17*, 597–603. [CrossRef]
26. Lieberthal, W.; Triaca, V.; Levine, J. Mechanisms of death induced by cisplatin in proximal tubular epithelial cells: Apoptosis vs. necrosis. *Am. J. Physiol.* **1996**, *270*, F700–F708. [CrossRef]
27. Borch, R.F.; Pleasants, M.E. Inhibition of cis-platinum nephrotoxicity by diethyldithiocarbamate rescue in a rat model. *Proc. Natl. Acad. Sci. USA* **1979**, *76*, 6611–6614. [CrossRef]
28. Zhou, H.; Kato, A.; Yasuda, H.; Miyaji, T.; Fujigaki, Y.; Yamamoto, T.; Yonemura, K.; Hishida, A. The induction of cell cycle regulatory and DNA repair proteins in cisplatin-induced acute renal failure. *Toxicol. Appl. Pharm.* **2004**, *200*, 111–120. [CrossRef]
29. Kashiwagi, E.; Tonomura, Y.; Kondo, C.; Masuno, K.; Fujisawa, K.; Tsuchiya, N.; Matsushima, S.; Torii, M.; Takasu, N.; Izawa, T.; et al. Involvement of neutrophil gelatinase-associated lipocalin and osteopontin in renal tubular regeneration and interstitial fibrosis after cisplatin-induced renal failure. *Exp. Toxicol. Pathol.* **2014**, *66*, 301–311. [CrossRef]
30. Molitoris, B.A.; Marrs, J. The role of cell adhesion molecules in ischemic acute renal failure. *Am. J. Med.* **1999**, *106*, 583–592. [CrossRef]
31. Bonventre, J.V.; Kelly, K.J. Adhesion molecules and acute renal failure. *Adv. Nephrol. Necker Hosp.* **1996**, *25*, 159–176. [PubMed]
32. Kruidering, M.; van de Water, B.; Zhan, Y.; Baelde, J.J.; Heer, E.; Mulder, G.J.; Stevens, J.L.; Nagelkerke, J.F. Cisplatin effects on F-actin and matrix proteins precede renal tubular cell detachment and apoptosis in vitro. *Cell Death Differ.* **1998**, *5*, 601–614. [CrossRef] [PubMed]
33. Jung, M.; Hotter, G.; Vinas, J.L.; Sola, A. Cisplatin upregulates mitochondrial nitric oxide synthase and peroxynitrite formation to promote renal injury. *Toxicol. Appl. Pharm.* **2009**, *234*, 236–246. [CrossRef] [PubMed]
34. Curmi, P.A.; Gavet, O.; Charbaut, E.; Ozon, S.; Lachkar-Colmerauer, S.; Manceau, V.; Siavoshian, S.; Maucuer, A.; Sobel, A. Stathmin and its phosphoprotein family: General properties, biochemical and functional interaction with tubulin. *Cell Struct. Funct.* **1999**, *24*, 345–357. [CrossRef]
35. Peschanski, M.; Hirsch, E.; Dusart, I.; Doye, V.; Marty, S.; Manceau, V.; Sobel, A. Stathmin: Cellular localization of a major phosphoprotein in the adult rat and human CNS. *J. Comp. Neurol.* **1993**, *337*, 655–668. [CrossRef]
36. Mertens, C.; Akam, E.A.; Rehwald, C.; Brune, B.; Tomat, E.; Jung, M. Intracellular Iron Chelation Modulates the Macrophage Iron Phenotype with Consequences on Tumor Progression. *PLoS ONE* **2016**, *11*, e0166164. [CrossRef]
37. Recalcati, S.; Locati, M.; Marini, A.; Santambrogio, P.; Zaninotto, F.; De Pizzol, M.; Zammataro, L.; Girelli, D.; Cairo, G. Differential regulation of iron homeostasis during human macrophage polarized activation. *Eur. J. Immunol.* **2010**, *40*, 824–835. [CrossRef]
38. Rehwald, C.; Schnetz, M.; Urbschat, A.; Mertens, C.; Meier, J.K.; Bauer, R.; Baer, P.; Winslow, S.; Roos, F.C.; Zwicker, K.; et al. The iron load of lipocalin-2 (LCN-2) defines its pro-tumour function in clear-cell renal cell carcinoma. *Br. J. Cancer* **2019**, *122*, 421–433. [CrossRef]
39. Mertens, C.; Mora, J.; Oren, B.; Grein, S.; Winslow, S.; Scholich, K.; Weigert, A.; Malmstrom, P.; Forsare, C.; Ferno, M.; et al. Macrophage-derived lipocalin-2 transports iron in the tumor microenvironment. *Oncoimmunology* **2018**, *7*, e1408751. [CrossRef]
40. Baer, P.C.; Nockher, W.A.; Haase, W.; Scherberich, J.E. Isolation of proximal and distal tubule cells from human kidney by immunomagnetic separation. Technical note. *Kidney Int.* **1997**, *52*, 1321–1331. [CrossRef]

41. Dekel, B.; Zangi, L.; Shezen, E.; Reich-Zeliger, S.; Eventov-Friedman, S.; Katchman, H.; Jacob-Hirsch, J.; Amariglio, N.; Rechavi, G.; Margalit, R.; et al. Isolation and characterization of nontubular sca-1+lin-multipotent stem/progenitor cells from adult mouse kidney. *J. Am. Soc. Nephrol.* **2006**, *17*, 3300–3314. [CrossRef]
42. Dasari, S.; Tchounwou, P.B. Cisplatin in cancer therapy: Molecular mechanisms of action. *Eur. J. Pharm.* **2014**, *740*, 364–378. [CrossRef]
43. Volarevic, V.; Djokovic, B.; Jankovic, M.G.; Harrell, C.R.; Fellabaum, C.; Djonov, V.; Arsenijevic, N. Molecular mechanisms of cisplatin-induced nephrotoxicity: A balance on the knife edge between renoprotection and tumor toxicity. *J. Biomed. Sci.* **2019**, *26*, 25. [CrossRef] [PubMed]
44. Zahedi, K.; Wang, Z.; Barone, S.; Tehrani, K.; Yokota, N.; Petrovic, S.; Rabb, H.; Soleimani, M. Identification of stathmin as a novel marker of cell proliferation in the recovery phase of acute ischemic renal failure. *Am. J. Physiol. Cell Physiol.* **2004**, *286*, C1203–C1211. [CrossRef] [PubMed]
45. Miura, K.; Goldstein, R.S.; Pasino, D.A.; Hook, J.B. Cisplatin nephrotoxicity: Role of filtration and tubular transport of cisplatin in isolated perfused kidneys. *Toxicology* **1987**, *44*, 147–158. [CrossRef]
46. Witzgall, R.; Brown, D.; Schwarz, C.; Bonventre, J.V. Localization of proliferating cell nuclear antigen, vimentin, c-Fos, and clusterin in the postischemic kidney. Evidence for a heterogenous genetic response among nephron segments, and a large pool of mitotically active and dedifferentiated cells. *J. Clin. Investig.* **1994**, *93*, 2175–2188. [CrossRef] [PubMed]
47. Caracausi, M.; Piovesan, A.; Antonaros, F.; Strippoli, P.; Vitale, L.; Pelleri, M.C. Systematic identification of human housekeeping genes possibly useful as references in gene expression studies. *Mol. Med. Rep.* **2017**, *16*, 2397–2410. [CrossRef] [PubMed]
48. Jung, M.; Weigert, A.; Tausendschon, M.; Mora, J.; Oren, B.; Sola, A.; Hotter, G.; Muta, T.; Brune, B. Interleukin-10-induced neutrophil gelatinase-associated lipocalin production in macrophages with consequences for tumor growth. *Mol. Cell Biol.* **2012**, *32*, 3938–3948. [CrossRef]
49. Tanase, D.M.; Gosav, E.M.; Radu, S.; Costea, C.F.; Ciocoiu, M.; Carauleanu, A.; Lacatusu, C.M.; Maranduca, M.A.; Floria, M.; Rezus, C. The Predictive Role of the Biomarker Kidney Molecule-1 (KIM-1) in Acute Kidney Injury (AKI) Cisplatin-Induced Nephrotoxicity. *Int. J. Mol. Sci.* **2019**, *20*, 5238. [CrossRef]
50. Mitobe, M.; Yoshida, T.; Sugiura, H.; Shirota, S.; Tsuchiya, K.; Nihei, H. Oxidative stress decreases klotho expression in a mouse kidney cell line. *Nephron Exp. Nephrol.* **2005**, *101*, e67–e74. [CrossRef]
51. Sugiura, H.; Yoshida, T.; Tsuchiya, K.; Mitobe, M.; Nishimura, S.; Shirota, S.; Akiba, T.; Nihei, H. Klotho reduces apoptosis in experimental ischaemic acute renal failure. *Nephrol. Dial. Transpl.* **2005**, *20*, 2636–2645. [CrossRef] [PubMed]
52. Hu, M.C.; Shi, M.; Zhang, J.; Quinones, H.; Kuro-o, M.; Moe, O.W. Klotho deficiency is an early biomarker of renal ischemia-reperfusion injury and its replacement is protective. *Kidney Int.* **2010**, *78*, 1240–1251. [CrossRef] [PubMed]
53. Duffield, J.S. Macrophages in kidney repair and regeneration. *J. Am. Soc. Nephrol.* **2011**, *22*, 199–201. [CrossRef] [PubMed]

International Journal of
*Molecular Sciences*

MDPI

*Review*

# The Influence of Inflammation on Anemia in CKD Patients

**Anna Gluba-Brzózka [1,*], Beata Franczyk [1], Robert Olszewski [2] and Jacek Rysz [1]**

[1] Department of Nephrology, Hypertension and Family Medicine, Medical University of Lodz, 90-549 Lodz, Poland; bfranczyk-skora@wp.pl (B.F.); jacek.rysz@umed.lodz.pl (J.R.)

[2] Department of Geriatrics, National Institute of Geriatrics Rheumatology and Rehabilitation and Department of Ultrasound, Institute of Fundamental Technological Research, Polish Academy of Sciences, Warsaw, Poland (IPPT PAN), 02-106 Warsaw, Poland; robert.olszewski@me.com

* Correspondence: aniagluba@yahoo.pl

Received: 18 November 2019; Accepted: 19 January 2020; Published: 22 January 2020

**Abstract:** Anemia is frequently observed in the course of chronic kidney disease (CKD) and it is associated with diminishing the quality of a patient's life. It also enhances morbidity and mortality and hastens the CKD progression rate. Patients with CKD frequently suffer from a chronic inflammatory state which is related to a vast range of underlying factors. The results of studies have demonstrated that persistent inflammation may contribute to the variability in Hb levels and hyporesponsiveness to erythropoietin stimulating agents (ESA), which are frequently observed in CKD patients. The understanding of the impact of inflammatory cytokines on erythropoietin production and hepcidin synthesis will enable one to unravel the net of interactions of multiple factors involved in the pathogenesis of the anemia of chronic disease. It seems that anti-cytokine and anti-oxidative treatment strategies may be the future of pharmacological interventions aiming at the treatment of inflammation-associated hyporesponsiveness to ESA. The discovery of new therapeutic approaches towards the treatment of anemia in CKD patients has become highly awaited. The treatment of anemia with erythropoietin (EPO) was associated with great benefits for some patients but not all.

**Keywords:** inflammation; chronic kidney disease; anemia; anemia of inflammation; ESA hyporesponsiveness

## 1. Introduction

Anemia is frequently observed in the course of chronic kidney disease (CKD) and it is associated with a diminished quality of patients' life. It also enhances morbidity and mortality and hastens the CKD progression rate [1]. Patients with CKD frequently suffer from a chronic inflammatory state which is related to the vast range of underlying factors, such as higher incidence of infections, increased levels of proinflammatory cytokines, the uremic milieu, the widespread presence of arteriosclerosis, and others [2]. The results of animal studies demonstrated that serum half-lives of proinflammatory cytokines, including TNF- and IL-1 are higher in animals without renal function [3]. Deterioration of renal function may also influence the level of other inflammatory molecules, such as serum C-reactive protein (CRP) or IL-6, which concentration inversely correlated with creatinine clearance [4,5].

The discovery of new therapeutic approaches towards the treatment of anemia in CKD patients has become highly awaited. Treatment of anemia with erythropoietin (EPO) was associated with great benefits for some patients but not all. Clinical and experimental evidence indicates the important role of inflammation in poor response to EPO therapy. Therefore, anti-inflammatory agents seem to be beneficial in the therapy of patients who are EPO bad responders as well as drugs that could antagonize the effects of hepcidin [6].

## 2. Anemia in CKD Patients

Anemia is a frequent problem in CKD patients [7]. In CKD, it is typically normocytic, normochromic, and hypoproliferative [8]. According to large-scale population studies the incidence of anemia (hemoglobin <12 g/dL) is less than 10% in patients with CKD stages I and II, 20%–40% in stage III, 50–60% in stage IV, and it exceeds 70% in patients with end-stage renal disease (stage V) [9–11]. Other studies indicate that in the dialysis population anemia incidence is as high as 90% [12,13].

The prevalence of more severe anemia (hemoglobin ≤ 10 g/dL) is much less common: 5.6% in stage 3 CKD and 27.2% in stage 5 non-dialysis CKD patients [13,14]. These data clearly show that anemia appears early in the course of CKD and its occurrence is increasing along with the declining glomerular filtration rate [11]. Data from the National Health and Nutrition Examination Survey (NHANES) in 2007–2008 and 2009–2010 [13] demonstrates that despite anemia being very common in patients with advanced CKD, patients in the United States were relatively rarely receiving treatment for it (only 20% of patients with CKD stage 4 and 42% of those with stage 5). Anemia in this study was defined using gender-specific thresholds (<12 g/dL for female patients and <13 g/dL for male patients). Glomerular filtration rate, gender, age, race, comorbidities are considered as the predictors of CKD anemia [15].

Anemia in patients with CKD is a multifactorial process, in which chronic inflammation, erythropoietin deficiency, iron metabolism disorders, blood loss on hemodialysis sessions, uncontrolled hyperparathyroidism, deficiency of essential nutrients like iron, folic acid, and vitamin B12, the use of some drugs, including ACE inhibitors and uremic toxins play the most important role [7,8,16,17]. The understanding of underlying mechanisms of anemia in CKD is important due to the fact that in some patients erythropoietin stimulating agents (ESA) treatment might be least ineffective or even deleterious [17,18].

*Pre-dialysis CKD patients.* According to studies, the relative deficiency in erythropoietin (EPO) production by the peritubular cells of kidneys is responsible for defective erythropoiesis in CKD patients [17,19]. Erythropoietin deficiency is associated with disturbances in the differentiation and maturation of red blood cell precursors [20]. The results of some studies imply that circulating uremic-induced inhibitors of erythropoiesis may contribute to the development of anemia [8,21]. Sera from uremic patients have been showed to inhibit hematopoietic progenitor's growth [22]. Chiang et al. [23] demonstrated that indoxyl sulfate (IS), which is a protein-bound uremic toxin, impaired erythropoiesis in a hydroxylase inhibitor (HIF)-dependent manner and limited EPO gene transcription during hypoxia. It seems that IS stimulates hepcidin production via a pathway that involves both aryl hydrocarbon receptor (AhR) and oxidative stress, which in consequence leads to iron sequestration and impaired iron utilization in CKD [24]. Wu et al. [25] found that IS removal improved the impact of ESA on anemia in late-stage CKD patients confirming that IS mediates renal anemia via EPO regulation. Moreover, Ahmed et al. [26] suggested that indoxyl sulfate triggered suicidal erythrocyte death in renal failure. Radioisotope labeling studies confirmed shortened red blood cell survival due to metabolic and mechanical factors in CKD [21,27]. In CKD, it was shown that intra- and extracellular factors diminished red blood cell survival by 30% to 50%, probably due to the red blood cell membrane failure to pump sodium to the extracellular medium [28].

Apart from true iron deficiency, in many CKD patients, functional iron deficiency has been observed. It is characterized by disturbed iron release from body stores, which makes meeting the demand for erythropoiesis impossible. Low serum transferrin saturation (a parameter informing the amount of circulating iron) and normal or high serum ferritin (a marker of body iron stores) were shown in this group of patients. Secondary hyperparathyroidism, which is frequently observed in CKD, contributes to the development of anemia and greater resistance to erythropoietin [29]. Finally, hepcidin, which is a key regulator of circulating iron absorption, has been found to be involved in the etiology of anemia in CKD [30,31]. Its concentrations were demonstrated to be influenced by inflammation [32]. The fact that anemia develops in spite of elevated EPO levels in CKD suggests that peripheral resistance or hyporesponsiveness to EPO may be the factual reason for its occurrence [11].

*Dialysis CKD patients.* Apart from the aforementioned mechanisms, anemia in dialysis patients can be associated with iron losses. According to Besarab et al. [21], the losses of iron in hemodialysis patients reach 1–3 g per year and they are associated with chronic bleeding related to platelet dysfunction and also frequent phlebotomy, hemolysis, and blood retained in the extracorporeal circulation during dialysis. Additionally, patients undergoing dialysis show impaired dietary iron absorption [33,34]. HD patients with high CRP levels (>8 mg/L) have been shown to have lower iron absorption than patients with lower CRP levels [35]. According to studies, inflammation (via cytokines and bacterial lipopolysaccharide, LPS) regulates hepcidin expression and production in response to liver iron levels, hypoxia and anemia, which results in functional iron deficiency or enhanced ferritin and diminished transferrin production, shunting iron to the reticuloendothelial storage pool instead of delivery to erythrocyte precursors [36–38]. Inflammation acting together with uremic toxicity and hepcidin exacerbates anemia at different stages. Tozoni et al. [39] suggested that in HD patients, hypoxemia and uremic toxins may act synergistically and decrease red blood cell life span (RBCLS). They provided evidence that even in the case of healthy red blood cells, hypoxia, and uremia stimulated eryptosis and disturbances in redox balance. These two stimuli together have been demonstrated to increase PS exposure, stimulate cellular shrinkage, and enhance calcium influx into the RBC [39]. Bonomini et al. [40] revealed that the RBC life span in CKD patients was related to enhanced erythrocyte deformability and abnormalities of plasma membrane symmetry and cytoskeleton. These alterations and the destruction of the membrane were shown to be hastened by the uremic environment, inflammation, and oxidative stress [41]. However, Bataille et al. [17] failed to find any correlation between plasmatic concentrations of uremic toxins, such as indole 3-acetic acid (IAA), sulfate (IS), and paracresyl sulfate (PCS), and any parameter related to anemia in hemodialysis patients. Therefore, they suggested that indolic uremic toxins and PCS may have no or a very slight impact on anemia parameters, i.e., Hb concentrations or ESA hyporesponsiveness in this population [17].

*KDIGO Recommendations*

KDIGO guidelines recommend hemoglobin level measurement in patients with CKD without diagnosed anemia when clinically indicated but at least once a year in subjects with CKD stage 3, at least 2 times a year in those with CKD stage 4–5 who are not on dialysis and at least every 3 months in those with stage 5 CKD undergoing either hemodialysis (HD) or peritoneal dialysis (PD) (Not Graded) [42]. In case of CKD patients with anemia, who are not treated with ESA, Hb levels should be measured when clinically indicated (Not Graded)—at least every 3 months in patients with CKD stage 3–5 who are not on dialysis (CKD-ND) or stage 5D on PD and every month in patients with CKD 5D in HD. In turn, in patients with anemia on ESA treatment, Hb levels should be measured when clinically indicated—in the correction phase once in a month and in the maintenance phase: at least every 3 months in patients with CKD (not on dialysis), monthly in patients with CKD-5D (hemodialysis), and every 2 months in patients with CKD patients on peritoneal dialysis [42].

The administration of vitamin D analogs has been linked with the amelioration of anemia and/or the reduction in EPO needs [29,43]. The beneficial effect of vitamin D may be associated with its impact on the suppressive effect of PTH and/or the stimulation of erythrocyte progenitor cells [29,43].

Clinical observations indicate that anemia in patients with end-stage renal disease (ESRD) and non–dialyzed CKD subjects is associated with poor outcomes, including higher mortality [14,44,45]. Large, retrospective studies carried by Yang et al. [46] and Brunelli et al. [47] have demonstrated the association between greater Hb variability and decreased survival. Another retrospective study of HD patients revealed a visible trend of increased mortality with increasing time below Hb target of 11 g/dL level [48]. In the case of patients whose Hb levels were <11 g/dL for 80%–100% of the time, mortality risk was ~1.8 times as high as in patients with no time below this level. The Dialysis Outcomes and Practice Patterns Study (DOPPS) demonstrated that mortality and hospitalization risk declined by 5% and 6% per 1-g/dL higher patient baseline Hb level ($p$ < or = 0.003 each), respectively. Moreover, risks of mortality and hospitalization risks were 10% to 12% lower for every 1-g/dL increased facility mean

Hb level [49]. The results of these studies suggest that the maintenance of the target Hb range in CKD patients is an important goal in the treatment of renal anemia.

## 3. Inflammation in CKD and Anemia of Inflammation

The prevalence of inflammation in CKD patients varies between populations [50]. According to estimations, more than 30%–50% of patients with ESRD have serological evidence of an active inflammatory state, as indicated by elevated levels of CRP and pro-inflammatory cytokines, including IL-1, IL-6, and tumor necrosis factor (TNF-$\alpha$) [51–55]. Among factors that are associated with the persistence of low-grade inflammation in CKD patients, there are oxidative stress, infectious complications, diminished clearance of cytokines, and dialysis-related factors [51]. The presence of more elevated levels of inflammatory markers, including serum ferritin and C-reactive protein was observed in patients with malnutrition in comparison to those without malnutrition (301.2 ± 127.1 mg/dL vs. 212.7 ± 124.9 mg/dL, $p < 0.05$; 63% vs. 33%, $p < 0.05$) [56]. Numerous studies indicated that the inflammatory state influences the development of renal anemia. de Francisco et al. [38] demonstrated that lower average CRP values were associated with better Hb control ($p < 0.0001$). Moreover, Agarwal et al. [57] revealed that serum albumin (an alternative inflammatory marker) was also a vital predictor of baseline Hb and sensitivity to ESAs. Proinflammatory cytokines have been shown to simultaneously affect erythropoiesis at several levels, including the suppression of erythroid progenitor cell proliferation [11]. Allen et al. [58] showed inhibition of erythroid colony formation by soluble factors in serum from patients with both end-stage renal disease and inflammatory disease. In vivo studies confirmed that the administration of TNF-$\alpha$ promotes hypoproliferative anemia through a direct effect on erythroid progenitor cells and indirect stimulation of IFN-$\gamma$ production [59]. However, some other studies have provided contradictory results and suggested that TNF-$\alpha$ and IL-1 promoted the growth of early progenitors (burst-forming units) but they inhibited the growth at later stages of erythropoiesis, i.e., erythroid colony-forming units [60]. Inflammatory state affects erythropoiesis also via the inhibition of hypoxia-induced EPO production in Hep3B cells [61]. It seems that the key pathway through which inflammation promotes the development of anemia is the modulation of iron metabolism. Elevated ferritin levels, diminished iron, and iron-binding capacity, as well as higher abundance of iron in the bone marrow, are the characteristic features of inflammation-associated anemia [38]. These features imply iron sequestration in reticuloendothelial cells and the state of inadequate plasma iron levels to support erythropoiesis [62]. The exact mechanism of the influence of the inflammatory state on the development of anemia may be related to hepcidin which affects iron homeostasis via the binding of the cell surface iron transporter ferroportin [63]. Consequently, the phosphorylation, internalization, ubiquitination, and degradation of ferroportin in the lysosomes is triggered [11,62]. This results in decreased iron efflux from duodenal enterocytes into the circulation (reduced iron absorption) as well as the diminished release of iron from macrophages into the reticuloendothelial system and finally in hypoferremia. The results of animal studies have indicated that in transgenic mouse models hepcidin is a key negative regulator of iron absorption in the small intestine, and iron release from macrophages [64]. Wrighting and Andrews [65] demonstrated that interleukin-6 induced hepcidin expression through signal transducer and activator of transcription 3 (STAT3). It has been shown that during inflammation increased hepcidin levels limited iron release from enterocytes, hepatocytes, and macrophages thus decreasing its availability for bacteria [2,64]. Dallalio et al. [66] indicated that the influence of hepcidin on the development of anemia of inflammation involved not only the impact on iron metabolism but also the inhibition of erythroid progenitor proliferation and survival. Numerous studies confirmed the causal role of hepcidin in the process of anemia of inflammation [11,67–69]. Sasu BJ indicated [68] that neutralizing monoclonal antibodies to hepcidin along with ESA restored normal hemoglobin levels in a mouse model of bacteria-induced anemia of inflammation, while ESA administration alone was not effective. The administration of exogenous EPO has been suggested to reduce hepcidin levels and therefore to ameliorate anemia of inflammation and iron sequestration [70]. Marked suppression was observed after 24 h from the administration of EPO and it persisted for a week.

Higher levels of inflammatory markers have been found to be related to decreased survival of CKD patients. Kalantar-Zadeh et al. [71] demonstrated 1.14 [95% confidence interval (CI) 1.03–1.26, $p = 0.01$] adjusted hazard ratio for death for each 1000 pmol/L increase in serum levels of myeloperoxidase (MPO) in 356 patients on maintenance HD. In the Modification of Diet in Renal Disease (MDRD) study involving stage 3 and 4 CKD patients, high CRP (≥0.3 mg/dL) was an independent predictor of both all-cause mortality and cardiovascular mortality in comparison to low CRP <0.3 mg/dL groups [72]. Other studies confirmed the relation between significantly increased overall mortality and cardiovascular mortality of HD patients and elevated CRP levels when compared to normal CRP levels ($p < 0.0001$) [73,74]. Increased concentrations of IL-6 in incident dialysis patients were also found to be considerably associated with poor outcome [53].

## 4. Anemia Treatment

### 4.1. Anemia Treatment with Iron

Anemia treatment in CKD patients should be based on drugs that enhance the synthesis of erythrocytes and provide adequate levels of iron for hemoglobin formation [75,76]. According to National Institute for Health and Care Excellence (NICE) the treatment of anemia in CKD patients requires the use of either iron or erythropoiesis-stimulating agents, their combination in order to address both absolute and functional iron deficiency [77,78]. According to the KDIGO guideline 2012, the correction of iron deficiency with oral or intravenous iron supplementation can reduce the severity of anemia in patients with CKD [42]. Physician prescribing iron therapy should balance the potential benefits of avoiding or minimizing blood transfusions, ESA therapy, and anemia-related symptoms against the risks of harm in individual patients, such as anaphylactoid and other acute reactions, unknown long-term risks) (Not Graded) [42]. Improving Global Outcomes (KDIGO) guidelines also suggest that in adult CKD patients with anemia who are not on iron or ESA therapy but also in adult CKD patients on ESA therapy who are not receiving iron supplementation, a trial of IV iron or alternatively 1–3 month trial of oral iron therapy (in non-dialysis CKD patients) (2C) should be introduced if patients require an increase in Hb concentration without starting ESA treatment or TSAT is ≤30% and ferritin is ≤500 ng/mL (≤500 mg/L) [42]. The route of iron administration should be selected on the basis of the severity of the iron deficiency, availability of venous access, response to prior oral iron therapy, side effects with prior oral or IV iron therapy, patient compliance, and cost. (Not Graded) [42]. The supplementation of oral iron is the simplest and cheapest iron deficiency therapy; however, it is frequently ineffective in CKD patients [79]. Oral preparations of iron (e.g., ferrous sulfate) are not appropriate in CKD patients due to impaired intestinal iron absorption and side-effect in the form of abdominal discomfort, constipation, and nausea [42]. In turn, IV iron improves medication adherence and the efficacy of iron deficiency treatment but requires IV access and is associated with infrequent but severe adverse reactions [42].

In patients with CKD ND, IV iron administration is preferred due to the fact the available evidence supports its better efficacy in comparison to oral administration of iron; however, due to the fact that the difference in the effect is rather small, in these patients, the route of iron administration can be either IV or oral [42,80–82]. Oral iron is typically prescribed to provide approximately 200 mg of elemental iron daily. However, in some patients, smaller daily doses may be useful and better tolerated. If the goals of iron supplementation are not met with a 1–3-month course of oral iron, IV iron supplementation should be considered [42]. The evidence derived from RCTs and other studies comparing IV iron with oral iron and placebo supports IV iron administration in CKD 5HD patients as it is associated with a greater increase in Hb concentration, a lower ESA dose, or both [42,83,84]. IV iron administration has been demonstrated to boost erythropoiesis, effectively replenish iron stores and enable the decrease of required ESA dose, however, it also promotes oxidative stress, atherosclerotic plaque development, and increases cardiovascular mortality [85]. Iron overload itself might be a cause of inflammation and contribute to ESA resistance. It has been showed to increase the synthesis of hepcidin which may be the link between inflammation and anemia [38,86].

### 4.2. Anemia Treatment with ESA

The exclusion of other than CKD causes of anemia, including iron and other hematinic deficiencies, chronic inflammation, malignancy, and drugs should be performed before the initiation of appropriate treatment [87]. Following the ruling out reversible causes of anemia, supplementary erythropoietin (epoetin) administration can be considered. Before the initiation and maintaining of ESA therapy, the potential benefits of reducing blood transfusions and anemia-related symptoms should be weighed against the risks of harm in individual patients (e.g., stroke, vascular access loss, hypertension) (1B) [88]. The decision concerning the initiation of ESA therapy in adult CKD ND patients with Hb concentration <10.0 g/dL (100 g/L) should be based on the rate of fall of Hb concentration, prior response to iron therapy, the risk of needing a transfusion, the risks related to ESA therapy, and the presence of symptoms attributable to anemia (2C) [88]. In case of adult CKD 5D patients, ESA therapy should be used to avoid Hb concentrations falling below 9.0 g/dL (90 g/L) by starting ESA therapy when the hemoglobin is between 9.0–10.0 g/dL (90–100 g/L) (2B) [88]. In the rest of CKD patients, ESA treatment is recommended in a dose enabling the maintenance of hemoglobin levels no higher than 11.5 g/dL (2B) [88]. According to recommendations, in all adult patients, ESAs should not be used to intentionally increase the Hb concentration above 13 g/dL (130 g/L) (1A), as it may increase the risk of stroke [18], hypertension [89], vascular access thrombosis (in case of hemodialysis patients) [90], and it can be associated with higher mortality [89]. The re-adjustment of ESA dose is required in patients suffering from ESA-related adverse events, in those with comorbidities resulting in ESA hyporesponsiveness or when Hb target range has been reached [88]. Numerous randomized clinical trials have demonstrated that Hg values ≥ 11.5 g/dL (≤115 g/L) in adult CKD patients may bring more harm than benefit [88]. Standard anemia treatment in CKD patients involves the administration of recombinant human erythropoietin, including epoetin $\alpha$ and epoetin $\beta$, due to the fact that a decrease in erythropoietin production in the kidneys is the key reason which underlines anemia [91]. Continuous erythropoiesis receptor activators which are a pegylated form of recombinant human erythropoietin with extended serum half-life allowing for longer dosing intervals (every 2 weeks) is currently gaining popularity in the community of dialysis patients [92]. Generally, the initial doses of epoetin-alfa or epoetin-beta dosing are from 20 to 50 IU/kg body weight three times a week. Darbepoetin-alfa doses usually start from 0.45 μg/kg body weight once weekly (subcutaneous or intravenous administration), or 0.75 μg/kg body weight once every 2 weeks (SC administration). In turn, CERA dosing starts at 0.6 μg/kg body weight once every 2 weeks by SC (CKD ND) or IV administration (CKD 5D patients), or 1.2 μg/kg body weight once every 4 weeks by SC administration for CKD ND patients [88]. Moreover, when a downward adjustment of Hb concentration is needed the decreasing of ESA dose instead of its withholding is suggested (2C). The frequency of ESA administration should be based on the CKD stage, patient tolerance, treatment setting, efficacy, and type of ESA. According to recommendations, during the initiation phase of ESA therapy, Hb concentration should be measured at least monthly. Later, during the maintenance phase, Hb level in non-dialysis CKD patients should be measured at least every 3 months, while in HD patients at least monthly. Treatment with ESA has been demonstrated to alleviate fatigue, weakness and headaches, improve quality of life and neurocognitive function as well as to lower the frequency of necessary blood transfusions [88]. A randomized, controlled trial performed by the Canadian Erythropoietin Study Group which included HD patients randomized to three groups to receive placebo ($n$ = 40), erythropoietin to achieve a hemoglobin concentration of 95–110 g/L ($n$ = 40), or erythropoietin to achieve a hemoglobin concentration of 115–130 g/L ($n$ = 38) demonstrated significant improvements in fatigue, physical function, moderate improvements in exercise tolerance and depression in ESA treated patients in comparison to patients not receiving erythropoietin. No differences were found in the abovementioned parameters between high and low hemoglobin groups [93]. However, three large randomized controlled trials (The Normal Hematocrit Study (NHCT) [90], The Correction of Hemoglobin and Outcomes in Renal Insufficiency (CHOIR) trial [94], and The Trial to Reduce Cardiovascular Events with Aranesp Therapy (TREAT) [18] demonstrated that establishing and reaching higher hemoglobin targets may be harmful to patients [92]. The re-analysis of results obtained in two large trials (CHOIR and the Cardiovascular Risk Reduction by Early Anemia Treatment (CREATE)) trials revealed that patients who despite receiving higher doses did not achieve their target hemoglobin had worse outcomes [95,96]. The use of too high doses of EPO was associated with an increased risk of cardiovascular incidents, stroke, rapid malignant progression in cancer patients, pure red blood cell aplasia, and increased mortality in other patients [90,97]. The abovementioned results of randomized controlled trials resulted in establishing KDIGO guidelines, which suggest that ESA should be administered with great caution in the case of CKD patients with active malignancy (1B), a history of stroke (1B), or a history of malignancy (2C) [88]. Patients treated with epoetin frequently require supplementation with oral or intravenous iron to maintain sufficient iron stores during the correction and the maintenance phases of management [14]. ESA treatment enhances erythropoiesis which leads to the exhaustion of iron pool, resulting in a relative iron deficiency [8]. The inflammatory state observed in CKD hinders erythropoiesis and reduces iron availability by the production of hepcidin [98,99]. Due to the fact that CKD patients also suffer from greater blood loss and diminished intestinal absorption of dietary iron, the supplementation of this compound is important to prevent absolute iron deficiency [76].

### 4.3. *New Strategies of Anemia Treatment*

New therapies targeted at inhibiting hepcidin production are being investigated as potential anemia treatment [76]. Studies are performed to assess the efficacy and safety of anti-IL-6 antibodies such as Tocilizumab and IL-6 monoclonal antibodies such as sultuximab. The latter one has been shown to increase hemoglobin levels, however, at the same time, it enhanced the risk of infections [100]. The administration of Atorvastatin to CKD was shown to significantly lower serum hepcidin levels and improved hematological parameters [101]. It has been demonstrated that activin type-II receptor (ActRII) IgG-Fc fusion proteins, including sotatercept and luspatercept, increase red blood cell numbers and hemoglobin levels in humans [102]. Activins are soluble ligands belonging to a large transforming growth factor-β (TGF-β) family and their expression is observed in bone marrow cells, including erythroid cells [103]. They are involved in the proliferation and differentiation of embryonic/hematopoietic stem and erythropoietic cells. Sotatercept is a fusion protein comprising of an extracellular chain of activin receptor IIA and the Fc domain of human IgG1. It inhibits the activation of endogenic, membranous receptors (ActRIIA) of activin by binding circulating activin and related proteins (e.g., BMP 10 and BMP 11) [104] Moreover, it influences the expression of angiotensin II which can promote erythropoiesis directly and indirectly via EPO production [105]. Sotatercept also stimulates the release of the mature erythrocyte forms, decreases the expression of the vascular endothelial growth factor (VEGF), which is an inhibitor of erythropoiesis and inhibits hepcidin transcription in the liver [106]. The results of preliminary studies with sotatercept in dialysis patients have demonstrated a dose-dependent increase in Hb and a decrease in extraosseous calcification [107]. Luspatercept ACE-536; Acceleron/Celgene Corp) is another ligand-trapping fusion protein that contains the extracellular domain of human activin receptor type IIB (ACTRIIB) modified to diminish activin binding [108]. In vivo, it has been shown to exert erythropoietic activity and stimulate the maturation of late-stage erythroid precursors in vivo [109]. The treatment with EPO and luspatercept provides a synergistic erythropoietic response [109]. In a phase 1, randomized, double-blind, placebo-controlled, clinical trial of ACE-536, it increased Hb levels in a dose-dependent mode 7 days after treatment initiation, and this effect was maintained for several weeks following treatment in postmenopausal women [110]. These observations are supported by an ongoing phase 2 clinical trials of ACE-536 in patients with β-thalassemia and myelodysplastic syndromes [108]. In clinical trials, these novel compounds were found to be well tolerated by healthy volunteers and patients suffering from anemia due to CKD, however, they have not been approved for sale as therapeutics as their long-term efficacy and safety especially the issues of immunogenicity and antifibrotic effects, still needs to be confirmed. Sasu et al. [111] using human hepcidin (hHepc) knock-in mice as a model of inflammation-induced anemia showed that high-affinity antibodies specific for hHepc neutralized hHepc in vitro and in vivo and facilitated anemia treatment due to the fact that they enhanced the absorption of dietary iron and stimulated its mobilization from iron stores for use in erythropoiesis [112]. In the treatment of anemia, CKD also compounds targeting hypoxia-inducible factor prolyl hydroxylase inhibitor (Hif1$\alpha$ inhibitors), including Vadustat, Daprodustat, and Roxadustat, have been studied. HIF1$\alpha$ seems to be an interesting target as it regulates renal EPO production and erythropoiesis [76]. The results of phase 2 trials involving CKD patients indicate that roxadustat enhanced levels of endogenous erythropoietin to within or near the physiologic range, and also it increased hemoglobin levels and improved iron homeostasis [113–117]. A single-blind, placebo-controlled study of ND-CKD stage 3 or 4 patients randomized to receive four escalating doses (0.7, 1.0, 1.5, 2.0 mg/kg) of roxadustat either twice or thrice weekly over 28 days demonstrated that this drug increased Hb in a dose-dependent manner [114]. Oral administration of 1 mg/kg roxadustat twice-weekly resulted in the increase in endogenous EPO (eEPO) levels after 4 h, with its peak at ~10 h, and the return to baseline within 24–48 h. In a subsequent phase IIa open-label study, analyzing various roxadustat dose regimens for 16 and 24 weeks in NDD-CKD participants, 92% of patients achieved hemoglobin response [116]. The rise in the hemoglobin level was independent of baseline C-reactive protein levels and iron repletion status. 16-week treatment with roxadustat resulted in the reduction in hepcidin levels by 16.9% ($p$ = 0.004) and the increase in hemoglobin level by a mean (±SD) of 1.83 (±0.09) g/dL ($p < 0.001$), while reticulocyte Hb content remained the same [116]. TSAT and ferritin levels diminishing was observed during the initial weeks of treatment with roxadustat, however, later they were stabilized [116]. These results were similar to those obtained in an open-label, phase IIb study, ESA-naïve incident PD and HD participants with severe anemia (mean Hb 8.3 g/dL at baseline) who were randomized to receive no iron, oral iron, or IV iron during the treatment with roxadustat for 12 weeks [115]. In this study, in 96% of patients, the Hb response (increase in Hb of ≥1.0 g/dL from baseline) was observed. Roxadustat treatment resulted in Hb elevation of ≥2 g/dL within 7 weeks of treatment, which was independent of baseline Hb level, iron repletion status, inflammatory status, and dialysis modality. A greater Hb response was found in groups of patients receiving also iron in comparison to those not receiving iron. Mean serum hepcidin was decreased significantly after 4 weeks of study [115]. Third phase trial in which CKD patients with Hg levels of 7.0 to 10.0 g/dL were randomly assigned to receive roxadustat or placebo three times a week for 8 weeks an increase of 1.9 ± 1.2 g/dL in the roxadustat group and a decrease of 0.4 ± 0.8 g/dL in the placebo group ($p < 0.001$) was observed. Moreover, a reduction from baseline in the hepcidin level by 56.14 ± 63.40 ng/mL in the roxadustat group and 15.10 ± 48.06 ng/mL in the placebo group was seen [113]. However, in the group receiving roxadustat, hyperkalemia, and metabolic acidosis were more frequent than in the placebo group. The beneficial impact of roxadustat on hemoglobin level maintained during the 18-week open-label period. According to the authors, the stability of serum iron levels in the roxadustat group may have been related to reductions in hepcidin levels, which enabled gut absorption of iron and improved the release of macrophage iron onto transferrin [113,118]. Other studies of non-dialyzed CKD patients have demonstrated that roxadustat increased hemoglobin levels with stable serum iron levels, despite robust erythropoiesis in the absence of intravenous administration of iron [116,119]. Moreover, it has been revealed that roxadustat is superior to the placebo in correcting anemia in non-dialysis CKD patients, it is non-inferior to erythropoietin-$\alpha$ for treatment of anemia in long-term dialysis patients.

Molidustat is another potential alternative to the standard treatment of anemia associated with CKD as it increases erythropoietin production and improves iron availability. This HIF-PH inhibitor mimics hypoxia by stabilizing HIF-$\alpha$ subunits and it shows high relative selectivity for the induction of EPO gene expression, predominately in the kidney [120,121]. Molidustat enables the accumulation of HIF, which is then transported to the nucleus where it promotes the transcription of EPO and other hypoxia-inducible genes and thus leading to the elevation of endogenous EPO levels [122].

In preclinical studies, molidustat restored renal EPO production with minor stimulation of hepatic EPO [121,123]. Moreover, it heightened plasma EPO and EPO mRNA in the kidney prevented the reduction in hematocrit and corrected Hb level [121]. A single-center, randomized, single-blind, placebo-controlled, group-comparison, dose-escalation 1 phase study demonstrated that oral administration of molidustat to healthy volunteers elicited a dose-dependent increase in endogenous EPO and that all doses of molidustat were well tolerated [124]. In three randomized, controlled, phase 2 studies, which are the part of the DIALOGUE (DaIly orAL treatment increasing endOGenoUs Erythropoietin) program, molidustat diminished transferrin saturation (TSAT), hepcidin, ferritin, and iron concentrations and increased total iron-binding capacity (TIBC) in treatment-naïve patients not on dialysis [125]. In these studies, the efficacy, safety, and tolerability of molidustat were compared with placebo or alternative ESA therapy in patients with anemia of CKD. In the first fixed-dose, placebo-controlled study (DIALOGUE 1), molidustat was shown to increase hemoglobin levels in patients not on dialysis [121]. The efficacy of molidustat was confirmed in DIALOGUE 2, in which patients were switched from darbepoetin to molidustat or continued with darbepoetin. Molidustat in all dose arms enabled maintaining hemoglobin levels within the pre-specified target range of 10.0–12.0 g/dL. The results indicate that starting dose of 25 or 50 mg once daily seems to be appropriate for CKD patients, since higher doses (i.e., 75 mg once daily) may increase the probability that hemoglobin levels will rise above the pre-specified limits [121]. In turn, in dialysis patients (DIALOGUE 4), only starting doses of molidustat of 75 and 150 mg once daily effectively maintained hemoglobin levels within the target range after switching from epoetin. Despite the level of kidney function impairment and disturbed hepatic erythropoietin production in included patients, molidustat mainly addresses kidney erythropoietin production [121]. In this study, patients treated with molidustat starting doses of 75 or 150 mg once daily had lower response rates, spent less time within the target hemoglobin range, and were more likely to have hemoglobin levels above the pre-specified limit in comparison to epoetin group [120,121]. Therefore, it seems that molidustat is an effective alternative to rhEPO and its analogs in the long-term management of anemia associated with CKD [122].

However, the treatment with HIF-PH inhibitors raises some safety concerns, due to the fact that these agents may stimulate tumorigenesis and angiogenesis which may exert a negative effect on retinal diseases or cancer [126]. Moreover, in phase 2 studies of these drugs, cases of hyperkalemia, hyperglycemia, and hyperuricemia were reported. It seems that adverse events in CKD patients may be related to the pharmacokinetics and dosing of HIF-PHIs. Finally, it has been suggested that these drugs may promote the development of thromboembolic complications such as pulmonary hypertension as well as the progression of CKD and polycystic kidney disease [126].

Pentoxifylline (methylxanthine derivative, PTX) is another drug which efficacy in the treatment has been tested in the CKD population [79]. Cooper et al. [127] hypothesized that pentoxifylline, which is traditionally used in the treatment of peripheral vascular disease, might improve the response to ESAs in anemic CKD patients via the inhibition pro-inflammatory cytokine production and thus the enhanced erythropoiesis. In their study, the use of oral pentoxifylline for 4 months in patients with ESRD and ESA-resistant anemia considerably increased the Hb concentration ($p = 0.0001$). Benbernou et al. [128] studied the effect of pentoxifylline on T-helper cell-derived cytokine production in human blood cells. Their study indicated that at an appropriate concentration ($5 \times 10^{-4}$ M concentration), PTX selectively suppressed interleukin-2 (IL-2), and interferon-gamma (INF-$\gamma$), while high levels of this drug ($1 \times 10^{-3}$ M) inhibited both TH1- and TH2-derived cytokines.

The results of phase 2 placebo-controlled studies in patients with CKD treated with vadadustat [129] as well as placebo-controlled [130] and dose-ranging [131] study of daprodustat in CKD population have demonstrated that such treatment was associated with the increase in hemoglobin level and its maintaining.

Vadadustat (AKB-6548) has been shown to restore baseline eEPO levels within 24 h following its oral administration [132]. In a phase IIa, double-blind, placebo-controlled trial of CKD patients who were randomized to receive escalating doses (240, 370, 500, 630 mg) of vadadustat or placebo orally once daily for 6 weeks, vadadustat significantly enhanced Hb levels in a dose-dependent manner. Moreover, it increased the total iron-binding capacity and decreased concentrations of ferritin and hepcidin. A phase IIb double-blind, placebo-controlled trial of non-dialyzed CKD patients randomized to receive a titratable dose of vadadustat (initial dose 450 mg) or placebo once daily for 20 weeks assessed efficacy and safety of once-daily vadadustat [129]. In this study, 54.9% of patients on vadadustat and 10.3% of patients on placebo achieved or maintained either a mean hemoglobin level of 11.0 g/dL or more or a mean increase in hemoglobin of 1.2 g/dL or more over the pre-dose average. Moreover, reticulocytes and total iron-binding capacity increased considerably in patients receiving vadadustat, while serum hepcidin and ferritin levels were reduced in comparison to patients on placebo. The authors concluded that vadadustat raised and maintained hemoglobin levels in a predictable and controlled manner while enhancing iron mobilization in patients with nondialysis-dependent CKD [129].

The effectiveness of daprodustat in the treatment of CKD-related anemia has been evaluated. In a 28-day, double-blind, phase IIa study of CKD stage 3–5 patients ($n = 73$) randomized to receive fixed daprodustat doses 0.5 mg, 2 mg, and 5 mg once daily or placebo [130], the treatment resulted in a dose-dependent increase in Hb and also dose-dependent decrease in hepcidin concentrations. In a second, parallel phase IIa conversion study comprising 83 HD participants maintained on stable doses of rhEPO who were randomized to receive the same doses of daprodustat as the prior study or to continue rhEPO [130], only the administration of 5 mg of daprodustat allowed maintaining Hb levels similarly to rhEPO; however, in groups receiving lower doses a reduction of Hb levels at 4 weeks was observed. Moreover, hepcidin levels increase was demonstrated in daprodustat low doses groups. Its concentration remained the same in patients receiving 5 mg of the drug and decreased in the rhEPO arm at 4 weeks.

New drugs in the treatment of anemia have been summarized in Table 1.

**Table 1.** The summary of trials concerning the use of new drugs in the treatment of anemia in CKD patients.

| Study Name | Study Type | Drug Name | Most Important Findings | Ref |
|---|---|---|---|---|
| DIALOGUE 1 (D1) ($n$ = 121) | 3 phase 2b, 16-week, randomized, double-blind, placebo-controlled, fixed-dose trial (25, 50, and 75 mg once daily; 25 and 50 mg twice daily) study of molidustat for the treatment of anemia in patients with CKD not previously treated with an analog of rhEPO, and who were not receiving dialysis treatment | Molidustat | Molidustat treatment was associated with estimated increases in mean hemoglobin levels of 1.4–2.0 g/dl | [120] |
| DIALOGUE 2 ($n$ = 124) | Open-label, variable-dose trials, in which treatment was switched from darbepoetin to molidustat or continued with the original agents. Starting molidustat doses ranged between 25–75 mg daily | Molidustat | Hemoglobin levels were maintained within the target range after switching to molidustat, with an estimated difference in mean change in hemoglobin levels between molidustat and darbepoetin treatments of up to 0.6 g/dL. | [120] |

**Table 1.** *Cont.*

| Study Name | Study Type | Drug Name | Most Important Findings | Ref |
|---|---|---|---|---|
| DIALOGUE 4 ($n$ = 199) | Open-label, variable-dose trials, in which treatment was switched from epoetin to molidustat or continued with the original agents. Starting molidustat ranged between 25–150 mg daily | Molidustat | Hemoglobin levels were maintained within the target range after switching to molidustat 75 and 150 mg, with estimated differences in mean change between molidustat and epoetin treatment of −0.1 and 0.4 g/dL. Molidustat was generally well tolerated, and most adverse events were mild or moderate in severity. | [120] |
| ($n$ = 116) | Randomized placebo-controlled dose-ranging and pharmacodynamics study of roxadustat (FG-4592) to treat anemia in nondialysis-dependent chronic kidney disease (NDD-CKD) patients | Roxadustat | In roxadustat-treated subjects, Hb levels increased from baseline in a dose-related manner. Maximum ΔHb within the first 6 weeks was significantly higher in the 1.5 and 2.0 mg/kg groups than in the placebo subjects. Hb responder rates were dose dependent and ranged from 30% in the 0.7 mg/kg BIW group to 100% in the 2.0 mg/kg BIW and TIW groups versus 13% in placebo. | [114] |
| ($n$ = 143) | Randomized, cohort study with varying roxadustat starting doses and frequencies followed by hemoglobin maintenance with roxadustat one to three times weekly. Treatment duration was 16 or 24 weeks. | Roxadustat | 92% of patients achieved hemoglobin response. Higher compared with lower starting doses led to earlier achievement of hemoglobin response. Roxadustat-induced Hb increases were independent of baseline C-reactive protein levels and iron repletion status. Over the first 16 treatment weeks, hepcidin levels decreased by 16.9% ($p$ = 0.004), reticulocyte hemoglobin content was maintained, and hemoglobin increased by a mean (±SD) of 1.83 (±0.09) g/dl ($p < 0.001$). | [116] |

**Table 1.** *Cont.*

| Study Name | Study Type | Drug Name | Most Important Findings | Ref |
| --- | --- | --- | --- | --- |
| ($n$ = 60) | Open-label, phase IIb study of ESA-naïve incident PD and HD participants (total $n$ = 60) with severe anemia (mean Hb 8.3 g/dl at baseline) who were randomized to receive no iron, oral iron, or IV iron during the treatment with roxadustat for 12 weeks | Roxadustat | Roxadustat at titrated doses increased mean Hb by ≥2.0 g/dL within 7 weeks regardless of baseline iron repletion status, C-reactive protein level, iron regimen, or dialysis modality. In groups receiving oral or IV iron, ΔHb(max) was similar and larger than in the no-iron group. Hb response (increase in Hb of ≥1.0 g/dL from baseline) was achieved in 96% of efficacy-evaluable patients. Mean serum hepcidin decreased significantly 4 weeks into study: by 80% in HD patients receiving no iron ($n$ = 22), 52% in HD and PD patients receiving oral iron ($n$ = 21), and 41% in HD patients receiving IV iron ($n$ = 9). | [115] |
| ($n$ = 154) | Phase 3 trial, CKD patients randomly assigned to receive roxadustat or placebo three times a week for 8 weeks in a double-blind manner. The randomized phase of the trial was followed by an 18-week open-label period in which all the patients received roxadustat. | Roxadustat | Hemoglobin level increased by 1.9 ± 1.2 g/dL in the roxadustat group and decreased by 0.4 ± 0.8 g/dl in the placebo group ($p < 0.001$). The mean reduction from baseline in the hepcidin level was 56.14 ± 63.40 ng/mL in the roxadustat group and 15.10 ± 48.06 ng/mL in the placebo group. Hyperkalemia and metabolic acidosis occurred more frequently in the roxadustat group than in the placebo group. | [113] |
| ($n$ = 93) | Phase 2a, multicenter, randomized, double-blind, placebo-controlled, dose-ranging trial (NCT01381094) of adults with anemia secondary to CKD stage 3 or 4. Patients were randomized to 5 groups: 240, 370, 500, or 630 mg of once-daily oral vadadustat or placebo for 6 weeks. All of them received low-dose supplemental oral iron (50 mg daily). | Vadadustat | Vadadustat significantly increased Hb after 6 weeks in a dose-dependent manner in comparison to placebo ($p < 0.0001$). It also increased total iron-binding capacity and reduced ferritin and hepcidin levels. | [132] |

**Table 1.** *Cont.*

| Study Name | Study Type | Drug Name | Most Important Findings | Ref |
| --- | --- | --- | --- | --- |
| | 20-week, double-blind, randomized, placebo-controlled, phase 2b study of efficacy and safety of once-daily vadadustat in patients with stages 3a to 5 non-dialysis-dependent CKD | Vadadustat | 54.9% of patients on vadadustat and 10.3% of patients on placebo achieved or maintained either a mean hemoglobin level of 11.0 g/dL or more or a mean increase in hemoglobin of 1.2 g/dL or more. Significant rise in reticulocytes and total iron-binding capacity and significant drop in serum hepcidin and ferritin levels were observed in patients on vadadustat compared with placebo. The incidence of adverse events was comparable between the 2 groups. | [129] |
| (non-dialysis $n$ = 71; HD $n$ = 80) | Two phase 2a studies to explore the relationship between the dose of daprodustat and hemoglobin response in: - patients with anemia of CKD (baseline hemoglobin 8.5–11.0 g/dL) not undergoing dialysis and not receiving recombinant human erythropoietin (non-dialysis study) - patients with anemia of CKD (baseline hemoglobin 9.5–12.0 g/dL) on hemodialysis and being treated with stable doses of recombinant human erythropoietin (hemodialysis study). Patients were randomized to a once-daily oral dose of daprodustat (0.5 mg, 2 mg, or 5 mg) or placebo for the non-dialysis study; continuing on recombinant human erythropoietin for the hemodialysis study) for 4 weeks, with a 2-week follow-up | Daprodustat | In the non-dialysis study, daprodustat influenced hemoglobin in a dose-dependent (administration of the highest dose resulted in a mean increase of 1 g/dL at week 4)In the hemodialysis study, treatment with daprodustat mean hemoglobin concentrations were maintained in the 5-mg arm after the switch from recombinant human erythropoietin; in lower-dose arms mean hemoglobin decreased. In both studies, the effects on hemoglobin occurred with elevations in endogenous erythropoietin within the range usually observed in the respective populations and markedly lower than those in the recombinant human erythropoietin control arm in the hemodialysis study, and without clinically significant elevations in plasma vascular endothelial growth factor concentrations. | [130] |

According to studies, also vitamin D has also decreased hepcidin gene transcription, reduced serum levels by 50% in healthy individuals within 24 h, stimulated erythropoiesis and limited inflammation [133]. Zughaier et al. [134] confirmed that in early-stage CKD patients, vitamin D3 supplementation lowered the hepcidin level after three months of the administration. However, this effect was not observed when the calcitriol form of vitamin D was used in patients with mild to moderate CKD [135]. Therefore, further studies are needed to confirm the effects of vitamin D in CKD patients. The use of vitamin E-modified dialysis membranes in ESA-treated HD patients was also shown to improve anemia. This phenomenon was associated with concentration-dependent vitamin E-related improvement of red blood cell survival [136].

Apart from new drugs, the improvement of anemia may be achieved in HD patients by greater adequacy of hemodialysis measured by Kt/V (which mirrors the clearance of urea and it is a surrogate marker for the clearance of small, but not middle or large-sized, uremic toxins [79]). Equilibrated Kt/V A is a more accurate measure of the dialysis dose due to the fact that it corrects for urea rebound. Adequate dialysis has been shown to ameliorate anemia and decrease ESA dosage required for anemia correction in patients with ESRD [137–139]. Such an approach enables the correction of oxidative stress and the removal of molecules that inhibit erythropoiesis and erythrocyte G6PD activity [140]. Therefore, patients with adequate HD ($Kt/V \geq 1.2$) have significantly higher erythrocyte G6PD activity and hemoglobin levels in comparison to patients who received inadequate HD [137]. Locatelli et al. [141] demonstrated that the use of a large-pore biocompatible membrane for a fixed 12-week follow-up improved anemia in hemodialysis patients in comparison with the use of a conventional cellulose membrane. Pedrini et al. [142] analyzed retrospectively the courses of hemoglobin levels and monthly ESA consumption in patients on mixed-HDF (hemodiafiltration) and on post-HDF. In Mixed-HDF, pre- and post-dilution substitution rates are adjusted by means of a feedback control system to obtain the maximal filtration fraction within safe pressure and hydraulic conditions, thus preventing progressive hemoconcentration [142–144]. Pedrini et al. [142] suggest that patients on mixed-HDF may have clinical benefits in terms of anemia management, including the requirement of lower ESA doses to maintain hemoglobin (Hb) levels within the recommended range. The use of Mixed-HDF enabled the maintaining of stable hemoglobin values with lower ESA doses when compared to Post-HDF patients. In their study, the monthly median ESA consumption of patients on Mixed-HDF at the end of the observation period was 50% lower than those of patients on Post-HDF. Authors suggested that this finding might be associated with the efficient removal of middle and large sized uremic toxins contributing to impaired erythropoiesis in dialysis patients. Maduell et al. [145] demonstrated a considerable amelioration of anemia when the substitution rate was substantially enhanced as a result of a better removal of uremic toxins. It seems that hepcidin is one of the important metabolites removed in such a dialysis. Stefansson et al. [146] confirmed that HDF removes hepcidin more efficiently than conventional HD, which results in clinical benefits related to anemia observed in HDF-treated patients. Moreover, the removal of proinflammatory cytokines also has been shown to be of high importance in the improvement of anemia as inflammatory cytokines can impair erythropoiesis and contribute to ESA resistance in CKD [142,147,148]. Some studies have demonstrated that HDF has the potential to reduce inflammation [149,150]. Other studies indicated lower ESA resistance index (ERI; (ESA/weight)/Hb [UI/kg/week/hb]) in patients treated with convective dialysis technique in comparison to patients treated with conventional HD [151,152]. However, some studies provided conflicting results in the context of anemia management and treatment modality is as other studies did not find improved anemia parameters in patients treated with convective dialysis technique [153,154]. Finally, a randomized clinical study designed to examine the effects of removal of inhibitors of erythropoiesis on anemia and EPO requirements in patients who could not reach target hemoglobin (Hb) levels ($\geq$11 g/dL) despite treatment with subcutaneous EPO revealed significantly lower EPO doses in polysulphone high-flux dialyzer (HF-HD), and considerably increased Hb levels in comparison to polysulphone low-flux dialyzer (LF-HD) group [155]. In the HF-HD group, the reduction of beta2-microglobulin (b2-MG) and phosphorus levels during dialysis was significantly higher in comparison to the low-flux group ($p < 0.001$). The authors suggested that the beneficial effects of high-flux dialysis may be mediated by greater clearance of moderate and high molecular weight toxins.

## 5. The Impact of Inflammation on Response to Iron Supplementation and ESAs

As it has been mentioned above, anemia of inflammation is characterized by increased ferritin levels, diminished iron and iron-binding capacity (transferrin) and the presence of iron in bone marrow macrophages, which indicate disturbed mobilization of iron from stores [57]. According to studies inflammation diminishes predictive values of ferritin and hepcidin for iron status and responsiveness to iron therapy [156]. Inflammation-mediated elevation in hepcidin concentration results in iron trapping within the macrophages and hepatocytes, resulting in functional iron deficiency (FID) and the requirement of a higher dose of IV iron to maintain Hb targets [157,158]. On the other hand, too aggressive intravenous iron therapy (IIT) may boost inflammation in patients with end-stage renal disease (ESRD) and lead to subsequent disturbances of iron metabolism [159]. Moreover, it has been demonstrated that in HD patients with high CRP levels intestinal iron absorption is lower, probably as a result of an inflammation-induced increase in ferritin and hepcidin that block iron absorption [35,160].

Numerous studies have demonstrated that some CKD patients treated with ESAs respond poorly or not at all [161,162]. Hyporesponsiveness to erythropoiesis-stimulating agents occurs in approximately 5–10% of patients receiving ESA and it poses an important diagnostic and management challenge [163]. Among the most frequent causes of ESA resistance, there are non-compliance, absolute or functional iron deficiency, and inflammation. According to NKF-KDOQI guidelines, hyporesponsiveness to erythropoietin can be defined as the presence of at least one of the following three conditions: a major decrease in Hb level at a constant ESA dose, a considerable increase in the ESA dose requirement to maintain a given Hb level, or a failure to increase Hb level to greater than 11 g/dl despite an ESA equivalent to erythropoietin greater than 500 IU/kg/week [164]. The reason for poor responding to ESA may be associated with an enhanced inflammatory state with elevated levels of inflammatory markers, including C reactive protein (CRP), IL-1, IL-6, and TNF-$\alpha$ in CKD patients [165]. Cytokines may impair iron metabolism, which results in functional iron deficiency [38]. They also directly influence different erythropoiesis stages and mediate apoptosis induction, which implies that the cytokine-mediated pro-inflammatory signaling also affects EPO activity [166]. Cytokines inhibit the expression and regulation of specific transcription factors that are involved in the control of erythrocyte differentiation [166]. Immune activation results in the production of TNF-$\alpha$ and IFN-$\gamma$ by T cells and TNF-$\alpha$ and IL-6 by monocytes. These pro-inflammatory cytokines were shown to hamper the proliferation of erythrocyte progenitor cells and to antagonize the antiapoptotic activities of EPO. According to studies, the responsiveness of erythrocyte progenitor cells to EPO seems to be inversely correlated with CKD severity as well as the amount of circulating cytokines. EPO requirement to restore the formation of erythrocyte colony-forming units is higher in the presence of elevated levels of IFN-gamma or TNF-$\alpha$ [6]. The inflammatory state contributes to poor response to treatment with EPO which finally leads to cachexia, a higher percentage of patients with cardiovascular disease and reduced quality of life [167,168]. According to studies, the interactions between different inflammatory mediators and ESA responses are complex and it seems that the type of cytokine and its signaling pathway is more important than plasma levels [38]. In the study of hemodialysis patients, epoetin responsiveness was associated with the concentration of IL-6, TNF-$\alpha$, and IL-12 [59]. Patients in whom levels of TNF-$\alpha$ were $\geq$2 ng/mL and IL-6 were $\geq$40 ng/mL required much higher doses of epoetin than patients with lower levels of these cytokines (128 U/kg/week versus 57 U/kg/week; $p = 0.0024$). A negative correlation between IL-12 production and epoetin doses were observed ($p = 0.029$). In turn, Bárány et al. [169] found the relationship between serum C-reactive protein (s-CRP) and the dose of recombinant human EPO required to maintain hemoglobin levels. In their study, weekly EPO dose used in patients with sCRP $\geq$ 20 mg/L was, on average, 80% higher than in patients with sCRP below that level. Moreover, EPO doses and sCRP inversely correlated with serum albumin and serum iron levels, which imply that the key mechanism through which inflammatory cytokines hamper erythropoiesis is coupled to iron metabolism. A cross-sectional study of maintenance HD outpatients demonstrated a positive correlation between serum concentrations of hs-CRP, IL-6, and TNF-$\alpha$ and both the required epoetin dose and an index of epoetin responsiveness [170]. Large multicenter studies assessing weekly epoetin dose requirement in HD patients categorized into four groups (untreated, hyperresponders, normoresponders, and hyporesponders) on the basis of weekly epoetin dose requirement showed that the median CRP level was higher in the hyporesponders than in the other groups (1.9 versus 0.8 mg/dL; $p = 0.004$) [171]. The median weekly epoetin dose ranged from 30 IU/kg/week in the hyperresponsive group to 263 IU/kg/week in the hyporesponsive group. Ferritin levels were lower in the hyporesponders in comparison to other patients (median 318 versus 445 ng/mL; $p = 0.01$). The results of this analysis support a clear relationship between epoetin hyporesponsiveness and either increased levels of CRP or iron deficiency in HD patients. According to studies, resistance to ESA seems to be related to increased mortality of HD patients, probably due to the fact that are those requiring higher doses of ESA usually have some concomitant infectious, inflammatory, or malignant conditions [170]. Potential strategies targeted at eliminating hyporesponsiveness to ESA in CKD patients with the systemic inflammatory state include selective anticytokine therapy with anti-TNF-$\alpha$ antibodies, IL-1 or IL-6 receptor antagonists, and statins [162,163]. Pentoxifylline, which is a nonselective phosphodiesterase inhibitor exhibiting anti-TNF alpha properties, has been shown to significantly inhibit hemoglobin within six months and reduced serum TNF-$\alpha$ concentration in patients with erythropoietin resistant anemia [172]. Other studies have demonstrated that pentoxifylline decreased other inflammatory parameters, including hsCRP, erythrocyte sedimentation rate (ESR), serum fibrinogen, and TNF-$\alpha$ in patients of CKD [173,174].

## 6. Conclusions

The results of studies have demonstrated that persistent inflammation may contribute to the variability in Hb levels and hyporesponsiveness to ESA which are frequently observed in CKD patients. It seems that variability in Hb values which are often below the target range may contribute to higher morbidity and mortality in these patients [175]. Available evidence implies that chronic kidney disease is a state of the enhanced inflammatory state with high activity of cytokines, which may suppress erythroid progenitor cell production resulting in hyporesponsiveness to ESAs and poor treatment outcomes. The understanding of the impact of inflammatory cytokines on erythropoietin production and hepcidin synthesis will enable to unravel the net of interactions of multiple factors involved in the pathogenesis of the anemia of chronic disease. It seems that anticytokine and antioxidative treatment strategies may be the future of pharmacological interventions aiming at the treatment of inflammation-associated hyporesponsiveness to ESA.

**Author Contributions:** A.G.-B., B.F., and R.O. searched for appropriate articles and prepared the draft version, J.R.—review and editing. All authors have read and agreed to the published version of the manuscript.

**Funding:** This research received no external funding.

**Conflicts of Interest:** The authors declare no conflict of interest.

## References

1. Cases, A.; Egocheaga, M.I.; Tranche, S.; Pallarés, V.; Ojeda, R.; Górriz, J.L.; Portolés, J.M. Anemia of chronic kidney disease: Protocol of study, management and referral to Nephrology. *Nefrologia* **2018**, *38*, 8–12. [CrossRef]
2. Malyszko, J.; Mysliwiec, M. Hepcidin in anemia and inflammation in chronic kidney disease. *Kidney Blood Press Res.* **2007**, *30*, 15–30. [CrossRef] [PubMed]
3. Poole, S.; Bird, T.A.; Selkirk, S.; Gaines-Das, R.E.; Choudry, Y.; Stephenson, S.L.; Kenny, A.J.; Saklatvaa, J. Fate of injected interleukin-1 in rats: Sequestration and degradation in the kidney. *Cytokine* **1990**, *2*, 416–422. [CrossRef]
4. Panichi, V.; Migliori, M.; De Pietro, S.; Taccola, D.; Bianchi, A.M.; Norpoth, M.; Metelli, M.R.; Giovannini, L.; Tetta, C.; Palla, R. C-reactive protein in patients with chronic renal diseases. *Ren. Fail.* **2001**, *23*, 551–562. [PubMed]

5. Stenvinkel, P.; Heimburger, O.; Wang, T.; Lindholm, B.; Bergstrom, J.; Elinder, C.G. High serum hyaluronan indicates poor survival in renal replacement therapy. *Am. J. Kidney Dis.* **1999**, *34*, 1083–1088. [CrossRef]
6. De Oliveira Júnior, W.V.; Sabino Ade, P.; Figueiredo, R.C.; Rios, D.R. Inflammation and poor response to treatment with erythropoietin in chronic kidney disease. *J. Bras. Nefrol.* **2015**, *37*, 255–263. [CrossRef]
7. Căldăraru, C.D.; Tarta, D.I.; Gliga, M.L.; Tarta, C.; Caraşca, E.; Albu, S.; Huţanu, A.; Dogaru, M.; Dogaru, G. Comparative Analysis of Hepcidin-25 and Inflammatory Markers in Patients with Chronic Kidney Disease with and without Anemia. *Acta Med. Marisiensis* **2017**, *63*, 10–14. [CrossRef]
8. Babitt, J.L.; Lin, H.Y. Mechanisms of anemia in CKD. *J. Am. Soc. Nephrol.* **2012**, *23*, 1631–1634. [CrossRef]
9. Hsu, C.Y.; McCulloch, C.E.; Curhan, G.C. Epidemiology of anemia associated with chronic renal insufficiency among adults in the United States: Results from the Third National Health and Nutrition Examination Survey. *J. Am. Soc. Nephrol.* **2002**, *13*, 504–510.
10. Astor, B.C.; Muntner, P.; Levin, A.; Eustace, J.A.; Coresh, J. Association of kidney function with anemia: The Third National Health and Nutrition Examination Survey (1988–1994). *Arch. Intern. Med.* **2002**, *162*, 1401–1408. [CrossRef]
11. Yilmaz, M.I.; Solak, Y.; Covic, A.; Goldsmith, D.; Kanbay, M. Renal Anemia of Inflammation: The Name Is Self-Explanatory. *Blood Purif.* **2011**, *32*, 220–225. [CrossRef] [PubMed]
12. McFarlane, S.I.; Chen, S.C.; Whaley-Connell, A.T.; Sowers, J.R.; Vassalotti, J.A.; Salifu, M.O.; Kidney Early Evaluation Program Investigators; Li, S.; Wang, C.; Bakris, G.; et al. Prevalence and associations of anemia of CKD: Kidney Early Evaluation Program (KEEP) and National Health and Nutrition Examination Survey (NHANES) 1999–2004. *Am. J. Kidney Dis.* **2008**, *51*, S46–S55.
13. Stauffer, M.E.; Fan, T. Prevalence of anemia in chronic kidney disease in the United States. *PLoS ONE* **2014**, *9*, e84943. [CrossRef] [PubMed]
14. Coyne, D.W.; Goldsmith, D.; Macdougall, I.C. New options for the anemia of chronic kidney disease. *Kidney Int. Suppl.* **2017**, *7*, 157–163. [CrossRef]
15. Gilbertson, D.; Peng, Y.; Bradbury, B.; Ebben, J.; Collins, A. Hemoglobin level variability: Anemia management among variability groups. *Am. J. Nephrol.* **2009**, *30*, 491–498. [PubMed]
16. Zadrazil, J.; Horak, P. Pathophysiology of anemia in chronic kidney diseases: A review. *Biomed. Pap. Med. Fac. Univ. Olomouc. Czech Repub.* **2015**, *159*, 197–202. [CrossRef] [PubMed]
17. Bataille, S.; Pelletier, M.; Sallée, M.; Berland, Y.; McKay, N.; Duval, A.; Gentile, S.; Mouelhi, Y.; Brunet, P.; Burtey, S. Indole 3-acetic acid, indoxyl sulfate and paracresyl-sulfate do not influence anemia parameters in hemodialysis patients. *BMC Nephrol. BioMed. Cent.* **2017**, *18*, 251. [CrossRef]
18. Pfeffer, M.A.; Burdmann, E.A.; Chen, C.Y.; Cooper, M.E.; de Zeeuw, D.; Eckardt, K.U.; Feyzi, J.M.; Ivanovich, P.; Kewalramani, R.; Levey, A.S.; et al. TREAT Investigators; A trial of darbepoetin alfa in type 2 diabetes and chronic kidney disease. *N. Engl. J. Med.* **2009**, *361*, 2019–2032. [CrossRef]
19. Macdougall, I.C. Role of uremic toxins in exacerbating anemia in renal failure. *Kidney Int. Suppl.* **2001**, *78*, S67–S72.
20. Cotes, P.M. Erythropoietin: The developing story. *Br. Med. J. (Clin. Res. Ed.)* **1988**, *296*, 805–806.
21. Besarab, A.; Ayyoub, F. Anemia in renal disease. In *Diseases of the Kidney and Urinary Tract*, 8th ed.; Schrier, R.W., Ed.; Lippincott Williams and Wilkins: Philadelphia, Pennsylvania, USA, 2007; pp. 2406–2430.
22. Kushner, D.S.; Beckman, B.; Nguyen, L.; Chen, S.; Della Santina, C.; Husserl, F.; Rice, J.; Fisher, J.W. Polyamines in the anemia of end-stage renal disease. *Kidney Int.* **1991**, *39*, 725–732. [CrossRef] [PubMed]
23. Chiang, C.K.; Tanaka, T.; Inagi, R.; Fujita, T.; Nangaku, M. Indoxyl sulfate, a representative uremic toxin, suppresses erythropoietin production in a HIF-dependent manner. *Lab. Investig.* **2011**, *91*, 1564–1571. [CrossRef] [PubMed]
24. Hamano, H.; Ikeda, Y.; Watanabe, H.; Horinouchi, Y.; Izawa-Ishizawa, Y.; Imanishi, M.; Zamami, Y.; Takechi, K.; Miyamoto, L.; Ishizawa, K.; et al. The uremic toxin indoxyl sulfate interferes with iron metabolism by regulating hepcidin in chronic kidney disease. *Nephrol. Dial. Transpl.* **2018**, *33*, 586–597. [CrossRef] [PubMed]
25. Wu, I.-W.; Hsu, K.-H.; Sun, C.-Y.; Wu, M.S.; Lee, C.C.; Tsai, C.J. Oral adsorbent AST-120 potentiates the effect of erythropoietin-stimulating agents on Stage 5 chronic kidney disease patients: A randomized crossover study. *Nephrol. Dial. Transplant.* **2014**, *29*, 1719–1727. [CrossRef] [PubMed]
26. Ahmed, M.S.; Abed, M.; Voelkl, J.; Lang, F. Triggering of suicidal erythrocyte death by uremic toxin indoxyl sulfate. *BMC Nephrol.* **2013**, *4*, 14–244. [CrossRef] [PubMed]

27. Vos, F.E.; Schollum, J.B.; Coulter, C.V.; Doyle, T.C.; Duffull, S.B.; Walker, R.J. Red blood cell survival in long-term dialysis patients. *Am. J. Kidney Dis.* **2011**, *58*, 591–598. [CrossRef]
28. Bandeira, M.F.S. Consequências hematológicas da uremia. In *Riella MC. Princípios de Nefrologia e Distúrbios Eletrolíticos*, 4th ed.; Guanabara Koogan: Rio de Janeiro, Brazil, 2003; pp. 691–701.
29. Weiss, G. Pathogenesis and treatment of anaemia of chronic disease. *Blood Rev.* **2002**, *16*, 87–96. [CrossRef]
30. Wagner, M.; Ashby, D. Hepcidin—A well-known iron biomarker with prognostic implications in chronic kidney disease. *Nephrol. Dial. Transpl.* **2013**, *28*, 2936–2939. [CrossRef]
31. Atkinson, M.; Kim, J.; Roy, C.; Warady, B.; White, C.T.; Furth, S. Hepcidin and risk for anemia in CKD: A cross-sectional and longitudinal analysis in the CKiD Cohort. *Pediatr. Nephrol.* **2015**, *30*, 635–643. [CrossRef]
32. Gupta, J.; Mitra, N.; Kanetsky, P.A.; Devaney, J.; Wing, M.R.; Reilly, M.; Shah, V.O.; Balakrishnan, V.S.; Guzman, N.J.; Girndt, M.; et al. Association between Albuminuria, Kidney Function, and Inflammatory Biomarker Profile in CKD in CRIC. *Clin. J. Am. Soc. Nephrol.* **2012**, *7*, 1938–1946. [CrossRef]
33. Fudin, R.; Jaichenko, J.; Shostak, A.; Bennett, M.; Gotloib, L. Correction of uremic iron deficiency anemia in hemodialyzed patients: A prospective study. *Nephron* **1998**, *79*, 299–305. [CrossRef] [PubMed]
34. Macdougall, I.C.; Tucker, B.; Thompson, J.; Tomson, C.R.; Baker, L.R.; Raine, A.E. A randomized controlled study of iron supplementation in patients treated with erythropoietin. *Kidney Int.* **1996**, *50*, 1694–1699. [CrossRef] [PubMed]
35. Kooistra, M.P.; Niemantsverdriet, E.C.; van Es, A.; Mol-Beerman, N.M.; Struyvenberg, A.; Marx, J.J. Iron absorption in erythropoietin-treated haemodialysis patients: Effects of iron availability, inflammation and aluminium. *Nephrol. Dial. Transpl.* **1998**, *13*, 82–88. [CrossRef] [PubMed]
36. Bowry, S.K.; Gatti, E. Impact of Hemodialysis Therapy on Anemia of Chronic Kidney Disease: The Potential Mechanisms. *Blood Purif.* **2011**, *32*, 210–219. [CrossRef] [PubMed]
37. Eleftheriadis, T.; Liaopoulos, V.; Antoniadi, G.; Kartsios, C.; Stefanidis, I. The role of hepcidin in iron homeostasis and anemia in hemodialysis patients. *Semin. Dial.* **2009**, *22*, 70–77. [CrossRef] [PubMed]
38. De Francisco, A.L.M.; Stenvinkel, P.; Vaulot, S. Inflammation and its impact on anemia in chronic kidney disease: From haemoglobin variability to hyporesponsiveness. *Nephrol. Dial. Transpl. Plus* **2009**, *2*, i18–i26.
39. Tozoni, S.S.; Dias, G.F.; Bohnen, G.; Grobe, N.; Pecoits-Filho, R.; Kotanko, P.; Moreno-Amaral, A.N. Uremia and Hypoxia Independently Induce Eryptosis and Erythrocyte Redox Imbalance. *Cell. Physiol. Biochem.* **2019**, *53*, 794–804.
40. Bonomini, M.; Sirolli, V. Uremic toxicity and anemia. *J. Nephrol.* **2003**, *16*, 21–28.
41. Kruse, A.; Uehlinger, D.E.; Gotch, F.; Kotanko, P.; Levin, N.W. Red blood cell lifespan, erythropoiesis and haemoglobin control. *Contrib. Nephrol.* **2008**, *161*, 247–254.
42. KDIGO. Clinical Practice Guideline for anemia in chronic kidney disease. *Kidney Int. Suppl.* **2012**, *2*, 279–335.
43. Icardi, A.; Paoletti, E.; De Nicola, L.; Mazzaferro, S.; Russo, R.; Cozzolino, M. Renal anaemia and EPO hyporesponsiveness associated with vitamin D deficiency: The potential role of inflammation. *Nephrol. Dial. Transpl.* **2013**, *28*, 1672–1679. [CrossRef] [PubMed]
44. Regidor, D.L.; Kopple, J.D.; Kovesdy, C.P. Associations between changes in hemoglobin and administered erythropoiesis-stimulating agent and survival in hemodialysis patients. *J. Am. Soc. Nephrol.* **2006**, *17*, 1181–1191. [CrossRef] [PubMed]
45. Kovesdy, C.P.; Trivedi, B.K.; Kalantar-Zadeh, K. Association of anemia with outcomes in men with moderate and severe chronic kidney disease. *Kidney Int.* **2006**, *69*, 560–564. [CrossRef]
46. Yang, W.; Israni, R.K.; Brunelli, S.M.; Joffe, M.M.; Fishbane, S.; Feldman, H.I. Hemoglobin Variability and Mortality in ESRD. *J. Am. Soc. Nephrol.* **2007**, *18*, 3164–3170. [CrossRef]
47. Brunelli, S.M.; Joffe, M.M.; Israni, R.K.; Yang, W.; Fishbane, S.; Berns, J.S.; Feldman, H.I. History-adjusted marginal structural analysis of the association between hemoglobin variability and mortality among chronic hemodialysis patients. *Clin. J. Am. Soc. Nephrol.* **2008**, *3*, 777–782. [CrossRef] [PubMed]
48. Ishani, A.; Solid, C.A.; Weinhandl, E.D.; Gilbertson, D.T.; Foley, R.N.; Collins, A.J. Association between number of months below K/DOQI haemoglobin target and risk of hospitalization and death. *Nephrol. Dial. Transplant.* **2008**, *23*, 1682–1689. [CrossRef]
49. Pisoni, R.L.; Bragg-Gresham, J.L.; Young, E.W.; Akizawa, T.; Asano, Y.; Locatelli, F.; Bommer, J.; Cruz, J.M.; Kerr, P.G.; Mendelssohn, D.C.; et al. Anemia management and outcomes from 12 countries in the Dialysis Outcomes and Practice Patterns Study (DOPPS). *Am. J. Kidney Dis.* **2004**, *44*, 94–111. [CrossRef]

50. Aggarwal, H.K.; Jain, D.; Chauda, R.; Bhatia, S.; Sehgal, R. Assessment of Malnutrition Inflammation Score in Different Stages of Chronic Kidney Disease. *Pril. (Makedon. Akad. Nauk. Umet. Odd. Med. Nauk.)* **2018**, *39*, 51–61. [CrossRef]
51. Stenvinkel, P.; Alvestrand, A. Inflammation in end-stage renal disease: Sources, consequences, and therapy. *Semin. Dial.* **2002**, *15*, 329–337. [CrossRef]
52. Owen, W.F.; Lowrie, E.G. C-reactive protein as an outcome predictor for maintenance hemodialysis patients. *Kidney Int.* **1998**, *54*, 627–636. [CrossRef]
53. Stenvinkel, P.; Barany, P.; Heimbürger, O.; Pecoits-Filho, R.; Lindholm, B. Mortality, malnutrition, and atherosclerosis in ESRD: What is the role of interleukin-6? *Kidney Int.* **2002**, *61*, S103–S108. [CrossRef] [PubMed]
54. Yeun, J.Y.; Levine, R.A.; Mantadilok, V.; Kaysen, G.A. C-Reactive protein predicts all-cause and cardiovascular mortality in hemodialysis patients. *Am. J. Kidney Dis.* **2000**, *35*, 469–476. [CrossRef]
55. Kimmel, P.L.; Phillips, T.M.; Simmens, S.J.; Peterson, R.A.; Weihs, K.L.; Alleyne, S.; Cruz, I.; Yanovski, J.A.; Veis, J.H. Immunologic function and survival in hemodialysis patients. *Kidney Int.* **1998**, *54*, 236–244. [CrossRef] [PubMed]
56. Prakash, J.; Raja, R.; Mishra, R.N.; Vohra, R.; Sharma, N.; Wani, I.A.; Parekh, A. High prevalence of malnutrition and inflammation in undialyzed patients with chronic renal failure in developing countries: A single center experience from eastern India. *Ren. Fail.* **2007**, *29*, 811–816. [CrossRef] [PubMed]
57. Agarwal, R.; Davis, J.L.; Smith, L. Serum albumin is strongly associated with erythropoietin sensitivity in hemodialysis patients. *Clin. J. Am. Soc. Nephrol.* **2008**, *3*, 98–104. [CrossRef] [PubMed]
58. Allen, D.A.; Breen, C.; Yaqoob, M.M.; Macdougall, I.C. Inhibition of CFU-E colony formation in uremic patients with inflammatory disease: Role of IFN-γ and TNF-α. *J. Investig. Med.* **1999**, *47*, 204–211.
59. Goicoechea, M.; Martin, J.; de Sequera, P.; Quiroga, J.A.; Ortiz, A.; Carreno, V.; Caramelo, C. Role of cytokines in the response to erythropoietin in hemodialysis patients. *Kidney Int.* **1998**, *54*, 1337–1343. [CrossRef]
60. Trey, J.E.; Kushner, I. The acute phase response and the hematopoietic system: The role of cytokines. *Crit. Rev. Oncol. Hematol.* **1995**, *21*, 1–18. [CrossRef]
61. Faquin, W.C.; Schneider, T.J.; Goldberg, M.A. Effect of inflammatory cytokines on hypoxia-induced erythropoietin production. *Blood* **1992**, *79*, 1987–1994. [CrossRef]
62. Ganz, T. Iron in innate immunity: Starve the invaders. *Curr. Opin. Immunol.* **2009**, *21*, 63–67. [CrossRef]
63. De Domenico, I.; Ward, D.M.; Langelier, C.; Vaughn, M.B.; Nemeth, E.; Sundquist, W.I.; Ganz, T.; Musci, G.; Kaplan, J. The molecular mechanism of hepcidin-mediated ferroportin down-regulation. *Mol. Biol. Cell* **2007**, *18*, 2569–2578. [CrossRef]
64. Ganz, T. Hepcidin, a key regulator of iron metabolism and mediator of anemia of inflammation. *Blood* **2003**, *102*, 783–788. [CrossRef]
65. Wrighting, D.M.; Andrews, N.C. Interleukin-6 induces hepcidin expression through STAT3. *Blood* **2006**, *108*, 3204–3209. [CrossRef]
66. Dallalio, G.; Law, E.; Means, T. Hepcidin inhibits in vitro erythroid colony formation at reduced erythropoietin. *Blood* **2006**, *107*, 2702–2704. [CrossRef]
67. Roy, C.N.; Mak, H.H.; Akpan, I.; Losyev, G.; Zurakowski, D.; Andrews, N.C. Hepcidin antimicrobial peptide transgenic mice exhibit features of the anemia of inflammation. *Blood* **2007**, *109*, 4038–4044. [CrossRef]
68. Sasu, B.J.; Haniu, M.; Boone, T.C.; Bi, X.-J.; Lee, G.K.J.; Arvedson, T.; Winters, A.G.; Cooke, K.; Sheng, J.Z. Hepcidin, Hepcidin Antagonists and Methods of Use. U.S. Patent US2008213277 A1, 4 September 2008.
69. Song, S.N.; Tomosugi, N.; Kawabata, H.; Ishikawa, T.; Nishikawa, T.; Yoshizaki, K. Down-regulation of hepcidin resulting from long-term treatment with an anti-IL-6 receptor antibody (tocilizumab) improves anemia of inflammation in multicentric Castleman's disease (MCD). *Blood* **2010**, *116*, 3627–3634. [CrossRef]
70. Ashby, D.R.; Gale, D.P.; Busbridge, M.; Murphy, K.G.; Duncan, N.D.; Cairns, T.D.; Taube, D.H.; Bloom, S.R.; Tam, F.W.; Chapman, R.; et al. Erythropoietin administration in humans causes a marked and prolonged reduction in circulating hepcidin. *Haematologica* **2010**, *95*, 505–508. [CrossRef]
71. Kalantar-Zadeh, K.; Brennan, M.L.; Hazen, S.L. Serum myeloperoxidase and mortality in maintenance hemodialysis patients. *Am. J. Kidney Dis.* **2006**, *48*, 59–68. [CrossRef]
72. Menon, V.; Greene, T.; Wang, X.; Pereira, A.A.; Marcovina, S.M.; Beck, G.J.; Kusek, J.W.; Collins, A.J.; Levey, A.S.; Sarnak, M.J. C-reactive protein and albumin as predictors of all-cause and cardiovascular mortality in chronic kidney disease. *Kidney Int.* **2005**, *68*, 766–772. [CrossRef]

73. Zimmermann, J.; Herrlinger, S.; Pruy, A.; Metzger, T.; Wanner, C. Inflammation enhances cardiovascular risk and mortality in hemodialysis patients. *Kidney Int.* **1999**, *55*, 648–658. [CrossRef]
74. Qureshi, A.R.; Alvestrand, A.; Divino-Filho, J.C.; Gutierrez, A.; Heimbürger, O.; Lindholm, B.; Bergström, J. Inflammation, malnutrition, and cardiac disease as predictors of mortality in hemodialysis patients. *J. Am. Soc. Nephrol.* **2002**, *13*, S28–S36.
75. Besarab, A.; Coyne, D.W. Iron supplementation to treat anemia in patients with chronic kidney disease. *Nat. Rev. Nephrol.* **2010**, *6*, 699–710. [CrossRef]
76. Begum, S.; Latunde-Dada, G.O. Anemia of Inflammation with An Emphasis on Chronic Kidney Disease. *Nutrients* **2019**, *11*, 2424. [CrossRef]
77. National Institute for Health and Care Excellence. *Chronic Kidney Disease: Managing Anaemia*; NICE Guideline: London, UK, 2015.
78. Gupta, N.; Wish, J.B. Hypoxia-Inducible Factor Prolyl Hydroxylase Inhibitors: A Potential New Treatment for Anemia in Patients With CKD. *Am. J. Kidney Dis.* **2017**, *69*, 815–826. [CrossRef]
79. Karkar, A. *Advances in Hemodialysis Techniques*; Suzuki, H., Ed.; IntechOpen: London, UK, 2013; Available online: https://www.intechopen.com/books/hemodialysis/advances-in-hemodialysis-techniques#B31 (accessed on 20 April 2019). [CrossRef]
80. Agarwal, R.; Rizkala, A.R.; Bastani, B.; Kaskas, M.O.; Leehey, D.J.; Besarab, A. A randomized controlled trial of oral versus intravenous iron in chronic kidney disease. *Am. J. Nephrol.* **2006**, *26*, 445–454. [CrossRef]
81. Schaefer, R.M.; Schaefer, L. Iron monitoring and supplementation: How do we achieve the best results. *Nephrol. Dial. Transpl.* **1998**, *13* (Suppl. 2), 9–12. [CrossRef]
82. Besarab, A.; Amin, N.; Ahsan, M.; Vogel, S.E.; Zazuwa, G.; Frinak, S.; Zazra, J.J.; Anandan, J.V.; Gupta, A. Optimization of epoetin therapy with intravenous iron therapy in hemodialysis patients. *J. Am. Soc. Nephrol.* **2000**, *11*, 530–538.
83. Besarab, A.; Kaiser, J.W.; Frinak, S. A study of parenteral iron regimens in hemodialysis patients. *Am. J. Kidney Dis.* **1999**, *34*, 21–28. [CrossRef]
84. Ford, B.A.; Coyne, D.W.; Eby, C.S.; Scott, M.G. Variability of ferritin measurements in chronic kidney disease; implications for iron management. *Kidney Int.* **2009**, *75*, 104–110. [CrossRef]
85. Cançado, R.D.; Muñoz, M. Intravenous iron therapy: How far have we come? *Rev. Bras. Hematol. Hemoter.* **2011**, *33*, 461–469. [CrossRef]
86. Pigeon, C.; Ilyin, G.; Courselaud, B.; Leroyer, P.; Turlin, B.; Brissot, P.; Loréal, O. A new mouse liver specific gene, encoding a protein homologous to human antimicrobial peptide hepcidin, is overexpressed during iron overload. *J. Biol. Chem.* **2001**, *276*, 7811–7819. [CrossRef] [PubMed]
87. Roger, S.D. Managing the anaemia of chronic kidney disease. *Aust. Prescr.* **2009**, *32*, 129–131. [CrossRef]
88. KDIGO. Use of ESAs and other agents to treat anemia in CKD. *Kidney Int. Sup.* **2012**, *2*, 299–310. [CrossRef]
89. Palmer, S.C.; Navaneethan, S.D.; Craig, J.C.; Johnson, D.W.; Tonelli, M.; Garg, A.X.; Pellegrini, F.; Ravani, P.; Jardine, M.; Perkovic, V.; et al. Meta-analysis: Erythropoiesis-stimulating agents in patients with chronic kidney disease. *Ann. Intern. Med.* **2010**, *153*, 23–33. [CrossRef]
90. Besarab, A.; Bolton, W.K.; Browne, J.K.; Egrie, J.C.; Nissenson, A.R.; Okamoto, D.M.; Schwab, S.J.; Goodkin, D.A. The effects of normal as compared with low hematocrit values in patients with cardiac disease who are receiving hemodialysis and epoetin. *N. Engl. J. Med.* **1998**, *339*, 584–590. [CrossRef]
91. Hayat, A.; Haria, D.; Salifu, M.O. Erythropoietin stimulating agents in the management of anemia of chronic kidney disease. Patient Prefer. *Adherence* **2008**, *2*, 195–200.
92. Nakhoul, G.; Simon, J.F. Anemia of chronic kidney disease: Treat it, but not too aggressively. *Clevel. Clin. J. Med.* **2016**, *83*, 613–624. [CrossRef]
93. Association between recombinant human erythropoietin and quality of life and exercise capacity of patients receiving haemodialysis. Canadian Erythropoietin Study Group. *BMJ* **1990**, *300*, 573–578.
94. Singh, A.K.; Szczech, L.; Tang, K.L.; Barnhart, H.; Sapp, S.; Wolfson, M.; Reddan, D.; CHOIR Investigators. Correction of anemia with epoetin alfa in chronic kidney disease. *N. Engl. J. Med.* **2006**, *355*, 2085–2098. [CrossRef]
95. Solomon, S.D.; Uno, H.; Lewis, E.F.; Eckardt, K.U.; Lin, J.; Burdmann, E.A.; de Zeeuw, D.; Ivanovich, P.; Levey, A.S.; Parfrey, P. Trial to Reduce Cardiovascular Events with Aranesp Therapy (TREAT) Investigators. Erythropoietic response and outcomes in kidney disease and type 2 diabetes. *N. Engl. J. Med.* **2010**, *363*, 1146–1155. [CrossRef]

96. Szczech, L.A.; Barnhart, H.X.; Inrig, J.K.; Reddan, D.N.; Sapp, S.; Califf, R.M.; Patel, U.D.; Singh, A.K. Secondary analysis of the CHOIR trial epoetin-alpha dose and achieved hemoglobin outcomes. *Kidney Int.* **2008**, *74*, 791–798. [CrossRef]
97. Horl, W.H. Clinical aspects of iron use in the anemia of kidney disease. *J. Am. Soc. Nephrol.* **2007**, *18*, 382–393. [CrossRef]
98. Silverstein, D.M. Inflammation in chronic kidney disease: Role in the progression of renal and cardiovascular disease. *Pediatr. Nephrol.* **2009**, *24*, 1445–1452. [CrossRef]
99. Atkinson, M.A.; White, C.T. Hepcidin in anemia of chronic kidney disease: Review for the pediatric nephrologist. *Pediatr. Nephrol.* **2012**, *27*, 33–40. [CrossRef]
100. Lang, V.R.; Englbrecht, M.; Rech, J.; Nusslein, H.; Manger, K.; Schuch, F.; Tony, H.P.; Fleck, M.; Manger, B.; Schett, G.; et al. Risk of infections in rheumatoid arthritis patients treated with tocilizumab. *Rheumatology* **2012**, *51*, 852–857. [CrossRef]
101. Masajtis-Zagajewska, A.; Nowicki, M. Effect of atorvastatin on iron metabolism regulation in patients with chronic kidney disease—A randomized double blind crossover study. *Ren. Fail.* **2018**, *40*, 700–709. [CrossRef]
102. Jelkmann, W. Activin receptor ligand traps in chronic kidney disease. *Curr. Opin. Nephrol. Hypertens.* **2018**, *27*, 351–357. [CrossRef]
103. Breda, L.; Rivella, S. Modulators of erythropoiesis: Emerging therapies for hemoglobinopathies and disorders of red cell production. *Hematol. Clin. N. Am.* **2014**, *28*, 375–386. [CrossRef]
104. Biggar, P.; Kim, G.H. Treatment of renal anemia: Erythropoiesis stimulating agents and beyond. *Kidney Res. Clin. Pr.* **2017**, *36*, 209–223. [CrossRef]
105. Iancu-Rubin, C.; Mosoyan, G.; Wang, J.; Kraus, T.; Sung, V.; Hoffman, R. Stromal cell-mediated inhibition of erythropoiesis can be attenuated by Sotatercept (ACE-011), an activin receptor type II ligand trap. *Exp. Hematol.* **2013**, *41*, 155–166. [CrossRef]
106. Finberg, K.E.; Whittlesey, R.L.; Fleming, M.D.; Andrews, N.C. Down-regulation of Bmp/Smad signaling by Tmprss6 is required for maintenance of systemic iron homeostasis. *Blood* **2010**, *115*, 3817–3826. [CrossRef] [PubMed]
107. A Phase 2 Study of Intravenous or Subcutaneous Dosing of Sotatercept (ACE-011) in Patients with End-Stage Kidney Disease on Hemodialysis 2013. Available online: https://www.clinicaltrials.gov/ct2/show/NCT01999582 (accessed on 2 January 2020).
108. Bonomini, M.; Del Vecchio, L.; Sirolli, V.; Locatelli, F. New Treatment Approaches for the Anemia of CKD. *Am. J. Kidney Dis.* **2016**, *67*, 133–142. [CrossRef] [PubMed]
109. Suragani, R.N.; Cadena, S.M.; Cawley, S.M.; Sako, D.; Mitchell, D.; Li, R.; Davies, M.V.; Alexander, M.J.; Devine, M.; Loveday, K.S.; et al. Transforming growth factor-β superfamily ligand trap ACE-536 corrects anemia by promoting late-stage erythropoiesis. *Nat. Med.* **2014**, *20*, 408–414. [CrossRef]
110. Attie, K.M.; Allison, M.J.; McClure, T.; Boyd, I.E.; Wilson, D.M.; Pearsall, A.E.; Sherman, M.L. A phase 1 study of ACE-536, a regulator of erythroid differentiation, in healthy volunteers. *Am. J. Hematol.* **2014**, *89*, 766–770. [CrossRef]
111. Sasu, B.J.; Cooke, K.S.; Arvedson, T.L.; Plewa, C.; Ellison, A.R.; Sheng, J.; Winters, A.; Juan, T.; Li, H.; Begley, C.G.; et al. Antihepcidin antibody treatment modulates iron metabolism and is effective in a mouse model of inflammation-induced anemia. *Blood* **2010**, *115*, 3616–3624. [CrossRef]
112. Bolignano, D.; D'Arrigo, G.; Pisano, A.; Coppolino, G. Pentoxifylline for Anemia in Chronic Kidney Disease: A Systematic Review and Meta-Analysis. *PLoS ONE* **2015**, *10*, e0134104. [CrossRef]
113. Chen, N.; Hao, C.; Peng, X.; Lin, H.; Yin, A.; Hao, L.; Tao, Y.; Liang, X.; Liu, Z.; Xing, C. Roxadustat for Anemia in Patients with Kidney Disease Not Receiving Dialysis. *N. Engl. J. Med.* **2019**, *381*, 1001–1010. [CrossRef]
114. Besarab, A.; Provenzano, R.; Hertel, J.; Zabaneh, R.; Klaus, S.J.; Lee, T.; Leong, R.; Hemmerich, S.; Yu, K.H.; Neff, T.B. Randomized placebo-controlled dose-ranging and pharmacodynamics study of roxadustat (FG-4592) to treat anemia in nondialysis-dependent chronic kidney disease (NDD-CKD) patients. *Nephrol. Dial. Transpl.* **2015**, *30*, 1665–1673. [CrossRef]
115. Besarab, A.; Chernyavskaya, E.; Motylev, I.; Shutov, E.; Kumbar, L.M.; Gurevich, K.; Chan, D.T.; Leong, R.; Poole, L.; Zhong, M. Roxadustat (FG-4592): Correction of anemia in incident dialysis patients. *J. Am. Soc. Nephrol.* **2016**, *27*, 1225–1233. [CrossRef]

116. Provenzano, R.; Besarab, A.; Sun, C.H.; Diamond, S.A.; Durham, J.H.; Cangiano, J.L.; Aiello, J.R.; Novak, J.E.; Lee, T.; Leong, R.; et al. Oral hypoxia-inducible factor prolyl hydroxylase inhibitor roxadustat (FG-4592) for the treatment of anemia in patients with CKD. *Clin. J. Am. Soc. Nephrol.* **2016**, *11*, 982–991. [CrossRef]
117. Provenzano, R.; Besarab, A.; Wright, S.; Dua, S.; Zeig, S.; Nguyen, P.; Poole, L.; Saikali, K.G.; Saha, G.; Hemmerich, S.; et al. Roxadustat (FG-4592) versus epoetin alfa for anemia in patients receiving maintenance hemodialysis: A phase 2, randomized, 6- to 19-week, open-label, active-comparator, dose-ranging, safety and exploratory efficacy study. *Am. J. Kidney Dis.* **2016**, *67*, 912–924. [CrossRef]
118. Ganz, T.; Nemeth, E. Hepcidin and iron homeostasis. *Biochim. Biophys. Acta* **2012**, *1823*, 1434–1443. [CrossRef]
119. Chen, N.; Qian, J.; Chen, J.; Yu, X.; Mei, C.; Hao, C.; Jiang, G.; Lin, H.; Zhang, X.; Zuo, L.; et al. Phase 2 studies of oral hypoxia-inducible factor prolyl hydroxylase inhibitor FG-4592 for treatment of anemia in China. *Nephrol. Dial. Transpl.* **2017**, *32*, 1373–1386. [CrossRef]
120. Macdougall, I.C.; Akizawa, T.; Berns, J.S.; Bernhardt, T.; Krueger, T. Effects of Molidustat in the Treatment of Anemia in CKD. *Clin. J. Am. Soc. Nephrol.* **2019**, *14*, 1524. [CrossRef]
121. Flamme, I.; Oehme, F.; Ellinghaus, P.; Jeske, M.; Keldenich, J.; Thuss, U. Mimicking hypoxia to treat anemia: HIF-stabilizer BAY 85-3934 (Molidustat) stimulates erythropoietin production without hypertensive effects. *PLoS ONE* **2014**, *9*, e111838. [CrossRef]
122. Akizawa, T.; Macdougall, I.C.; Berns, J.S.; Bernhardt, T.; Staedtler, G.; Taguchi, M.; Iekushi, K.; Krueger, T. Long-Term Efficacy and Safety of Molidustat for Anemia in Chronic Kidney Disease: DIALOGUE Extension Studies. *Am. J. Nephrol.* **2019**, *49*, 271–280. [CrossRef]
123. Akizawa, T.; Taguchi, M.; Matsuda, Y.; Iekushi, K.; Yamada, T.; Akizawa, T. Molidustat for the treatment of renal anaemia in patients with dialysis-dependent chronic kidney disease: Design and rationale of three phase III studies. *BMJ Open* **2019**, *9*, e026602. [CrossRef]
124. Böttcher, M.; Lentini, S.; Arens, E.R.; Kaiser, A.; van der Mey, D.; Thuss, U.; Kubitza, D.; Wensing, G. First-in-man-proof of concept study with molidustat: A novel selective oral HIF-prolyl hydroxylase inhibitor for the treatment of renal anaemia. *Br. J. Clin. Pharm.* **2018**, *84*, 1557–1565. [CrossRef]
125. Akizawa, T.; Macdougall, I.C.; Berns, J.S.; Yamamoto, H.; Taguchi, M.; Iekushi, K.; Bernhardt, T. Iron Regulation by Molidustat, a Daily Oral Hypoxia-Inducible Factor Prolyl Hydroxylase Inhibitor, in Patients with Chronic Kidney Disease. *Nephron* **2019**, *143*, 243–254. [CrossRef]
126. Sanghani, N.S.; Haase, V.H. Hypoxia-inducible factor activators in renal anemia: Current clinical experience. *Adv. Chronic Kidney Dis.* **2019**, *26*, 253–266. [CrossRef]
127. Ramirez, R.; Carracedo, J.; Merino, A.; Nogueras, S.; Alvarez-Lara, M.A.; Rodríguez, M.; Martin-Malo, A.; Tetta, C.; Aljama, P. Microinflammation induces endothelial damage in hemodialysis patients: The role of convective transport. *Kidney Int.* **2007**, *72*, 108–113. [CrossRef]
128. Benbernou, N.; Esnault, S.; Potron, G.; Guenounou, M. Regulatory effects of pentoxifylline on T-helper cell-derived cytokine production in human blood cells. *J. Cardiovas. Pharm.* **1995**, *25*, 75–79. [CrossRef]
129. Pergola, P.E.; Spinowitz, B.S.; Hartman, C.S.; Maroni, B.J.; Haase, V.H. Vadadustat, a novel oral HIF stabilizer, provides effective anemia treatment in nondialysis-dependent chronic kidney disease. *Kidney Int.* **2016**, *90*, 1115–1122. [CrossRef]
130. Holdstock, L.; Meadowcroft, A.M.; Maier, R.; Johnson, B.M.; Jones, D.; Rastogi, A.; Zeig, S.; Lepore, J.J.; Cobitz, A.R. Four-week studies of oral hypoxia-inducible factor-prolyl hydroxylase inhibitor GSK1278863 for treatment of anemia. *J. Am. Soc. Nephrol.* **2016**, *27*, 1234–1244. [CrossRef]
131. Brigandi, R.A.; Johnson, B.; Oei, C.; Westerman, M.; Olbina, G.; de Zoysa, J.; Roger, S.D.; Sahay, M.; Cross, N.; McMahon, L.; et al. A novel hypoxia-inducible factor-prolyl hydroxylase inhibitor (GSK1278863) for anemia in CKD: A 28-day, phase 2A randomized trial. *Am. J. Kidney Dis.* **2016**, *67*, 861–871. [CrossRef]
132. Martin, E.R.; Smith, M.T.; Maroni, B.J.; Zuraw, Q.C.; deGoma, E.M. Clinical trial of Vadadustat in patients with anemia secondary to stage 3 or 4 chronic kidney disease. *Am. J. Nephrol.* **2017**, *45*, 380–388. [CrossRef]
133. Bacchetta, J.; Zaritsky, J.; Lisse, T.; Sea, J.; Chun, R.; Nemeth, E.; Ganz, T.; Westerman, M.; Hewison, M. Vitamin D as a New Regulator of Iron Metabolism: Vitamin D Suppresses Hepcidin in Vitro and In Vivo. *J. Am. Soc. Nephrol.* **2011**, *22*, 564–572.
134. Zughaier, S.M.; Alvarez, J.A.; Sloan, J.H.; Konrad, R.J.; Tangpricha, V. The role of vitamin D in regulating the iron-hepcidin-ferroportin axis in monocytes. *J. Clin. Transl. Endocrinol.* **2014**, *1*, 19–25. [CrossRef]

135. Panwar, B.; McCann, D.; Olbina, G.; Westerman, M.; Gutierrez, O.M. Effect of calcitriol on serum hepcidin in individuals with chronic kidney disease: A randomized controlled trial. *BMC Nephrol.* **2018**, *19*, 35. [CrossRef]
136. Usberti, M.; Gerardi, G.; Micheli, A.; Tira, P.; Bufano, G.; Gaggia, P.; Movilli, E.; Cancarini, G.C.; De Marinis, S.; D'Avolio, G.; et al. Effects of a vitamin E-bonded membrane and of glutathione on anemia and erythropoietin requirements in hemodialysis patients. *J. Nephrol.* **2002**, *15*, 558–564.
137. Ayesh Haj Yousef, M.H.; Bataineh, A.; Elamin, E.; Khader, Y.; Alawneh, K.; Rababah, M. Adequate hemodialysis improves anemia by enhancing glucose-6-phosphate dehydrogenase activity in patients with end-stage renal disease. *BMC Nephrol.* **2014**, *15*, 155. [CrossRef]
138. Ifudu, O.; Uribarri, J.; Rajwani, I.; Vlacich, V.; Reydel, K.; Delosreyes, G.; Friedman, E.A. Adequacy of dialysis and differences in haematocrit among dialysis facilities. *Am. J. Kidney Dis.* **2000**, *36*, 1166–1174. [CrossRef] [PubMed]
139. Movilli, E.; Cancarini, G.C.; Zani, R.; Camerini, C.; Sandrini, M.; Maiorca, R. Adequacy of dialysis reduces the dose of recombinant erythropoietin independently from the use biocompatible membranes in haemodialysis patients. *Nephrol. Dial. Transplant.* **2001**, *16*, 111–114. [CrossRef] [PubMed]
140. National Kidney Foundation. Kidney Dialysis Outcome Quality Initiative (K/DOQI): Clinical Practice Guidelines for Hemodialysis Adequacy: Update 2000. Available online: http://www.kidney.org/professionals/kdoqi/guidelines_updates/doqi_uptoc.html#hd (accessed on 5 September 2019).
141. Locatelli, F.; Andrulli, S.; Pecchini, F.; Pedrini, L.; Agliata, S.; Lucchi, L.; Farina, M.; La Milia, V.; Grassi, C.; Borghi, M.; et al. Effect of high-flux dialysis on the anaemia of haemodialysis patients. *Nephrol. Dial. Transpl.* **2000**, *15*, 1399–1409. [CrossRef] [PubMed]
142. Pedrini, L.A.; Zawada, A.M.; Winter, A.C.; Pham, J.; Klein, G.; Wolf, M.; Feuersenger, A.; Ruggiero, P.; Feliciani, A.; Barbieri, C.; et al. Effects of high-volume online mixed-hemodiafiltration on anemia management in dialysis patients. *PLoS ONE* **2019**, *14*, e0212795. [CrossRef] [PubMed]
143. Pedrini, L.A.; Cozzi, G.; Faranna, P.; Mercieri, A.; Ruggiero, P.; Zerbi, S.; Feliciani, A.; Riva, A. Transmembrane pressure modulation in high-volume mixed hemodiafiltration to optimize efficiency and minimize protein loss. *Kidney Int.* **2006**, *69*, 573–579. [CrossRef]
144. Pedrini, L.A.; Wiesen, G. Overcoming the limitations of post-dilution on-line hemodiafiltration: Mixed dilution hemodiafiltration. *Contrib. Nephrol.* **2011**, *175*, 129–140. [CrossRef]
145. Maduell, F.; del Pozo, C.; Garcia, H.; Sanchez, L.; Hdez-Jaras, J.; Albero, M.D.; Calvo, C.; Torregrosa, I.; Navarro, V. Change from conventional haemodiafiltration to on-line haemodiafiltration. *Nephrol. Dial. Transpl.* **1999**, *14*, 1202–1207. [CrossRef]
146. Stefansson, B.V.; Abramson, M.; Nilsson, U.; Haraldsson, B. Hemodiafiltration improves plasma 25-hepcidin levels: A prospective, randomized, blinded, cross-over study comparing hemodialysis and hemodiafiltration. *Nephron Extra* **2012**, *2*, 55–65. [CrossRef]
147. Adamson, J.W. Hyporesponsiveness to erythropoiesis stimulating agents in chronic kidney disease: The many faces of inflammation. *Adv. Chronic Kidney Dis.* **2009**, *16*, 76–82. [CrossRef]
148. Wiecek, A.; Piecha, G. Is haemodiafiltration more favourable than haemodialysis for treatment of renal anaemia? *Nephrol. Dial. Transpl.* **2015**, *30*, 523–525. [CrossRef] [PubMed]
149. den Hoedt, C.H.; Bots, M.L.; Grooteman, M.P.; van der Weerd, N.C.; Mazairac, A.H.; Penne, E.L.; Levesque, R.; ter Wee, P.M.; Nubé, M.J.; Blankestijn, P.J.; et al. Online hemodiafiltration reduces systemic inflammation compared to low-flux hemodialysis. *Kidney Int.* **2014**, *86*, 423–432. [CrossRef] [PubMed]
150. Panichi, V.; Rizza, G.M.; Paoletti, S.; Bigazzi, R.; Aloisi, M.; Barsotti, G.; Rindi, P.; Donati, G.; Antonelli, A.; Panicucci, E.; et al. Chronic inflammation and mortality in haemodialysis: Effect of different renal replacement therapies. Results from the RISCAVID study. *Nephrol. Dial. Transpl.* **2008**, *23*, 2337–2343. [CrossRef] [PubMed]
151. Marcelli, D.; Bayh, I.; Merello, J.I.; Ponce, P.; Heaton, A.; Kircelli, F.; Chazot, C.; Di Benedetto, A.; Marelli, C.; Ladanyi, E.; et al. Dynamics of the erythropoiesis stimulating agent resistance index in incident hemodiafiltration and high-flux hemodialysis patients. *Kidney Int.* **2016**, *90*, 192–202. [CrossRef] [PubMed]
152. Panichi, V.; Scatena, A.; Rosati, A.; Giusti, R.; Ferro, G.; Malagnino, E.; Capitanini, A.; Piluso, A.; Conti, P.; Bernabini, G.; et al. High-volume online haemodiafiltration improves erythropoiesis-stimulating

agent (ESA) resistance in comparison with low-flux bicarbonate dialysis: Results of the REDERT study. *Nephrol. Dial. Transpl.* **2015**, *30*, 682–689. [CrossRef]
153. Oates, T.; Pinney, J.H.; Davenport, A. Haemodiafiltration versus high-flux haemodialysis: Effects on phosphate control and erythropoietin response. *Am. J. Nephrol.* **2011**, *33*, 70–75. [CrossRef]
154. van der Weerd, N.C.; Den Hoedt, C.H.; Blankestijn, P.J.; Bots, M.L.; van den Dorpel, M.A.; Levesque, R.; Mazairac, A.H.; Nubé, M.J.; Penne, E.L.; ter Wee, P.M.; et al. Resistance to erythropoiesis stimulating agents in patients treated with online hemodiafiltration and ultrapure low-flux hemodialysis: Results from a randomized controlled trial (CONTRAST). *PLoS ONE* **2014**, *9*, e94434. [CrossRef]
155. Ayli, D.; Ayli, M.; Azak, A.; Yüksel, C.; Kosmaz, G.P.; Atilgan, G.; Dede, F.; Abayli, E.; Camlibel, M. The effect of high-flux hemodialysis on renal anemia. *J. Nephrol.* **2004**, *17*, 701–706.
156. Ueda, N.; Takasawa, K. Impact of Inflammation on Ferritin, Hepcidin and the Management of Iron Deficiency Anemia in Chronic Kidney Disease. *Nutrients* **2018**, *10*, 1173. [CrossRef]
157. Gangat, N.; Wolanskyj, A.P. Anemia of chronic disease. *Semin. Hematol* **2013**, *50*, 232–238. [CrossRef]
158. Susantitaphong, P.; Alqahtani, F.; Jaber, B.L. Efficacy and safety of intravenous iron therapy for functional iron deficiency anemia in hemodialysis patients: A meta-analysis. *Am. J. Nephrol.* **2014**, *39*, 130–141. [CrossRef] [PubMed]
159. Jairam, A.; Das, R.; Aggarwal, P.K.; Kohli, H.S.; Gupta, K.L.; Sakhuja, V.; Jha, V. Iron status, inflammation and hepcidin in ESRD patients: The confounding role of intravenous iron therapy. *Indian J. Nephrol.* **2010**, *20*, 125–131. [PubMed]
160. Nakanishi, T.; Kuragano, T.; Kaibe, S.; Nagasawa, Y.; Hasuike, Y. Should we reconsider iron administration based on prevailing ferritin and hepcidin concentrations? *Clin. Exp. Nephrol.* **2012**, *16*, 819–826. [CrossRef] [PubMed]
161. Gunnell, J.; Yeun, J.Y.; Depner, T.A.; Kaysen, G.A. Acute-phase response predicts erythropoietin resistance in haemodialysis and PD patients. *Am. J. Kidney Dis.* **1999**, *33*, 63–72. [CrossRef]
162. Stenvinkel, P. Inflammation in end-stage renal failure: Could it be treated? *Nephrol. Dial. Transpl.* **2002**, *17*, 33–38. [CrossRef] [PubMed]
163. Nand, N.; Chauhan, V.; Seth, S.; Batra, N.; Dsouza, S. Inflammation and erythropoietin hyporesponsiveness: Role of pentoxifylline, an anti TNF-$\alpha$ agent. *JIACM* **2016**, *17*, 16–20.
164. National Kidney Foundation. KDOQI clinical practice guidelines for chronic kidney disease, evaluation, classification, and stratification. *Am. J. Kidney Dis.* **2002**, *39*, 1–266.
165. Santos, E.J.F.; Hortegal, E.V.; Serra, H.O.; Lages, J.S.; Salgado-Filho, N.; dos Santos, A.M. Epoetin alfa resistance in hemodialysis patients with chronic kidney disease: A longitudinal study. *Braz. J. Med. Biol. Res.* **2018**, *51*, e7288. [CrossRef]
166. Macdougall, I.C.; Cooper, A.C. Erythropoietin resistance: The role of inflammation and pro-inflammatory cytokines. *Nephrol. Dial. Transpl.* **2002**, *17*, 39–43. [CrossRef]
167. Kalantar-Zadeh, K.; McAllister, C.J.; Lehn, R.S.; Lee, G.H.; Nissenson, A.R.; Kopple, J.D. Effect of malnutrition-inflammation complex syndrome on EPO hyporesponsiveness in maintenance hemodialysis patients. *Am. J. Kidney Dis.* **2003**, *42*, 761–773. [CrossRef]
168. Agarwal, N.; Prchal, J.T. Anemia of chronic disease (anemia of inflammation). *Acta Haematol.* **2009**, *122*, 103–108. [CrossRef] [PubMed]
169. Barany, P.; Divino, J.C.; Bergström, J. High C-reactive protein is a strong predictor of resistance to erythropoietin in hemodialysis patients. *Am. J. Kidney Dis.* **1997**, *29*, 565–568. [CrossRef]
170. Hung, S.C.; Lin, Y.P.; Tarng, D.C. Erythropoiesis-stimulating agents in chronic kidney disease: What have we learned in 25 years? *J. Med. Assoc.* **2014**, *113*, 3–10. [CrossRef] [PubMed]
171. Locatelli, F.; Andrulli, S.; Memoli, B.; Maffei, C.; Del Vecchio, L.; Aterini, S.; De Simone, W.; Mandalari, A.; Brunori, G.; Amato, M.; et al. Nutritional-inflammation status and resistance to erythropoietin therapy in haemodialysis patients. *Nephrol. Dial. Transpl.* **2006**, *21*, 991–998. [CrossRef] [PubMed]
172. Navarro, J.F.; Mora, C.; Garcia, J. Rivero, A.; Macía, M.; Gallego, E.; Méndez, M.L.; Chahin, J.. Effects of pentoxifylline on the hematologic status in anaemic patients with advanced renal failure. *J. Urol. Nephrol.* **1999**, *33*, 121–125.
173. Goicoechea, M.; de Vinuesa, S.G.; Quiroga, B.; Verdalles, U.; Barraca, D.; Yuste, C.; Panizo, N.; Verde, E.; Muñoz, M.A.; Luño, J. Effects of pentoxifylline on inflammatory parameters in chronic kidney disease patients: A randomised trial. *J. Nephrol.* **2012**, *25*, 969–975. [CrossRef]

174. Tavazoe, M.; Balali, A.; Shahbazian, H.; Ghorbani, A. Pentoxifylline and Improvement of Anaemia in End-Stage Renal Disease. *Iran. J. Kidney Dis.* **2009**, *3*, 302.
175. Locatelli, F.; Aljama, P.; Barany, P.; Canaud, B.; Carrera, F.; Eckardt, K.U.; Hörl, W.H.; Macdougal, I.C.; Macleod, A.; Wiecek, A.; et al. Revised European best practice guidelines for the management of anaemia in patients with chronic renal failure. *Nephrol. Dial. Transplant.* **2004**, *19* (Suppl. 2), ii1–ii47.

MDPI
St. Alban-Anlage 66
4052 Basel
Switzerland
Tel. +41 61 683 77 34
Fax +41 61 302 89 18
www.mdpi.com

*International Journal of Molecular Sciences* Editorial Office
E-mail: ijms@mdpi.com
www.mdpi.com/journal/ijms